Recent Advances in Obesity Research
(Volume 1)

Understanding Obesity: From its Causes to Impact on Life

Edited by
Rosário Monteiro

Department of Biomedicine, Biochemistry Unit,
Faculty of Medicine, University of Porto, Porto, Portugal

i3S - Instituto de Investigação e Inovação em Saúde,
University of Porto, Porto, Portugal

Unidade de Saúde Familiar Pedras Rubras,
Agrupamento de Centros de Saúde Maia-Valongo, Maia,
Northern Regional Health Administration, Portugal

&

Maria João Martins

Department of Biomedicine, Biochemistry Unit,
Faculty of Medicine, University of Porto, Porto, Portugal

Recent Advances in Obesity Research

Volume # 1

Understanding Obesity: From its Causes to Impact on Life

Editors: Rosário Monteiro and Maria João Martins

Associate Editor: Hervé Dutau

ISBN (Online): 9789811442636

ISBN (Print): 9789811442612

ISBN (Paperback): 978-1-68108-770-2

Published by Bentham Science Publishers Pte. Ltd. Singapore. All Rights Reserved.

need for a court order if at any point you breach any terms of this License Agreement. In no event will any delay or failure by Bentham Science Publishers in enforcing your compliance with this License Agreement constitute a waiver of any of its rights.

3. You acknowledge that you have read this License Agreement, and agree to be bound by its terms and conditions. To the extent that any other terms and conditions presented on any website of Bentham Science Publishers conflict with, or are inconsistent with, the terms and conditions set out in this License Agreement, you acknowledge that the terms and conditions set out in this License Agreement shall prevail.

Bentham Science Publishers Pte. Ltd.
80 Robinson Road #02-00
Singapore 068898
Singapore
Email: subscriptions@benthamscience.net

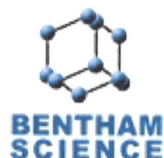

BENTHAM SCIENCE

CONTENTS

FOREWORD

While under-nutrition still is a serious problem in less wealthy countries, currently the obesity pandemic is the major health concern worldwide, especially in industrialized and developing countries. Easy access to comparatively inexpensive, palatable and energy-dense food combined with the sedentary lifestyle favors development of overweight and obesity. Social status has a major impact on development of obesity, most likely by influencing key behavioral factors but also through its prominent contribution to stress exposure.

Age is a primary risk factor for weight gain. Overweight and obesity-related morbidities, *e.g.* primarily cardiovascular disease and type 2 diabetes, but also cancer, are the major cause of reduced healthy life-span. Their incidence correlates with duration of obesity. Therefore, a serious concern is the increase in obesity in youth. Feeding behavior, which is acquired in early childhood, is maintained life-long. Therefore, it is important to identify critical and sensitive periods for obesity development. Triggers for obesity development may, however, act even earlier in life: the nutritional and metabolic status of the mother may impact the development of an obese phenotype in the offspring by fetal programing.

Obesity-related diseases are a consequence of dysfunctional adipose tissue. Excess storage of fat in adipose tissue results in remodeling that encompasses hypertrophy and hyperplasia of white adipocytes, loss of "fat burning" brown adipocytes, white adipocyte metabolic stress and, eventually, white adipocyte death. A shift from an anti-inflammatory to a proinflammatory profile of resident adipose macrophages results in the increased release of proinflammatory cytokines. Adipose tissue insulin resistance gives rise to an increased release of fatty acids, which are stored as ectopic fat in skeletal muscle and liver. An imbalance in adipokine formation affects metabolism in their target organs. As a rule, the chronic subacute inflammation that underlies these changes is more pronounced in abdominal adipose tissue than in subcutaneous adipose tissue, explaining the tight correlation of waist circumference rather than BMI with obesity-related diseases. Since adipose tissue dysfunction does not strictly correlate with its mass, it is important to identify easily detectable blood surrogate markers for its functional status.

Even though excessive caloric intake is, beyond any doubt, the major driving factor for obesity development, environmental xenobiotics causing endocrine disruption may contribute to obesity by causing reduced energy expenditure, hormone receptor-driven changes in adipocyte function and epigenetic reprogramming. Similarly, the gut microbiota appears to play a role in the development of overweight. Gut sterilization and microbiome transplantation affect diet-induced obesity development in mice. However, presently, no reliable data are available for humans. Current studies analyze the benefit of pro- or prebiotic diets to improve weight control by influencing the microbiome.

Caloric restriction is key to weight reduction. Many diets with varying proportions of macronutrients have been proposed to improve healthy weight loss. However, evidence that extreme reduction or exclusion of one macronutrient from the diet might improve the outcome appears to be scarce. Similarly, the impact of minor food constituents, such as secondary plant metabolites, *e.g.* polyphenols, is still a matter of debate. Besides caloric restriction, an increase in physical activity is an essential life-style intervention for weight reduction. There is increasing evidence that physical activity not only increases energy expenditure but also positively reprograms metabolism both in skeletal muscle and systemically by modulating hormone, myokine and cytokine homeostasis.

While life-style intervention is the most logical approach to prevent or treat obesity, lack of compliance also makes it the most ineffective. Several pharmacological targets, peripheral and central, have been identified to treat obesity or obesity-related comorbid conditions with varying short term efficacy and long term success. Strong interpatient variations call for a more individualized approach. Bariatric surgery, once thought to be an *ultima ratio* to combat extreme obesity, has proved to improve metabolic health prior to major weight reduction and has recently gained much attention as "metabolic surgery".

The 17 chapters of this book approach the obesity problem from the molecular, mechanistic, epidemiological and clinical point of view.

Gerhard P. Püschel
Institute of Nutritional Science,
Department of Nutritional Biochemistry,
University of Potsdam,
Nuthetal,
Germany

PREFACE

Obesity, defined as excessive fat accumulation that may impair health, has seen its prevalence increase to unprecedented levels globally, being projected to continue to rise. Obesity meets all accepted criteria of a medical disease, including a known etiology, recognized signs and symptoms, and a range of structural and functional changes that culminate in pathologic consequences.

The major concern about the alarming increase of obesity numbers relates to its association with risk to develop cardiovascular diseases, diabetes, some cancers and highly disabling musculoskeletal disorders, which are among the leading causes of death and morbidity in the world. In fact, currently, in most countries of the world, overweight and obesity are linked to more deaths than underweight. This is particularly important when we acknowledge that obesity is becoming a problem in increasingly early ages and that childhood obesity is associated with a higher chance of obesity, premature death and disability in adulthood.

Before this scenario, it is not surprising that obesity, being a preventable disease, has become a major priority for global health policies. Decreasing obesity incidence requires the effort of different social and health care structures and a constant update on the scientific knowledge about its determinants, prevention and management strategies as well as consequences.

Given multifactorial nature of obesity etiology, dealing with obesity requires a similar multitude of approaches. This book overviews the main contributing factors to obesity: from social and behavioral determinants throughout the life course, influences from before we are born to what we eat (not only nutrients and non-nutrient compounds with impact on body weight but also food contaminants), which bacteria colonize our gut, and how and how much we spend energy we accumulate. The dynamic role of the adipose tissue during obesity development, the pressure put on to its remodeling and differences in obesity phenotypes regarding association with pathological outcomes are also presented as well as the latest advances made on finding biological markers of adipose tissue dysfunction. The latest treatment options for obesity from medical, pharmacological and surgical areas are reviewed, also recognizing educational, social and psychological issues as central when handling obesity. Associations with chronic and disabling diseases, like cancer, diabetes and cardiovascular diseases that place heavy tolls on human societies, are debated, highlighting how obesity predisposes to their development and how obesity treatments might improve their outcome. The bidirectional relationship of stress with obesity is discussed, as are the changes in adipose tissue accretion along the aging process, also outlining the obesity paradox.

Perhaps obesity prevention should have been the main focus of this book, as some advocate that obesity is a chronic disease, treatment options have only limited success, and obesity predisposition may be determined as far as three generations back. But while the necessary changes in society, mentalities and attitudes are in delay, we expect health researchers, practitioners, as well as decision-makers, may find this book a useful tool gathering the latest updates on obesity research, with involvement of experts from different backgrounds, which contribute with findings from their own research on obesity but also with personal views onto how the complex nature of the obesity problem should be dealt with.

Rosário Monteiro and Maria João Martins
Department of Biomedicine,
Biochemistry Unit,

Faculty of Medicine,
i3S - Instituto de Investigação e Inovação em Saúde,
University of Porto,
Porto,
Portugal

List of Contributors

Adriana R. Rodrigues Department of Biomedicine, Experimental Biology Unit, Faculty of Medicine, University of Porto, Porto, Portugal
IBMC - Instituto de Biologia Molecular e Celular, University of Porto, Porto, Portugal
i3S - Instituto de Investigação e Inovação em Saúde, University of Porto, Porto, Portugal

Alexandra M. Gouveia Department of Biomedicine, Experimental Biology Unit, Faculty of Medicine, University of Porto, Porto, Portugal
IBMC - Instituto de Biologia Molecular e Celular, University of Porto, Porto, Portugal
i3S - Instituto de Investigação e Inovação em Saúde, University of Porto, Porto, Portugal
Faculty of Nutrition and Food Sciences, University of Porto, Porto, Portugal

Alejandro Santos Faculty of Nutrition and Food Sciences, University of Porto, Porto, Portugal
i3S - Instituto de Investigação e Inovação em Saúde, University of Porto, Porto, Portugal

Ana Faria Nutrição e Metabolismo, NOVA Medical School, Faculdade de Ciências Médicas, Universidade Nova de Lisboa, Lisboa, Portugal
CINTESIS - Center for Health Technology and Services Research, ProNutri - Clinical Nutrition & Disease Programming, University of Porto, Porto, Portugal

Andreia Oliveira EPIUnit - Institute of Public Health, University of Porto, Porto, Portugal
Faculty of Medicine, University of Porto, Porto, Portugal

António Ascensão CIAFEL - Research Center in Physical Activity, Health and Leisure, Faculty of Sport, University of Porto, Porto, Portugal
LaMetEx - Laboratory of Metabolism and Exercise, Faculty of Sport, University of Porto, Porto, Portugal

Cátia Braga-Pontes School of Health Sciences, Polytechnic of Leiria,, Health Research Unit, Polytechnic of Leiria, Leiria, Portugal

Célia Candeias Unidade de Saúde Familiar Pedras Rubras, Agrupamento de Centros de Saúde Maia-Valongo, Maia, Portugal

Conceição Calhau Nutrição e Metabolismo, NOVA Medical School, Faculdade de Ciências Médicas, Universidade Nova de Lisboa, Lisboa, Portugal
CINTESIS - Center for Health Technology and Services Research, ProNutri - Clinical Nutrition & Disease Programming, University of Porto, Porto, Portugal

Catarina Durão EPIUnit - Institute of Public Health, University of Porto, Porto, Portugal
Faculty of Medicine, University of Porto, Porto, Portugal
NOVA Medical School, Faculdade de Ciências Médicas,, Universidade Nova de Lisboa, Lisboa, Portugal

Carla Lopes EPIUnit - Institute of Public Health, University of Porto, Porto, Portugal
Faculty of Medicine, University of Porto, Porto, Portugal

Cláudia Marques

Nutrição e Metabolismo, NOVA Medical School, Faculdade de Ciências Médicas, Universidade Nova de Lisboa, Lisboa, Portugal
CINTESIS - Center for Health Technology and Services Research, ProNutri - Clinical Nutrition & Disease Programming, University of Porto, Porto, Portugal

Cidália D. Pereira

School of Health Sciences, Polytechnic of Leiria, Health Research Unit, Polytechnic of Leiria, Leiria, Portugal

Cristina Pereira-Wilson

Department of Biology, University of Minho, University of Minho, Braga, Portugal
CITAB-UM - Center for the Research and Technology of Agro-Environmental and Biological Sciences, University of Minho, Braga, Portugal
Center for Biological Engineering, University of Minho, Braga, Portugal

Davide Carvalho

Department of Endocrinology, Diabetes, and Metabolism, Faculty of Medicine, University of Porto, Porto, Portugal
i3S - Instituto de Investigação e Inovação em Saúde, University of Porto, Porto, Portugal
Department of Endocrinology, Diabetes and Metabolism, Centro Hospitalar S. João, Porto, Portugal

Delminda Neves

Department of Biomedicine, Experimental Biology Unit, Faculty of Medicine, University of Porto, Porto, Portugal
i3S - Instituto de Investigação e Inovação em Saúde, University of Porto, Porto, Portugal

Diogo Pestana

Nutrição e Metabolismo, NOVA Medical School, Faculdade de Ciências Médicas, Universidade Nova de Lisboa, Lisboa, Portugal
CINTESIS - Center for Health Technology and Services Research, ProNutri - Clinical Nutrition & Disease Programming,, Universidade Nova de Lisboa, Porto, Portugal

Diana Teixeira

Nutrição e Metabolismo, NOVA Medical School, Faculdade de Ciências Médicas, Universidade Nova de Lisboa, Lisboa, Portugal
CINTESIS - Center for Health Technology and Services Research, ProNutri - Clinical Nutrition & Disease Programming,, Universidade Nova de Lisboa, Porto, Portugal

Elisa Keating

Department of Biomedicine, Biochemistry Unit, Faculty of Medicine, University of Porto, Porto, Portugal
CINTESIS - Center for Research in Health Technologies and Information Systems, University of Porto, Porto, Portugal

Elisabete Ramos

EPIUnit - Institute of Public Health, University of Porto, Porto, Portugal
Faculty of Medicine, University of Porto, Porto, Portugal

Fátima Martel

Department of Biomedicine, Biochemistry Unit, Faculty of Medicine, University of Porto, Porto, Portugal
i3S - Instituto de Investigação e Inovação em Saúde, University of Porto, Porto, Portugal

Gil Faria

ULS Matosinhos/Hospital de Pedro Hispano, Serviço de Cirurgia Geral, Matosinhos, Polytechnic Institute of Porto, Portugal
CINTESIS - Center for Health Technology and Services Research, Faculty of Medicine, University of Porto, Porto, Portugal

Gerhard P. Püschel   Department of Nutritional Biochemistry, University of Potsdam, Institute of Nutritional Science, Nuthetal, Germany

Henrique Almeida   Department of Biomedicine, Experimental Biology Unit, Faculty of Medicine, University of Porto, Porto, Portugal
i3S - Instituto de Investigação e Inovação em Saúde, University of Porto, Porto, Portugal

Isabel Azevedo   Department of Biomedicine, Biochemistry Unit, Faculty of Medicine, University of Porto, Porto, Portugal

Inês Brandão   Department of Biomedicine, Biochemistry Unit, Faculty of Medicine, University of Porto, Porto, Portugal
i3S - Instituto de Investigação e Inovação em Saúde, University of Porto, Porto, Portugal

Joana Araújo   EPIUnit - Institute of Public Health, University of Porto, Porto, Portugal
Faculty of Medicine, University of Porto, Porto, Portugal

Jorge Beleza   CIAFEL - Research Center in Physical Activity, Health and Leisure, Faculty of Sport, University of Porto, Porto, Portugal
LaMetEx - Laboratory of Metabolism and Exercise, Faculty of Sport, University of Porto, Porto, Portugal

João T. Guimarães   Serviço de Patologia Clínica, Centro Hospitalar São João, Porto, Portugal
Department of Biomedicine, Biochemistry Unit, Faculty of Medicine, University of Porto, Porto, Portugal
Institute of Public Health, University of Porto, University of Porto, Porto, Portugal

José Magalhães   CIAFEL - Research Center in Physical Activity, Health and Leisure, Faculty of Sport, University of Porto, Porto, Portugal
LaMetEx - Laboratory of Metabolism and Exercise, Faculty of Sport, University of Porto, Porto, Portugal

Margaria Faria   Serviço de Patologia Clínica, Centro Hospitalar São João, Porto, Portugal

Maria J. Martins   Department of Biomedicine, Biochemistry Unit, Faculty of Medicine, University of Porto, Porto, Portugal
i3S - Instituto de Investigação e Inovação em Saúde, University of Porto, Porto, Portugal

Maria J. Salazar   Department of Biomedicine, Experimental Biology Unit, Faculty of Medicine, University of Porto, Porto, Portugal
IBMC - Instituto de Biologia Molecular e Celular, University of Porto, Porto, Portugal
i3S - Instituto de Investigação e Inovação em Saúde, University of Porto, Porto, Portugal

Marco Assunção   Serviço de Patologia Clínica, Centro Hospitalar São João, Porto, Portugal
CBQF - Centro de Biotecnologia e Química Fina - Laboratório Associado, Escola Superior de Biotecnologia, Universidade Católica Portuguesa, Porto, Portugal

Nuno Borges   Faculty of Nutrition and Food Sciences, University of Porto, Porto, Portugal
CINTESIS - Center for Health Technology and Services Research, University of Porto, Porto, Portugal

Pedro Coelho

Department of Biomedicine, Biochemistry Unit, Faculty of Medicine, University of Porto, Porto, Portugal
i3S - Instituto de Investigação e Inovação em Saúde, University of Porto, Porto, Portugal

Paula Freitas

Department of Endocrinology, Diabetes, and Metabolism, Faculty of Medicine, University of Porto, Porto, Portugal
i3S - Instituto de Investigação e Inovação em Saúde, University of Porto, Porto, Portugal
Department of Endocrinology, Diabetes and Metabolism, Centro Hospitalar S. João, Porto, Portugal

Raquel Costa

Department of Biomedicine, Biochemistry Unit, Faculty of Medicine, University of Porto, Porto, Portugal
i3S - Instituto de Investigação e Inovação em Saúde, University of Porto, Porto, Portugal

Rosário Monteiro

Department of Biomedicine, Biochemistry Unit, Faculty of Medicine, University of Porto, Porto, Portugal
i3S - Instituto de Investigação e Inovação em Saúde, University of Porto, Porto, Portugal
Unidade de Saúde Familiar Pedras Rubras, Agrupamento de Centros de Saúde Maia-Valongo, Maia, Portugal

Rita Negrão

Department of Biomedicine, Biochemistry Unit, Faculty of Medicine, University of Porto, Porto, Portugal
i3S - Instituto de Investigação e Inovação em Saúde, University of Porto, Porto, Portugal

Raquel Soares

Department of Biomedicine, Biochemistry Unit, Faculty of Medicine, University of Porto, Porto, Portugal
i3S - Instituto de Investigação e Inovação em Saúde, University of Porto, Porto, Portugal

Sara Andrade

Department of Biomedicine, Biochemistry Unit, Faculty of Medicine, University of Porto, Porto, Portugal
i3S - Instituto de Investigação e Inovação em Saúde, University of Porto, Porto, Portugal

Susana G. Guerreiro

Department of Biomedicine, Biochemistry Unit, Faculty of Medicine, University of Porto, Porto, Portugal
i3S - Instituto de Investigação e Inovação em Saúde, University of Porto, Porto, Portugal

Sílvia Rocha-Rodrigues

CIAFEL - Research Center in Physical Activity, Health and Leisure, Faculty of Sport, University of Porto, Porto, Portugal
LaMetEx - Laboratory of Metabolism and Exercise, Faculty of Sport, University of Porto, Porto, Portugal

Vanessa Guerreiro

Department of Endocrinology, Diabetes, and Metabolism, Faculty of Medicine, University of Porto, Porto, Portugal
i3S - Instituto de Investigação e Inovação em Saúde, University of Porto, Porto, Portugal
Department of Endocrinology, Diabetes and Metabolism, Centro Hospitalar S. João, Porto, Portugal

Vânia S. Ribeiro School of Health Sciences, Polytechnic of Leiria, Leiria, Portugal
Health Research Unit, Polytechnic of Leiria, Leiria, Portugal

CHAPTER 1

A Life Course Approach to Obesity and Cardio-vascular Disease

Joana Araújo[1,2] and **Elisabete Ramos**[1,2,*]

[1] *EPI Unit - Institute of Public Health, University of Porto, Porto, Portugal*

[2] *Faculty of Medicine, University of Porto, Porto, Portugal*

Abstract: The increasing prevalence of childhood obesity, as well as the recognition of the role of early factors for the development of cardiovascular disease, called the attention to the impact of the dynamics of adiposity across pediatric age on adult health outcomes, highlighting the potential application of life course frameworks in this context. Therefore, there is increasing interest in identifying critical and sensitive periods for obesity development and to identify how to summarize lifetime exposure to adiposity/obesity to measure its impact on cardiovascular disease. The discussion of the application of the life course approach to the study of obesity determinants and its relation with cardiometabolic health is presented in this chapter. Additionally, different methods to summarize the cumulative exposure to adiposity are described as well as the challenges of measuring direct and indirect effects of childhood adiposity on adult cardiovascular disease.

Keywords: Adolescence, Cardiovascular disease, Childhood, Chronic disease, Critical periods, Duration, Growth trajectories, Life course, Lifetime risk, Obesity, Pediatric obesity, Sensitive periods.

INTRODUCTION

There has been increasing interest in changing the focus from the adult risk factors model of chronic disease etiology to a life course framework, in which biological, behavioral and psychological factors acting across the individual's life span influence the risk of the disease. The life course approach is not a recent thinking, but it has gained more attention in epidemiology with the recognition of the role of early life factors in cardiovascular and other chronic diseases [1, 2]. Therefore, the paradigm has changed from the adult lifestyle model of chronic disease, with adult health-related behaviors, such as smoking, alcohol intake, diet, and physical activity, assuming an important effect on adult-onset diseases [3, 4],

---

[*] **Corresponding author Elisabete Ramos:** Institute of Public Health, University of Porto, Porto, Portugal; Tel/Fax: +351 222061820; E-mail: eliramos@med.up.pt

Rosário Monteiro and Maria João Martins (Eds.)

to the life course approach that also recognizes the importance of early exposures for the lifetime risk of disease [5].

The life course epidemiology is defined as the study of the long-term effects of different exposures at different phases of the life cycle on health or on the risk of disease [6, 7]. In addition to the study of factors to which the individual is exposed across the life span, the life course epidemiology also addresses the influence of exposures across generations, with previous studies suggesting intergenerational effects of prenatal exposures, which may not be limited to the first generation offspring [8]. Although in the last few decades much more attention has been given to the effect of early life factors, life course epidemiology should not be seen as a polarization of early life factors, on one hand, and adult lifestyle factors, on the other hand, but instead the influence of various factors operating across all life span, that independently, cumulatively and interactively influence the risk of disease [5]. Additionally, both time and timing are recognized as important for establishing causality between exposures and outcomes [9]. Many chronic diseases, such as cardiovascular disease, have long latency periods, and early exposures may be involved in the initial processes of the disease, long before their clinical manifestations. On the other hand, the timing of occurrence of the exposures is also important since exposures occurring at specific periods may have higher impact on disease risk. Specifically, critical and sensitive periods have been identified in the context of life course epidemiology [6], namely those for the development of obesity and cardiometabolic outcomes [10, 11].

The life course framework is useful to conceptualize and study the complex net of determinants of obesity, since there are individual risk factors and more systemic drivers [12, 13], and factors also act at different phases of the life cycle, from gestation to adult life [11, 14, 15]. Those factors include exposures during fetal life, or even preconception exposures of the mother, as well as rapid weight growth during infancy or early adiposity rebound, among others [10, 11, 16]. On the other hand, the life course approach may also allow a better understanding of the lifetime risk for cardiovascular disease, resulting from the accumulation of risk with age, influenced by the exposures occurring at all stages of the life span [17 - 19]. Among those factors, obesity is one of the most important determinants [20] and its association with cardiovascular risk has been shown for all ages [17, 21, 22]. Therefore, a life course framework applied to the study of the obesity determinants and its relation with cardiometabolic outcomes may provide useful insights into the comprehension of the disease etiology and to inform prevention and intervention strategies.

LIFE COURSE THEORETICAL MODELS

Different theoretical models have been proposed to guide research in life course epidemiology, as summarized in Table **1**. The proposed models are a simplistic illustration of the effect of the exposures across the life course, and should be adapted to the study of different outcomes and exposures. Additionally, the proposed models are not mutually exclusive, and features from different models may coexist.

Table 1. Theoretical models in life course epidemiology.

Critical Period Model	
Gives emphasis to the timing of exposure. *Exposures acting during specific periods may irreversibly affect the risk of later disease.*	
- without later effect modifiers	The exposures act during critical periods and have effects on anatomical structure or physiological functioning, which may be long-lasting and irreversible.
- with later effect modifiers	In sensitive period models there is greater scope for reversibility of the effects, with later effect modifiers.
Accumulation of Risk Model	
Exposure effect accumulates over the life course. *The total amount,i.e., number, severity and duration of the exposures, and/or sequence of the events affect the risk of the disease.*	
- independent and uncorrelated exposures	Effect of exposures accumulate over time, but exposure risk is independent.
- correlated exposures (clustering or chains of risk)	Risk factors tend to cluster (*accumulation model with risk clustering*), or form chains of risk, where one exposure leads to another, with additive or trigger effects (*pathway model*).

One of the life course models is based on the concepts of critical and sensitive periods. This *critical period model* emphasizes the timing of the exposure – the effect of the exposure to a factor at a specific period may have irreversible effects on anatomical structure or physiological functioning [6, 7]. Critical periods are phases of the development characterized by permanent anatomical or functioning changes resulting from exposure to specific environmental stimuli, which may confer additional long-term risk for specific health outcomes [6, 7, 10]. During these specific timespans, exposure to the factors may result in increased risk of disease, but exposure outside those periods seems not to confer additional risk. It is known that during mammalian development, exposure to specific environmental stimuli is essential for the development of anatomical structures and their functioning. However, exposure to specific factors during specific periods, for example during intrauterine period, may origin irreversible changes and predict long-term outcomes. Other periods not characterized by this level of structural or functional development are described as sensitive. Sensitive periods are also periods of rapid development, when stronger effects of exposure to some factor is observed, in comparison to exposure outside that time frame. However, as opposed to what occurs in critical periods, that effect may be modified or reversed [6, 7]. For example, although adolescence is often described in the literature as a critical period for obesity development, it would rather be a sensitive period since there is a variety of different developmental stages that take place at variable time periods, instead one specific critical period. Although differences in the deterministic features between the critical and sensitive periods exist, both concepts have in common the importance of the timing of exposures for the risk of outcomes occurring later in life, which is the main characteristic of the critical period model. These concepts have their roots in the hypothesis of the fetal origins of adult disease, and the model is also known as 'biological programming' or as 'latency model'. Additionally, it incorporates the idea of sensitive periods, applied to exposures acting during sensitive periods, whose effect in the later risk of disease may be changed by later physiological or psychological stressors [6].

Another main class of the life course models is the *accumulation of risk model* (Table **1**). This model suggests that effects of exposures, such as environmental, socioeconomic and behavioral, gradually accumulate over time and may cause long-term damage [6, 7]. The number, severity and duration of the insults over the life course may impact the risk of the disease, with a dose-response effect. The accumulation of risk may follow different models, depending on the disease, with exposures being independent, clustered exposures or occurring in chains of risk [6, 7]. In the accumulation of risk model with independent and uncorrelated exposures, the development of the disease is dependent on the accumulation of risk over time, that could be influenced by several factors, but each risk factor acts independently of the others [6]. Alternatively, exposures may be correlated; for example, health-related behaviors, or adverse social circumstances tend to cluster. This is known as an *accumulation model with risk clustering* [7]. Finally, in the model based on chains of risk, one adverse exposure may increase the probability of being exposed to another factor and so on, increasing the risk of the disease. The relation between the exposures is not deterministic, but each exposure increases (or decreases) the probability of another exposure. Chains of risk could be of two different types; in one model, in addition to the effect on subsequent exposures, the risk factor also have an 'additive effect' on the risk of the disease, independently of the later exposure [6]. If each exposure only influences the risk of the subsequent exposure, with no additional direct effect on disease risk, is the final exposure in the chain that has a marked effect and precipitates disease onset – this is described as a 'trigger effect' [6].

In the context of non-communicable diseases, risk clustering is possibly the most common model, since health-related behaviors tend to cluster. However, the recognition of the potential effect of early exposures would also support the critical period model. As these theoretical models – critical period and accumulation of risk – are not necessarily mutually exclusive, in the accumulation risk models, the timing could also be important, with exposures that act during specific periods having greater impact on risk of disease and also accumulating with other exposures. Therefore, the development of chronic diseases is complex and it is probably a consequence of the interaction of both the critical period and accumulation risk models [9, 19].

OBESITY DEVELOPMENT: CRITICAL AND SENSITIVE PERIODS

Critical or sensitive periods for obesity development have been identified across the life course [10, 11, 16]. Fetal life is recognized as a critical period, because of profound development of tissues and organs. Exposure to specific factors during this period may "programme" physiological functioning, and therefore may play a role in disease etiology [10, 23, 24]. Other sensitive or critical periods include infancy, childhood, namely the period of the adiposity rebound, and also adolescence, related to puberty and behavioral changes [10, 16, 25].

Prenatal Period and Infancy

The potential effect of exposures occurring in the prenatal period and infancy was firstly described in the 1970s in the Dutch Hunger Winter Study [26]. In this study, changes in maternal nutrition because of severe food rationing during the Second World War were associated with offspring obesity. Prevalence of obesity in the 19-year-old males who had been exposed to famine in the first two trimesters of gestation was higher, compared to exposure in the third trimester only [26]. Later, Barker *et al* [1, 2, 27] showed an association between rates of infant mortality and adult deaths (ecological analysis) and in other study found an association between birthweight and adult ischemic heart disease mortality. These studies led to the "Barker's hypothesis" or developmental origins theory, which proposed that gestational undernutrition may promote fetal programming that changes body's structure, function and metabolism, which is implicated in the etiology of adult coronary heart disease [28]. This theory was later expanded to the Developmental Origins of Health and Disease (DOHaD) [29, 30]. The DOHaD refers to the effect of broader environmental exposures in pregnancy, such as maternal nutrition, or exposure to environmental chemicals, drugs, infections or stress, not only on coronary heart disease, and extends the period of interest to preconception and infancy. This effect that takes place in these diffe-rent periods may be explained by developmental plasticity, and has widespread consequences for later health, namely obesity and cardiovascular disease.

As discussed elsewhere in this book, some studies have shown that exposure to some factors during pregnancy (chemicals, maternal stress, nutrition or obesity), as well as rapid postnatal weight gain are associated with offspring obesity [31, 32]. Additionally, studies have suggested that these associations are observed across at least three generations [33], supporting that the inter-generational effects for disease susceptibility are not restricted to one generation. Underlying mechanisms that increase susceptibility for later disease might include epigenetic processes that alter gene expression, such as the DNA methylation [7, 31, 32]. However, the influence of maternal exposures on the offspring metabolic profile is still under investigation and debate, at least regarding the effect and the mechanisms of some exposures. A recent study including data from three birth cohorts, analysed whether the effect of maternal pregnancy adiposity on offspring metabolic traits was due to intrauterine mechanisms or shared familial characteristics [34]. Authors found similar associations of both maternal and paternal BMI with the offspring metabolism at 16, 17 or 31 years, suggesting that the relationship is likely to be explained by shared genetic or familial lifestyle factors [34].

Childhood

Another critical period for obesity development is the adiposity rebound occurring at mid-childhood [10, 11]. There is an increase in adiposity during the first year of life, followed by a decline until a minimum (nadir) is reached at approximately 6 years of age. The "adiposity rebound" is defined as the increase in adiposity registered after that nadir, and it was firstly described in 1984 by Rolland-Cachera *et al* [35]. The timing of the adiposity rebound has been associated with later adiposity, with earlier age at adiposity rebound being associated with greater degree of adiposity in adolescence and in young adulthood [35, 36]. Other studies have also found a significant association of early adiposity rebound with obesity later in life [10, 37].

However, some methodological issues make the identification of adiposity rebound difficult. One of those limitations is the requirement of at least 3 serial BMI measurements, including measurements before and after the nadir, and therefore it can only be recognized after it had occurred. Moreover, since adiposity rebound occurs during a period of intense growth characterized by changes in height and it is based on BMI measurements, it does not necessarily indicate changes in body fat [37, 38]. In addition to the methodological limitations related to its measurement, the utility of adiposity rebound to predict later adiposity is also discussable. The association between timing of adiposity rebound and later adiposity may be biased by reverse causation, because early adiposity rebound is a marker of early high BMI [39, 40] and of accelerated maturation [35, 39]. Supporting the idea that age at adiposity rebound may be less relevant than childhood adiposity levels, in two studies BMI level at age 7 and age at adiposity rebound presented the same predictive value for later adiposity identification [39, 40]. These findings reinforce that, independently of the age at adiposity rebound, higher adiposity in childhood seems to be related to obesity in adulthood.

Adolescence

Adolescence is characterized by intense growth [41], being the second period of life, after infancy, with more marked changes. It is also one of the most complex periods in human growth, with marked changes in body composition and morphological signs of maturation, in addition to increases in size [10, 41]. Reinforcing the relevance of this period, fat cell number seems to be determined by the end of adolescence with no reversal in adult life [25, 42]. In addition to changes in the amount of body fat, changes in body fat distribution in adolescence may also be critical for the obesity development [10, 11, 25]. Sex-differences are modest before puberty, but during pubertal development, sex hormones promote changes in body fat that lead to sexual dimorphism in body composition and fat distribution [43, 44]. While females have an increase in fat mass, especially peripherally, but a relatively low fat-free mass, males experience a substantial gain of fat-free mass during this period, but fat mass remains relatively stable [43, 44]. These changes in the absolute levels of fat and fat-free mass lead to opposite trends in the percentage of body fat during adolescence – an increase in females and a decrease in males. In adulthood, the body fat percentage is, on average, 25% in females and 13% in males [41, 43], and females present a gynecoid shape due to higher accumulation of peripheral fat, especially on the hips and thighs, during puberty, while males have an android body shape, represented by higher accumulation of central fat, and relatively stable peripheral fat [43, 44].

The relevance of adolescence for obesity development is not independent of the relevance of puberty, since this is the trigger for most of the changes happening during adolescence. Studies have suggested an inverse association between pubertal timing and obesity. In females, earlier age at menarche has been linked to higher risk of later obesity [45, 46]. A systematic review investigated the association between age at menarche and adult BMI, and found that 30 out of the 34 studies examined reported an inverse association [47]. The pooled data from the 10 cohort studies identified, showed an increase of adult BMI by 0.34 kg/m^2 (95% CI 0.33-0.34) in girls with early age at menarche (< 12 years) [47]. In boys, there was also an inverse association between timing of maturation and later adiposity, in studies that used age at peak height velocity as an indicator of maturation [46, 48]. Pubertal timing has also been linked to body fat distribution, although evidence is still scarce and inconsistent. In the Amsterdam Growth and Health Study, there was an association between early age at menarche in girls and a trunk-oriented fat distribution pattern, but in boys age at peak height velocity was not associated with fat distribution [49]. In that study, differences in the association between girls and boys may be explained by the different indicators of pubertal timing. However, another study using the same indicator in males (age at peak height velocity) showed that early onset of puberty and higher central fat mass were significantly associated [48]. The inconsistent findings for the association with fat distribution may be related to the difficulty of distinguishing the effects of body fat distribution from those of total fat amount.

However, such as for the adiposity rebound, the association between pubertal timing and later adiposity is not immune to reverse causation bias. Higher BMI at early childhood was shown to be associated with earlier pubertal onset in some studies [50, 51], and therefore, earlier maturation may be induced by higher adiposity, and pubertal timing may be a mediator between early and later adiposity, or simply an indicator of early adiposity levels.

In addition to the effect of physiological changes that characterize this period of life, behavioral changes taking place during adolescence may also increase the risk of obesity. Behavioral changes include changes in dietary, physical and sedentary habits that occur throughout adolescence and may influence obesity development [25]. Psychosocial and cognitive changes during adolescence lead to increased autonomy and adolescents progressively feel capable of managing themselves on their own, which involves making decisions and solving their own problems [52]. Additionally, the focus of the adolescents changes from the family to the peers [53, 54], which decreases the influence of the family on adolescents' choices. New behavior acquisition, including the initiation of health-related behaviors such as smoking, alcohol consumption, drug use or sexual behaviors [55], may happen during this period, as well as changes in dietary and physical activity patterns [56, 57]. In general, studies showed an increase in unhealthy behaviors during adolescence, for instance, there is an increase in sedentary behavior and a decrease in physical activity [56], and it is more pronounced in adolescent girls [58, 59], with implications for weight gain [60]. Most studies also showed an increase in unhealthy food choices during adolescence, for example, a decrease in the frequency of breakfast consumption and an increase in snacking and fast-food consumption [57, 61]. Since most of the habits formed during adolescence are very likely to track into adulthood [62], behavioral changes in adolescence will have not only short-term but also long-term effects on weight gain and obesity.

LIFE-TIME OBESITY AND CARDIOVASCULAR DISEASE

Obesity increases the risk of a variety of disorders from cardiovascular, endocrine, pulmonary, gastrointestinal, and psychosocial systems [63, 64], and the mortality risk [65 - 68]. Overweight and obesity were estimated to have caused 3.4 million deaths worldwide in 2010 [67], and the upward trend in obesity may revert progresses in life expectancy [69].

There is a stronger association of obesity with cardiovascular disease and diabetes mortality, in comparison to other diseases [65, 69]. The Prospective Studies Collaboration [69] examined data from almost 900000 participants from 57 prospective studies, and showed that vascular mortality was about 40% higher (HR=1.41, 95% CI 1.37-1.45) and diabetes mortality 120% higher (HR=2.16, 1.89-2.46), per each 5 kg/m^2 increase in BMI. Risk estimates were 10% for neoplastic and 20% for respiratory mortality. Abdullah *et al* also found a significant direct association between the number of years lived with obesity and the mortality risk, and this association was stronger for cardiovascular disease mortality than for cancer mortality [65]. Obesity, along with diabetes, elevated serum cholesterol levels, smoking and physical inactivity are usually described as classical or traditional risk factors of cardiovascular disease [70, 71], as firstly identified in the research from the Framingham Heart Study. Other factors more recently identified and denominated as novel cardiovascular risk factors are low-grade chronic inflammation, abnormal blood coagulation, homocysteine, among many others [70 - 72]. Although the list of independent cardiovascular risk factors identified so far is extensive [70], the predictive ability and clinical implications of the novel risk factors is not so well understood yet, and traditional risk factors seem to explain most part of the incidence of cardiovascular disease and mortality [67, 71, 73]. Among the traditional risk factors, obesity is one of the major determinants of cardiovascular disease. According to the Global Burden of Metabolic Risk Factors for Chronic Diseases Collaboration, in 2010 63% of deaths due to cardiovascular diseases, chronic kidney disease and diabetes were attributable to the combined effect of four cardiometabolic risk factors: high BMI, high blood pressure, high glucose and high cholesterol values [20].

Although there is a strong association between obesity and cardiovascular disease, there is some potential for the reversibility of the effect. Most of the evidence on the reversibility of cardiovascular risk related to obesity comes from weight-loss interventions. Generally studies have shown that weight loss, achieved through either bariatric surgery or lifestyle interventions, was associated with improvements in cardiovascular risk factors [74 - 76]. Observational studies have also shown that cardiovascular risk factors of individuals that were obese as children but changed to non-obesity categories in adulthood were similar to risk factors of those who were never obese [77]. Other studies have also found that groups of individuals presenting a declining trajectory of adiposity across pediatric age also showed a reduction in cardiovascular risk in adulthood [78 - 82]. Therefore, it seems to be a potential for the attenuation of the cardiovascular risk if obesity is reverted.

From a public health perspective, the study of the association of obesity with cardiovascular diseases is of great relevance, because of the strong association between obesity and cardiovascular-related mortality, as well as the high prevalence of obesity and burden of cardiovascular diseases worldwide. The association between adult obesity and cardiovascular disease incidence and mortality seems to be well established [20]. However, there is limited evidence on the effect of childhood obesity on adult cardiovascular events from longitudinal studies, due to the difficult operationalization of cohort studies with long follow-up periods. Additionally, childhood obesity increased mainly from 1980s onwards, changing from 16.9% in 1980 to 23.8% in 2013 in boys, and from 16.2% to 22.6% in girls [83]. On the other hand, cardiovascular acute events (for example, stroke and ischemic heart disease) are more frequent from the fifth decade of life onwards [84, 85]. Therefore, the first generation that experienced high prevalence of obesity since childhood have not reached the life decades of higher incidence of cardiovascular events yet. Therefore, the magnitude of the consequences of childhood obesity, in general and specifically for cardiovascular diseases, is not fully understood yet. There is also particular interest on clarifying the effects of childhood obesity on early markers of cardiovascular disease.

Despite the difficulties in evaluating the real association between childhood obesity and adult outcomes, available data support a strong association. Studies have shown that childhood obesity increases the risk of cardiovascular risk factors as early as in preschool aged children [86, 87]. In general, studies have examined the association for obesity at specific ages, and consistently showed that higher obesity level or adiposity at any age is associated with higher risk of cardiovascular risk factors, events and mortality [68, 88, 89]. However, the dynamics of adiposity/BMI across the pediatric age, such as changes in the grade of adiposity and the duration of obesity, have not been explored in most studies. Therefore, there is increasing interest in the study of pediatric obesity effect on adult outcomes, taking into account the cumulative exposure to adiposity across the life course.

Measuring Life-time Obesity

The focus of research on the association of obesity with cardiovascular disease has changed from measuring the impact of adult obesity, to the effect of obesity at earlier ages and its cumulative effect. Changes in the pattern of the exposures, namely across age strata, with higher prevalence of exposures at younger ages led to the development of methodologies that capture the cumulative effect of exposures. Different approaches have been used to summarize the exposure to obesity across the life course – from simple constructs such as duration of obesity, to more sophisticated methods such as growth trajectories.

Studies testing the effect of obesity duration on cardiovascular disease or risk factors have generally used the age of obesity onset as an indicator of obesity duration [22, 90 - 95]. However, the identification of obesity onset is difficult and depends on the total duration of follow-up and number of examinations across the period under study or, if self-reported, it may be influenced by potential biases. Since length of follow-up, age at baseline and number of measurements greatly varies across studies, this may in part explain conflicting results between studies, with some studies showing that subjects with higher duration of obesity were more likely to have a worst cardiovascular risk profile in adulthood [22, 90, 93, 95], while other studies found no association [91, 92, 94]. The main limitation of this construct is the restriction to the duration concept, not taking into account the degree of obesity. For example, two subjects living with obesity for ten years would be attributed the same exposure, independently of one having a BMI of 32 kg/m^2 and the other a BMI of 40 kg/m^2.

A construct that summarizes both duration and grade of obesity was proposed by Abdullah *et al* [96]. The variable "obese-years" is calculated multiplying the number of units above the obesity cut-off by the number of years lived with that BMI [96]. For example, a person living two years with a BMI of 32 kg/m^2 and five years with a BMI of 35 kg/m^2 would be exposed to 36 obese-years [(32-29)*2 + (35-29)*5]. The obese-years was shown to be associated with increased incidence of diabetes [96, 97] and cardiovascular disease [98], and was suggested as a better indicator of the health risks, in comparison to BMI or duration of obesity alone [96]. Although this measure takes into account fluctuations in BMI, in contrast to duration of obesity alone, both constructs account only for time lived with adiposity above a certain level (BMI at or above 30 kg/m^2 for adults, or equivalent cut-offs for children and adolescents), and do not consider BMI fluctuations within normal ranges. However, previous evidence does not support the assumption that health risks are associated only to BMI values above a specific threshold. For example, Twig *et al* used data from 2.3 million Israeli adolescents examined from 1967 through 2010, and showed that higher BMI during adolescence even within the normal range (50th to 75th percentiles) was associated with higher cardiovascular and all-cause mortality in adulthood [68]. Therefore, new methodologies to summarize exposure to adiposity within the entire BMI spectrum are warranted. In this line, the area under the curve of BMI

(BMI$_{AUC}$) has recently been proposed as a way of summarizing the duration and grade of BMI, considering fluctuations within the entire BMI range [99]. The BMI$_{AUC}$ is calculated using BMI repeated measurements across age, and computing a cubic spline interpolation; then the area under the curve is calculated using the composite trapezoid rule, and a higher BMI$_{AUC}$ represents higher cumulative exposure to BMI for the number of years of follow-up. The advantages of this measure are the quantification of both duration and degree of obesity, considering fluctuations in the degree of BMI, not only those above a specific threshold (the obesity cut-off) but within the entire spectrum of values [99].

The identification of adiposity trajectories over the life course is another available methodology to study the lifetime risk associated with obesity. The study of growth trajectories in pediatric age is of great relevance for surveillance and for clinical practice, as well as for etiology research [100]. Different methods are available to compute growth modeling, such as mixed-effects models or group-based methods. Some studies have applied mixed-effects models, where random effects capture individual variation across time, to identify individual growth trajectories [101 - 113]. Other studies have used group-based statistical methods, which allow the identification of subpopulations characterized by distinct developmental trajectories [78 - 82, 114 - 133]. In the mixed-effects models, the trajectory of each subject is identified, however, several parameters (for example, intercept and slope) are needed to describe the trajectory and, therefore, the information about all parameters is needed to study the association with the outcomes. Also, the interpretation of the parameters may be more difficult, in comparison to the previous methods described. In the group-based methods, the individual trajectory is also estimated, but a second step is applied in order to group individuals with similar trajectories. The probability of belonging to each group is estimated for each subject and the subject can be allocated to the group with higher probability of membership. The group-based methods can be of easier interpretation, with each subject being assigned a group trajectory, instead of being characterized by several parameters. However, one of the problems may be identification of the number of groups so that all patterns of development trajectories in a given population are represented, and it may be influenced by some researcher subjectivity. Group trajectories with low prevalence in the population are more difficult to be represented, and there may be some heterogeneity within each group. Additionally, the groups identified may be population-specific, not representing all existing trajectories in other populations.

Some studies have specifically applied growth modeling to study the effect of growth trajectories on cardiovascular risk factors or metabolic outcomes [78 - 82, 127]. In general, studies showed that the most adverse cardiovascular outcomes were found in individuals with growth trajectories characterized by higher adiposity, and especially with early obesity onset. For example, Ventura *et al* [81] examined trajectories from 5 to 15 years in girls and showed that the 'upward percentile crossing' trajectory had the highest metabolic risk factors at 15 years, compared to the '50th percentile tracking', while the 'delayed downward percentile crossing' presented similar levels. In the Raine Study [79], subjects in increasing trajectories from birth to 14 years had the highest levels of insulin resistance at 14 years, while insulin resistance levels in declining trajectories and in the reference trajectory ('Optimal growth') were similar. In the Isle of Wight birth cohort, systolic and diastolic blood pressure at 18 years were higher in the delayed overweight trajectory, compared to the 'normal' trajectory, but still lower than the values found in the early persistent obesity trajectory [82]. In the EPITeen cohort, from Porto, Portugal, the 'High, increasing' BMI trajectory identified for the period between 13 and 21 years [78], presented the most unfavorable cardiovascular risk profile at 21 years. In trajectories identified from 5 to 18 years in the Birth to Twenty (Bt20) cohort, the trajectories of early onset obesity or overweight had higher blood pressure levels in late adolescence [80]. On the other hand, in several studies trajectories characterized by a decline in adiposity/obesity presented in general intermediate levels of cardiovascular risk factors, in comparison to stable high adiposity or increasing adiposity, and the normal/optimal growth trajectories [78 - 82].

Studies have shown that the increasing trajectories tend to present risk factors similar to individuals with consistently high levels of adiposity. This may be because the increase in adiposity increases the cardiovascular risk or because the risk factors at a given moment are more influenced by adiposity levels at that same moment, and to a lesser extent by cumulative exposure to adiposity. Also for the declining trajectories, reduction in the risk factors may be due to reduction of adiposity over time or because the attained final levels of adiposity are lower. Therefore, it is difficult to understand to what extent the association with cardiovascular risk factors and events is a consequence of the cumulative exposure to adiposity or is explained by the final attained adiposity levels.

Direct or Mediated Effects of Early Obesity

One of the problems to fully understand the role of childhood obesity on adult health is related with the strong correlation between childhood and adulthood adiposity. Three systematic reviews consistently showed a moderate to strong tracking of obesity from childhood into adulthood [134 - 136]. The first systematic review on this topic was published in 1993 and included studies from 1970 to 1992 [134]. It concluded that, despite a high variation in the correlation between BMI in childhood and adulthood, obese children were at least two times more likely to be obese in adulthood, in comparison to nonobese children [134]. Singh *et al* in a systematic review published in 2008 also showed an increased risk of overweight in adulthood for overweight or obese youth [136]. The most recent systematic review and meta-analysis from 2016 included fifteen prospective cohort studies. The risk of being obese in adulthood was estimated to be about five times higher for obese children and adolescents, when compared to nonobese children and adolescents [135]. Additionally, all systematic reviews support that the association with adult obesity is stronger for adolescent than for childhood obesity [134 - 136]. Giving as example the results from the Fels Longitudinal Study, the probability of being obese at 35 years of age was higher for those with obesity at older pediatric ages: below 30% for obese children aged 5 years; ranged from 30% to 60% for obese girls aged 5-12 years, and for boys 5-18 years; and above 60% for older obese adolescents [137]. However, these differences may partly result from the shorter time interval between adolescent and adult BMI measurements, which may influence the magnitude of the association.

Therefore, if most of the obese children become obese adults, it is difficult to quantify how much of the health events in adulthood are explained by current adiposity or by childhood adiposity. This may partly explain inconsistent results from the studies addressing the role of childhood obesity, independently of adult obesity [22, 138 - 143]. One study did not find an association between childhood BMI and risk of coronary heart disease later in life [138], but in general studies have reported direct significant associations, but also suggested a mediation of the effect by adult obesity [22, 141]. Two other studies also found an association between childhood obesity and adult outcomes, but they did not explore the potential mediation by adult obesity [142, 143]. A systematic review of 16 studies showed that the association observed between childhood obesity and adult cardiovascular disease risk was dependent on the tracking of BMI from childhood to adulthood, and therefore concluded that there was little evidence for an independent effect of childhood obesity [140]. A similar conclusion was reached by Park *et al* in a systematic review published in 2012 [144]. From the few studies analysing the effects independently of adult BMI, there was a lack of evidence for the independent association of childhood obesity on adult cardiovascular risk factors or events [144]. A systematic review analysing the ability capacity of childhood BMI for the prediction of obesity-related morbidities in adulthood included 37 studies and concluded that childhood BMI was not a good predictor of adult morbidity, since most of the adults with obesity-related morbidity were normal weight children [139]. However, studies included in this review were mostly from older cohort studies with relatively low prevalence of childhood obesity. The most recent systematic review on this topic included 23 studies and showed that childhood obesity was associated with adult cardiovascular risk factors, but also suggested that the effect was potentially mediated by adult BMI [89]. It also concluded that there is still a need for higher-quality studies on this topic to evaluate direct and indirect effects of childhood obesity.

The measurement of the independent effects of childhood obesity on morbidity is methodologically challenging. Several studies have used standard regression models to measure the association between childhood obesity and adult outcomes, adjusting for adult adiposity/obesity. Nonetheless, this adjustment may introduce over-adjustment biases [145] and collinearity problems [146]. Additionally, the adjusted models are of difficult interpretation since the adjusted estimates reflect the effect of adiposity change between measurements, and not only the effect of childhood adiposity adjusted for adult adiposity [147]. Therefore, other statistical techniques, such as structural equation models, may have great application to study the effect of childhood obesity on adult outcomes. For example, in path analysis models, both direct and indirect effects can be estimated and results are easily interpretable [148, 149]. Other methodologies may also be potentially applicable in this context, although still underexplored, such as causal mediation analysis [150] or Mendelian randomization [151], in order to study the causal effects of childhood obesity on the development of cardiovascular disease.

CONCLUDING REMARKS

The available evidence supports that the cumulative exposure to adiposity and its dynamics across the life span influence the cardiovascular outcomes in adulthood. However, the classical methods do not respond fully to the challenges of measuring the long-term effects of adiposity, and to disentangle the direct effects of childhood adiposity from those mediated by adult adiposity. The frameworks based on the life course epidemiology, although complex, have a high potential to measure the lifetime risk of obesity and to develop methodologies that better clarify the associations with chronic disease, namely cardiovascular disease. Additionally, the study of younger birth cohorts experiencing higher levels of adiposity since earlier ages will provide further insights on the investigation of the long-term association between obesity and cardiovascular disease, with implications for public health.

CONSENT FOR PUBLICATION

Not applicable.

CONFLICT OF INTEREST

The authors confirm that this chapter contents have no conflict of interest.

ACKNOWLEDGEMENTS

Declared none.

REFERENCES

[1]   Barker DJ, Gluckman PD, Godfrey KM, Harding JE, Owens JA, Robinson JS. Fetal nutrition and cardiovascular disease in adult life. Lancet 1993; 341(8850): 938-41.
[http://dx.doi.org/10.1016/0140-6736(93)91224-A] [PMID: 8096277]

[2]   Barker DJ, Osmond C. Infant mortality, childhood nutrition, and ischaemic heart disease in England and Wales. Lancet 1986; 1(8489): 1077-81.
[http://dx.doi.org/10.1016/S0140-6736(86)91340-1] [PMID: 2871345]

[3]   Dobson AJ, Evans A, Ferrario M, *et al.* Changes in estimated coronary risk in the 1980s: data from 38 populations in the WHO MONICA Project. World Health Organization. Monitoring trends and determinants in cardiovascular diseases. Ann Med 1998; 30(2): 199-205.
[http://dx.doi.org/10.3109/07853899808999404] [PMID: 9667799]

[4]   Robinson RJ. Is the child father of the man? BMJ 1992; 304(6830): 789-90.
[http://dx.doi.org/10.1136/bmj.304.6830.789] [PMID: 1392701]

[5]   Kuh D, Shlomo YB. A life course approach to chronic disease epidemiology. 2nd ed., Oxford: Oxford University Press 2004.
[http://dx.doi.org/10.1093/acprof:oso/9780198578154.001.0001]

[6]   Kuh D, Ben-Shlomo Y, Lynch J, Hallqvist J, Power C. Life course epidemiology. J Epidemiol Community Health 2003; 57(10): 778-83.
[http://dx.doi.org/10.1136/jech.57.10.778] [PMID: 14573579]

[7]   Ben-Shlomo Y, Kuh D. A life course approach to chronic disease epidemiology: conceptual models, empirical challenges and interdisciplinary perspectives. Int J Epidemiol 2002; 31(2): 285-93.
[http://dx.doi.org/10.1093/ije/31.2.285] [PMID: 11980781]

[8]   Drake AJ, Walker BR. The intergenerational effects of fetal programming: non-genomic mechanisms for the inheritance of low birth weight and cardiovascular risk. J Endocrinol 2004; 180(1): 1-16.
[http://dx.doi.org/10.1677/joe.0.1800001] [PMID: 14709139]

[9]   Lynch J, Smith GD. A life course approach to chronic disease epidemiology. Annu Rev Public Health 2005; 26: 1-35.
[http://dx.doi.org/10.1146/annurev.publhealth.26.021304.144505] [PMID: 15760279]

[10]   Cameron N, Demerath EW. Critical periods in human growth and their relationship to diseases of aging. Am J Phys Anthropol 2002; 119 (Suppl. 35): 159-84.
[http://dx.doi.org/10.1002/ajpa.10183] [PMID: 12653312]

[11]   Dietz WH. Periods of risk in childhood for the development of adult obesity--what do we need to learn? J Nutr 1997; 127(9): 1884S-6S.
[http://dx.doi.org/10.1093/jn/127.9.1884S] [PMID: 9278575]

[12]   Glass TA, McAtee MJ. Behavioral science at the crossroads in public health: extending horizons, envisioning the future. Social science & medicine (1982) 2006; 62(7): 1650-71.
[http://dx.doi.org/10.1016/j.socscimed.2005.08.044]

[13]   Swinburn BA, Sacks G, Hall KD, *et al.* The global obesity pandemic: shaped by global drivers and local environments. Lancet 2011; 378(9793): 804-14.
[http://dx.doi.org/10.1016/S0140-6736(11)60813-1] [PMID: 21872749]

[14]   Pérez-Escamilla R, Kac G. Childhood obesity prevention: a life-course framework. Int J Obes Suppl 2013; 3 (Suppl. 1): S3-5.
[http://dx.doi.org/10.1038/ijosup.2013.2] [PMID: 25018875]

[15]   Butland B, Jebb S, Kopelman P, *et al.* Foresight Tackling Obesities: Future Choices - Project report. 2nd ed., UK: Government's Foresight Programme 2007.

[16]   Adair LS. Child and adolescent obesity: epidemiology and developmental perspectives. Physiol Behav 2008; 94(1): 8-16.
[http://dx.doi.org/10.1016/j.physbeh.2007.11.016] [PMID: 18191968]

[17]   Ayer J, Charakida M, Deanfield JE, Celermajer DS. Lifetime risk: childhood obesity and cardiovascular risk. Eur Heart J 2015; 36(22): 1371-6.
[http://dx.doi.org/10.1093/eurheartj/ehv089] [PMID: 25810456]

[18]   Dulloo AG, Jacquet J, Seydoux J, Montani JP. The thrifty 'catch-up fat' phenotype: its impact on insulin sensitivity during growth trajectories to obesity and metabolic syndrome. Int J Obes 2006; 30 (Suppl. 4): S23-35.
[http://dx.doi.org/10.1038/sj.ijo.0803516] [PMID: 17133232]

[19]   Aboderin I, Kalache A, Ben-Shlomo Y, *et al.* Life Course Perspectives on Coronary Heart Disease, Stroke and Diabetes: Key Issues and Implications for Policy and Research. Geneva: World Health Organization 2001.

[20]   Global Burden of Metabolic Risk Factors for Chronic Diseases Collaboration. Cardiovascular disease, chronic kidney disease, and diabetes mortality burden of cardiometabolic risk factors from 1980 to 2010: a comparative risk assessment. Lancet Diabetes Endocrinol 2014; 2(8): 634-47.
[http://dx.doi.org/10.1016/S2213-8587(14)70102-0] [PMID: 24842598]

[21]   Shashaj B, Bedogni G, Graziani MP, *et al.* Origin of cardiovascular risk in overweight preschool children: a cohort study of cardiometabolic risk factors at the onset of obesity. JAMA Pediatr 2014; 168(10): 917-24.
[http://dx.doi.org/10.1001/jamapediatrics.2014.900] [PMID: 25111132]

[22]   Power C, Thomas C. Changes in BMI, duration of overweight and obesity, and glucose metabolism: 45 years of follow-up of a birth cohort. Diabetes Care 2011; 34(9): 1986-91.
[http://dx.doi.org/10.2337/dc10-1482] [PMID: 21775760]

[23]   Galjaard S, Devlieger R, Van Assche FA. Fetal growth and developmental programming. J Perinat Med 2013; 41(1): 101-5.
[http://dx.doi.org/10.1515/jpm-2012-0020] [PMID: 23314514]

[24]   Tarantal AF, Berglund L. Obesity and lifespan health--importance of the fetal environment. Nutrients 2014; 6(4): 1725-36.
[http://dx.doi.org/10.3390/nu6041725] [PMID: 24763115]

[25]   Alberga AS, Sigal RJ, Goldfield G, Prud'homme D, Kenny GP. Overweight and obese teenagers: why is adolescence a critical period? Pediatr Obes 2012; 7(4): 261-73.
[http://dx.doi.org/10.1111/j.2047-6310.2011.00046.x] [PMID: 22461384]

[26]   Ravelli G-P, Stein ZA, Susser MW. Obesity in young men after famine exposure in utero and early infancy. N Engl J Med 1976; 295(7): 349-53.
[http://dx.doi.org/10.1056/NEJM197608122950701] [PMID: 934222]

[27]   Barker DJ, Winter PD, Osmond C, Margetts B, Simmonds SJ. Weight in infancy and death from ischaemic heart disease. Lancet 1989; 2(8663): 577-80.
[http://dx.doi.org/10.1016/S0140-6736(89)90710-1] [PMID: 2570282]

[28]   Barker DJ. The origins of the developmental origins theory. J Intern Med 2007; 261(5): 412-7.
[http://dx.doi.org/10.1111/j.1365-2796.2007.01809.x] [PMID: 17444880]

[29]   Wadhwa PD, Buss C, Entringer S, Swanson JM. Developmental origins of health and disease: brief history of the approach and current focus on epigenetic mechanisms. Semin Reprod Med 2009; 27(5): 358-68.
[http://dx.doi.org/10.1055/s-0029-1237424] [PMID: 19711246]

[30] Gillman MW, Barker D, Bier D, *et al.* Meeting report on the 3rd International Congress on Developmental Origins of Health and Disease (DOHaD). Pediatr Res 2007; 61(5 Pt 1): 625-9.
[http://dx.doi.org/10.1203/pdr.0b013e3180459fcd] [PMID: 17413866]

[31] Inadera H. Developmental origins of obesity and type 2 diabetes: molecular aspects and role of chemicals. Environ Health Prev Med 2013; 18(3): 185-97.
[http://dx.doi.org/10.1007/s12199-013-0328-8] [PMID: 23382021]

[32] Benyshek DC. The developmental origins of obesity and related health disorders--prenatal and perinatal factors. Coll Antropol 2007; 31(1): 11-7.
[PMID: 17598381]

[33] Nielsen LA, Nielsen TR, Holm JC. The Impact of Familial Predisposition to Obesity and Cardiovascular Disease on Childhood Obesity. Obes Facts 2015; 8(5): 319-28.
[http://dx.doi.org/10.1159/000441375] [PMID: 26465142]

[34] Santos Ferreira DL, Williams DM, Kangas AJ, *et al.* Association of pre-pregnancy body mass index with offspring metabolic profile: Analyses of 3 European prospective birth cohorts. PLoS Med 2017; 14(8)e1002376
[http://dx.doi.org/10.1371/journal.pmed.1002376] [PMID: 28829768]

[35] Rolland-Cachera MF, Deheeger M, Bellisle F, Sempé M, Guilloud-Bataille M, Patois E. Adiposity rebound in children: a simple indicator for predicting obesity. Am J Clin Nutr 1984; 39(1): 129-35.
[http://dx.doi.org/10.1093/ajcn/39.1.129] [PMID: 6691287]

[36] Rolland-Cachera MF, Deheeger M, Guilloud-Bataille M, Avons P, Patois E, Sempé M. Tracking the development of adiposity from one month of age to adulthood. Ann Hum Biol 1987; 14(3): 219-29.
[http://dx.doi.org/10.1080/03014468700008991] [PMID: 3662424]

[37] Taylor RW, Grant AM, Goulding A, Williams SM. Early adiposity rebound: review of papers linking this to subsequent obesity in children and adults. Curr Opin Clin Nutr Metab Care 2005; 8(6): 607-12.
[http://dx.doi.org/10.1097/01.mco.0000168391.60884.93] [PMID: 16205460]

[38] Campbell MW, Williams J, Carlin JB, Wake M. Is the adiposity rebound a rebound in adiposity? IJPO : an official journal of the International Association for the Study of Obesity 2011; 6(2-2): e207-15.
[http://dx.doi.org/10.3109/17477166.2010.526613]

[39] Williams S, Davie G, Lam F. Predicting BMI in young adults from childhood data using two approaches to modelling adiposity rebound. International journal of obesity and related metabolic disorders : journal of the International Association for the Study of Obesity 1999; 23(4): 348-54.
[http://dx.doi.org/10.1038/sj.ijo.0800824]

[40] Freedman DS, Kettel Khan L, Serdula MK, Srinivasan SR, Berenson GS. BMI rebound, childhood height and obesity among adults: the Bogalusa Heart Study. International journal of obesity and related metabolic disorders : journal of the International Association for the Study of Obesity 2001; 25(4): 543-9.
[http://dx.doi.org/10.1038/sj.ijo.0801581]

[41] Veldhuis JD, Roemmich JN, Richmond EJ, *et al.* Endocrine control of body composition in infancy, childhood, and puberty. Endocr Rev 2005; 26(1): 114-46.
[http://dx.doi.org/10.1210/er.2003-0038] [PMID: 15689575]

[42] Spalding KL, Arner E, Westermark PO, *et al.* Dynamics of fat cell turnover in humans. Nature 2008; 453(7196): 783-7.
[http://dx.doi.org/10.1038/nature06902] [PMID: 18454136]

[43] Loomba-Albrecht LA, Styne DM. Effect of puberty on body composition. Curr Opin Endocrinol Diabetes Obes 2009; 16(1): 10-5.
[http://dx.doi.org/10.1097/MED.0b013e328320d54c] [PMID: 19115520]

[44] Wells JC. Sexual dimorphism of body composition. Best Pract Res Clin Endocrinol Metab 2007; 21(3): 415-30.

[http://dx.doi.org/10.1016/j.beem.2007.04.007] [PMID: 17875489]

[45]   Bralić I, Tahirović H, Matanić D, *et al.* Association of early menarche age and overweight/obesity. J Pediatr Endocrinol Metab 2012; 25(1-2): 57-62.
[http://dx.doi.org/10.1515/jpem-2011-0277] [PMID: 22570951]

[46]   van Lenthe FJ, Kemper CG, van Mechelen W. Rapid maturation in adolescence results in greater obesity in adulthood: the Amsterdam Growth and Health Study. Am J Clin Nutr 1996; 64(1): 18-24.
[http://dx.doi.org/10.1093/ajcn/64.1.18] [PMID: 8669409]

[47]   Prentice P, Viner RM. Pubertal timing and adult obesity and cardiometabolic risk in women and men: a systematic review and meta-analysis. Int J Obes 2013; 37(8): 1036-43.
[http://dx.doi.org/10.1038/ijo.2012.177] [PMID: 23164700]

[48]   Kindblom JM, Lorentzon M, Norjavaara E, *et al.* Pubertal timing is an independent predictor of central adiposity in young adult males: the Gothenburg osteoporosis and obesity determinants study. Diabetes 2006; 55(11): 3047-52.
[http://dx.doi.org/10.2337/db06-0192] [PMID: 17065341]

[49]   van Lenthe FJ, Kemper HC, van Mechelen W, *et al.* Biological maturation and the distribution of subcutaneous fat from adolescence into adulthood: the Amsterdam Growth and Health Study. International journal of obesity and related metabolic disorders : journal of the International Association for the Study of Obesity 1996; 20(2): 121-9.

[50]   Lee JM, Appugliese D, Kaciroti N, Corwyn RF, Bradley RH, Lumeng JC. Weight status in young girls and the onset of puberty. Pediatrics 2007; 119(3): e624-30.
[http://dx.doi.org/10.1542/peds.2006-2188] [PMID: 17332182]

[51]   Kaplowitz PB, Slora EJ, Wasserman RC, Pedlow SE, Herman-Giddens ME. Earlier onset of puberty in girls: relation to increased body mass index and race. Pediatrics 2001; 108(2): 347-53.
[http://dx.doi.org/10.1542/peds.108.2.347] [PMID: 11483799]

[52]   Steinberg L, Silverberg SB. The vicissitudes of autonomy in early adolescence. Child Dev 1986; 57(4): 841-51.
[http://dx.doi.org/10.2307/1130361] [PMID: 3757604]

[53]   Laursen B, Bukowski WM. A Developmental Guide to the Organisation of Close Relationships. Int J Behav Dev 1997; 21(4): 747-70.
[http://dx.doi.org/10.1080/016502597384659] [PMID: 20090927]

[54]   De Goede IH, Branje SJ, Meeus WH. Developmental changes in adolescents' perceptions of relationships with their parents. J Youth Adolesc 2009; 38(1): 75-88.
[http://dx.doi.org/10.1007/s10964-008-9286-7] [PMID: 19636793]

[55]   Warren CW, Kann L, Small ML, Santelli JS, Collins JL, Kolbe LJ. Age of initiating selected health-risk behaviors among high school students in the United States. J Adolesc Health 1997; 21(4): 225-31.
[http://dx.doi.org/10.1016/S1054-139X(97)00112-2] [PMID: 9304453]

[56]   Dumith SC, Gigante DP, Domingues MR, Kohl HW III. Physical activity change during adolescence: a systematic review and a pooled analysis. Int J Epidemiol 2011; 40(3): 685-98.
[http://dx.doi.org/10.1093/ije/dyq272] [PMID: 21245072]

[57]   Feeley A, Musenge E, Pettifor JM, Norris SA. Changes in dietary habits and eating practices in adolescents living in urban South Africa: the birth to twenty cohort. Nutrition 2012; 28(7-8): e1-6.
[http://dx.doi.org/10.1016/j.nut.2011.11.025] [PMID: 22465902]

[58]   Collings PJ, Wijndaele K, Corder K, *et al.* Magnitude and determinants of change in objectively-measured physical activity, sedentary time and sleep duration from ages 15 to 17.5y in UK adolescents: the ROOTS study. Int J Behav Nutr Phys Act 2015; 12: 61.
[http://dx.doi.org/10.1186/s12966-015-0222-4] [PMID: 25971606]

[59]   Metcalf BS, Hosking J, Jeffery AN, Henley WE, Wilkin TJ. Exploring the Adolescent Fall in Physical Activity: A 10-yr Cohort Study (EarlyBird 41). Med Sci Sports Exerc 2015; 47(10): 2084-92.

[http://dx.doi.org/10.1249/MSS.0000000000000644] [PMID: 25706294]

[60]   Must A, Tybor DJ. Physical activity and sedentary behavior: a review of longitudinal studies of weight and adiposity in youth. Int J Obes 2005; 29 (Suppl. 2): S84-96.
[http://dx.doi.org/10.1038/sj.ijo.0803064] [PMID: 16385758]

[61]   Alexy U, Wicher M, Kersting M. Breakfast trends in children and adolescents: frequency and quality. Public Health Nutr 2010; 13(11): 1795-802.
[http://dx.doi.org/10.1017/S1368980010000091] [PMID: 20236559]

[62]   Craigie AM, Lake AA, Kelly SA, Adamson AJ, Mathers JC. Tracking of obesity-related behaviours from childhood to adulthood: A systematic review. Maturitas 2011; 70(3): 266-84.
[http://dx.doi.org/10.1016/j.maturitas.2011.08.005] [PMID: 21920682]

[63]   Reilly JJ, Methven E, McDowell ZC, *et al.* Health consequences of obesity. Arch Dis Child 2003; 88(9): 748-52.
[http://dx.doi.org/10.1136/adc.88.9.748] [PMID: 12937090]

[64]   Daniels SR. Complications of obesity in children and adolescents. Int J Obes 2009; 33 (Suppl. 1): S60-5.
[http://dx.doi.org/10.1038/ijo.2009.20] [PMID: 19363511]

[65]   Abdullah A, Wolfe R, Stoelwinder JU, *et al.* The number of years lived with obesity and the risk of all-cause and cause-specific mortality. Int J Epidemiol 2011; 40(4): 985-96.
[http://dx.doi.org/10.1093/ije/dyr018] [PMID: 21357186]

[66]   Twig G, Afek A, Shamiss A, *et al.* Adolescence BMI and trends in adulthood mortality: a study of 2.16 million adolescents. J Clin Endocrinol Metab 2014; 99(6): 2095-103.
[http://dx.doi.org/10.1210/jc.2014-1213] [PMID: 24601695]

[67]   Lim SS, Vos T, Flaxman AD, *et al.* A comparative risk assessment of burden of disease and injury attributable to 67 risk factors and risk factor clusters in 21 regions, 1990-2010: a systematic analysis for the Global Burden of Disease Study 2010. Lancet 2012; 380(9859): 2224-60.
[http://dx.doi.org/10.1016/S0140-6736(12)61766-8] [PMID: 23245609]

[68]   Twig G, Yaniv G, Levine H, *et al.* Body-Mass Index in 2.3 Million Adolescents and Cardiovascular Death in Adulthood. N Engl J Med 2016; 374(25): 2430-40.
[http://dx.doi.org/10.1056/NEJMoa1503840] [PMID: 27074389]

[69]   Whitlock G, Lewington S, Sherliker P, *et al.* Prospective Studies Collaboration. Body-mass index and cause-specific mortality in 900 000 adults: collaborative analyses of 57 prospective studies. Lancet 2009; 373(9669): 1083-96.
[http://dx.doi.org/10.1016/S0140-6736(09)60318-4] [PMID: 19299006]

[70]   Brotman DJ, Walker E, Lauer MS, O'Brien RG. In search of fewer independent risk factors. Arch Intern Med 2005; 165(2): 138-45.
[http://dx.doi.org/10.1001/archinte.165.2.138] [PMID: 15668358]

[71]   O'Donnell CJ, Elosua R. [Cardiovascular risk factors. Insights from Framingham Heart Study]. Rev Esp Cardiol 2008; 61(3): 299-310.
[http://dx.doi.org/10.1157/13116658] [PMID: 18361904]

[72]   Mack M, Gopal A. Epidemiology, traditional and novel risk factors in coronary artery disease. Cardiol Clin 2014; 32(3): 323-32.
[http://dx.doi.org/10.1016/j.ccl.2014.04.003] [PMID: 25091961]

[73]   Forouzanfar MH, Alexander L, Anderson HR, *et al.* GBD 2013 Risk Factors Collaborators. Global, regional, and national comparative risk assessment of 79 behavioural, environmental and occupational, and metabolic risks or clusters of risks in 188 countries, 1990-2013: a systematic analysis for the Global Burden of Disease Study 2013. Lancet 2015; 386(10010): 2287-323.
[http://dx.doi.org/10.1016/S0140-6736(15)00128-2] [PMID: 26364544]

[74]   Schwingshackl L, Dias S, Hoffmann G. Impact of long-term lifestyle programmes on weight loss and

cardiovascular risk factors in overweight/obese participants: a systematic review and network meta-analysis. Syst Rev 2014; 3: 130.
[http://dx.doi.org/10.1186/2046-4053-3-130] [PMID: 25358395]

[75] Zomer E, Gurusamy K, Leach R, *et al*. Interventions that cause weight loss and the impact on cardiovascular risk factors: a systematic review and meta-analysis. Obes Rev 2016; 17(10): 1001-11.
[http://dx.doi.org/10.1111/obr.12433] [PMID: 27324830]

[76] Batsis JA, Romero-Corral A, Collazo-Clavell ML, Sarr MG, Somers VK, Lopez-Jimenez F. Effect of bariatric surgery on the metabolic syndrome: a population-based, long-term controlled study. Mayo Clin Proc 2008; 83(8): 897-907.
[http://dx.doi.org/10.1016/S0025-6196(11)60766-0] [PMID: 18674474]

[77] Juonala M, Magnussen CG, Berenson GS, *et al*. Childhood adiposity, adult adiposity, and cardiovascular risk factors. N Engl J Med 2011; 365(20): 1876-85.
[http://dx.doi.org/10.1056/NEJMoa1010112] [PMID: 22087679]

[78] Araújo J, Barros H, Ramos E, Li L. Trajectories of total and central adiposity throughout adolescence and cardiometabolic factors in early adulthood. Int J Obes 2016; 40(12): 1899-905.
[http://dx.doi.org/10.1038/ijo.2016.170] [PMID: 27677621]

[79] Huang RC, de Klerk NH, Smith A, *et al*. Lifecourse childhood adiposity trajectories associated with adolescent insulin resistance. Diabetes Care 2011; 34(4): 1019-25.
[http://dx.doi.org/10.2337/dc10-1809] [PMID: 21378216]

[80] Munthali RJ, Kagura J, Lombard Z, Norris SA. Childhood adiposity trajectories are associated with late adolescent blood pressure: birth to twenty cohort. BMC Public Health 2016; 16: 665.
[http://dx.doi.org/10.1186/s12889-016-3337-x] [PMID: 27473865]

[81] Ventura AK, Loken E, Birch LL. Developmental trajectories of girls' BMI across childhood and adolescence. Obesity (Silver Spring) 2009; 17(11): 2067-74.
[http://dx.doi.org/10.1038/oby.2009.123] [PMID: 19424165]

[82] Ziyab AH, Karmaus W, Kurukulaaratchy RJ, Zhang H, Arshad SH. Developmental trajectories of Body Mass Index from infancy to 18 years of age: prenatal determinants and health consequences. J Epidemiol Community Health 2014; 68(10): 934-41.
[http://dx.doi.org/10.1136/jech-2014-203808] [PMID: 24895184]

[83] Ng M, Fleming T, Robinson M, *et al*. Global, regional, and national prevalence of overweight and obesity in children and adults during 1980-2013: a systematic analysis for the Global Burden of Disease Study 2013. Lancet 2014; 384(9945): 766-81.
[http://dx.doi.org/10.1016/S0140-6736(14)60460-8] [PMID: 24880830]

[84] Krishnamurthi RV, Feigin VL, Forouzanfar MH, *et al*. Global Burden of Diseases, Injuries, Risk Factors Study 2010 (GBD 2010); GBD Stroke Experts Group. Global and regional burden of first-ever ischaemic and haemorrhagic stroke during 1990-2010: findings from the Global Burden of Disease Study 2010. Lancet Glob Health 2013; 1(5): e259-81.
[http://dx.doi.org/10.1016/S2214-109X(13)70089-5] [PMID: 25104492]

[85] Moran AE, Forouzanfar MH, Roth GA, *et al*. Temporal trends in ischemic heart disease mortality in 21 world regions, 1980 to 2010: the Global Burden of Disease 2010 study. Circulation 2014; 129(14): 1483-92.
[http://dx.doi.org/10.1161/CIRCULATIONAHA.113.004042] [PMID: 24573352]

[86] Anderson LN, Lebovic G, Hamilton J, *et al*. TARGet Kids Collaboration. Body Mass Index, Waist Circumference, and the Clustering of Cardiometabolic Risk Factors in Early Childhood. Paediatr Perinat Epidemiol 2016; 30(2): 160-70.
[http://dx.doi.org/10.1111/ppe.12268] [PMID: 26645704]

[87] Messiah SE, Vidot DC, Gurnurkar S, Alhezayen R, Natale RA, Arheart KL. Obesity is significantly associated with cardiovascular disease risk factors in 2- to 9-year-olds. J Clin Hypertens (Greenwich) 2014; 16(12): 889-94.

[http://dx.doi.org/10.1111/jch.12427] [PMID: 25307314]

[88]   Reilly JJ, Kelly J. Long-term impact of overweight and obesity in childhood and adolescence on morbidity and premature mortality in adulthood: systematic review. Int J Obes 2011; 35(7): 891-8.
[http://dx.doi.org/10.1038/ijo.2010.222] [PMID: 20975725]

[89]   Umer A, Kelley GA, Cottrell LE, Giacobbi P Jr, Innes KE, Lilly CL. Childhood obesity and adult cardiovascular disease risk factors: a systematic review with meta-analysis. BMC Public Health 2017; 17(1): 683.
[http://dx.doi.org/10.1186/s12889-017-4691-z] [PMID: 28851330]

[90]   Abdullah A, Stoelwinder J, Shortreed S, *et al.* The duration of obesity and the risk of type 2 diabetes. Public Health Nutr 2011; 14(1): 119-26.
[http://dx.doi.org/10.1017/S1368980010001813] [PMID: 20587115]

[91]   Hekimsoy Z, Oktem IK. Duration of obesity is not a risk factor for type 2 diabetes mellitus, arterial hypertension and hyperlipidemia. Diabetes Obes Metab 2003; 5(6): 432-7.
[http://dx.doi.org/10.1046/j.1463-1326.2003.00298.x] [PMID: 14617229]

[92]   Pinto Pereira SM, Power C. Life course body mass index, birthweight and lipid levels in mid-adulthood: a nationwide birth cohort study. Eur Heart J 2013; 34(16): 1215-24.
[http://dx.doi.org/10.1093/eurheartj/ehs333] [PMID: 23234645]

[93]   Pontiroli AE, Galli L. Duration of obesity is a risk factor for non-insulin-dependent diabetes mellitus, not for arterial hypertension or for hyperlipidaemia. Acta Diabetol 1998; 35(3): 130-6.
[http://dx.doi.org/10.1007/s005920050117] [PMID: 9840448]

[94]   Tanamas SK, Wong E, Backholer K, *et al.* Duration of obesity and incident hypertension in adults from the Framingham Heart Study. J Hypertens 2015; 33(3): 542-5.
[http://dx.doi.org/10.1097/HJH.0000000000000441] [PMID: 25479024]

[95]   The NS, Richardson AS, Gordon-Larsen P. Timing and duration of obesity in relation to diabetes: findings from an ethnically diverse, nationally representative sample. Diabetes Care 2013; 36(4): 865-72.
[http://dx.doi.org/10.2337/dc12-0536] [PMID. 23223352]

[96]   Abdullah A, Wolfe R, Mannan H, Stoelwinder JU, Stevenson C, Peeters A. Epidemiologic merit of obese-years, the combination of degree and duration of obesity. Am J Epidemiol 2012; 176(2): 99-107.
[http://dx.doi.org/10.1093/aje/kwr522] [PMID: 22759723]

[97]   Abdullah A, Amin FA, Hanum F, *et al.* Estimating the risk of type-2 diabetes using obese-years in a contemporary population of the Framingham Study. Glob Health Action 2016; 9(1): 30421.
[http://dx.doi.org/10.3402/gha.v9.30421] [PMID: 27369220]

[98]   Abdullah A, Amin FA, Stoelwinder J, *et al.* Estimating the risk of cardiovascular disease using an obese-years metric. BMJ Open 2014; 4(9)e005629
[http://dx.doi.org/10.1136/bmjopen-2014-005629] [PMID: 25231490]

[99]   Araújo J, Severo M, Barros H, Ramos E. Duration and degree of adiposity: effect on cardiovascular risk factors at early adulthood. Int J Obes 2017; 41(10): 1526-30.
[http://dx.doi.org/10.1038/ijo.2017.133] [PMID: 28584300]

[100] Regnault N, Gillman MW. Importance of characterizing growth trajectories. Ann Nutr Metab 2014; 65(2-3): 110-3.
[http://dx.doi.org/10.1159/000365893] [PMID: 25413648]

[101] Buyken AE, Karaolis-Danckert N, Remer T, Bolzenius K, Landsberg B, Kroke A. Effects of breastfeeding on trajectories of body fat and BMI throughout childhood. Obesity (Silver Spring) 2008; 16(2): 389-95.
[http://dx.doi.org/10.1038/oby.2007.57] [PMID: 18239649]

[102] Eissa MA, Dai S, Mihalopoulos NL, Day RS, Harrist RB, Labarthe DR. Trajectories of fat mass index,

fat free-mass index, and waist circumference in children: Project HeartBeat! Am J Prev Med 2009; 37(1) (Suppl.): S34-9.
[http://dx.doi.org/10.1016/j.amepre.2009.04.005] [PMID: 19524154]

[103] Howe LD, Tilling K, Galobardes B, *et al.* Socioeconomic disparities in trajectories of adiposity across childhood. International journal of pediatric obesity : IJPO : an official journal of the International Association for the Study of Obesity 2011; 6(2-2): e144-53.
[http://dx.doi.org/10.3109/17477166.2010.500387]

[104] Sherar LB, Eisenmann JC, Chilibeck PD, *et al.* Relationship between trajectories of trunk fat mass development in adolescence and cardiometabolic risk in young adulthood. Obesity (Silver Spring) 2011; 19(8): 1699-706.
[http://dx.doi.org/10.1038/oby.2010.340] [PMID: 21273991]

[105] Burdette AM, Needham BL. Neighborhood environment and body mass index trajectories from adolescence to adulthood. J Adolesc Health 2012; 50(1): 30-7.
[http://dx.doi.org/10.1016/j.jadohealth.2011.03.009] [PMID: 22188831]

[106] Albrecht SS, Gordon-Larsen P. Ethnic differences in body mass index trajectories from adolescence to adulthood: a focus on Hispanic and Asian subgroups in the United States. PLoS One 2013; 8(9)e72983
[http://dx.doi.org/10.1371/journal.pone.0072983] [PMID: 24039835]

[107] Bae D, Wickrama KA, O'Neal CW. Social consequences of early socioeconomic adversity and youth BMI trajectories: gender and race/ethnicity differences. J Adolesc 2014; 37(6): 883-92.
[http://dx.doi.org/10.1016/j.adolescence.2014.06.002] [PMID: 24971847]

[108] Boyer BP, Nelson JA, Holub SC. Childhood body mass index trajectories predicting cardiovascular risk in adolescence. J Adolesc Health 2015; 56(6): 599-605.
[http://dx.doi.org/10.1016/j.jadohealth.2015.01.006] [PMID: 25746172]

[109] Jones A. Residential mobility and trajectories of adiposity among adolescents in urban and non-urban neighborhoods. J Urban Health 2015; 92(2): 265-78.
[http://dx.doi.org/10.1007/s11524-015-9952-5] [PMID: 25801487]

[110] Nau C, Schwartz BS, Bandeen-Roche K, *et al.* Community socioeconomic deprivation and obesity trajectories in children using electronic health records. Obesity (Silver Spring) 2015; 23(1): 207-12.
[http://dx.doi.org/10.1002/oby.20903] [PMID: 25324223]

[111] Aarestrup J, Gamborg M, Tilling K, Ulrich LG, Sørensen TI, Baker JL. Childhood body mass index growth trajectories and endometrial cancer risk. Int J Cancer 2017; 140(2): 310-5.
[http://dx.doi.org/10.1002/ijc.30464] [PMID: 27718528]

[112] Cohen-Manheim I, Doniger GM, Sinnreich R, *et al.* Body Mass Index, Height and Socioeconomic Position in Adolescence, Their Trajectories into Adulthood, and Cognitive Function in Midlife. J Alzheimers Dis 2017; 55(3): 1207-21.
[http://dx.doi.org/10.3233/JAD-160843] [PMID: 27814299]

[113] Howe LD, Tilling K, Benfield L, *et al.* Changes in ponderal index and body mass index across childhood and their associations with fat mass and cardiovascular risk factors at age 15. PLoS One 2010; 5(12)e15186
[http://dx.doi.org/10.1371/journal.pone.0015186] [PMID: 21170348]

[114] Li C, Goran MI, Kaur H, Nollen N, Ahluwalia JS. Developmental trajectories of overweight during childhood: role of early life factors. Obesity (Silver Spring) 2007; 15(3): 760-71.
[http://dx.doi.org/10.1038/oby.2007.585] [PMID: 17372328]

[115] Nonnemaker JM, Morgan-Lopez AA, Pais JM, Finkelstein EA. Youth BMI trajectories: evidence from the NLSY97. Obesity (Silver Spring) 2009; 17(6): 1274-80.
[http://dx.doi.org/10.1038/oby.2009.5] [PMID: 19584884]

[116] Balistreri KS, Van Hook J. Trajectories of overweight among US school children: a focus on social and economic characteristics. Matern Child Health J 2011; 15(5): 610-9.

[http://dx.doi.org/10.1007/s10995-010-0622-7] [PMID: 20535537]

[117]   Pryor LE, Tremblay RE, Boivin M, *et al.* Developmental trajectories of body mass index in early childhood and their risk factors: an 8-year longitudinal study. Arch Pediatr Adolesc Med 2011; 165(10): 906-12.
[http://dx.doi.org/10.1001/archpediatrics.2011.153] [PMID: 21969392]

[118]   Smith AJ, O'Sullivan PB, Beales DJ, de Klerk N, Straker LM. Trajectories of childhood body mass index are associated with adolescent sagittal standing posture. International journal of pediatric obesity : IJPO : an official journal of the International Association for the Study of Obesity 2011; 6(2-2): e97-106.
[http://dx.doi.org/10.3109/17477166.2010.530664]

[119]   Carter MA, Dubois L, Tremblay MS, Taljaard M, Jones BL. Trajectories of childhood weight gain: the relative importance of local environment versus individual social and early life factors. PLoS One 2012; 7(10)e47065
[http://dx.doi.org/10.1371/journal.pone.0047065] [PMID: 23077545]

[120]   Chen X, Brogan K. Developmental trajectories of overweight and obesity of US youth through the life course of adolescence to young adulthood. Adolesc Health Med Ther 2012; 3: 33-42.
[http://dx.doi.org/10.2147/AHMT.S30178] [PMID: 24600285]

[121]   Garden FL, Marks GB, Simpson JM, Webb KL. Body mass index (BMI) trajectories from birth to 11.5 years: relation to early life food intake. Nutrients 2012; 4(10): 1382-98.
[http://dx.doi.org/10.3390/nu4101382] [PMID: 23201761]

[122]   Haga C, Kondo N, Suzuki K, *et al.* Developmental trajectories of body mass index among Japanese children and impact of maternal factors during pregnancy. PLoS One 2012; 7(12)e51896
[http://dx.doi.org/10.1371/journal.pone.0051896] [PMID: 23272187]

[123]   Jun HJ, Corliss HL, Boynton-Jarrett R, Spiegelman D, Austin SB, Wright RJ. Growing up in a domestic violence environment: relationship with developmental trajectories of body mass index during adolescence into young adulthood. J Epidemiol Community Health 2012; 66(7): 629-35.
[http://dx.doi.org/10.1136/jech.2010.110932] [PMID: 21296904]

[124]   Huang DY, Lanza HI, Wright-Volel K, Anglin MD. Developmental trajectories of childhood obesity and risk behaviors in adolescence. J Adolesc 2013; 36(1): 139-48.
[http://dx.doi.org/10.1016/j.adolescence.2012.10.005] [PMID: 23199644]

[125]   Lane SP, Bluestone C, Burke CT. Trajectories of BMI from early childhood through early adolescence: SES and psychosocial predictors. Br J Health Psychol 2013; 18(1): 66-82.
[http://dx.doi.org/10.1111/j.2044-8287.2012.02078.x] [PMID: 22574894]

[126]   von Bonsdorff MB, Tormakangas T, Rantanen T, *et al.* Early life body mass trajectories and mortality in older age: Findings from the Helsinki Birth Cohort Study. Ann Med 2014; 1-6.
[PMID: 25307361]

[127]   Araújo J, Severo M, Barros H, Mishra GD, Guimarães JT, Ramos E. Developmental trajectories of adiposity from birth until early adulthood and association with cardiometabolic risk factors. Int J Obes 2015; 39(10): 1443-9.
[http://dx.doi.org/10.1038/ijo.2015.128] [PMID: 26155921]

[128]   Brault MC, Aimé A, Bégin C, Valois P, Craig W. Heterogeneity of sex-stratified BMI trajectories in children from 8 to 14 years old. Physiol Behav 2015; 142: 111-20.
[http://dx.doi.org/10.1016/j.physbeh.2015.02.001] [PMID: 25656690]

[129]   Giles LC, Whitrow MJ, Davies MJ, Davies CE, Rumbold AR, Moore VM. Growth trajectories in early childhood, their relationship with antenatal and postnatal factors, and development of obesity by age 9 years: results from an Australian birth cohort study. Int J Obes 2015; 39(7): 1049-56.
[http://dx.doi.org/10.1038/ijo.2015.42] [PMID: 26008137]

[130]   Chen YC, Liou TH, Chen PC, *et al.* Growth trajectories and asthma/rhinitis in children: a longitudinal

study in Taiwan. Eur Respir J 2017; 49(1)1600741
[http://dx.doi.org/10.1183/13993003.00741-2016] [PMID: 27824597]

[131] Ford ND, Martorell R, Mehta NK, Ramirez-Zea M, Stein AD. Life-Course Body Mass Index Trajectories Are Predicted by Childhood Socioeconomic Status but Not Exposure to Improved Nutrition during the First 1000 Days after Conception in Guatemalan Adults. J Nutr 2016; 146(11): 2368-74.
[http://dx.doi.org/10.3945/jn.116.236075] [PMID: 27655759]

[132] Koning M, Hoekstra T, de Jong E, Visscher TL, Seidell JC, Renders CM. Identifying developmental trajectories of body mass index in childhood using latent class growth (mixture) modelling: associations with dietary, sedentary and physical activity behaviors: a longitudinal study. BMC Public Health 2016; 16(1): 1128.
[http://dx.doi.org/10.1186/s12889-016-3757-7] [PMID: 27793201]

[133] Nesbit KC, Low JA, Sisson SB. Adolescent BMI trajectories with clusters of physical activity and sedentary behaviour: an exploratory analysis. Obes Sci Pract 2016; 2(2): 115-22.
[http://dx.doi.org/10.1002/osp4.36] [PMID: 27840687]

[134] Serdula MK, Ivery D, Coates RJ, Freedman DS, Williamson DF, Byers T. Do obese children become obese adults? A review of the literature. Prev Med 1993; 22(2): 167-77.
[http://dx.doi.org/10.1006/pmed.1993.1014] [PMID: 8483856]

[135] Simmonds M, Llewellyn A, Owen CG, Woolacott N. Predicting adult obesity from childhood obesity: a systematic review and meta-analysis. Obes Rev 2016; 17(2): 95-107.
[http://dx.doi.org/10.1111/obr.12334] [PMID: 26696565]

[136] Singh AS, Mulder C, Twisk JW, van Mechelen W, Chinapaw MJ. Tracking of childhood overweight into adulthood: a systematic review of the literature. Obes Rev 2008; 9(5): 474-88.
[http://dx.doi.org/10.1111/j.1467-789X.2008.00475.x] [PMID: 18331423]

[137] Guo SS, Wu W, Chumlea WC, Roche AF. Predicting overweight and obesity in adulthood from body mass index values in childhood and adolescence. Am J Clin Nutr 2002; 76(3): 653-8.
[http://dx.doi.org/10.1093/ajcn/76.3.653] [PMID: 12198014]

[138] Lawlor DA, Leon DA. Association of body mass index and obesity measured in early childhood with risk of coronary heart disease and stroke in middle age: findings from the aberdeen children of the 1950s prospective cohort study. Circulation 2005; 111(15): 1891-6.
[http://dx.doi.org/10.1161/01.CIR.0000161798.45728.4D] [PMID: 15837941]

[139] Llewellyn A, Simmonds M, Owen CG, Woolacott N. Childhood obesity as a predictor of morbidity in adulthood: a systematic review and meta-analysis. Obes Rev 2016; 17(1): 56-67.
[http://dx.doi.org/10.1111/obr.12316] [PMID: 26440472]

[140] Lloyd LJ, Langley-Evans SC, McMullen S. Childhood obesity and adult cardiovascular disease risk: a systematic review. Int J Obes 2010; 34(1): 18-28.
[http://dx.doi.org/10.1038/ijo.2009.61] [PMID: 19434067]

[141] Law CM, Shiell AW, Newsome CA, *et al.* Fetal, infant, and childhood growth and adult blood pressure: a longitudinal study from birth to 22 years of age. Circulation 2002; 105(9): 1088-92.
[http://dx.doi.org/10.1161/hc0902.104677] [PMID: 11877360]

[142] Li L, Law C, Power C. Body mass index throughout the life-course and blood pressure in mid-adult life: a birth cohort study. J Hypertens 2007; 25(6): 1215-23.
[http://dx.doi.org/10.1097/HJH.0b013e3280f3c01a] [PMID: 17563534]

[143] Sovio U, Kaakinen M, Tzoulaki I, *et al.* How do changes in body mass index in infancy and childhood associate with cardiometabolic profile in adulthood? Findings from the Northern Finland Birth Cohort 1966 Study. Int J Obes 2014; 38(1): 53-9.
[http://dx.doi.org/10.1038/ijo.2013.165] [PMID: 24080793]

[144] Park MH, Falconer C, Viner RM, Kinra S. The impact of childhood obesity on morbidity and

mortality in adulthood: a systematic review. Obes Rev 2012; 13(11): 985-1000.
[http://dx.doi.org/10.1111/j.1467-789X.2012.01015.x] [PMID: 22731928]

[145] Schisterman EF, Cole SR, Platt RW. Overadjustment bias and unnecessary adjustment in epidemiologic studies. Epidemiology 2009; 20(4): 488-95.
[http://dx.doi.org/10.1097/EDE.0b013e3181a819a1] [PMID: 19525685]

[146] De Stavola BL, Nitsch D, dos Santos Silva I, *et al.* Statistical issues in life course epidemiology. Am J Epidemiol 2006; 163(1): 84-96.
[http://dx.doi.org/10.1093/aje/kwj003] [PMID: 16306313]

[147] Lucas A, Fewtrell MS, Cole TJ. Fetal origins of adult disease-the hypothesis revisited. BMJ 1999; 319(7204): 245-9.
[http://dx.doi.org/10.1136/bmj.319.7204.245] [PMID: 10417093]

[148] Loehlin JC. Latent variable models: An introduction to factor, path, and structural equation analysis. 4th ed., New Jersey: Psychology Press 2004.
[http://dx.doi.org/10.4324/9781410609823]

[149] Gamborg M, Andersen PK, Baker JL, *et al.* Life course path analysis of birth weight, childhood growth, and adult systolic blood pressure. Am J Epidemiol 2009; 169(10): 1167-78.
[http://dx.doi.org/10.1093/aje/kwp047] [PMID: 19357327]

[150] Zhang Z, Zheng C, Kim C, Van Poucke S, Lin S, Lan P. Causal mediation analysis in the context of clinical research. Ann Transl Med 2016; 4(21): 425.
[http://dx.doi.org/10.21037/atm.2016.11.11] [PMID: 27942516]

[151] Smith GD, Ebrahim S. Mendelian randomization: genetic variants as instruments for strengthening causal inference in observational studies.National Research Council - Biosocial Surveys. Washington, DC: The National Academies Press 2008.

CHAPTER 2

Social and Health Behavior Determinants of Obesity

Andreia Oliveira[1,2,*], **Catarina Durão**[1,3] and **Carla Lopes**[1,2]

[1] *EPI Unit - Institute of Public Health, University of Porto, Porto, Portugal*

[2] *Faculty of Medicine, University of Porto, Porto, Portugal*

[3] *NOVA Medical School, Faculdade de Ciências Médicas, Universidade Nova de Lisboa, Lisboa, Portugal*

Abstract: The understanding of obesity's etiology has broadened from an individual to a more comprehensive perspective of environmental influences, based in social ecological models. Interventions to tackle obesity are dependent on understanding interactions within complex systems and on changing modifiable risk factors with high impact at the population level. In this chapter, literature on social and behavioral factors associated with obesity was reviewed. Socioeconomic factors seem to be main drivers of obesity. This effect may act indirectly through mediators such as diet and physical activity. The transgenerational profile of both socioeconomic conditions and obesity should also be highlighted. Thus, these influences should be taken from a life-course perspective. The establishment of obesity is nested in early life and the family context, including feeding practices, parents' dietary habits and lifestyles, and parental obesity, are proximal determinants of childhood obesity. Pregnancy, breastfeeding and weaning are identified as sensitive periods for establishing eating habits and therefore obesity development. Research has focused extensively on the effects of diet and physical activity on the energy balance; however, there seems to exist a lack of consistent associations. Evidence is more robust regarding the protective effects of vegetables, whole grains and the Mediterranean Diet, and the detrimental effect of sugar-sweetened beverages and sedentary behaviors, namely television viewing, particularly in children. Smoking and moderate alcohol drinking have been negatively associated with obesity, but a confounding effect of a general lifestyle profile cannot be excluded. The influence of smoking during pregnancy on later childhood obesity is supported by more robust evidence.

Keywords: Alcohol drinking, Body mass index, Childhood obesity, Diet, Energy balance, Epidemiologic factors, Epidemiologic studies, Family characteristics, Feeding behavior, Health behavior, Meta-analysis, Obesity, Physical activity, Smoking, Social determinants of health, Socioeconomic status, Weight gain.

* **Corresponding author Andreia Oliveira:** Institute of Public Health, University of Porto, Porto, Portugal; Tel/Fax: +351 222061820; E-mail: acmatos@ispup.up.pt

Rosário Monteiro and Maria João Martins (Eds.)

INTRODUCTION

Obesity rates are massive throughout the world [1, 2]. Although genetics may explain differences between individuals, it cannot explain the temporal upward trend of obesity at the population level [3, 4]. The epidemiologic transition occurred in the last decades, *i.e.*, a shift from a pattern of prevailing infectious diseases to prevalent chronic and degenerative diseases associated with urban-industrial lifestyles is in line with a nutritional transition phenomenon [5]. According to this, the increasingly permissive obesogenic environment is believed to be a main driver for the current obesity epidemic.

It is believed that obesity results from an interplay between a large range of determinants set within wider social and environmental contexts [6]. Traditionally, studies lack comprehensive models examining the environment in which the individual is placed. More recently, some studies have tried to clarify the interplay of factors associated with the development of obesity, considering those at the individual level but also trying to incorporate a broader understanding of important environmental factors [7]. This knowledge on the determinants of obesity and, in particular, those with a modifiable profile, is essential for a better understanding of the necessary components to support intervention actions and prevention efforts on obesity.

Conceptual Frameworks for Defining Obesity Determinants

For obesity research and prevention, it is consensual that multidimensional approaches focusing on multiple levels of influence are needed. These multilevel approaches to obesity determinants have been conceptualized using the Ecological Systems Theory, which considers the contexts, or ecological niche, in which an individual is placed in order to understand the development of a particular characteristic [8]. Accordingly, a change in a certain characteristic cannot be effectively understood without taking into account their distal and proximal ecological contexts. For example, in the case of a child, proximal contexts include the family and the school, both included in a broader social context. Child's individual risk factors, such as diet, interact with individual's characteristics, such as sex and age, and are shaped by contextual factors, influenced by more distal ones such as the community characteristics [8].

For a better definition of obesity determinants, the interrelationship between several factors must be considered in more comprehensive models. Conceptual frameworks able to enhance knowledge about possible causal mechanisms and a better understanding of upstream and downstream factors, as well as which factors are more influential, are specially warranted [9, 10].

The complexity of the obesogenic environment demands for the definition of a comprehensive framework for understanding and describing determinants that are believed to be dynamic and act at multiple levels [7, 11]. Individuals are embedded in environments that have become increasingly more permissive (increased opportunity to eat) and are more prone to sedentary behaviors. The importance of promoting supportive environments was recognized many years ago in the Ottawa Charter [12], and since then sophisticated environmental models have been developed to deal with key determinants of obesity, such as diet and physical activity.

The ANGELO (Analysis Grid for Environments Linked to Obesity) framework seems to be an useful tool for characterizing the environment across multiple levels of influence [11]. It dissects the environment into micro- and macro-levels and four types of environment: physical (what is available), economic (what are the costs), political (what are the rules) and sociocultural (what is the social and cultural background) [11]. Individuals interact with the environment in several micro-environmental settings, such as schools, workplaces, homes and neighbourhoods, which are influenced by wider macro-environmental sectors, such as health systems and the food industry. This approach seems to be promising, since interventions mainly based on educational, behavioral or pharmacological measures have limited success on obesity prevention or treatment [6].

A model for health promotion focuses attention on both individual and social environmental factors as targets for health promotion interventions [13]. This socioecological model provides a framework for defining different levels of health determinants: individual (*e.g.*, gender, ethnicity), family (*e.g.*, parenting style, family structure), organizational (*e.g.,* school or workplace policies), community/neighbourhood (*e.g.*, food retails, parks), and public policy (*e.g.*, taxation, campaigns, marketing), and their interaction. It addresses the importance of interventions directed at changing interpersonal, organizational, community, and public policy, which support and maintain unhealthy behaviors.

Another framework for determinants of physical activity and eating behaviors [14] was proposed by defining three types of influences, conceptualized in a hierarchical approach: behavior settings (including psychobiological, cultural, social and lifestyles factors), proximal leverage points that control behavior settings (including familial and community influences), and distal leverage points (including political and policy determinants), which have indirect effects on behavior settings.

The Environmental Research framework for weight Gain prevention (EnRG framework) has also proposed a dual-process model to understand the most important determinants of energy balance-related behaviors as well as the causal mechanisms underlying these behaviors [15]. According to this model, environmental influences are hypothesized to influence behavior by a dual-process view, *i.e.*, both directly (the automatic, unconscious influence of the environment on behavior) and indirectly (assuming mediating roles). Six factors are proposed as potential moderators in the framework: demographic factors, personality, awareness of personal behavior, involvement/motivation, habit strength and engagement in clustered behavior. The application of this framework may guide research towards causal mechanisms linking environmental factors to energy balance-related behaviors. It also advocates that the behavioral determinants of a positive energy balance will be different according to age groups, such as children [15].

Given the recognition that habits are formed early in life and track into adulthood, and because of the current increasing rates of childhood obesity, several studies have focused on determinants of obesity-related dietary and physical activity behaviors in children and their families. Some studies have also focused on determining the population attributable fraction of factors associated with obesity, *i.e.*, determining the impact of factors in the population. This approach is particularly interesting to identify the most relevant and preventable factors associated with obesity to guide future interventions. For childhood overweight, the family and the social environment (parental obesity, parental smoking and parental education) seems to be the most important [16].

In literature, several factors at different levels have been described as determinants of obesity or its mediators. This book chapter will focus on social and health behavioral factors associated with obesity. Obesity will be approached as the main outcome, and dietary intake and physical activity will be considered as 'intermediate' obesogenic outcomes as well as main proximal exposures of obesity.

SOCIAL DETERMINANTS OF OBESITY

Social environment is broadly defined as the surroundings that influence an individual's behavior by promoting a sense of social control through the creation of social norms, although there is no consensual definition [17]. It includes potentially modifiable social determinants of health, defined as the conditions where people are born, live, work, grow and age [18]. This complex environment includes both physical (*e.g.*, green spaces) and social (*e.g.*, income) determinants [19].

In the context of obesity, many factors may be discussed within the cluster of social determinants, such as socioeconomic status (SES), education, health literacy, residential conditions, access to health care, social support or working conditions. In turn, these circumstances are shaped by the distribution of money, power and resources at other levels (*i.e.*, local, national or global). Social determinants of health are mostly responsible for health inequities (unfair and avoidable differences in health status) within and between countries [18]. Specifically in Europe, large socioeconomic inequities in terms of obesity were reported. The inequity gradient varies between countries and may show increased steepness at lower education levels, meaning that obese people in lower socioeconomic groups are getting heavier at a faster rate especially if they have low education level. Much of the premature mortality and loss of healthy years observed in lower socioeconomic groups can be explained by obesity-related diseases [20].

A systematic review published in 2011 [21] showed that the most studied sociodemographic factor was the socioeconomic level. Low socioeconomic level area was significantly associated with increased obesity (in 42 out of 56 studies), although in the four longitudinal studies identified only one found an association between living in a poor neighbourhood and increased body mass index (BMI) over 10 years. In 2012 another systematic review [22] highlighted that obesity in developing countries is a problem of the rich for both men and women. Recently, in 2016 [23], a review added that collective efficacy (*e.g.*, the extent to which residents share norms or trust one another), social capital (*e.g.*, belonging to neighborhood associations), and social support were negatively associated with BMI/obesity, while social cohesion (*e.g.*, sense of community involvement) showed inconsistent associations.

It should also be emphasised that there are differences on the association between social determinants and obesity according to ethnicity and gender.

Inequities according to ethnicity have been reported in obesity prevalence in many European countries. In the United Kingdom, although the relationship between obesity and ethnicity is not straightforward, prevalence in women appears to be higher among Black African, Black Caribbean and Pakistani groups and lower for those of Chinese ethnicity when compared with their White counterparts [20]. It should also be pointed out that ethnic differences in the prevalence of adult and childhood obesity may be explained by socioeconomic deprivation [24].

Additionally, women are at higher risk of obesity due to higher propensity to gain fat [25]. Indeed, considering the World Health Organization (WHO) European Region [26], prevalence of obesity is higher among females. Also, 26% of obesity in men and 50% in women can be attributed to inequities in education level. In middle-income countries, obesity in women is becoming a disproportionate problem of the poor and future research should try to better understand why the shift in the burden of obesity from higher to lower SES occurs faster among women compared with men [22].

It should also be highlighted that not only SES is associated with health and obesity, but also childhood SES is correlated with adulthood socioeconomic conditions. Moreover, SES is not expected to play, by itself, a role in adult obesity, but rather it is expected to exert its effects through other determinants such as later social determinants and/or behavioral characteristics that exert a more proximal effect on obesity [27].

Keeping in mind SES trajectories from childhood into adult life, obesity prevalence in women especially those with low SES, as well as the worldwide prevalence of overweight and obesity in children [28], and that the foundation for obesity is nested in early life, the family context is crucial as it is the first social structure to which children are exposed. Hence, we propose a theoretical model for obesity development considering conceptual levels of determinants of children's behaviors within the social and family context Fig. (1).

The family's Social Environment

The family context is critical in children's general socialization. Within this social structure, parenting affects children's social development, being crucial for survival and well-being of the offspring [29, 30]. The act of parenting may be defined as caring for the young, including aspects such as food provision, nursing, protection, and skills' teaching [29]. Family environments include parental behaviors such as parenting styles, parenting child-feeding practices or parental diet that influence child's weight indirectly through the effect on the child's diet [31].

Parenting Styles and Parenting Child-feeding Practices

General parenting style refers to all domains of the parent-child relation, while feeding styles refer to the specific domain of feeding children. The typology of parenting styles is operationalized in two dimensions: demandingness (number /types of control and expectations parents place on the child) and responsiveness (extent to which parents demonstrate consideration for child's emotional needs). From these, four styles emerge: Authoritative, Authoritarian, Indulgent, and Neglectful [31].

As highlighted in a narrative review published in 2015 [32], authoritative parents were consistently found to have healthier children in terms of weight-related outcome measures (nutrition, physical activity, and weight status). In 2014 [33], a meta-analysis reported that positive parent-child relationship and higher levels of parental responsiveness were associated with lower weight but that most effect sizes were small, concluding that general parenting styles should not be made main targets of preventing and treating strategies for obesity. On the other hand, some evidence suggests that general parenting sets the context in which food parenting practices are performed. In fact, depending on the context, food parenting practices might have a stronger or weaker influence on children's dietary behavior and weight status [32].

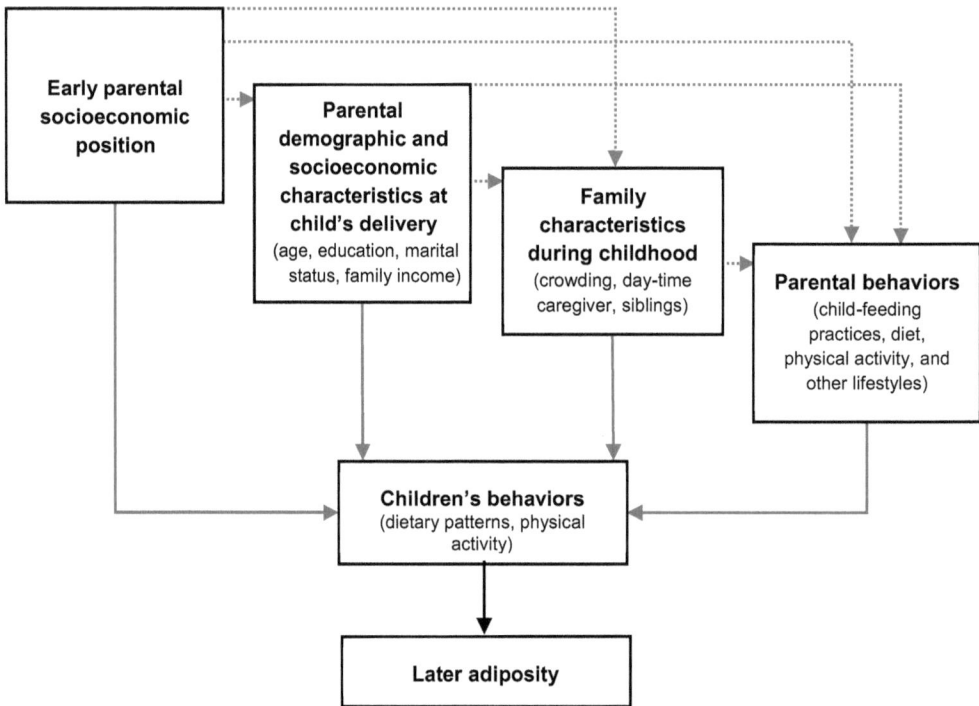

Fig. (1). Conceptual framework for examining determinants of children's behaviors and association with later adiposity. Arrows represent theoretical relationships of determinants of children's behaviors and adiposity during early childhood and later in life. Dotted grey lines indicate possible indirect effects in the pathway between levels of determinants; Solid grey lines represent possible direct effects. The solid black line represents the association between children's behaviors and later adiposity. Upstream factors influence downstream ones that, in turn, influence the child's behaviors which - ultimately - may exert its effect on subsequent adiposity.

Parenting child-feeding practices are defined as specific strategies used by parents to control what, when and how much their children eat, such as pressuring the child to eat (pressure-to-eat), restricting access to certain foods and monitoring children's diet [31]. Parenting child-feeding practices have been studied mainly regarding the central topic of parental control and its association with children's dietary behavior, while the association with overweight in childhood has been less examined and has shown controversial findings.

According to a narrative review published in 2015 [32], greater parental control seems to lead to either lower adiposity in the long-term or to have minimal impact on children's weight. Parental restriction has been the most studied practice. In contrast, there is less evidence on pressure-to-eat and monitoring. Considering longitudinal studies, some have found no effect of restriction and pressure-to-eat [34], while others have found no effect between restriction and later BMI after controlling for a baseline marker of adiposity or for maternal BMI [35, 36], and others have reported positive associations between restriction and adiposity [31, 32]. Monitoring has been associated with both higher overweight [37] and lower BMI [38].

The conflicting and rather confusing literature about parental control can be explained by several aspects, such as the complex nature of the construct of parental control or lack of distinction between practices and styles, being important to notice that conflicting findings might also be related to the possibility that practices are dependent on parenting style. Conflicting findings may also be related with methodological issues. Most studies have been cross-sectional not enabling to examine if parenting child-feeding practices are having an effect on child's weight or if it is the other way around [32, 39], and a bidirectional effect may even exist. Recent prospective analysis [40] showed that higher BMI at the age of 4 years significantly positively increased later maternal restriction, and not the other way around.

Most studies on parenting child-feeding practices focus on the role of mothers. A systematic review published in 2014 [41] addressed fathers' child-feeding practices and concluded that evidence was scarce, although some differences between mothers' and fathers' practices were noted. Fathers were less likely to monitor children's dietary intake and were more likely to use pressure-to-eat. Also, fathers were more likely to pressure the child to eat or to restrict food for reasons related to child's adiposity [41].

Parental Diet and Parental Characteristics

The family social environment may influence children's obesity also through parents' characteristics (*e.g.*, income, education, marital status, work status, weight status), the home food environment, parental nurturing and parents' own dietary intake [42]. Evidence supports that the home food environment, shared family meals, and electronic media use are associated with childhood obesity, mostly through the effect exerted on child's behavior [42].

Evidence suggests that food availability and/or accessibility are associated with child eating habits; a higher availability of healthy foods are associated with healthier diets in children. However, evidence on the association between food availability and weight is still under discussion [31].

Similarly, studies on parental dietary intake also focused predominantly on children's dietary intake, showing consistent positive associations between parents' and children's consumption of fruit and vegetables, milk, sugar-sweetened beverages and energy-dense foods [42]. Considering that parents act as social role models, these findings would be expected. Still, studies on broader ranges of foods are scarce and those with overall dietary measures, such as dietary patterns of both parents and children, are even scarcer, especially among preschool children. This is surprising, particularly if we consider that parental influence at this age is likely to be especially important as they are starting to respond to environmental familial cues, dietary habits are still being established, and prevalence of obesity is high even before the school environment started to exert its effect.

Concerning children's weight, research from multiple countries shows a strong association between parental and child obesity [43]. Similarities in weight between mothers and their offspring are observed in distinct ethnicities and it may be simply related to the fact that both share the same environment. Yet, genetics may also predispose both the mother and the child to obesity. Moreover, it is also possible that epigenetic mechanisms interfere with gene expression and, in result, overweight/obese women deliver babies with higher propensity to store excessive amounts of fat since early infancy [44]. On the other hand, it has also been proposed that the mother-offspring similarity may occur particularly when the foetus is a female and that the association between fatness and reproductive success in women may start at birth. Data suggests that the ability to produce fatter female infants and children (within our evolutionary past context) may have had reproductive benefits such as earlier menarche and more resilient ovarian function of these offspring when adults. However, in today's environment this adaptive pattern may have gone beyond its evolved function, into disease [45].

Other Psychosocial Characteristics within the Family Context

Children's dietary habits are also modified under the influence of other caregivers, peers and siblings [8]. In turn, dietary intake may exert an effect on adiposity, possibly resulting in obesity. Indeed, the child is routinely fed by someone other than a parent, namely grandparents, other relatives or caregivers in organized childcare [46]. Limited evidence has reported family composition and peer's diet to be associated with children's dietary intake, while sibling's intake has been reported to be associated with obesity among adolescents. Moreover, within the home environment, children from higher SES families benefit from better quality residential space, are more likely to have sufficient space to accommodate their needs, are less likely to be exposed to crowding or to unhealthy foods which - in the long-term - can contribute to childhood and adult obesity [27].

Also, it has been stressed how much family's SES can influence its functioning [27]. Families with higher SES show lower levels of conflicts, are more likely to show warm and attentive relationships, and are more likely to belong to families with consistent parenting.

Also, there is evidence that psychosocial stress is associated with obesity in children. Negative life events, maltreatment, impaired family communication, as well as parental stress have been reported as environmental stressors associated with childhood obesity. Furthermore, depression and obesity are co-morbid in children and adults and a bi-directional association is plausible. Likewise, mothers' emotional and mental well-being has been associated with childhood obesity [42].

EARLY-LIFE DETERMINANTS OF DIETARY HABITS AND ADIPOSITY

Evidence on how perinatal and postnatal exposures influence later dietary intake and eating behaviors, and how they could impact on child's growth and adiposity, has been previously discussed. A review of systematic reviews [47] including evidence on determinants of obesity from conception to 5 years of age described as main factors associated with infant and childhood overweight and obesity: gestational diabetes, maternal smoking, rapid infant growth and obesity in infancy, short-sleep duration, less than 30 minutes of daily physical activity, and consumption of sugar-sweetened beverages. Breastfeeding was described as a possible protective factor of obesity.

These factors could influence adiposity development directly through metabolic pathways or by influencing the establishment of children's eating behaviors. The influence of maternal gestational weight gain, diabetes and smoking on child's body fat at pre-school age seems to be mainly through intrauterine programming, instead of having indirect effect through birthweight [48]. However, it has been described that low birth weight children have a compensatory accelerated growth in the first months of life, described as catch-up-growth, gaining more fat rather than muscle that leads to high fat mass later in life, and consequently to adverse metabolic outcomes [49]. Low birth weight or pre-term children could also have more problematic eating behaviors at different stages of life, which in turn could be mediators to a worse health profile in future [50].

Additionally, parents of low birth weight children or with children who lost an excessive amount of weight after birth, or grow slowly, may be more likely to implement feeding practices that result in higher later dietary intake. Early parental feeding practices could also influence children's food preferences and acceptance [51]. Children have innate preferences to sweet flavors and naturally reject sour or bitter tastes. Early exposure to non-innate preferred flavors, first *in utero*, *via* amniotic fluid, and later through breastmilk or during the weaning period could be fundamental for better acceptance of more healthy foods, such as vegetables, and could promote variety in children's diet [52]. Never or short-breastfeeding duration has been consistently related to lower fruit and vegetables intake in young children [53]. Moderate protective effects of breastfeeding when compared with milk formula against childhood overweight have been suggested [54], but no strong evidence could be pointed out [55, 56]. The complementary feeding period is a 'window of opportunity' for the acceptance of a variety of foods with different flavors and textures. Some practices, such as repeated exposure, introduction of a variety of foods, and the right timing of introduction of weaning foods is fundamental for increasing food acceptance in children [57].

Additionally, other parental feeding practices could influence food intake regulation. For instance, parents who used 'Food as a reward' are more likely to have children (aged 3-6 years) who eat in the absence of hunger. When energy-dense foods are available freely after a meal, children eat in the absence of hunger and consume extra energy [58]. Food should be offered to children in response to their feelings of hunger, and not used as reward for a good behavior or for any other reason [59].

The effects of early feeding practices on child's growth and obesity development have been more difficult to establish. However, it seems that weight trajectories could be influenced or influence eating habits in early childhood. Children in a "persistent weight gain" trajectory had higher odds of following a dietary pattern rich in energy-dense foods, at 4 years of age [60].

Studying early life exposures of dietary habits and obesity development across the life span is a challenging task and suitable methodological strategies plus robust research structures, such as population-based birth cohorts with large sample sizes, are needed in order to better clarify the associations and the strength of causal inference.

DIETARY INFLUENCES OF OBESITY

Foods

Consumption of several specific foods or food groups has been related with obesity development. Research has mainly focused on fruit, vegetables, whole grains and sugar-sweetened beverages, while investigation of other food groups has been more limited.

Fruit and vegetables intake has been proposed to be protective against obesity, mainly due to their low-energy density and high content in fibre, vitamins and phytochemicals, their satiating effects and the possibility of replacing energy-denser foods from the diet [61]. However, earlier reviews, particularly focused on childhood obesity [62, 63], do not suggest a protective effect of fruit and vegetables or plant-based diets, based on limited evidence. In fact, a paradoxical effect of fruit on obesity was previously discussed [64]. Besides its antiobesity potential effects, they also contain large amounts of simple sugars (glucose, fructose, sucrose), which are likely to induce obesity [64]. In middle-aged adults, a review published in 2017 concluded that the consumption of whole fruits is inversely associated with long-term weight gain [65]. Another previous review has concluded that most evidence points towards a possible inverse association between fruit intake and overweight [66].

Whole grains have been also linked to body weight [67, 68]. A comprehensive review suggests that there is strong evidence that a diet high in whole grains is associated with lower BMI [67]. On the other hand, there is no evidence that low-carbohydrate diets that restrict cereal intakes offer long-term advantages for sustained weight loss. However, a latter review [68] highlighted that epidemiological studies and clinical trials are providing diverging results. While all the prospective epidemiological studies (reviewed until 2011) showed that a higher intake of whole grains is associated with lower BMI and body weight gain, the results of few clinical trials do not confirm that a whole grain low-calorie diet is more effective in reducing body weight than a refined cereal diet. Although further studies with adequate methodology are needed to clarify this effect, there is biological plausibility supporting it, *i.e.*, whole grains have lower energy density, promote the fermentation of non-digestible carbohydrates (satiety signals), modulate intestinal microflora, and have lower glycemic index.

Sugar-sweetened beverages and their relationship with weight gain, particularly in childhood, cover probably the large body of evidence, allowing even for a review of systematic literature reviews [69]. Among thirteen reviews and meta-analyses described, most (n=9) concluded that there was a direct association between sugar-sweetened beverages and obesity in children and adolescents. Nonetheless, methodological inconsistences preclude definite conclusions. There is also evidence that the intake of free sugars or sugar-sweetened beverages among free living people, both children and adults, is a determinant of body weight [70]. Although more research is needed, sufficient evidence seems to exist for supporting public health strategies to limit the consumption of soft drinks as part of a healthy diet.

With much more limited evidence, dairy products have been associated with a decreased risk of obesity [71, 72], and also higher quantities of red and processed meats were positively associated with obesity risk [73], both in meta-analysis of observational studies.

Nutrients

A recent systematic review and meta-analysis concluded that dietary energy density, as a determinant of energy intake, was directly associated with adiposity and BMI [74]. The macronutrient distribution of diets may also have a role on obesity development, independently of total energy intake. However, the complex interrelation between macronutrients and its co-occurrence in several foods and meals have limited the understanding of its independent role [62]. According to a commentary by the Committee on Nutrition of the European Society for Pediatric Gastroenterology Hepatology and Nutrition (ESPGHAN) [75], no single nutrient has been unequivocally associated with the development of obesity in children, and no specific recommendations for macronutrient intakes to prevent obesity can be made.

As fat is twice as energy-dense compared to carbohydrates and protein, much attention has been devoted to its study. Still, no conclusive results have been found. Most relations between nutritional intake and obesity have been assessed in experimental studies testing controlled diets for weight loss. High-fat diets, due to their high-energy density and high-palatability, stimulate voluntary energy intake. Nonetheless, in a systematic review of clinical trials with 6-18 year-old subjects, low-fat diets, compared to isocaloric low-carbohydrate diets, fail to show weight reductions [76]. In fact, summary evidence suggests that fat-restricted diets are no better than calorie-restricted diets in attaining long-term weight loss in overweight or obese individuals [77]. Another systematic review and meta-analysis [78] has also compared the effect of standard-protein and low-fat diets on weight loss of adults, compared with isocaloric high-protein, low-fat diets. The latter showed only modest benefits in reducing body weight and fat mass.

The lack of effectiveness of low-fat diets in weight reduction alongside with the increasing obesity prevalence worldwide has refocused research on the potential role of low-carbohydrate and low-glycemic diets in obesity etiology. Dietary glycemic load quantifies the overall glycemic effect of a given food, including both quality (*i.e.,* glycemic index) and quantity of carbohydrates from diet [79]. A review of randomized controlled trials concluded that individuals following diets with low-glycemic index or load lost more weight and had more improvement in lipid profiles than those receiving a higher glycemic index or load diets [80]. Nevertheless, the long-term effects of low-glycemic diets should be further explored. In Portuguese children, the effect of dietary glycemic load on adiposity was prospectively assessed in the Portuguese birth cohort Generation XXI, and boys with high-glycemic load diets at 4 years of age had more adiposity at 7 years of age [81]. It was also concluded in boys that the glycemic load seems to interact with protein intake, enhancing even more increased adiposity. In both girls and boys, protein intake at preschool age was positively associated with later BMI, and positively associated with a fat mass index in boys [81]. This finding may be reflecting the role that both amino acids and glucose (along with growth factors such as insulin) play in signaling pathways that regulate cell growth, and may be related to higher sensitivity to central insulin in boys.

Actually, high-protein intake has been positively associated with adiposity in other studies. The "early protein hypothesis", proposed by Koletzko *et al* [82], suggests that a high-protein intake in the first year of life, namely provided by milk formula, could predispose infants to a rapid weight gain in the first few months of life and an increased obesity risk in later life, corroborated by further studies [83, 84].

Dietary Patterns

Dietary patterns represent a more innovative methodological approach to study the complex effect of diet on health outcomes. They account for cumulative and interactive effects of several nutrients and/or foods, and are particularly useful for diseases for which multiple dietary components are established, such as obesity. Hypothesis-oriented dietary patterns (often named as *a priori* patterns, indexes or scores) are defined as a composite score from various food items or nutrients, and have been defined to assess the adherence to guidelines or specific eating habits [85]. This type of approach has been much more commonly associated with obesity than *a posteriori* dietary patterns, which explore *post hoc* dietary data, identifying relevant dietary patterns of the study population by statistical techniques.

Some studies have suggested optimal diets for obesity prevention. These would be high in fibre-rich cereals, fruit, vegetables [86, 87], fish, olive oil and nuts; and fat-reduced and low in meat, processed meat foods and trans-fatty acids [86, 87] as well as restricted in energy-containing drinks [86]. Studies also indicate that vegetarian diets are associated with a lower BMI and a lower prevalence of obesity in adults and children [88].

Both perspectives fill in the concept of the Mediterranean diet, which has been extensively negatively associated with obesity-related outcomes. Previous systematic reviews [89, 90], examining results from prospective cohort and cross-sectional studies, as well as clinical trials, have concluded that although not all studies show a protective effect of the Mediterranean diet on body weight and obesity, the evidence suggests a possible beneficial role of this dietary pattern. The antiobesity effects of the Mediterranean diet have been extensively highlighted in the literature [91, 92]. Its beneficial effects are likely due to the high consumption of plant-based foods that provide a large quantity of fibre, low-energy density and low-glycemic load. Monounsaturated fats (mainly from olive oil) also help to improve glucose metabolism, increase postprandial fat oxidation, enhance diet-induced thermogenesis and therefore increase the overall daily energy expenditure. Other dietary factors may contribute to the potential antiobesity effects, such as n-3 fatty acids, phenolic compounds, dietary fibre and dietary antioxidants, such as resveratrol [91, 92].

Beyond the Mediterranean Diet, other dietary patterns have been also studied in relation to obesity. A systematic review and meta-analysis of observational studies failed to show an association between the dietary diversity score and obesity occurrence, which was partly attributed to different methodological options for assessing dietary intake and defining the composite score [93].

Dietary patterns identified using an *a posteriori* approach, *i.e.*, by using statistical methods, and their prospective association with an obesity-related outcome were also focus of a systematic review in childhood [94]. Only seven studies met the eligibility criteria, and despite differences between studies, a common dietary pattern high in energy-dense, high-fat and low-fibre foods seems to predispose young people to later overweight and obesity. In children from the Portuguese birth cohort Generation XXI, out of three dietary patterns identified, the one high in energy-dense foods at 4 years of age was positively associated with BMI and other adiposity indicators at 7 years of age in girls [95]. In the Avon Longitudinal Study of Parents and Children (ALSPAC cohort), dietary patterns with high-energy density were also associated with increasing fat mass from mid-childhood until adolescence [96].

In adults, a recent meta-analysis has also tried to summarize the association between *a posteriori* healthy dietary patterns (frequently called as the 'Prudent' dietary pattern) and central obesity using data from 13 studies (most cross-sectional) [97], but no significant association was found, when compared with the effects of the Westernized dietary pattern. Probably because *a posteriori* dietary patterns are data driven and specific of each population, consensual results are more difficult to achieve.

PHYSICAL ACTIVITY AND OBESITY

The direct effect of the different components of physical activity (type, frequency, intensity and duration) on obesity is still under research. Physical activity has been studied in terms of leisure-time physical activity (including sedentary behaviors), transportation-, occupation-, and domestic-related physical activities. In relation to obesity prevention, most focus has been given to leisure-time physical activity, especially the sedentary ones. Several interventional studies have been also performed testing primarily weight loss and weight management outcomes.

Leisure-time physical activity includes activities that are energy intense, such as running, cycling, and swimming, but also those that require minimal energy expenditure, such as television viewing or reading, and for that reason seen as sedentary activities as well. Studies exploring the relation between sedentary behaviors and obesity have been increasingly prevalent in the literature, particularly in children. An overview of systematic reviews described 14 systematic reviews examining whether sedentary behavior was associated with BMI, weight gain, overweight/obesity and adiposity in children, adolescents and adults [98]. Time of television viewing (more than 120 minutes per day) has been positively related with childhood obesity, probably explained by simple displacement of physical activity and increased intake of more unhealthy foods due to advertisement, automatic eating and distraction. Other sedentary activities such as computer/internet use, video game playing, sitting at work/school, have not been studied as extensively as television viewing, but there is evidence that they may also contribute to obesity. Nonetheless, in adolescents and adults, two systematic reviews published in 2017 concluded that a small dose-response association exists between sedentary behavior and adiposity, but there is no evidence for a causal association [99, 100].

The daily number of steps could also be seen as marker of sedentary behaviors. Active choices in the daily living, such as parking further away or using stairs as opposed to using elevators to intentional walking for continuous periods of time are good alternatives to increase physical activity and have been increasingly associated with obesity prevention. A meta-analysis was conducted to examine the effect of a walking programme on the risk factors of cardiovascular disease in an inactive population, and concluded that there is a modest weight loss associated with walking interventions [101].

Sleep seems to be the only "sedentary" activity with protective effects on weight gain. Sleep is an important modulator of neuroendocrine function and glucose metabolism, and epidemiological data have linked short-sleep duration and poor-sleep quality to obesity risk [102, 103].

Epidemiological studies suggest that increasing physical activity will have beneficial effects in general health, but this relation seems to be curvilinear, with softening effects as physical activity increases. It has been also described that multiple sessions or short-duration sessions (for example of 10 minutes) have similar effects in the improvement of some health indicators as continuous periods with a similar duration. In a randomized controlled trial with overweight women, short-bouts of exercise enhanced weight loss and produced similar changes in cardiorespiratory fitness when compared to long-bouts of exercise [104]. From a practical perspective, it may be preferred when prescribing exercise to obese adults.

Intervention studies have also been conducted to evaluate the effectiveness of exercise interventions without calorie restriction or the combination of diet and exercise in weight loss or weight management. Although the latter seems to be the most effective, moderate-intensity to high-intensity aerobic exercise-only interventions without prescribed diet, conducted at a frequency of at least three to five times per week, showed also weight loss results [105]. Indeed, a systematic review of randomized controlled trials concluded that exercise is an effective weight loss intervention, particularly when combined with dietary change. Even if no weight is lost, exercise is associated with improved cardiovascular disease risk factors [106].

The relation between weight status and commute time (or vehicle miles of travel), as an indicator of transportation, has been also described. Individuals reporting high levels of auto use have higher BMI scores [107]. Occupation and domestic activities are also believed to have a decreasing contribution to total energy expenditure along time due to mechanization of job-related tasks, and labor-saving devices. Most time potentially saved due to domestic devices may be spent in sedentary activities, and for that reason may be related with weight gain over time.

ALCOHOL AND SMOKING EFFECTS ON OBESITY

Alcoholic beverages are an important source of energy intake (7.1 kcal for each gram). Due to their liquid form, there is evidence towards a process of poor diet compensation, but data from observational and intervention studies have been contradictory, with a few studies suggesting a positive association between alcoholic beverages intake and obesity development [108 - 112]. It has been also in debate that both the quantity and type of alcoholic drink may contribute to different findings, and whether the alcohol is consumed with meals or not [113].

Recent prospective studies show that light-to-moderate alcohol intake is not associated with adiposity gain while heavy drinking [114], and also binge drinking [109], have been more consistently related to weight gain. Some epidemiological data even suggests that moderate alcohol intake may even protect against obesity, since a J-shaped association was observed [111, 115]. However, evidence shows contradictory results [114]. The confounding effect with a general healthier lifestyle profile of those who have moderate alcohol intake was proposed has an explanation for findings' heterogeneity.

Smoking is another health behavior associated with obesity development in previous research. In general, studies have reported an inverse relation between smoking and body weight [116 - 119]. A study from the WHO [117] including almost 70,000 participants aged 35-64 years from 42 populations concluded that regular smokers had significantly lower median BMI, when compared to never smokers. In the short-term, nicotine seems to increase energy expenditure [120] which may help to explain the lower body weight status of smokers compared to non-smokers and the common weight-regain after smoking cessation [121]. On the other hand, heavy smokers seem to have higher BMI than do light smokers [116, 118, 122, 123], and it is worthy to highlight the clustering of cigarette smoking with risk behaviors [124]. Smoking has been also associated with central fat accumulation [119, 122].

These smoking effects on body fat were assessed in the short-term. When smoking effects were assessed in a longitudinal cohort from baseline to 7 years of follow-up, smoking had a minimal effect on body weight [125]. Thus, longitudinal studies and more up-to-date are needed to disentangle the effect of smoking on body weight.

An extensive research has been focused on smoking during pregnancy and its effects on child's health outcomes, namely obesity. Just recently, a meta-analyses of 39 observational studies concluded that smoking during sensitive periods, like pregnancy, is related to later childhood overweight and obesity [126]. A similar review was conducted in 2008 with the same conclusions [127].

CONCLUDING REMARKS

There is a wide range of study limitations when examining determinants of obesity development. Different conceptualizations and measurement methods of both determinants and obesity outcomes may contribute to heterogeneous findings across studies. There is also a lack of appropriate control of confounders in some studies (overestimation of the strength or significance of the associations), while others may have 'overcorrected' for factors such as dietary intake and weight status, diminishing the magnitude or significance of the reported associations. In addition, several studies have a cross-sectional design, making it difficult to establish time precedence, and thus prospective studies are warranted.

Obesity is a complex outcome, for which multiple exposures have been studied along time. Comprehensive models incorporating an interplay of factors at both the individual level and the surrounding environment seem to be the best approach to understand the complexity of obesity etiology and to identify the best interventions to discontinue further increases in the obesity epidemic.

In this book chapter, evidence on the influence of social and health behavioral factors for obesity development was summarized. Putting it into perspective, social determinants seem to play a central role, as they seem to have an indirect influence on a wide range of factors also indicated as obesity determinants. Since early life, the family and the social environment shape individual's lifestyles choices, namely dietary intake and physical activity, which in turn will increase their likelihood for later weight gain. Pregnancy, and the breastfeeding and weaning periods are identified as sensitive periods for establishing eating habits and therefore obesity development.

Overall, there is a lack of evidence on the effect of diet on weight status, probably due to the complex nature of both, as well as due to methodological challenges for assessing them. The antiobesity effects of vegetables, whole-grains, and the Mediterranean diet have been more researched, as well as the effect of sugar-sweetened beverages in increasing body weight, particularly during childhood.

Sedentary behaviors are drivers for childhood obesity, but in adolescents and adults, recent reviews concluded that there is no evidence for a causal association.

Smoking and moderate alcohol drinking have been negatively associated with obesity, but long-term prospective studies should confirm these associations, and a confounding effect of a general lifestyle profile cannot be excluded. On the other hand, smoking during pregnancy has more robust evidence suggesting that it increases the risk of overweight and obesity in later childhood.

The creation of environments supportive of healthier behaviors may be a promising approach to tackle the obesity epidemics. Interventions should also consider factors within the family context and should consider early life determinants.

CONSENT FOR PUBLICATION

Not applicable.

CONFLICT OF INTEREST

The authors confirm that this chapter contents have no conflict of interest.

ACKNOWLEDGEMENTS

Andreia Oliveira receives funds from the FCT Investigator contract (IF/01350/2015), with FEDER funds through the Operational Programme Competitiveness and Internationalization and national funding from the Foundation for Science and Technology - FCT (Portuguese Ministry of Science, Technology and Higher Education), co-funded by the FCT and the POPH/FSE Program.

REFERENCES

[1]   NCD Risk Factor Collaboration (NCD-RisC). Trends in adult body-mass index in 200 countries from 1975 to 2014: a pooled analysis of 1698 population-based measurement studies with 19·2 million participants. Lancet 2016; 387(10026): 1377-96.
        [http://dx.doi.org/10.1016/S0140-6736(16)30054-X] [PMID: 27115820]

[2]   Ng M, Fleming T, Robinson M, *et al.* Global, regional, and national prevalence of overweight and obesity in children and adults during 1980-2013: a systematic analysis for the Global Burden of Disease Study 2013. Lancet 2014; 384(9945): 766-81.
        [http://dx.doi.org/10.1016/S0140-6736(14)60460-8] [PMID: 24880830]

[3]   Wardle J, Carnell S, Haworth CM, Plomin R. Evidence for a strong genetic influence on childhood adiposity despite the force of the obesogenic environment. Am J Clin Nutr 2008; 87(2): 398-404.
        [http://dx.doi.org/10.1093/ajcn/87.2.398] [PMID: 18258631]

[4]   Llewellyn C, Wardle J. Behavioral susceptibility to obesity: Gene-environment interplay in the development of weight. Physiol Behav 2015; 152(Pt B): 494-501.

[5]   Popkin BM. Contemporary nutritional transition: determinants of diet and its impact on body composition. Proc Nutr Soc 2011; 70(1): 82-91.
        [http://dx.doi.org/10.1017/S0029665110003903] [PMID: 21092363]

[6]   Government Office for Science Tackling Obesities: Future Choices - Project Report. UK. 2007.

[7]   Kirk SF, Penney TL, McHugh TL. Characterizing the obesogenic environment: the state of the evidence with directions for future research. Obes Rev 2010; 11(2): 109-17.
        [http://dx.doi.org/10.1111/j.1467-789X.2009.00611.x] [PMID: 19493302]

[8]   Davison KK, Birch LL. Childhood overweight: a contextual model and recommendations for future research. Obes Rev 2001; 2(3): 159-71.
        [http://dx.doi.org/10.1046/j.1467-789x.2001.00036.x] [PMID: 12120101]

[9]   de Vet E, de Ridder DT, de Wit JB. Environmental correlates of physical activity and dietary behaviours among young people: a systematic review of reviews. Obes Rev 2011; 12(5): e130-42.
        [http://dx.doi.org/10.1111/j.1467-789X.2010.00784.x] [PMID: 20630024]

[10]   van der Horst K, Oenema A, Ferreira I, *et al.* A systematic review of environmental correlates of obesity-related dietary behaviors in youth. Health Educ Res 2007; 22(2): 203-26.

[http://dx.doi.org/10.1093/her/cyl069] [PMID: 16861362]

[11] Swinburn B, Egger G, Raza F. Dissecting obesogenic environments: the development and application of a framework for identifying and prioritizing environmental interventions for obesity. Prev Med 1999; 29(6 Pt 1): 563-70.
[http://dx.doi.org/10.1006/pmed.1999.0585] [PMID: 10600438]

[12] World Health Organization and Welfare Canada Canadian Public Health Association. Ottawa Charter for Health Promotion. Ottava 1986.

[13] McLeroy KR, Bibeau D, Steckler A, Glanz K. An ecological perspective on health promotion programs. Health Educ Q 1988; 15(4): 351-77.
[http://dx.doi.org/10.1177/109019818801500401] [PMID: 3068205]

[14] Booth SL, Sallis JF, Ritenbaugh C, *et al.* Environmental and societal factors affect food choice and physical activity: rationale, influences, and leverage points. Nutr Rev 2001; 59(3 Pt 2): S21-39.
[http://dx.doi.org/10.1111/j.1753-4887.2001.tb06983.x] [PMID: 11330630]

[15] Kremers SP, de Bruijn GJ, Visscher TL, *et al.* Environmental influences on energy balance-related behaviors: a dual-process view. Int J Behav Nutr Phys Act 2006; 3: 9.
[http://dx.doi.org/10.1186/1479-5868-3-9] [PMID: 16700907]

[16] Plachta-Danielzik S, Kehden B, Landsberg B, *et al.* Attributable risks for childhood overweight: evidence for limited effectiveness of prevention. Pediatrics 2012; 130(4): e865-71.
[http://dx.doi.org/10.1542/peds.2011-3296] [PMID: 22945402]

[17] Institute of Medicine. The Future of the Public's Health in the 21st Century. Washington, DC: National Academies Press 2003.

[18] World Health Organization. World conference on social determinants of health: meeting report, Rio de Janeiro, Brazil, 19-21 October 2011. Geneva

[19] Arroyo-Johnson C, Mincey KD. Obesity Epidemiology Worldwide. Gastroenterol Clin North Am 2016; 45(4): 571-9.
[http://dx.doi.org/10.1016/j.gtc.2016.07.012] [PMID: 27837773]

[20] Loring B, Robertson A. Obesity and inequities Guidance for addressing inequities in overweight and obesity Copenhagen. 2014.

[21] Leal C, Chaix B. The influence of geographic life environments on cardiometabolic risk factors: a systematic review, a methodological assessment and a research agenda. Obes Rev 2011; 12(3): 217-30.
[http://dx.doi.org/10.1111/j.1467-789X.2010.00726.x] [PMID: 20202135]

[22] Dinsa GD, Goryakin Y, Fumagalli E, Suhrcke M. Obesity and socioeconomic status in developing countries: a systematic review. Obes Rev 2012; 13(11): 1067-79.
[http://dx.doi.org/10.1111/j.1467-789X.2012.01017.x] [PMID: 22764734]

[23] Glonti K, Mackenbach JD, Ng J, *et al.* Psychosocial environment: definitions, measures and associations with weight status-a systematic review. Obes Rev 2016; 17 (Suppl. 1): 81-95.
[http://dx.doi.org/10.1111/obr.12383] [PMID: 26879116]

[24] Dixon B, Peña MM, Taveras EM. Lifecourse approach to racial/ethnic disparities in childhood obesity. Adv Nutr 2012; 3(1): 73-82.
[http://dx.doi.org/10.3945/an.111.000919] [PMID: 22332105]

[25] Wells JC. Sexual dimorphism of body composition. Best Pract Res Clin Endocrinol Metab 2007; 21(3): 415-30.
[http://dx.doi.org/10.1016/j.beem.2007.04.007] [PMID: 17875489]

[26] World Health Organization and Directorate General for Health and Consumers. Strategy for Europe on nutrition, overweight and obesity related health issues: Implementation progress report Geneva. 2010.

[27] Cohen S, Janicki-Deverts D, Chen E, Matthews KA. Childhood socioeconomic status and adult health.

Ann N Y Acad Sci 2010; 1186: 37-55.
[http://dx.doi.org/10.1111/j.1749-6632.2009.05334.x] [PMID: 20201867]

[28]   UNICEF, WHO Levels and trends in child malnutrition Geneva. 2016.

[29]   Dulac C, O'Connell LA, Wu Z. Neural control of maternal and paternal behaviors. Science 2014; 345(6198): 765-70.
[http://dx.doi.org/10.1126/science.1253291] [PMID: 25124430]

[30]   Rilling JK, Young LJ. The biology of mammalian parenting and its effect on offspring social development. Science 2014; 345(6198): 771-6.
[http://dx.doi.org/10.1126/science.1252723] [PMID: 25124431]

[31]   Ventura AK, Birch LL. Does parenting affect children's eating and weight status? Int J Behav Nutr Phys Act 2008; 5: 15.
[http://dx.doi.org/10.1186/1479-5868-5-15] [PMID: 18346282]

[32]   Gerards SM, Kremers SP. The Role of Food Parenting Skills and the Home Food Environment in Children's Weight Gain and Obesity. Curr Obes Rep 2015; 4(1): 30-6.
[http://dx.doi.org/10.1007/s13679-015-0139-x] [PMID: 25741454]

[33]   Pinquart M. Associations of general parenting and parent-child relationship with pediatric obesity: a meta-analysis. J Pediatr Psychol 2014; 39(4): 381-93.
[http://dx.doi.org/10.1093/jpepsy/jst144] [PMID: 24756228]

[34]   Gregory JE, Paxton SJ, Brozovic AM. Maternal feeding practices, child eating behaviour and body mass index in preschool-aged children: a prospective analysis. Int J Behav Nutr Phys Act 2010; 7: 55.
[http://dx.doi.org/10.1186/1479-5868-7-55] [PMID: 20579397]

[35]   Rifas-Shiman SL, Sherry B, Scanlon K, *et al.* Does maternal feeding restriction lead to childhood obesity in a prospective cohort study? Arch Dis Child 2011; 96(3): 265-9.
[http://dx.doi.org/10.1136/adc.2009.175240] [PMID: 21081589]

[36]   Campbell K, Andrianopoulos N, Hesketh K, *et al.* Parental use of restrictive feeding practices and child BMI z-score. A 3-year prospective cohort study. Appetite 2010; 55(1): 84-8.
[http://dx.doi.org/10.1016/j.appet.2010.04.006] [PMID: 20420869]

[37]   Moens E, Braet C, Soetens B. Observation of family functioning at mealtime: a comparison between families of children with and without overweight. J Pediatr Psychol 2007; 32(1): 52-63.
[http://dx.doi.org/10.1093/jpepsy/jsl011] [PMID: 16801324]

[38]   Faith MS, Berkowitz RI, Stallings VA, *et al.* Parental feeding attitudes and styles and child body mass index: prospective analysis of a gene-environment interaction. Pediatrics 2004; 114(4): e429-36.
[http://dx.doi.org/10.1542/peds.2003-1075-L] [PMID: 15466068]

[39]   Birch LL. Child feeding practices and the etiology of obesity. Obesity (Silver Spring) 2006; 14(3): 343-4.
[http://dx.doi.org/10.1038/oby.2006.45] [PMID: 16648602]

[40]   Afonso L, Lopes C, Severo M, *et al.* Bidirectional association between parental child-feeding practices and body mass index at 4 and 7 y of age. Am J Clin Nutr 2016; 103(3): 861-7.
[http://dx.doi.org/10.3945/ajcn.115.120824] [PMID: 26843159]

[41]   Khandpur N, Blaine RE, Fisher JO, Davison KK. Fathers' child feeding practices: a review of the evidence. Appetite 2014; 78: 110-21.
[http://dx.doi.org/10.1016/j.appet.2014.03.015] [PMID: 24667152]

[42]   Campbell MK. Biological, environmental, and social influences on childhood obesity. Pediatr Res 2016; 79(1-2): 205-11.
[http://dx.doi.org/10.1038/pr.2015.208] [PMID: 26484623]

[43]   Wang Y, Min J, Khuri J, Li M. A Systematic Examination of the Association between Parental and Child Obesity across Countries. Adv Nutr 2017; 8(3): 436-48.

[http://dx.doi.org/10.3945/an.116.013235] [PMID: 28507009]

[44]   Pérez-Escamilla R, Kac G. Childhood obesity prevention: a life-course framework. Int J Obes Suppl 2013; 3 (Suppl. 1): S3-5.
[http://dx.doi.org/10.1038/ijosup.2013.2] [PMID: 25018875]

[45]   Power ML, Schulkin J. Sex differences in fat storage, fat metabolism, and the health risks from obesity: possible evolutionary origins. Br J Nutr 2008; 99(5): 931-40.
[http://dx.doi.org/10.1017/S0007114507853347] [PMID: 17977473]

[46]   Savage JS, Fisher JO, Birch LL. Parental influence on eating behavior: conception to adolescence. J Law Med Ethics 2007; 35(1): 22-34.
[http://dx.doi.org/10.1111/j.1748-720X.2007.00111.x] [PMID: 17341215]

[47]   Monasta L, Batty GD, Cattaneo A, *et al.* Early-life determinants of overweight and obesity: a review of systematic reviews. Obes Rev 2010; 11(10): 695-708.
[http://dx.doi.org/10.1111/j.1467-789X.2010.00735.x] [PMID: 20331509]

[48]   Santos S, Severo M, Gaillard R, *et al.* The role of prenatal exposures on body fat patterns at 7 years: Intrauterine programming or birthweight effects? Nutr Metab Cardiovasc Dis 2016; 26(11): 1004-10.
[http://dx.doi.org/10.1016/j.numecd.2016.06.010] [PMID: 27461861]

[49]   Koletzko B, Brands B, Poston L, *et al.* Early nutrition programming of long-term health. Proc Nutr Soc 2012; 71(3): 371-8.
[http://dx.doi.org/10.1017/S0029665112000596] [PMID: 22703585]

[50]   Oliveira A, de Lauzon-Guillain B, Jones L, *et al.* Birth weight and eating behaviors of young children. J Pediatr 2015; 166(1): 59-65.
[http://dx.doi.org/10.1016/j.jpeds.2014.09.031] [PMID: 25444001]

[51]   Mennella JA, Nicklaus S, Jagolino AL, Yourshaw LM. Variety is the spice of life: strategies for promoting fruit and vegetable acceptance during infancy. Physiol Behav 2008; 94(1): 29-38.
[http://dx.doi.org/10.1016/j.physbeh.2007.11.014] [PMID: 18222499]

[52]   Maier AS, Chabanet C, Schaal B, *et al.* Breastfeeding and experience with variety early in weaning increase infants' acceptance of new foods for up to two months. Clin Nutr 2008; 27(6): 849-57.
[http://dx.doi.org/10.1016/j.clnu.2008.08.002] [PMID: 18838198]

[53]   de Lauzon-Guillain B, Jones L, Oliveira A, *et al.* The influence of early feeding practices on fruit and vegetable intake among preschool children in 4 European birth cohorts. Am J Clin Nutr 2013; 98(3): 804-12.
[http://dx.doi.org/10.3945/ajcn.112.057026] [PMID: 23864537]

[54]   Weng SF, Redsell SA, Swift JA, *et al.* Systematic review and meta-analyses of risk factors for childhood overweight identifiable during infancy. Arch Dis Child 2012; 97(12): 1019-26.
[http://dx.doi.org/10.1136/archdischild-2012-302263] [PMID: 23109090]

[55]   Marseglia L, Manti S, D'Angelo G, *et al.* Obesity and breastfeeding: The strength of association. Women Birth 2015; 28(2): 81-6.
[http://dx.doi.org/10.1016/j.wombi.2014.12.007] [PMID: 25595034]

[56]   Moschonis G, de Lauzon-Guillain B, Jones L, *et al.* The effect of early feeding practices on growth indices and obesity at preschool children from four European countries and UK schoolchildren and adolescents. Eur J Pediatr 2017; 176(9): 1181-92.
[http://dx.doi.org/10.1007/s00431-017-2961-5] [PMID: 28711955]

[57]   Nicklaus S. Children's acceptance of new foods at weaning. Role of practices of weaning and of food sensory properties. Appetite 2011; 57(3): 812-5.
[http://dx.doi.org/10.1016/j.appet.2011.05.321] [PMID: 21651933]

[58]   Remy E, Issanchou S, Chabanet C, *et al.* Impact of adiposity, age, sex and maternal feeding practices on eating in the absence of hunger and caloric compensation in preschool children. Int J Obes 2015; 39(6): 925-30.

[http://dx.doi.org/10.1038/ijo.2015.30] [PMID: 25777357]

[59]   Issanchou S. Determining Factors and Critical Periods in the Formation of Eating Habits: Results from the Habeat Project. Ann Nutr Metab 2017; 70(3): 251-6.
[http://dx.doi.org/10.1159/000471514] [PMID: 28407627]

[60]   Fonseca MJ, Durão C, Lopes C, Santos AC. Weight following birth and childhood dietary intake: A prospective cohort study. Nutrition 2017; 33: 58-64.
[http://dx.doi.org/10.1016/j.nut.2016.08.008] [PMID: 27908552]

[61]   Slavin JL, Lloyd B. Health benefits of fruits and vegetables. Adv Nutr 2012; 3(4): 506-16.
[http://dx.doi.org/10.3945/an.112.002154] [PMID: 22797986]

[62]   Newby PK. Are dietary intakes and eating behaviors related to childhood obesity? A comprehensive review of the evidence. J Law Med Ethics 2007; 35(1): 35-60.
[http://dx.doi.org/10.1111/j.1748-720X.2007.00112.x] [PMID: 17341216]

[63]   Newby PK. Plant foods and plant-based diets: protective against childhood obesity? Am J Clin Nutr 2009; 89(5): 1572S-87S.
[http://dx.doi.org/10.3945/ajcn.2009.26736G] [PMID: 19321559]

[64]   Sharma SP, Chung HJ, Kim HJ, Hong ST. Paradoxical Effects of Fruit on Obesity. Nutrients 2016; 8(10): 633.
[http://dx.doi.org/10.3390/nu8100633] [PMID: 27754404]

[65]   Hebden L, O'Leary F, Rangan A, *et al.* Fruit consumption and adiposity status in adults: A systematic review of current evidence. Crit Rev Food Sci Nutr 2017; 57(12): 2526-40.
[http://dx.doi.org/10.1080/10408398.2015.1012290] [PMID: 26115001]

[66]   Alinia S, Hels O, Tetens I. The potential association between fruit intake and body weight--a review. Obes Rev 2009; 10(6): 639-47.
[http://dx.doi.org/10.1111/j.1467-789X.2009.00582.x] [PMID: 19413705]

[67]   Williams PG, Grafenauer SJ, O'Shea JE. Cereal grains, legumes, and weight management: a comprehensive review of the scientific evidence. Nutr Rev 2008; 66(4): 171-82.
[http://dx.doi.org/10.1111/j.1753-4887.2008.00022.x] [PMID: 18366531]

[68]   Giacco R, Della Pepa G, Luongo D, Riccardi G. Whole grain intake in relation to body weight: from epidemiological evidence to clinical trials. Nutr Metab Cardiovasc Dis 2011; 21(12): 901-8.
[http://dx.doi.org/10.1016/j.numecd.2011.07.003] [PMID: 22036468]

[69]   Keller A, Bucher Della Torre S. Sugar-Sweetened Beverages and Obesity among Children and Adolescents: A Review of Systematic Literature Reviews. Child Obes 2015; 11(4): 338-46.
[http://dx.doi.org/10.1089/chi.2014.0117] [PMID: 26258560]

[70]   Te Morenga L, Mallard S, Mann J. Dietary sugars and body weight: systematic review and meta-analyses of randomised controlled trials and cohort studies. BMJ 2012; (346): e7492.
[http://dx.doi.org/10.1136/bmj.e7492] [PMID: 23321486]

[71]   Wang W, Wu Y, Zhang D. Association of dairy products consumption with risk of obesity in children and adults: a meta-analysis of mainly cross-sectional studies. Ann Epidemiol 2016; 26(12): 870-882..
[http://dx.doi.org/10.1016/j.annepidem.2016.09.005] [PMID: 27756684]

[72]   Lu L, Xun P, Wan Y, He K, Cai W. Long-term association between dairy consumption and risk of childhood obesity: a systematic review and meta-analysis of prospective cohort studies. Eur J Clin Nutr 2016; 70(4): 414-23.
[http://dx.doi.org/10.1038/ejcn.2015.226] [PMID: 26862005]

[73]   Rouhani MH, Salehi-Abargouei A, Surkan PJ, Azadbakht L. Is there a relationship between red or processed meat intake and obesity? A systematic review and meta-analysis of observational studies. Obes Rev 2014; 15(9): 740-8.
[http://dx.doi.org/10.1111/obr.12172] [PMID: 24815945]

[74] Rouhani MH, Haghighatdoost F, Surkan PJ, Azadbakht L. Associations between dietary energy density and obesity: A systematic review and meta-analysis of observational studies. Nutrition 2016; 32(10): 1037-47.
[http://dx.doi.org/10.1016/j.nut.2016.03.017] [PMID: 27238958]

[75] Agostoni C, Braegger C, Decsi T, *et al.* Role of dietary factors and food habits in the development of childhood obesity: a commentary by the ESPGHAN Committee on Nutrition. J Pediatr Gastroenterol Nutr 2011; 52(6): 662-9.
[http://dx.doi.org/10.1097/MPG.0b013e3182169253] [PMID: 21593641]

[76] Gow ML, Ho M, Burrows TL, *et al.* Impact of dietary macronutrient distribution on BMI and cardiometabolic outcomes in overweight and obese children and adolescents: a systematic review. Nutr Rev 2014; 72(7): 453-70.
[http://dx.doi.org/10.1111/nure.12111] [PMID: 24920422]

[77] Summerbell CD, Cameron C, Glasziou PP. WITHDRAWN: Advice on low-fat diets for obesity. Cochrane Database Syst Rev 2008; (3): CD003640
[PMID: 18646093]

[78] Wycherley TP, Moran LJ, Clifton PM, *et al.* Effects of energy-restricted high-protein, low-fat compared with standard-protein, low-fat diets: a meta-analysis of randomized controlled trials. Am J Clin Nutr 2012; 96(6): 1281-98.
[http://dx.doi.org/10.3945/ajcn.112.044321] [PMID: 23097268]

[79] Salmerón J, Ascherio A, Rimm EB, *et al.* Dietary fiber, glycemic load, and risk of NIDDM in men. Diabetes Care 1997; 20(4): 545-50.
[http://dx.doi.org/10.2337/diacare.20.4.545] [PMID: 9096978]

[80] Thomas DE, Elliott EJ, Baur L. Low glycaemic index or low glycaemic load diets for overweight and obesity. Cochrane Database Syst Rev 2007; 18(3)CD005105
[http://dx.doi.org/10.1002/14651858.CD005105.pub2] [PMID: 17636786]

[81] Durão C, Oliveira A, Santos AC, *et al.* Protein intake and dietary glycemic load of 4-year-olds and association with adiposity and serum insulin at 7 years of age: sex-nutrient and nutrient-nutrient interactions. Int J Obes 2017; 41(4): 533-41.
[http://dx.doi.org/10.1038/ijo.2016.240] [PMID: 28028320]

[82] Koletzko B, Broekaert I, Demmelmair H, *et al.* Protein intake in the first year of life: a risk factor for later obesity? The E.U. childhood obesity project. Adv Exp Med Biol 2005; 569: 69-79.
[http://dx.doi.org/10.1007/1-4020-3535-7_12] [PMID: 16137110]

[83] Koletzko B, von Kries R, Closa R, *et al.* Can infant feeding choices modulate later obesity risk? Am J Clin Nutr 2009; 89(5): 1502S-8S.
[http://dx.doi.org/10.3945/ajcn.2009.27113D] [PMID: 19321574]

[84] Weber M, Grote V, Closa-Monasterolo R, *et al.* Lower protein content in infant formula reduces BMI and obesity risk at school age: follow-up of a randomized trial. Am J Clin Nutr 2014; 99(5): 1041-51.
[http://dx.doi.org/10.3945/ajcn.113.064071] [PMID: 24622805]

[85] Hu FB. Dietary pattern analysis: a new direction in nutritional epidemiology. Curr Opin Lipidol 2002; 13(1): 3-9.
[http://dx.doi.org/10.1097/00041433-200202000-00002] [PMID: 11790957]

[86] Astrup A, Dyerberg J, Selleck M, Stender S. Nutrition transition and its relationship to the development of obesity and related chronic diseases. Obes Rev 2008; 9 (Suppl. 1): 48-52.
[http://dx.doi.org/10.1111/j.1467-789X.2007.00438.x] [PMID: 18307699]

[87] Bulló M, Casas-Agustench P, Amigó-Correig P, *et al.* Inflammation, obesity and comorbidities: the role of diet. Public Health Nutr 2007; 10(10A): 1164-72.
[http://dx.doi.org/10.1017/S1368980007000663] [PMID: 17903326]

[88] Sabaté J, Wien M. Vegetarian diets and childhood obesity prevention. Am J Clin Nutr 2010; 91(5):

1525S-9S.
[http://dx.doi.org/10.3945/ajcn.2010.28701F] [PMID: 20237136]

[89]   Kastorini CM, Milionis HJ, Goudevenos JA, Panagiotakos DB. Mediterranean diet and coronary heart disease: is obesity a link? - A systematic review. Nutr Metab Cardiovasc Dis 2010; 20(7): 536-51.
[http://dx.doi.org/10.1016/j.numecd.2010.04.006] [PMID: 20708148]

[90]   Buckland G, Bach A, Serra-Majem L. Obesity and the Mediterranean diet: a systematic review of observational and intervention studies. Obes Rev 2008; 9(6): 582-93.
[http://dx.doi.org/10.1111/j.1467-789X.2008.00503.x] [PMID: 18547378]

[91]   Kwan HY, Chao X, Su T, *et al.* The anticancer and antiobesity effects of Mediterranean diet. Crit Rev Food Sci Nutr 2017; 57(1): 82-94.
[http://dx.doi.org/10.1080/10408398.2013.852510] [PMID: 25831235]

[92]   Schröder H. Protective mechanisms of the Mediterranean diet in obesity and type 2 diabetes. J Nutr Biochem 2007; 18(3): 149-60.
[http://dx.doi.org/10.1016/j.jnutbio.2006.05.006] [PMID: 16963247]

[93]   Salehi-Abargouei A, Akbari F, Bellissimo N, Azadbakht L. Dietary diversity score and obesity: a systematic review and meta-analysis of observational studies. Eur J Clin Nutr 2016; 70(1): 1-9.
[http://dx.doi.org/10.1038/ejcn.2015.118] [PMID: 26220567]

[94]   Ambrosini GL. Childhood dietary patterns and later obesity: a review of the evidence. Proc Nutr Soc 2014; 73(1): 137-46.
[http://dx.doi.org/10.1017/S0029665113003765] [PMID: 24280165]

[95]   Durão C, Severo M, Oliveira A, *et al.* Association between dietary patterns and adiposity from 4 to 7 years of age. Public Health Nutr 2017; 20(11): 1973-82.
[http://dx.doi.org/10.1017/S1368980017000854] [PMID: 28534458]

[96]   Emmett PM, Jones LR. Diet, growth, and obesity development throughout childhood in the Avon Longitudinal Study of Parents and Children. Nutr Rev 2015; 73 (Suppl. 3): 175-206.
[http://dx.doi.org/10.1093/nutrit/nuv054] [PMID: 26395342]

[97]   Rezagholizadeh F, Djafarian K, Khosravi S, Shab-Bidar S. A posteriori healthy dietary patterns may decrease the risk of central obesity: findings from a systematic review and meta-analysis. Nutr Res 2017; 41: 1-13.
[http://dx.doi.org/10.1016/j.nutres.2017.01.006] [PMID: 28577788]

[98]   de Rezende LF, Rodrigues Lopes M, Rey-López JP, *et al.* Sedentary behavior and health outcomes: an overview of systematic reviews. PLoS One 2014; 9(8)e105620
[http://dx.doi.org/10.1371/journal.pone.0105620] [PMID: 25144686]

[99]   Biddle SJH, García Bengoechea E, Pedisic Z, *et al.* Screen Time, Other Sedentary Behaviours, and Obesity Risk in Adults: A Review of Reviews. Curr Obes Rep 2017; 6(2): 134-47.
[http://dx.doi.org/10.1007/s13679-017-0256-9] [PMID: 28421472]

[100]   Biddle SJ, Garcia Bengoechea E, Wiesner G. Sedentary behaviour and adiposity in youth: A systematic review of reviews and analysis of causality. Int J Behav Nutr Phys Act 2017; 14: 43.

[101]   Murtagh EM, Nichols L, Mohammed MA, *et al.* The effect of walking on risk factors for cardiovascular disease: an updated systematic review and meta-analysis of randomised control trials. Prev Med 2015; 72: 34-43.
[http://dx.doi.org/10.1016/j.ypmed.2014.12.041] [PMID: 25579505]

[102]   Chaput JP, Klingenberg L, Sjödin A. Do all sedentary activities lead to weight gain: sleep does not. Curr Opin Clin Nutr Metab Care 2010; 13(6): 601-7.
[http://dx.doi.org/10.1097/MCO.0b013e32833ef30e] [PMID: 20823775]

[103]   Beccuti G, Pannain S. Sleep and obesity. Curr Opin Clin Nutr Metab Care 2011; 14(4): 402-12.
[http://dx.doi.org/10.1097/MCO.0b013e3283479109] [PMID: 21659802]

[104] Jakicic JM, Wing RR, Butler BA, Robertson RJ. Prescribing exercise in multiple short bouts *versus* one continuous bout: effects on adherence, cardiorespiratory fitness, and weight loss in overweight women. Int J Obes Relat Metab Disord 1995; 19(12): 893-901.
[PMID: 8963358]

[105] Chin SH, Kahathuduwa CN, Binks M. Physical activity and obesity: what we know and what we need to know. Obes Rev 2016; 17(12): 1226-44.
[http://dx.doi.org/10.1111/obr.12460] [PMID: 27743411]

[106] Shaw K, Gennat H, O'Rourke P, Del Mar C. Exercise for overweight or obesity. Cochrane Database Syst Rev 2006; 18(4)CD003817
[PMID: 17054187]

[107] McCormack GR, Virk JS. Driving towards obesity: a systematized literature review on the association between motor vehicle travel time and distance and weight status in adults. Prev Med 2014; 66: 49-55.
[http://dx.doi.org/10.1016/j.ypmed.2014.06.002] [PMID: 24929196]

[108] Poppitt SD. Beverage Consumption: Are Alcoholic and Sugary Drinks Tipping the Balance towards Overweight and Obesity? Nutrients 2015; 7(8): 6700-18.
[http://dx.doi.org/10.3390/nu7085304] [PMID: 26270675]

[109] Yeomans MR. Alcohol, appetite and energy balance: is alcohol intake a risk factor for obesity? Physiol Behav 2010; 100(1): 82-9.
[http://dx.doi.org/10.1016/j.physbeh.2010.01.012] [PMID: 20096714]

[110] Suter PM. Is alcohol consumption a risk factor for weight gain and obesity? Crit Rev Clin Lab Sci 2005; 42(3): 197-227.
[http://dx.doi.org/10.1080/10408360590913542] [PMID: 16047538]

[111] Sayon-Orea C, Martinez-Gonzalez MA, Bes-Rastrollo M. Alcohol consumption and body weight: a systematic review. Nutr Rev 2011; 69(8): 419-31.
[http://dx.doi.org/10.1111/j.1753-4887.2011.00403.x] [PMID: 21790610]

[112] Lourenço S, Oliveira A, Lopes C. The effect of current and lifetime alcohol consumption on overall and central obesity. Eur J Clin Nutr 2012; 66(7): 813-8.
[http://dx.doi.org/10.1038/ejcn.2012.20] [PMID: 22378229]

[113] Wannamethee SG, Shaper AG, Whincup PH. Alcohol and adiposity: effects of quantity and type of drink and time relation with meals. Int J Obes 2005; 29(12): 1436-44.
[http://dx.doi.org/10.1038/sj.ijo.0803034] [PMID: 16077718]

[114] Traversy G, Chaput JP. Alcohol Consumption and Obesity: An Update. Curr Obes Rep 2015; 4(1): 122-30.
[http://dx.doi.org/10.1007/s13679-014-0129-4] [PMID: 25741455]

[115] Lukasiewicz E, Mennen LI, Bertrais S, *et al.* Alcohol intake in relation to body mass index and waist-to-hip ratio: the importance of type of alcoholic beverage. Public Health Nutr 2005; 8(3): 315-20.
[http://dx.doi.org/10.1079/PHN2004680] [PMID: 15918929]

[116] Chiolero A, Jacot-Sadowski I, Faeh D, *et al.* Association of cigarettes smoked daily with obesity in a general adult population. Obesity (Silver Spring) 2007; 15(5): 1311-8.
[http://dx.doi.org/10.1038/oby.2007.153] [PMID: 17495208]

[117] Molarius A, Seidell JC, Kuulasmaa K, *et al.* Smoking and relative body weight: an international perspective from the WHO MONICA Project. J Epidemiol Community Health 1997; 51(3): 252-60.
[http://dx.doi.org/10.1136/jech.51.3.252] [PMID: 9229053]

[118] Rásky E, Stronegger WJ, Freidl W. The relationship between body weight and patterns of smoking in women and men. Int J Epidemiol 1996; 25(6): 1208-12.
[http://dx.doi.org/10.1093/ije/25.6.1208] [PMID: 9027526]

[119] Kvaavik E, Meyer HE, Tverdal A. Food habits, physical activity and body mass index in relation to

smoking status in 40-42 year old Norwegian women and men. Prev Med 2004; 38(1): 1-5.
[http://dx.doi.org/10.1016/j.ypmed.2003.09.020] [PMID: 14672635]

[120]   Collins LC, Cornelius MF, Vogel RL, *et al.* Effect of caffeine and/or cigarette smoking on resting energy expenditure. Int J Obes Relat Metab Disord 1994; 18(8): 551-6.
[PMID: 7951476]

[121]   Eisenberg D, Quinn BC. Estimating the effect of smoking cessation on weight gain: an instrumental variable approach. Health Serv Res 2006; 41(6): 2255-66.
[http://dx.doi.org/10.1111/j.1475-6773.2006.00594.x] [PMID: 17116119]

[122]   Bamia C, Trichopoulou A, Lenas D, Trichopoulos D. Tobacco smoking in relation to body fat mass and distribution in a general population sample. Int J Obes Relat Metab Disord 2004; 28(8): 1091-6.
[http://dx.doi.org/10.1038/sj.ijo.0802697] [PMID: 15197410]

[123]   Istvan JA, Cunningham TW, Garfinkel L. Cigarette smoking and body weight in the Cancer Prevention Study I. Int J Epidemiol 1992; 21(5): 849-53.
[http://dx.doi.org/10.1093/ije/21.5.849] [PMID: 1468844]

[124]   Chiolero A, Wietlisbach V, Ruffieux C, *et al.* Clustering of risk behaviors with cigarette consumption: A population-based survey. Prev Med 2006; 42(5): 348-53.
[http://dx.doi.org/10.1016/j.ypmed.2006.01.011] [PMID: 16504277]

[125]   Klesges RC, Ward KD, Ray JW, *et al.* The prospective relationships between smoking and weight in a young, biracial cohort: The Coronary Artery Risk Development in Young Adults Study. J Consult Clin Psychol 1998; 66(6): 987-93.
[http://dx.doi.org/10.1037/0022-006X.66.6.987] [PMID: 9874912]

[126]   Rayfield S, Plugge E. Systematic review and meta-analysis of the association between maternal smoking in pregnancy and childhood overweight and obesity. J Epidemiol Community Health 2017; 71(2): 162-73.
[http://dx.doi.org/10.1136/jech-2016-207376] [PMID: 27480843]

[127]   Oken E, Levitan EB, Gillman MW. Maternal smoking during pregnancy and child overweight: Systematic review and meta-analysis. Int J Obes 2008; 32(2): 201-10.
[http://dx.doi.org/10.1038/sj.ijo.0803760] [PMID: 18278059]

CHAPTER 3

Obesity and Adipose Tissue Remodeling

Adriana R. Rodrigues[1,2,3,#], **Maria J. Salazar**[1,2,3,#] and **Alexandra M. Gouveia**[1,2,3,4,*]

[1] *Department of Biomedicine, Experimental Biology Unit, Faculty of Medicine, University of Porto, Porto, Portugal*

[2] *IBMC - Instituto de Biologia Molecular e Celular, University of Porto, Porto, Portugal*

[3] *i3S - Instituto de Investigação e Inovação em Saúde, University of Porto, Porto, Portugal*

[4] *Faculty of Nutrition and Food Sciences, University of Porto, Porto, Portugal*

Abstract: Adipose Tissue (AT) is an endocrine organ with a key role in the regulation of the energy homeostasis. White AT accumulates energy in the form of triglycerides within lipid droplets and, therefore, is particularly abundant in obesity. In contrast, brown AT is specialized for energy expenditure playing a pivotal role on thermogenesis control and its mass decreases with obesity. AT secretes a large number of adipokines that regulate the central control of appetite and the metabolism of diverse peripheral tissues. This secretion and also the anatomical features of AT are closely related with the nutritional status and, naturally, strongly differ between normal weight and obese individuals. AT remodeling is indeed an ongoing process, that is pathologically exacerbated in the obese state. This review will discuss and present updated data describing the main changes in AT that correlate with an obese status. In obesity, AT changes in mass, capacity for energy storage, distribution through the organism, cellular composition, endocrine role and signaling. In summary, the chronic excess of nutrient supply leads to adipocyte hyperplasia and hypertrophy, hypoxia, mitochondrial dysfunction, proinflammatory signaling, adipokine secretion and, ultimately, to cell death. The extent of AT remodeling is closely associated with the pathophysiological consequences of obesity, including insulin resistance, cardiovascular disease, hypertension and hepatic steatosis.

Keywords: Adipocyte, Adipogenesis, Adipokines, Adipose tissue, Angiogenesis, Beige adipocyte, Brown adipose tissue, Crown-like structure, Fat, Fibrosis, Hyperplasia, Hypertrophy, Hypoxia, Inflammation, Insulin resistance, Lipid, Obesity, Oxidative stress, Subcutaneous adipose tissue, Visceral adipose tissue, White adipose tissue.

* **Corresponding author Alexandra M. Gouveia:** Departamento de Biomedicina - Unidade de Biologia Experimental, Faculdade de Medicina, Universidade do Porto, Porto, Portugal; Tel: +351 225513600; Fax:+351 225513601; E-mail: agouveia@med.up.pt
# both authors equally contributed to the manuscript

Rosário Monteiro and Maria João Martins (Eds.)
All rights reserved-© 2020 Bentham Science Publishers

INTRODUCTION

Obesity has to be regarded as an epidemic health problem. The numbers are scaring, with alarming prevalence rates in many developing and developed countries. World Health Organization data reveals that in 2014, 15% of women and 11% of men aged 18 and over were obese worldwide [body mass index (BMI) $\geq$ 30 kg/m^2]. This "globesity" stands as one of the most serious health challenges of the early 21st century all over the world. Obesity is recognized as a chronic and systemic inflammatory disorder and is definitely a major risk factor for many diseases such as heart disease, stroke and other cardiovascular conditions, type 2 diabetes, osteoarthritis and some types of cancers [1]. Therefore, this morbid and potentially fatal entity ought to be taken seriously and efficient strategies to control obesity should be considered.

Environmental factors, such as the general consumption of high-calorie foods, lifestyle with reduced physical exercise, as well as genetic factors that predispose to weight gain, contribute to an imbalance between food intake and energy expenditure and consequently to an abnormal or excessive fat accumulation [2]. This increase in fat mass is accompanied by a total remodeling of the adipose tissue (AT), namely the increase of the number and/or size of the adipocytes, changes in vascular cells, the dysregulation of the pattern of secreted cytokines, increased inflammation and overproduction of the extracellular matrix (ECM). AT remodeling also considers the alteration of adipocyte morphology and function, which is able to transdifferentiate between white to beige/brown depending on various factors, including the metabolic status. AT alterations do not remain circumscribed to AT but are also reflected in other metabolic organs, such as pancreas, liver and muscle, in consequence of cell-cell communication and signaling mediated by adipose-secreted molecules.

However, it should be mentioned that some obese individuals are considered metabolically healthy, since they bypass the pathological consequences of AT remodeling. Furthermore, some AT alterations, such as white adipose tissue (WAT) "browning", are considered as potential therapeutic strategies to obesity. These findings highlight the importance of detailed studies on the molecular mechanisms underlying AT remodeling.

GENERAL COMPOSITION AND FUNCTION OF ADIPOSE TISSUE

Adipose Tissue Distribution in Humans and Rodents

The adipose organ can be classified in two main distinct types due to their singular functions and apparent color difference: WAT, specialized in energy storage, and brown adipose tissue (BAT), that dissipates energy in the form of heat, a proccss denominated thermogenesis. WAT is, in turn, separated in two major representative depots: the subcutaneous adipose tissue (SAT) and the visceral adipose tissue (VAT) [3]. It is also found in smaller amounts in the retro-orbital, periarticular, bone marrow, intermuscular and pericardial zones [4].

In humans and rodents, SAT is positioned under the dermis of the skin providing thermal insulation and mechanical cushioning to the body [5]. Although there are gender differences in human subcutaneous fat distribution, SAT is the larger adipose depot, occupying about 80% of all body fat, mainly spread in the abdominal and gluteofemoral areas [6]. In rodents, SAT is separated in two depots: the anterior and the posterior. The anterior corresponds to the interscapular, subscapular, axillary and cervical depots and the posterior is composed by the dorso-lumbar, gluteal and inguinal depots [7]. The inguinal subcutaneous region, located in the layer under the skin outside the abdominal cavity at the hips is the major SAT fat pad [8].

Mammalian VAT is located around the abdominal organs providing filling and protection. In humans, VAT depots are positioned in the omental, mesenteric and perirenal areas [9]. In rodents, two main VAT depots exist, one positioned in the thorax that includes the mediastinic depot, and the other located at the abdomen, including the omental, mesenteric, perirenal, retroperitoneal, parametrial, periovaric, epididymal and perivesical sub-depots [10]. The epididymal VAT, also termed gonadal AT, located in the perigonadal region is considered the greater VAT depot [8].

BAT is a unique organ found in all mammals, contributing throughout the evolutionary process to their survival in periods of night-time cold, hibernation and thermal stress at birth [11]. In humans, BAT was initially considered biologically active only in newborns and children with no relevant role in the adult energetic metabolism [12]. However, recent studies of Positron Emission Tomography - Computed Tomography (PET-CT), demonstrated that the adult human has functionally active BAT and that the amount of this tissue is inversely correlated with BMI, suggesting a role in metabolism during adulthood [13, 14]. In the human infant, BAT is located mainly in the interscapular area of the body, but is also present at the axillary, cervical, perirenal, periadrenal regions [4] and in the facial area, the Bichat's fat pad [15]. As it progresses into adulthood, BAT area regresses and is redistributed mainly to the interscapular, supraclavicular and cervical areas, being also found in smaller proportions in the axillary and paravertebral zones [16, 17]. In rodents, BAT is distributed in higher proportions on the interscapular and dorso-cervical regions, but is also found in the axillary and perirenal areas [18].

Adipose Tissue Composition and Plasticity

Adipocytes

WAT and BAT are mainly composed of white and brown adipocytes, respectively. Due to its extraordinary plasticity, over the last years, several authors have described and characterized two additional types of adipocytes, the beige and the pink, that arise through transdifferentiation of white adipocytes in response to a specific stimuli [19, 20].

White adipocytes comprise a single large spherical lipid droplet that occupies most of the cell area, which is why they are called unilocular cells. The reduced cytoplasm, positioned around the lipid droplet, contains the nucleus squeezed at the periphery. This adipocyte has a reduced number of mitochondria because its main function is to accumulate energy in the form of triglycerides (TGs) within the lipid droplet. The accumulation of TGs reflects the imbalance between energy intake and expenditure [21] and the more TGs accumulated, the greater the adipocyte becomes. Usually, this cell has a diameter of around 100 μm, but can vary from about 30 μm to 160 μm or more [10].

Brown adipocytes, also termed multilocular adipocytes, have a polygonal or ellipsoid shape and are smaller than the white ones, typically with a diameter between 15 to 50 μm. The nucleus is round shaped and situated at the center of the cell, surrounded by multiple lipid droplets distributed through the cytoplasm as well as numerous spherical mitochondria with laminar cristae [19]. It is due to the presence of these abundant organelles that these cells perform thermogenesis, a process that consists in burning energy to release heat in detriment of adenosine triphosphate (ATP) production. Brown adipocyte mitochondria express a unique protein with a fundamental role in the thermogenic process, the uncoupling protein 1 (UCP1) that uncouples the oxidation of fuel substrates from the synthesis of ATP, thus generating heat [22]. BAT activity is induced by a myriad of factors including cold exposure and β-adrenergic receptor agonists, mainly through stimulation of the sympathetic nervous system (SNS) that innervates BAT [23].

Beige adipocytes were identified for the first time in 1984 in the WAT of mice exposed to cold, at the time still designated brown adipocytes [24]. Later, these cells were denominated beige adipocytes since they contain characteristics of white and brown adipocytes and are highly differentiated from white adipocytes under external stimuli [25] in a process known as WAT "browning". These beige adipocytes arise in the WAT mass and, like the brown adipocytes, have numerous lipid droplets dispersed in the cytoplasm, increased mitochondrial biogenesis and UCP1 expression which provide them with thermogenic capacity [26]. In rodents, beige adipocytes are mainly located in SAT, in the anterior and inguinal areas [27]. The transcriptional program of beige cells has been characterized and considers UCP1, the peroxisome proliferator-activated receptor gamma coactivator 1 alpha (PGC1α), Cidea, deiodinase iodothyronine type 2 (DIO2) and PR domain containing 16 (PRDM16), all genes closely related to the main role of BAT [20].

Lastly, pink adipocytes were described in mouse subcutaneous fat depots [19]. They are mammary gland alveolar epithelial cells that arise during pregnancy through transdifferentiation of white adipocytes from the female SAT and play a key role during lactation to produce and secrete milk in the mammary gland [19].

Other Important Constituents of Adipose Tissue

Adipocytes are the most abundant cells in AT, but others have also a fundamental role in the structure and function of this organ. Considering WAT, it is also composed by preadipocytes, stem cells, fibroblasts, endothelial and immune cells [28]. Immune cells are found in the stromal vascular fraction (SFV) and contribute to AT homeostasis, maintaining the welfare of adipocytes and removing apoptotic cells. These immune system cells include macrophages, neutrophils, eosinophils, mast cells and several subtypes of T and B cells [29]. In turn, BAT consists of preadipocytes, endothelial and interstitial cells.

Additionally, AT structure is also composed by ECM components, capillaries and is also innervated by the SNS. In fact, AT is functionally linked to its vasculature, which is extensive, with a capillary network surrounding each adipocyte. The vasculature supply is responsible for the transport of oxygen, nutrients, hormones, growth factors, stem and inflammatory cells, waste products, fatty acids and adipokines [30].

The ECM of AT consists of interstitial fibers and pericellular membranes that are mainly composed by fibronectin, laminin, heparan sulphate proteoglycan and collagens, which in turn contribute for the maintenance and support of the structure and function of AT [31]. Type IV and I collagens are the major proteins that constitute the ECM but collagen type VI also contributes to its support and stability. Under certain circumstances, these collagen fibers can be digested by a family of neutral endopeptidases, the matrix metalloproteinases that enable the remodeling of ECM [32, 33].

BAT is vastly innervated by the SNS and highly vascularized comparing to WAT, since it has elevated oxygen consumption needs, because of its higher thermogenic activity, and the need to distribute heat throughout the body rapidly. Since the metabolism of the beige adipocyte is very similar to that of the brown adipocyte, requiring higher oxygen levels, when browning of WAT occurs, there is a switch to a proangiogenic phenotype in this tissue [34].

Adipose Tissue as a Secretion Organ

Adipocytes secrete a large number of bioactive mediators that signal to several organs such as the brain, liver or skeletal muscle, thereby modulating food intake, energy expenditure, blood pressure as well as lipid and glucose metabolism [35]. Examples of these adipokines are leptin, adiponectin, resistin, retinol binding protein 4 (RBP4), omentin and nesfatin.

Leptin is, so far, the best-studied adipokine and its discovery in 1994 as the responsible gene for hyperphagia and obesity of the ob/ob mice is perhaps one of the most-important findings related to obesity [36]. Since then, AT has been regarded as an endocrine organ instead of a mere fat deposit. Leptin is secreted from WAT in proportion to the total amount of fat in the body and signals the status of energy storage to the brain [37]. Therefore, plasma leptin levels strongly correlate with BMI and weight gain [38, 39]. At the central nervous system (CNS), this adipocyte-derived satiety hormone targets two distinct hypothalamic pathways: it inhibits the expression of the orexigenic peptides agouti-related peptide (AgRP) and neuropeptide Y (NPY) while stimulates the production of anorexigenic pro-opiomelanocortin-derived peptides such as the alpha melanocyte-stimulating hormone (αMSH). By increasing αMSH and decreasing AgRP release, leptin orchestrates the activation of satiety signals, which relays in a decrease of food intake and body weight [40]. Despite the enhanced circulating levels of leptin in obese individuals, the expected anorectic effects are not reached since the high and chronic levels of leptin usually lead to leptin resistance, which further exacerbate the obesity dynamics. Leptin resistance seems to be a complex process involving not only a decrease on leptin transport and signaling into the brain [38, 41] but also modifications of leptin responsiveness in adipocytes, since this hormone can bind directly to leptin receptors expressed in adipocytes to reduce fat pad size (by inhibiting lipogenesis and increasing lipolysis [42]). Thus, obesity-related leptin desensitization cannot be treated with exogenous leptin as demonstrated by many data collected over the last years [43].

Adiponectin, although being the most abundant protein released by AT, is substantially reduced in the circulating blood of animal models of obesity and insulin resistance [44, 45]. In contrast to leptin, plasma levels of adiponectin inversely correlate with BMI and increase with weight loss [46, 47]. This anti-obesity adipokine may act as a reliable predictor for metabolic dysfunction since it is secreted at higher levels by functional adipocytes from lean subjects while being downregulated in dysfunctional adipocytes from obese subjects [47].

Adiponectin increases glucose uptake and fat oxidation in the muscle, suppresses glucose production in the liver by upregulating the AMP-activated protein kinase pathway (AMPK) [48, 49] and stimulates insulin secretion by pancreatic islets [50]. In contrast to leptin, at the CNS, adiponectin acts as an appetite stimulator by enhancing hypothalamic AMPK activity and food intake [51]. Adiponectin was also described to inhibit BAT lipolysis and thermogenesis [52].

Omentin, mainly produced by human omental adipose depot, is negatively correlated with obesity and insulin resistance markers [53]. By contrast, resistin secretion increases with obesity, particularly in VAT where is mainly produced. Since administration of resistin in mice impairs glucose tolerance and insulin activity, it has been speculated that resistin may be responsible for the diabetic phenotype of obesity [54]. RBP4 is another adipokine upregulated in diabetic mice and humans that impairs insulin signaling in liver and muscle through inhibition of insulin receptor substrate 1 (IRS1). RBP4 is preferentially produced by VAT during obesity and diabetes being a marker for visceral obesity [47]. Nesfatin, mainly produced by SAT, is thought to have a role on nutrient sensing and appetite regulation, similarly to leptin [55].

In addition to peptide adipokines, AT also releases lipokines, lipid metabolites that also have a function on whole-body metabolism. The C16:1n7-palmitoleate, synthesized through stearoyl-CoA desaturase-1, improves insulin response in the muscle and inhibits fat accumulation in the liver [56].

OBESITY-MEDIATED ADIPOSE TISSUE REMODELING

During the progression of obesity, WAT undergoes several cellular and structural remodeling procedures. First, the tissue expands in terms of adipocyte size and number and then inflammatory cells are recruited. In an attempt to compensate the tissue expansion there is a remodeling of the vasculature and the ECM in order to mobilize nutrients and oxygen. But, once obesity and inflammation become chronic these mechanisms tend to fail and WAT becomes dysfunctional [57]. The sequential steps leading to AT dysfunction are far from being understood, but a decrease on tissue plasticity, caused by enhanced inflammatory and fibrotic pathways, relates to a vascular insufficiency and hypoxic status, among other stressful conditions, that ultimately leads to metabolic dysfunction Fig. (**1**).

Adipocyte Hyperplasia and Hypertrophy

Health problems associated to obesity have long been known to correlate with the pathological expansion of AT. It is believed that WAT becomes dysfunctional when it fails to expand properly in an attempt to store the excess energy in overnutrition circumstances. AT expansion is accomplished by an increment in fat mass that is largely determined by the increasing number (hyperplasia) and size (hypertrophy) of adipocytes. As obesity progresses, the chronic energy overflow will cause adipocyte hypertrophy rather than hyperplasia.

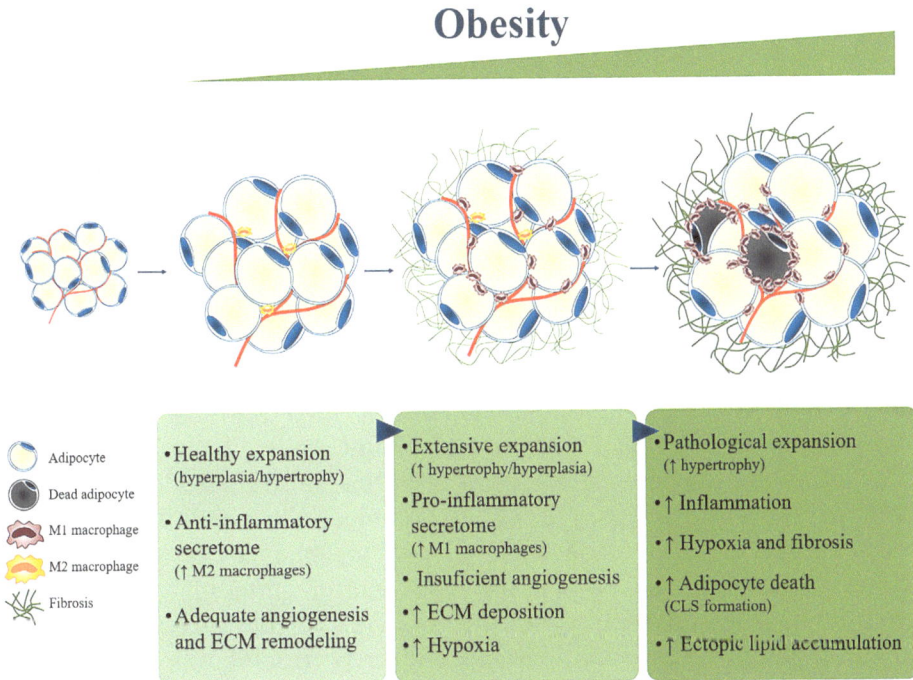

Fig. (1). Adipose tissue remodeling along obesity. In heathy conditions, adipose tissue expansion is mainly conveyed by adipocyte hyperplasia with an appropriate vasculature and extracellular matrix (ECM) remodeling. Resident M2 macrophages restrict inflammation by secretion of anti-inflammatory adipokines. Continuous expansion of adipose tissue along obesity by hypertrophy instead of hyperplasia will limit angiogenesis and oxygen supply that eventually enhance hypoxia. This will increase ECM deposition that further drives the development of adipose tissue fibrosis. Enlarged adipocytes are characterized by a proinflammatory secretome due to the massive recruitment of M1 macrophages responsible for the formation of "crown-like" structures (CLS) around dead adipocytes. Ultimately, dysfunctional adipose tissue is no longer able to accumulate properly the lipid surplus therefore causing ectopic lipid accumulation that is strongly associated with obesity comorbidities like cardiovascular diseases and diabetes.

AT expansion through hyperplasia requires an adipocyte precursor pool in WAT able to undergo differentiation. Data have shown a depletion of this preadipocyte pool in WAT from morbidly obese humans due to increased adipogenesis rate [58]. Other authors revealed that, although the total number of adipocytes found in obese is greater than in lean individuals, AT has a constant turnover rate of approximately 10% each year in adulthood independently from BMI [59]. This study also demonstrated that the total number of adipocytes is established during childhood or adolescence and does not change by a positive energy balance, in which new adipocytes can arise but are compensated with a higher apoptosis rate. It is also interesting to note that even after a significant weight loss program, the adipocyte number remains the same despite a reduced adipocyte volume [59]. Indeed, a decreased replicative potential and a premature cellular senescence also accounts for impairing hyperplasia [60]. This should encourage even further the AT expansion through hypertrophy as well as the ectopic accumulation of lipid surplus.

Adipocyte hypertrophy ultimately results in a reduced number of healthy small adipocytes in obesity, while large adipocytes persist as a continuous source of proinflammatory molecules [61]. In fact, adipocyte size is positively correlated with macrophage infiltration in obese mice and is accompanied by adipocyte death [62]. Also in human adipocytes, inflammation and susceptibility to cell death are both increased in adipose depots with larger adipocytes [63]. Enlarged adipocyte size, rather than obesity itself, predicts hyperinsulinemia and type 2 diabetes [64]. In fact, the adipocyte volume is quantitatively associated with insulin resistance. Recently, an adipocyte volume threshold has been described above which type 2 diabetes risk significantly raises [65]. Additionally, murine white adipocytes of the cell line 3T3-L1 overloaded with free fatty acids (FFA) to become enlarged revealed a decrease in glucose transporter type 4 (GLUT4) trafficking to cell surface, which disrupts insulin signaling [66]. Therefore, hypertrophy is correlated with serum insulin levels, insulin resistance and type 2 diabetes and, therefore, obese individuals with hypertrophic adipocytes are prone to be glucose intolerant and hyperinsulinemic as opposed to equally obese subjects with a smaller adipocyte pattern. Also, in women with comparable BMIs, adipocyte hypertrophy has a more adverse metabolic profile than cellular hyperplasia [67]. Evidence that large adipose cells in AT are associated with poor metabolic profiles has been accumulated for many years so it is now quite well accepted that adipocyte hypertrophy is a key characteristic of AT dysfunction [33, 68, 69].

Dynamics of WAT expandability during obesity differs among adipose depots. In mice fed a high-fat diet (HFD), the gonadal VAT is the primary fat depot that expands, followed by the SAT and mesenteric VAT. As the animals further gain body weight, gonadal VAT stops expanding in contrast to SAT and mesenteric VAT [70].

In general, under overnutrition circumstances, VAT expands predominantly by adipocyte hypertrophy being preferentially connected with central obesity while SAT grows more commonly through adipocyte hyperplasia [71]. Differences between SAT and VAT expansion may be explained by the fact that SAT has an increased number of preadipocytes with greater differentiation capacity compared to those from VAT. Besides, VAT adipocytes are more prone to cell death [57]. Given the positive correlation between hypertrophy and AT dysfunction, it is therefore not surprising that VAT, composed mainly by hypertrophic adipocytes, is generally related to insulin resistance, inflammation, and other metabolic abnormalities while SAT, formed mostly by newly formed adipocytes, usually predicts better outcomes and may have a protective role in obesity. Furthermore, lipolysis is elevated in hypertrophic adipocytes, which means that VAT is the main responsible for the huge elevation of FFA circulating levels in obesity [72].

Overall, these data suggest that SAT may be a critical factor for the pathological expansion of AT since circulating lipids may be predominantly stored in SAT depot before marked expansion of the VAT occurs. Once the SAT fails to appropriately expand through hyperplasia, VAT hypertrophy will lead to generalized ectopic fat deposition in other tissues, like the liver and the muscle, progressive insulin and leptin resistance and chronic systemic inflammation.

Macrophage Infiltration in Adipose Tissue and Inflammatory Profile

Healthy remodeling and expansion of AT requires a safe proinflammatory signaling that, when disrupted, impairs adipogenesis and enhances ectopic lipid accumulation [73]. The low-grade local inflammation may be thus an adaptive response for a proper storage of excess energy in AT, thereby protecting against metabolic and inflammatory disturbances. Notwithstanding, in obesity, AT becomes highly infiltrated with immune cells, particularly proinflammatory macrophages, that lead to a chronic production of inflammatory factors affecting overall adipocyte metabolism. An increase of macrophage infiltration has been widely described in rodent models of obesity but also in human obesity, particularly in visceral depots [74]. Increased inflammation in the AT is known to affect white, beige and brown adipogenesis [57] thus compromising fat storage and lipid homeostasis. The crosstalk between AT and other metabolic organs potentiates a shift from a low-grade local inflammatory profile to a systemic inflammatory state.

The unhealthy hypertrophic expansion of WAT during obesity occurs in parallel with alterations on adipokine secretory profile, which typically includes an increase of proinflammatory factors, such as tumor necrosis factor alpha (TNFα), interleukin 1β (IL1β), IL6, IL8, leptin, resistin, lipocalin 2 and monocyte chemoattractant protein 1 (MCP1), and a reduction of anti-inflammatory factors, such as IL4, IL10 and adiponectin [43, 75, 76].

The accumulation of proinflammatory cells, particularly in VAT, such as macrophages, mast cells, neutrophils, B and T cells adds to the burden of obesity-related complications. In an obese state, those who were previously anti-inflammatory macrophages - M2 population (present in lean individuals) - undergo a phenotypic change, adopting a proinflammatory phenotype - M1 population [77]. The proportion of the proinflammatory 'classically activated' M1 macrophages increases over the second population of macrophages residing in the AT, the anti-inflammatory 'alternatively activated' M2 macrophages [78]. M1 macrophages dysregulate adipocyte signaling and function [75, 76] not only through the secretion of proinflammatory cytokines but also by the formation of 'crown-like' structures (CLS), constituted by macrophage aggregation surrounding dead or dying adipocytes, which is considered a marker for macrophage infiltration [61]. CLS number is known to increase greater than 10-fold with obesity and to be significantly enriched in VAT comparing to SAT in both obese mice and humans [79].

Inflammatory cytokines are secreted from both WAT-resident immune cells and adipocytes themselves and in most cases it is not possible to distinguish their origin. This is, for example, the case of TNFα, IL6, RBP4, and lipocalin 2. Regarding resistin, data from mice and humans are controversial with the adipocytes being the exclusive source of resistin in mice whereas in humans it is mainly found in macrophages and monocytes [80]. By contrast, expression of leptin and adiponectin in AT is restricted to adipocytes [47].

In fact, besides its role on food intake regulation, leptin acts as a proinflammatory cytokine promoting the secretion of IL6 and TNFα by monocytes and CC-chemokine ligands by macrophages [47]. It also promotes the differentiation of helper T cells into a proinflammatory helper T cells (TH1) phenotype increasing IL2 and interferon gamma (IFNγ) and suppressing the release of IL4 by anti-inflammatory helper T cells (TH2) [81]. Resistin also exerts a proinflammatory role in AT by increasing the production of TNFα and IL6 by monocytes. On vascular endothelial cells, resistin enhances leukocyte adhesion by promoting the expression of the proinflammatory vascular cell adhesion molecule-1 (VCAM1) and intercellular adhesion molecule-1 (ICAM1) [47]. Adiponectin is thought to act as a protector of systemic inflammation in part by modulating macrophage phenotype and function [82]. Plasma adiponectin levels are negatively correlated with the proinflammatory marker C-reactive protein (CRP) in obese and diabetic patients. Adiponectin administrations in obese mice seem to restore metabolic profile ameliorating glucose metabolism and liver function apparently by reducing macrophage number and TNFα secretion [47, 83].

TNFα, which is increased in obesity has long been known to induce lipolysis, decrease adipogenesis and enhance insulin resistance by decreasing GLUT4 expression and IRS1 activation [84 - 87]. Blockage of TNFα signaling improves insulin-dependent glucose uptake [88]. More evidence, accumulated over the last years, argues that restoring the inflammatory profile of AT decreases adipocyte size and improves insulin sensitivity, lipid metabolism and overall metabolic function. Indeed, IL1β antagonists have reached clinical trials owing to its therapeutic potential on diabetic patients by restoring insulin signaling, glucose transport and fatty acid uptake [43].

IL6 and MCP1 are also upregulated in obesity. MCP1 is well-known by its role on attracting macrophages into the AT in obesity promoting insulin resistance and hepatic steatosis [89]. Similarly, IL6 increments on serum are related to the development of type 2 diabetes [47]. IL6 can also stimulate the production of CRP by the liver, a significant marker of systemic inflammation. Different fat depots have distinct contributions to the inflammatory status and metabolic profile of obesity, with VAT being more proinflammatory and SAT anti-inflammatory. Indeed, macrophages are more abundant and IL6 production is higher in VAT than in SAT. A higher energetic consumption also induces more visceral fat expression of TNFα and plasminogen activator inhibitor 1 (PAI1), a hemostatic factor associated with atherosclerosis [90, 91]. Differences between SAT and VAT relate to the inflammatory profile of hyperplasia and hypertrophy processes. Hypertrophic adipocytes, typical from VAT, secrete more proinflammatory cytokines whereas hyperplasic adipocytes, predominantly found in SAT, are more commonly characterized by an anti-inflammatory secretome.

Although adipocyte dysfunction in obesity has deleterious effects on metabolism, the lack of AT, especially SAT, is metabolically harmful as well. This is the case of lipodystrophies that are also linked to severe co-morbidities, apparently due to a lack of secretion of anti-inflammatory adipokines [92]. Furthermore, it was demonstrated that surgical removal of large amounts of SAT in obese subjects does not lead to any metabolic benefit in contrast to VAT excision [93, 94]. This, perhaps explain why metabolically healthy obese subjects have approximately 50% less VAT and more fat stored in their subcutaneous depot than the unhealthy obese individuals [95]. It is thus somehow encouraging to note, however, that weight loss by other methods such as caloric restriction or exercise can reverse the proinflammatory state of obesity switching toward to a healthy inflammatory profile [83].

Hypoxia and Angiogenesis

AT is the only organ able to grow throughout the entire life while retaining a relative high angiogenic activity. AT expansion in healthy conditions is supported by sufficient vasculature which appropriately supplies nutrients and oxygen. However, as AT expands in obesity through adipocyte hypertrophy, vasculature remodeling became relative deficient and a local AT hypoxia is assembled. Hypoxia accelerates obese AT fibrosis and increases local inflammatory response [72], which exacerbates the obese phenotype.

When hypoxia is established in hypertrophic AT, there is a compensatory mechanism by which AT enhances angiogenesis in attempt to counteract the low oxygen levels. In this context, the hypoxia-inducible factor 1 alpha (HIF1α), widely known as "the master regulator of oxygen homeostasis", is induced and alters the expression of many genes involved in a diverse array of functions, including angiogenesis, ECM remodeling and inflammation [96]. Hypoxia-induced HIF1α activation can directly upregulate the expression of the vascular endothelial growth factor (VEGF) [72, 97] which increases vascularization and ameliorates metabolic profile of HFD mice. Disruption of VEGF, by contrast, exacerbates insulin resistance and the inflammatory profile of obesity [98]. However, in energy surplus conditions, angiogenesis and VEGF production appears to be mediated by other factors than HIF1α since the compensatory angiogenic expansion derived from hypoxia becomes insufficient. Hypoxia-independent mechanisms of angiogenesis are also documented, namely the activation of angiogenic programs mediated by PGC1α, AMPK, and peroxisome proliferator-activated receptor gamma (PPARγ), a master regulator of adipocyte differentiation [97].

The importance of HIF1α in obesity has been supported by a large body of evidence. Indeed, selective deletion of HIF1α in AT decreases weight gain and improves insulin sensitivity in mice fed a HFD with a significant reduction in adipocyte size [99]. By contrast, transgenic overexpression of HIF1α in AT promotes weight gain and glucose intolerance in both lean and obese mice accompanied by an adipocyte enlargement [100]. Similarly, Sun *et al* (2013) demonstrated that HIF1α specific inhibition with PX-478 also improves metabolic function and reduces fibrosis and inflammatory profile of HFD mice. Additionally, PX-478 decreases adipocyte size and normalizes the elevated leptin expression induced by the HFD. Leptin was also suggested to be a target for HIF1α, which may explain why hypoxia correlates positively with adipocyte enlargement and leptin production [33, 96].

Similar to what happens with tissue expansion and inflammation, the angiogenic profile from different fat depots also varies. In non-obese individuals, the vascular density and angiogenic activity of endothelial cells is higher in SAT in comparison to VAT [101]. This feature decays along obesity, in which capillary rarefaction is thought to occur more rapidly in SAT than in VAT. Indeed, SAT becomes less vascularized and proangiogenic than VAT in obese subjects [102]. Despite having a higher vascular network, hypoxia and inflammatory-related genes are increasingly expressed in VAT when compared to the SAT. These inconsistent findings are explained by Villaret *et al* through an upregulation of senescence markers in endothelial cells from VAT compared to SAT [102]. Thus, loss of endothelial function in VAT seems to impair the rescue of the angiogenic potential that would outcome from the enhanced vascular network. There are, however, other contradictory results showing no differences in vascular density between the two depots in obese humans, although being higher in VAT than in SAT in lean individuals [103]. The consensus of these three studies is that capillary density is lower in both VAT and SAT of obese humans compared with lean subjects.

Consistent with Villaret *et al* [102], increased hypoxia has been correlated with elevated adipocyte death rate, which is more likely to be found in VAT than in SAT. Indeed, the inadequate supply of oxygen in face of expanding VAT may induce cell death and CLS formation.

Regarding BAT, since it is more highly vascularized than WAT, the obesity-associated increase in hypoxia and decrease in angiogenic potential have a strong impact on BAT function by impairing mitochondrial activity, thermogenesis and energy expenditure [104]. Indeed, vascular rarefaction is thought to be a main reason for the accumulation of lipid droplets and BAT "whitening" phenotype as obesity develops [105]. In this setting, Sun *et al* showed that adipocyte-specific VEGF-A overexpression improves vascularization and promotes the "browning" or "beiging" of WAT with upregulation of UCP1 and PGC1α, enhances energy expenditure and increases resistance to obesity [106].

Extracellular Matrix Deposition and Fibrosis

Alteration of ECM components occurs earlier in humans with moderate weight gain and increases further along obesity [107]. AT expansion depends on the ability of the ECM to remodel without losing flexibility, which requires a coordinated degradation of the existing and the production of new ECM components. The higher the flexibility of the ECM, the more lipids are endorsed in adipose depots. However, a metabolically dysfunctional AT produces excess matrix components causing the development of fibrosis and consequently a higher ECM rigidity that interferes with adipose plasticity [108]. Fibrosis is the pathological consequence of ECM dysregulation, characterized by an abundance of ECM proteins, particularly collagens. Indeed, it has been shown that increased fibrotic content, particularly collagen VI, is associated with compromised metabolism in obese humans [109]. Collagen fibers can accumulate around the adipocyte, forming the "periadipocyte collagens" and in AT vessels as well [33]. In line, blocking collagen synthesis in the ob/ob mouse prevents adipogenesis and decreases fat mass and body weight [108].

During obesity, evidence collected suggests that hypoxia precedes ECM accumulation in obesity. When the vasculature does not follow the increased volume achieved by adipocytes the blood flow is limited driving to the hypoxic state and HIF1α-induced enhanced deposition of ECM proteins, therefore promoting fibrosis. Recently, Sun *et al*, demonstrated that HIF1α inhibition prevents fibrotic response in AT from obese mice which contributes to metabolic improvement [33]. Yet, fibrosis can also improve rigidity of the vasculature, which inhibits angiogenesis and enhances even further the hypoxic process.

The unusual expression of ECM components found in obesity seems to dictate the recruitment and activation of immune cells, actively contributing to the obesity-related proinflammatory profile. Metabolic improvement on ob/ob mice caused by disruption of collagen VI is accomplished by a decrease on AT inflammation and CLS number [108]. In further support of this notion, an HFD challenge time course experiment in mice revealed that infiltration of macrophages and the associated inflammation initiates after the fibrotic environment is achieved [110].

Altogether, one can realize that deficient angiogenesis of AT during obesity leads to hypoxia and increments on HIF1α expression responsible for promoting inflammatory responses and ECM deposition, which in turn will impair vessel outgrowth and angiogenesis, decreasing even more the oxygen available to hypertrophied adipocytes.

The amount of collagen deposition increases with obesity in both VAT and SAT depots but, paradoxically, fibrosis is more abundant in SAT than in VAT where inflammation is increased. It is, however, speculated that fibrosis in VAT could have a protective role restricting adipocyte hypertrophy [57]. Notwithstanding, further studies are needed to understand the mechanisms and kinetics of fibrosis in both fat depots.

Transdifferentiation of Adipocytes in Obesity

The AT has revealed an enormous plasticity, modulated by a huge number of environmental and physiological factors, including different metabolic conditions. In this context, adipocytes have the ability to modify their structure and function, when physiologically required. One of the most well-described adipocyte transformation mechanism considers the transdifferentiation of white into beige adipocytes, designated as "browning" of WAT. In fact, several classical factors have been implicated in the formation of clusters of thermogenic beige adipocytes within the WAT, namely chronic cold exposure and activation of β3-adrenergic receptors [111]. Additionally, exercise and several endocrine and metabolic factors have also been implicated in the "browning" mechanism, namely fibroblast growth factor 21, cardiac natriuretic peptides and bone morphogenic protein [23]. Recent results from our group characterize the browning effects of a new group of molecules, the melanocortins, neuropeptides that impact directly on white adipocyte biology by stimulating lipolysis and impairing FFA re-esterification [112, 113]. In WAT from obese mice, the melanocortin αMSH is able to stimulate the appearance of multilocular adipocytes, and to increase the expression of BAT-hallmark genes, respiratory rate and mitochondrial biogenesis [114]. This ability of WAT to transdifferentiate some of their adipocytes into beige adipocytes is also dependent on BMI [115]. It was observed that human SAT increases thermogenic genes in response to a cold stimulus and this response is inhibited by obesity and inflammation. This data is in agreement with BAT activation since, in humans, reduced BAT function is closely associated with obesity, compromised metabolic health and cardiovascular risk [17, 116]. Consistently, mice genetically engineered to have less BAT gain more weight than control mice [117]. As already stated, a BAT "whitening" phenotype has also been observed through the development of obesity [105].

Adipose Tissue Remodeling as a Therapeutic Perspective to Obesity

An ideal treatment to obesity considers the degradation of the harmful fatty acids accumulated in the WAT without any deleterious effect to other tissues, such as lipotoxicity and metabolic and cardiovascular problems. In this context, the transdifferentiation of white into beige adipocytes or the activation of pre existent BAT constitutes a way to utilize the excess FFA and, consequently, can be considered as a therapeutic target to obesity. In fact, it was estimated that 50 g of human active BAT may be responsible for up to 5% of the basal metabolic rate [118]. Cold induced-human BAT significantly contributes to the increase of the resting energy expenditure [119, 120] and there is solid evidence demonstrating the benefits of an enhanced amount of BAT, by transplantation or in genetic mice models [121].

Evidence collected also indicates that restoring inflammatory profile by reversing the M1/M2 macrophage ratio ameliorates obesity-associated inflammation by decreasing adipocyte size and improving metabolic condition. Indeed, infusion of M2 macrophages into obese mice decreases adipocyte size and improves serum lipid profile and insulin resistance by rescuing inflammatory homeostasis through a rise on the ratio of M2 to M1 macrophages [122]. Furthermore, administration of IL4, which can polarize former M1 macrophages to the anti-inflammatory M2 phenotype, ameliorates diet-induced obesity and insulin resistance in obese mice [123]. The inhibition of IL1β signaling, which in opposite is thought to decrease polarization to the M1 phenotype, is also able to enhance insulin sensitivity and to reduce markers of systemic inflammation, like CPR and IL6, in type 2 diabetic patients treated with IL1β receptor antagonists [124]. Thus, several authors are advocating that restoring macrophages' homeostasis with a reversed M2/M1 ratio might be an effective approach to combat obesity.

An additional approach relies on the observation that some obese individuals are metabolically healthy. There are examples of obese persons with BMI over 30 kg/m^2 that are insulin sensitive and have normal metabolic parameters [125]. It was found that these individuals have smaller adipocytes in the AT and a lower number of immune cells. These small adipocytes still have capacity to store fatty acids excess, ameliorating insulin resistance. Additionally, antidiabetic thiazolidinedione derivatives, like rosiglitazone, induce the differentiation of small new adipocytes [126]. These observations and the full understanding of the adipocyte hypertrophy mechanisms could provide a new therapeutic solution for the metabolic complications associated with obesity.

CONCLUDING REMARKS

AT has no longer the concept of energy storage organ since it is now recognized to release many bioactive substances that have a crucial role in the integration of systemic metabolism.

Expansion of AT along obesity by hypertrophy instead of hyperplasia will limit angiogenesis and oxygen supply that eventually enhance hypoxia. This will increase ECM deposition and AT fibrosis. Enlarged adipocytes are characterized by a proinflammatory secretome and a dysregulated expression of adipokines. Ultimately, AT becomes dysfunctional and the excess of circulating fat starts to accumulate ectopically which strongly associates with obesity-comorbidities like cardiovascular diseases and diabetes Fig. (**1**).

Although obesity may seem like a no-return process and its knowledge very difficult to achieve, it is thus inspiring and challenging to note that some attempts to rescue any of these events may have a huge potential for obesity therapeutics.

CONSENT FOR PUBLICATION

Not applicable.

CONFLICT OF INTEREST

The authors confirm that this chapter contents have no conflict of interest.

ACKNOWLEDGEMENTS

This work was supported by FCT/MEC (PIDDAC) and FEDER-Fundo Europeu de Desenvolvimento Regional, COMPETE 2020-Programa Operacional Competitividade e Internacionalização (PTDC/BIM-MET/2123/2014); Adriana Rodrigues is supported by POPH/FSE and by FCT (SFRH/BPD/92868/2013).

REFERENCES

[1]   Pi-Sunyer FX. The medical risks of obesity. Obes Surg 2002; 12 (Suppl. 1): 6S-11S.
        [http://dx.doi.org/10.1007/BF03342140] [PMID: 11969107]

[2]   Chiesi M, Huppertz C, Hofbauer KG. Pharmacotherapy of obesity: targets and perspectives. Trends Pharmacol Sci 2001; 22(5): 247-54.
        [http://dx.doi.org/10.1016/S0165-6147(00)01664-3] [PMID: 11339976]

[3]   Wronska A, Kmiec Z. Structural and biochemical characteristics of various white adipose tissue depots. Acta Physiol (Oxf) 2012; 205(2): 194-208.
        [http://dx.doi.org/10.1111/j.1748-1716.2012.02409.x] [PMID: 22226221]

[4]   Gesta S, Tseng YH, Kahn CR. Developmental origin of fat: tracking obesity to its source. Cell 2007; 131(2): 242-56.
        [http://dx.doi.org/10.1016/j.cell.2007.10.004] [PMID: 17956727]

[5]   Driskell RR, Jahoda CA, Chuong CM, Watt FM, Horsley V. Defining dermal adipose tissue. Exp Dermatol 2014; 23(9): 629-31.
        [http://dx.doi.org/10.1111/exd.12450] [PMID: 24841073]

[6]   Arner P. Regional adipocity in man. J Endocrinol 1997; 155(2): 191-2.
        [http://dx.doi.org/10.1677/joe.0.1550191] [PMID: 9415044]

[7]   Cinti S. The adipose organ at a glance. Dis Model Mech 2012; 5(5): 588-94.
        [http://dx.doi.org/10.1242/dmm.009662] [PMID: 22915020]

[8]   Chusyd DE, Wang D, Huffman DM, Nagy TR. Relationships between Rodent White Adipose Fat Pads and Human White Adipose Fat Depots. Front Nutr 2016; 3(10)
        [http://dx.doi.org/10.3389/fnut.2016.00010]

[9]   Tchernof A, Després JP. Pathophysiology of human visceral obesity: an update. Physiol Rev 2013; 93(1): 359-404.
        [http://dx.doi.org/10.1152/physrev.00033.2011] [PMID: 23303913]

[10]   Cinti S. The adipose organ. Prostaglandins Leukot Essent Fatty Acids 2005; 73(1): 9-15.
        [http://dx.doi.org/10.1016/j.plefa.2005.04.010] [PMID: 15936182]

[11]   Cannon B, Nedergaard J. Brown adipose tissue: function and physiological significance. Physiol Rev 2004; 84(1): 277-359.
        [http://dx.doi.org/10.1152/physrev.00015.2003] [PMID: 14715917]

[12]   Lean ME. Brown adipose tissue in humans. Proc Nutr Soc 1989; 48(2): 243-56.
        [http://dx.doi.org/10.1079/PNS19890036] [PMID: 2678120]

[13]   Cypess AM, Lehman S, Williams G, *et al.* Identification and importance of brown adipose tissue in adult humans. N Engl J Med 2009; 360(15): 1509-17.
        [http://dx.doi.org/10.1056/NEJMoa0810780] [PMID: 19357406]

[14]   Virtanen KA, Lidell ME, Orava J, *et al.* Functional brown adipose tissue in healthy adults. N Engl J Med 2009; 360(15): 1518-25.
        [http://dx.doi.org/10.1056/NEJMoa0808949] [PMID: 19357407]

[15]   Ponrartana S, Patil S, Aggabao PC, Pavlova Z, Devaskar SU, Gilsanz V. Brown adipose tissue in the

buccal fat pad during infancy. PLoS One 2014; 9(2)e89533
[http://dx.doi.org/10.1371/journal.pone.0089533] [PMID: 24586852]

[16]   Nedergaard J, Bengtsson T, Cannon B. Unexpected evidence for active brown adipose tissue in adult humans. Am J Physiol Endocrinol Metab 2007; 293(2): E444-52.
[http://dx.doi.org/10.1152/ajpendo.00691.2006] [PMID: 17473055]

[17]   van Marken Lichtenbelt WD, Vanhommerig JW, Smulders NM, *et al.* Cold-activated brown adipose tissue in healthy men. N Engl J Med 2009; 360(15): 1500-8.
[http://dx.doi.org/10.1056/NEJMoa0808718] [PMID: 19357405]

[18]   Oelkrug R, Polymeropoulos ET, Jastroch M. Brown adipose tissue: physiological function and evolutionary significance. J Comp Physiol B 2015; 185(6): 587-606.
[http://dx.doi.org/10.1007/s00360-015-0907-7] [PMID: 25966796]

[19]   Giordano A, Smorlesi A, Frontini A, Barbatelli G, Cinti S. White, brown and pink adipocytes: the extraordinary plasticity of the adipose organ. Eur J Endocrinol 2014; 170(5): R159-71.
[http://dx.doi.org/10.1530/EJE-13-0945] [PMID: 24468979]

[20]   Wu J, Boström P, Sparks LM, *et al.* Beige adipocytes are a distinct type of thermogenic fat cell in mouse and human. Cell 2012; 150(2): 366-76.
[http://dx.doi.org/10.1016/j.cell.2012.05.016] [PMID: 22796012]

[21]   Henry SL, Bensley JG, Wood-Bradley RJ, Cullen-McEwen LA, Bertram JF, Armitage JA. White adipocytes: more than just fat depots. Int J Biochem Cell Biol 2012; 44(3): 435-40.
[http://dx.doi.org/10.1016/j.biocel.2011.12.011] [PMID: 22222895]

[22]   Schulz TJ, Tseng YH. Brown adipose tissue: development, metabolism and beyond. Biochem J 2013; 453(2): 167-78.
[http://dx.doi.org/10.1042/BJ20130457] [PMID: 23805974]

[23]   Bonet ML, Oliver P, Palou A. Pharmacological and nutritional agents promoting browning of white adipose tissue. Biochim Biophys Acta 2013; 1831(5): 969-85.
[http://dx.doi.org/10.1016/j.bbalip.2012.12.002] [PMID: 23246573]

[24]   Young P, Arch JR, Ashwell M. Brown adipose tissue in the parametrial fat pad of the mouse. FEBS Lett 1984; 167(1): 10-4.
[http://dx.doi.org/10.1016/0014-5793(84)80822-4] [PMID: 6698197]

[25]   Ishibashi J, Seale P. Medicine. Beige can be slimming. Science 2010; 328(5982): 1113-4.
[http://dx.doi.org/10.1126/science.1190816] [PMID: 20448151]

[26]   Giralt M, Villarroya F. White, brown, beige/brite: different adipose cells for different functions? Endocrinology 2013; 154(9): 2992-3000.
[http://dx.doi.org/10.1210/en.2013-1403] [PMID: 23782940]

[27]   Sidossis L, Kajimura S. Brown and beige fat in humans: thermogenic adipocytes that control energy and glucose homeostasis. J Clin Invest 2015; 125(2): 478-86.
[http://dx.doi.org/10.1172/JCI78362] [PMID: 25642708]

[28]   Esteve Ràfols M. Adipose tissue: cell heterogeneity and functional diversity. Endocrinol Nutr (English Edition) 2014; 61(2): 100-12.
[http://dx.doi.org/10.1016/j.endonu.2013.03.011] [PMID: 23834768]

[29]   Huh JY, Park YJ, Ham M, Kim JB. Crosstalk between adipocytes and immune cells in adipose tissue inflammation and metabolic dysregulation in obesity. Mol Cells 2014; 37(5): 365-71.
[http://dx.doi.org/10.14348/molcells.2014.0074] [PMID: 24781408]

[30]   Lemoine AY, Ledoux S, Larger E. Adipose tissue angiogenesis in obesity. Thromb Haemost 2013; 110(4): 661-8.
[http://dx.doi.org/10.1160/TH13-01-0073] [PMID: 23595655]

[31]   Divoux A, Clément K. Architecture and the extracellular matrix: the still unappreciated components of

the adipose tissue. Obes Rev 2011; 12(5): e494-503.
[http://dx.doi.org/10.1111/j.1467-789X.2010.00811.x] [PMID: 21366833]

[32]   Mariman EC, Wang P. Adipocyte extracellular matrix composition, dynamics and role in obesity. Cell Mol Life Sci 2010; 67(8): 1277-92.
[http://dx.doi.org/10.1007/s00018-010-0263-4] [PMID: 20107860]

[33]   Sun K, Tordjman J, Clément K, Scherer PE. Fibrosis and adipose tissue dysfunction. Cell Metab 2013; 18(4): 470-7.
[http://dx.doi.org/10.1016/j.cmet.2013.06.016] [PMID: 23954640]

[34]   Luo X, Jia R, Luo XQ, *et al.* Cold Exposure Differentially Stimulates Angiogenesis in BAT and WAT of Mice: Implication in Adrenergic Activation. Cell Physiol Biochem 2017; 42(3): 974-86.
[http://dx.doi.org/10.1159/000478680] [PMID: 28662501]

[35]   Deng Y, Scherer PE. Adipokines as novel biomarkers and regulators of the metabolic syndrome. Ann N Y Acad Sci 2010; 1212: (E1-e19..
[http://dx.doi.org/10.1111/j.1749-6632.2010.05875.x]

[36]   Zhang Y, Proenca R, Maffei M, Barone M, Leopold L, Friedman JM. Positional cloning of the mouse obese gene and its human homologue. Nature 1994; 372(6505): 425-32.
[http://dx.doi.org/10.1038/372425a0] [PMID: 7984236]

[37]   Coll AP. Effects of pro-opiomelanocortin (POMC) on food intake and body weight: mechanisms and therapeutic potential? Clin Sci (Lond) 2007; 113(4): 171-82.
[http://dx.doi.org/10.1042/CS20070105] [PMID: 17623013]

[38]   Caro JF, Kolaczynski JW, Nyce MR, *et al.* Decreased cerebrospinal-fluid/serum leptin ratio in obesity: a possible mechanism for leptin resistance. Lancet 1996; 348(9021): 159-61.
[http://dx.doi.org/10.1016/S0140-6736(96)03173-X] [PMID: 8684156]

[39]   Considine RV, Sinha MK, Heiman ML, *et al.* Serum immunoreactive-leptin concentrations in normal-weight and obese humans. N Engl J Med 1996; 334(5): 292-5.
[http://dx.doi.org/10.1056/NEJM199602013340503] [PMID: 8532024]

[40]   Cowley MA, Smart JL, Rubinstein M, *et al.* Leptin activates anorexigenic POMC neurons through a neural network in the arcuate nucleus. Nature 2001; 411(6836): 480-4.
[http://dx.doi.org/10.1038/35078085] [PMID: 11373681]

[41]   Münzberg H, Flier JS, Bjørbaek C. Region-specific leptin resistance within the hypothalamus of diet-induced obese mice. Endocrinology 2004; 145(11): 4880-9.
[http://dx.doi.org/10.1210/en.2004-0726] [PMID: 15271881]

[42]   Harris RB. Direct and indirect effects of leptin on adipocyte metabolism. Biochim Biophys Acta 2014; 1842(3): 414-23.
[http://dx.doi.org/10.1016/j.bbadis.2013.05.009] [PMID: 23685313]

[43]   Kusminski CM, Bickel PE, Scherer PE. Targeting adipose tissue in the treatment of obesity-associated diabetes. Nat Rev Drug Discov 2016; 15(9): 639-60.
[http://dx.doi.org/10.1038/nrd.2016.75] [PMID: 27256476]

[44]   Hu E, Liang P, Spiegelman BM. AdipoQ is a novel adipose-specific gene dysregulated in obesity. J Biol Chem 1996; 271(18): 10697-703.
[http://dx.doi.org/10.1074/jbc.271.18.10697] [PMID: 8631877]

[45]   Hotta K, Funahashi T, Bodkin NL, *et al.* Circulating concentrations of the adipocyte protein adiponectin are decreased in parallel with reduced insulin sensitivity during the progression to type 2 diabetes in rhesus monkeys. Diabetes 2001; 50(5): 1126-33.
[http://dx.doi.org/10.2337/diabetes.50.5.1126] [PMID: 11334417]

[46]   Lang HF, Chou CY, Sheu WH, Lin JY. Weight loss increased serum adiponectin but decreased lipid levels in obese subjects whose body mass index was lower than 30 kg/m². Nutr Res 2011; 31(5): 378-86.

[http://dx.doi.org/10.1016/j.nutres.2011.04.004] [PMID: 21636016]

[47]   Ouchi N, Parker JL, Lugus JJ, Walsh K. Adipokines in inflammation and metabolic disease. Nat Rev Immunol 2011; 11(2): 85-97.
[http://dx.doi.org/10.1038/nri2921] [PMID: 21252989]

[48]   Liu Q, Yuan B, Lo KA, Patterson HC, Sun Y, Lodish HF. Adiponectin regulates expression of hepatic genes critical for glucose and lipid metabolism. Proc Natl Acad Sci USA 2012; 109(36): 14568-73.
[http://dx.doi.org/10.1073/pnas.1211611109] [PMID: 22904186]

[49]   Yamauchi T, Kamon J, Waki H, *et al.* The fat-derived hormone adiponectin reverses insulin resistance associated with both lipoatrophy and obesity. Nat Med 2001; 7(8): 941-6.
[http://dx.doi.org/10.1038/90984] [PMID: 11479627]

[50]   Okamoto M, Ohara-Imaizumi M, Kubota N, *et al.* Adiponectin induces insulin secretion *in vitro* and *in vivo at* a low glucose concentration. Diabetologia 2008; 51(5): 827-35.
[http://dx.doi.org/10.1007/s00125-008-0944-9] [PMID: 18369586]

[51]   Kubota N, Yano W, Kubota T, *et al.* Adiponectin stimulates AMP-activated protein kinase in the hypothalamus and increases food intake. Cell Metab 2007; 6(1): 55-68.
[http://dx.doi.org/10.1016/j.cmet.2007.06.003] [PMID: 17618856]

[52]   Qiao L, Yoo Hs, Bosco C, *et al.* Adiponectin reduces thermogenesis by inhibiting brown adipose tissue activation in mice. Diabetologia 2014; 57(5): 1027-36.
[http://dx.doi.org/10.1007/s00125-014-3180-5] [PMID: 24531262]

[53]   de Souza Batista CM, Yang RZ, Lee MJ, *et al.* Omentin plasma levels and gene expression are decreased in obesity. Diabetes 2007; 56(6): 1655-61.
[http://dx.doi.org/10.2337/db06-1506] [PMID: 17329619]

[54]   Steppan CM, Bailey ST, Bhat S, *et al.* The hormone resistin links obesity to diabetes. Nature 2001; 409(6818): 307-12.
[http://dx.doi.org/10.1038/35053000] [PMID: 11201732]

[55]   Ramanjaneya M, Chen J, Brown JE, *et al.* Identification of nesfatin-1 in human and murine adipose tissue: a novel depot-specific adipokine with increased levels in obesity. Endocrinology 2010; 151(7): 3169-80.
[http://dx.doi.org/10.1210/en.2009-1358] [PMID: 20427481]

[56]   Cao H, Gerhold K, Mayers JR, Wiest MM, Watkins SM, Hotamisligil GS. Identification of a lipokine, a lipid hormone linking adipose tissue to systemic metabolism. Cell 2008; 134(6): 933-44.
[http://dx.doi.org/10.1016/j.cell.2008.07.048] [PMID: 18805087]

[57]   Pellegrinelli V, Carobbio S, Vidal-Puig A. Adipose tissue plasticity: how fat depots respond differently to pathophysiological cues. Diabetologia 2016; 59(6): 1075-88.
[http://dx.doi.org/10.1007/s00125-016-3933-4] [PMID: 27039901]

[58]   Maumus M, Peyrafitte JA, D'Angelo R, *et al.* Native human adipose stromal cells: localization, morphology and phenotype. Int J Obes 2011; 35(9): 1141-53.
[http://dx.doi.org/10.1038/ijo.2010.269] [PMID: 21266947]

[59]   Spalding KL, Arner E, Westermark PO, *et al.* Dynamics of fat cell turnover in humans. Nature 2008; 453(7196): 783-7.
[http://dx.doi.org/10.1038/nature06902] [PMID: 18454136]

[60]   Roldan M, Macias-Gonzalez M, Garcia R, Tinahones FJ, Martin M. Obesity short-circuits stemness gene network in human adipose multipotent stem cells. FASEB J 2011; 25(12): 4111-26.
[http://dx.doi.org/10.1096/fj.10-171439] [PMID: 21846837]

[61]   Cinti S, Mitchell G, Barbatelli G, *et al.* Adipocyte death defines macrophage localization and function in adipose tissue of obese mice and humans. J Lipid Res 2005; 46(11): 2347-55.
[http://dx.doi.org/10.1194/jlr.M500294-JLR200] [PMID: 16150820]

[62]   Strissel KJ, Stancheva Z, Miyoshi H, *et al.* Adipocyte death, adipose tissue remodeling, and obesity complications. Diabetes 2007; 56(12): 2910-8.
[http://dx.doi.org/10.2337/db07-0767] [PMID: 17848624]

[63]   Skurk T, Alberti-Huber C, Herder C, Hauner H. Relationship between adipocyte size and adipokine expression and secretion. J Clin Endocrinol Metab 2007; 92(3): 1023-33.
[http://dx.doi.org/10.1210/jc.2006-1055] [PMID: 17164304]

[64]   Weyer C, Foley JE, Bogardus C, Tataranni PA, Pratley RE. Enlarged subcutaneous abdominal adipocyte size, but not obesity itself, predicts type II diabetes independent of insulin resistance. Diabetologia 2000; 43(12): 1498-506.
[http://dx.doi.org/10.1007/s001250051560] [PMID: 11151758]

[65]   Klöting N, Blüher M. Adipocyte dysfunction, inflammation and metabolic syndrome. Rev Endocr Metab Disord 2014; 15(4): 277-87.
[http://dx.doi.org/10.1007/s11154-014-9301-0] [PMID: 25344447]

[66]   Kim JI, Huh JY, Sohn JH, *et al.* Lipid-overloaded enlarged adipocytes provoke insulin resistance independent of inflammation. Mol Cell Biol 2015; 35(10): 1686-99.
[http://dx.doi.org/10.1128/MCB.01321-14] [PMID: 25733684]

[67]   Arner E, Westermark PO, Spalding KL, *et al.* Adipocyte turnover: relevance to human adipose tissue morphology. Diabetes 2010; 59(1): 105-9.
[http://dx.doi.org/10.2337/db09-0942] [PMID: 19846802]

[68]   Goossens GH. The Metabolic Phenotype in Obesity: Fat Mass, Body Fat Distribution, and Adipose Tissue Function. Obes Facts 2017; 10(3): 207-15.
[http://dx.doi.org/10.1159/000471488] [PMID: 28564650]

[69]   Rosen ED, Spiegelman BM. What we talk about when we talk about fat. Cell 2014; 156(1-2): 20-44.
[http://dx.doi.org/10.1016/j.cell.2013.12.012] [PMID: 24439368]

[70]   van Beek L, van Klinken JB, Pronk AC, *et al.* The limited storage capacity of gonadal adipose tissue directs the development of metabolic disorders in male C57Bl/6J mice. Diabetologia 2015; 58(7): 1601-9.
[http://dx.doi.org/10.1007/s00125-015-3594-8] [PMID: 25962520]

[71]   Joe AW, Yi L, Even Y, Vogl AW, Rossi FM. Depot-specific differences in adipogenic progenitor abundance and proliferative response to high-fat diet. Stem Cells 2009; 27(10): 2563-70.
[http://dx.doi.org/10.1002/stem.190] [PMID: 19658193]

[72]   Choe SS, Huh JY, Hwang IJ, Kim JI, Kim JB. Adipose Tissue Remodeling: Its Role in Energy Metabolism and Metabolic Disorders Front Endocrinol (Lausanne) 2016; 7(30)

[73]   Wernstedt Asterholm I, Tao C, Morley TS, *et al.* Adipocyte inflammation is essential for healthy adipose tissue expansion and remodeling. Cell Metab 2014; 20(1): 103-18.
[http://dx.doi.org/10.1016/j.cmet.2014.05.005] [PMID: 24930973]

[74]   Cancello R, Tordjman J, Poitou C, *et al.* Increased infiltration of macrophages in omental adipose tissue is associated with marked hepatic lesions in morbid human obesity. Diabetes 2006; 55(6): 1554-61.
[http://dx.doi.org/10.2337/db06-0133] [PMID: 16731817]

[75]   Sun K, Kusminski CM, Scherer PE. Adipose tissue remodeling and obesity. J Clin Invest 2011; 121(6): 2094-101.
[http://dx.doi.org/10.1172/JCI45887] [PMID: 21633177]

[76]   Lackey DE, Olefsky JM. Regulation of metabolism by the innate immune system. Nat Rev Endocrinol 2016; 12(1): 15-28.
[http://dx.doi.org/10.1038/nrendo.2015.189] [PMID: 26553134]

[77]   Cildir G, Akıncılar SC, Tergaonkar V. Chronic adipose tissue inflammation: all immune cells on the

stage. Trends Mol Med 2013; 19(8): 487-500.
[http://dx.doi.org/10.1016/j.molmed.2013.05.001] [PMID: 23746697]

[78]　Lumeng CN, Bodzin JL, Saltiel AR. Obesity induces a phenotypic switch in adipose tissue macrophage polarization. J Clin Invest 2007; 117(1): 175-84.
[http://dx.doi.org/10.1172/JCI29881] [PMID: 17200717]

[79]　Patel PS, Buras ED, Balasubramanyam A. The role of the immune system in obesity and insulin resistance. J Obes 2013 2013; (616193):

[80]　Savage DB, Sewter CP, Klenk ES, *et al.* Resistin / Fizz3 expression in relation to obesity and peroxisome proliferator-activated receptor-gamma action in humans. Diabetes 2001; 50(10): 2199-202.
[http://dx.doi.org/10.2337/diabetes.50.10.2199] [PMID: 11574398]

[81]　Lord GM, Matarese G, Howard JK, Baker RJ, Bloom SR, Lechler RI. Leptin modulates the T-cell immune response and reverses starvation-induced immunosuppression. Nature 1998; 394(6696): 897-901.
[http://dx.doi.org/10.1038/29795] [PMID: 9732873]

[82]　Kumada M, Kihara S, Ouchi N, *et al.* Adiponectin specifically increased tissue inhibitor of metalloproteinase-1 through interleukin-10 expression in human macrophages. Circulation 2004; 109(17): 2046-9.
[http://dx.doi.org/10.1161/01.CIR.0000127953.98131.ED] [PMID: 15096450]

[83]　Forsythe LK, Wallace JM, Livingstone MB. Obesity and inflammation: the effects of weight loss. Nutr Res Rev 2008; 21(2): 117-33.
[http://dx.doi.org/10.1017/S0954422408138732] [PMID: 19087366]

[84]　Hauner H, Petruschke T, Russ M, Röhrig K, Eckel J. Effects of tumour necrosis factor alpha (TNF alpha) on glucose transport and lipid metabolism of newly-differentiated human fat cells in cell culture. Diabetologia 1995; 38(7): 764-71.
[http://dx.doi.org/10.1007/s001250050350] [PMID: 7556976]

[85]　Stephens JM, Pekala PH. Transcriptional repression of the GLUT4 and C/EBP genes in 3T3-L1 adipocytes by tumor necrosis factor-alpha. J Biol Chem 1991; 266(32): 21839-45.
[PMID: 1939208]

[86]　Hotamisligil GS, Peraldi P, Budavari A, Ellis R, White MF, Spiegelman BM. IRS-1-mediated inhibition of insulin receptor tyrosine kinase activity in TNF-alpha- and obesity-induced insulin resistance. Science 1996; 271(5249): 665-8.
[http://dx.doi.org/10.1126/science.271.5249.665] [PMID: 8571133]

[87]　Guilherme A, Virbasius JV, Puri V, Czech MP. Adipocyte dysfunctions linking obesity to insulin resistance and type 2 diabetes. Nat Rev Mol Cell Biol 2008; 9(5): 367-77.
[http://dx.doi.org/10.1038/nrm2391] [PMID: 18401346]

[88]　Hotamisligil GS, Shargill NS, Spiegelman BM. Adipose expression of tumor necrosis factor-alpha: direct role in obesity-linked insulin resistance. Science 1993; 259(5091): 87-91.
[http://dx.doi.org/10.1126/science.7678183] [PMID: 7678183]

[89]　Kanda H, Tateya S, Tamori Y, *et al.* MCP-1 contributes to macrophage infiltration into adipose tissue, insulin resistance, and hepatic steatosis in obesity. J Clin Invest 2006; 116(6): 1494-505.
[http://dx.doi.org/10.1172/JCI26498] [PMID: 16691291]

[90]　Einstein FH, Atzmon G, Yang XM, *et al.* Differential responses of visceral and subcutaneous fat depots to nutrients. Diabetes 2005; 54(3): 672-8.
[http://dx.doi.org/10.2337/diabetes.54.3.672] [PMID: 15734842]

[91]　Starr ME, Evers BM, Saito H. Age-associated increase in cytokine production during systemic inflammation: adipose tissue as a major source of IL-6. J Gerontol A Biol Sci Med Sci 2009; 64(7): 723-30.

[http://dx.doi.org/10.1093/gerona/glp046] [PMID: 19377014]

[92] Ma X, Lee P, Chisholm DJ, James DE. Control of adipocyte differentiation in different fat depots; implications for pathophysiology or therapy. Front Endocrinol (Lausanne) 2015; 6(1)

[93] Klein S, Fontana L, Young VL, *et al.* Absence of an effect of liposuction on insulin action and risk factors for coronary heart disease. N Engl J Med 2004; 350(25): 2549-57.
[http://dx.doi.org/10.1056/NEJMoa033179] [PMID: 15201411]

[94] Palmer AK, Kirkland JL. Aging and adipose tissue: potential interventions for diabetes and regenerative medicine. Exp Gerontol 2016; 86(97-105)
[http://dx.doi.org/10.1016/j.exger.2016.02.013]

[95] Primeau V, Coderre L, Karelis AD, *et al.* Characterizing the profile of obese patients who are metabolically healthy. Int J Obes 2011; 35(7): 971-81.
[http://dx.doi.org/10.1038/ijo.2010.216] [PMID: 20975726]

[96] Trayhurn P. Hypoxia and adipose tissue function and dysfunction in obesity. Physiol Rev 2013; 93(1): 1-21.
[http://dx.doi.org/10.1152/physrev.00017.2012] [PMID: 23303904]

[97] Corvera S, Gealekman O. Adipose tissue angiogenesis: impact on obesity and type-2 diabetes. Biochim Biophys Acta 2014; 1842(3): 463-72.
[http://dx.doi.org/10.1016/j.bbadis.2013.06.003] [PMID: 23770388]

[98] Sung HK, Doh KO, Son JE, *et al.* Adipose vascular endothelial growth factor regulates metabolic homeostasis through angiogenesis. Cell Metab 2013; 17(1): 61-72.
[http://dx.doi.org/10.1016/j.cmet.2012.12.010] [PMID: 23312284]

[99] Jiang C, Qu A, Matsubara T, *et al.* Disruption of hypoxia-inducible factor 1 in adipocytes improves insulin sensitivity and decreases adiposity in high-fat diet-fed mice. Diabetes 2011; 60(10): 2484-95.
[http://dx.doi.org/10.2337/db11-0174] [PMID: 21873554]

[100] Zhang X, Lam KS, Ye H, *et al.* Adipose tissue-specific inhibition of hypoxia-inducible factor 1alpha induces obesity and glucose intolerance by impeding energy expenditure in mice. J Biol Chem 2010; 285(43): 32869-77.
[http://dx.doi.org/10.1074/jbc.M110.135509] [PMID: 20716529]

[101] Gealekman O, Guseva N, Hartigan C, *et al.* Depot-specific differences and insufficient subcutaneous adipose tissue angiogenesis in human obesity. Circulation 2011; 123(2): 186-94.
[http://dx.doi.org/10.1161/CIRCULATIONAHA.110.970145] [PMID: 21200001]

[102] Villaret A, Galitzky J, Decaunes P, *et al.* Adipose tissue endothelial cells from obese human subjects: differences among depots in angiogenic, metabolic, and inflammatory gene expression and cellular senescence. Diabetes 2010; 59(11): 2755-63.
[http://dx.doi.org/10.2337/db10-0398] [PMID: 20713685]

[103] O'Rourke RW, White AE, Metcalf MD, *et al.* Hypoxia-induced inflammatory cytokine secretion in human adipose tissue stromovascular cells. Diabetologia 2011; 54(6): 1480-90.
[http://dx.doi.org/10.1007/s00125-011-2103-y] [PMID: 21400042]

[104] Fuster JJ, Ouchi N, Gokce N, Walsh K. Obesity-Induced Changes in Adipose Tissue Microenvironment and Their Impact on Cardiovascular Disease. Circ Res 2016; 118(11): 1786-807.
[http://dx.doi.org/10.1161/CIRCRESAHA.115.306885] [PMID: 27230642]

[105] Shimizu I, Aprahamian T, Kikuchi R, *et al.* Vascular rarefaction mediates whitening of brown fat in obesity. J Clin Invest 2014; 124(5): 2099-112.
[http://dx.doi.org/10.1172/JCI71643] [PMID: 24713652]

[106] Sun K, Wernstedt Asterholm I, Kusminski CM, *et al.* Dichotomous effects of VEGF-A on adipose tissue dysfunction. Proc Natl Acad Sci USA 2012; 109(15): 5874-9.
[http://dx.doi.org/10.1073/pnas.1200447109] [PMID: 22451920]

[107] Alligier M, Meugnier E, Debard C, *et al.* Subcutaneous adipose tissue remodeling during the initial phase of weight gain induced by overfeeding in humans. J Clin Endocrinol Metab 2012; 97(2): E183-92.
[http://dx.doi.org/10.1210/jc.2011-2314] [PMID: 22162470]

[108] Khan T, Muise ES, Iyengar P, *et al.* Metabolic dysregulation and adipose tissue fibrosis: role of collagen VI. Mol Cell Biol 2009; 29(6): 1575-91.
[http://dx.doi.org/10.1128/MCB.01300-08] [PMID: 19114551]

[109] Pasarica M, Gowronska-Kozak B, Burk D, *et al.* Adipose tissue collagen VI in obesity. J Clin Endocrinol Metab 2009; 94(12): 5155-62.
[http://dx.doi.org/10.1210/jc.2009-0947] [PMID: 19837927]

[110] Halberg N, Khan T, Trujillo ME, *et al.* Hypoxia-inducible factor 1alpha induces fibrosis and insulin resistance in white adipose tissue. Mol Cell Biol 2009; 29(16): 4467-83.
[http://dx.doi.org/10.1128/MCB.00192-09] [PMID: 19546236]

[111] Harms M, Seale P. Brown and beige fat: development, function and therapeutic potential. Nat Med 2013; 19(10): 1252-63.
[http://dx.doi.org/10.1038/nm.3361] [PMID: 24100998]

[112] Rodrigues AR, Almeida H, Gouveia AM. α-MSH signalling *via* melanocortin 5 receptor promotes lipolysis and impairs re-esterification in adipocytes. Biochim Biophys Acta 2013; 1831(7): 1267-75.
[http://dx.doi.org/10.1016/j.bbalip.2013.04.008] [PMID: 24046867]

[113] Rodrigues AR, Almeida H, Gouveia AM. Intracellular signaling mechanisms of the melanocortin receptors: current state of the art. Cell Mol Life Sci 2015; 72(7): 1331-45.
[http://dx.doi.org/10.1007/s00018-014-1800-3] [PMID: 25504085]

[114] Rodrigues AR, Salazar MJ, Rocha-Rodrigues S, *et al.* Peripherally administered melanocortins induce mice fat browning and prevent obesity. Int J Obes (Lond) 2019; 43(5): 1058-69.
[http://dx.doi.org/10.1038/s41366-018-0155-5] [PMID: 30018312]

[115] Saito M, Okamatsu-Ogura Y, Matsushita M, *et al.* High incidence of metabolically active brown adipose tissue in healthy adult humans: effects of cold exposure and adiposity. Diabetes 2009; 58(7): 1526-31.
[http://dx.doi.org/10.2337/db09-0530] [PMID: 19401428]

[116] Lowell BB, S-Susulic V, Hamann A, *et al.* Development of obesity in transgenic mice after genetic ablation of brown adipose tissue. Nature 1993; 366(6457): 740-2.
[http://dx.doi.org/10.1038/366740a0] [PMID: 8264795]

[117] van Marken Lichtenbelt WD, Schrauwen P. Implications of nonshivering thermogenesis for energy balance regulation in humans. Am J Physiol Regul Integr Comp Physiol 2011; 301(2): R285-96.
[http://dx.doi.org/10.1152/ajpregu.00652.2010] [PMID: 21490370]

[118] Chondronikola M, Volpi E, Børsheim E, *et al.* Brown adipose tissue improves whole-body glucose homeostasis and insulin sensitivity in humans. Diabetes 2014; 63(12): 4089-99.
[http://dx.doi.org/10.2337/db14-0746] [PMID: 25056438]

[119] Ouellet V, Labbé SM, Blondin DP, *et al.* Brown adipose tissue oxidative metabolism contributes to energy expenditure during acute cold exposure in humans. J Clin Invest 2012; 122(2): 545-52.
[http://dx.doi.org/10.1172/JCI60433] [PMID: 22269323]

[120] Kim SH, Plutzky J. Brown Fat and Browning for the Treatment of Obesity and Related Metabolic Disorders. Diabetes Metab J 2016; 40(1): 12-21.
[http://dx.doi.org/10.4093/dmj.2016.40.1.12] [PMID: 26912151]

[121] Zhang Q, Hao H, Xie Z, *et al.* M2 macrophages infusion ameliorates obesity and insulin resistance by remodeling inflammatory/macrophages' homeostasis in obese mice Mol Cell Endocrinol 2017; 443(63-71)

[122] Chang YH, Ho KT, Lu SH, Huang CN, Shiau MY. Regulation of glucose/lipid metabolism and insulin sensitivity by interleukin-4. Int J Obes 2012; 36(7): 993-8.
[http://dx.doi.org/10.1038/ijo.2011.168] [PMID: 21894160]

[123] Larsen CM, Faulenbach M, Vaag A, *et al.* Interleukin-1-receptor antagonist in type 2 diabetes mellitus. N Engl J Med 2007; 356(15): 1517-26.
[http://dx.doi.org/10.1056/NEJMoa065213] [PMID: 17429083]

[124] Navarro E, Funtikova AN, Fíto M, Schröder H. Can metabolically healthy obesity be explained by diet, genetics, and inflammation? Mol Nutr Food Res 2015; 59(1): 75-93.
[http://dx.doi.org/10.1002/mnfr.201400521] [PMID: 25418549]

[125] Koh YJ, Park BH, Park JH, *et al.* Activation of PPAR gamma induces profound multilocularization of adipocytes in adult mouse white adipose tissues. Exp Mol Med 2009; 41(12): 880-95.
[http://dx.doi.org/10.3858/emm.2009.41.12.094] [PMID: 19745605]

CHAPTER 4

Adipokines as Emerging Biomarkers of Adipocyte Dysfunction

Marco Assunção[1,2], João T. Guimarães[1,3,4], Margarida Faria[1] and Rosário Monteiro[3,5,6,*]

[1] *Serviço de Patologia Clínica, Centro Universitário Hospitalar São João, Porto, Portugal*

[2] *Universidade Católica Portuguesa, CBQF - Centro de Biotecnologia e Química Fina - Laboratório Associado, Escola Superior de Biotecnologia, Porto, Portugal*

[3] *Department of Biomedicine, Biochemistry Unit, Faculty of Medicine, University of Porto, Porto, Portugal*

[4] *Institute of Public Health, University of Porto, University of Porto, Portugal*

[5] *i3S - Instituto de Investigação e Inovação em Saúde, University of Porto, Porto, Portugal*

[6] *Unidade de Saúde Familiar Pedras Rubras, Agrupamento de Centros de Saúde Maia-Valongo, Maia, Portugal*

Abstract: The recognition that certain obese patients do not exhibit unfavorable metabolic changes, with a low risk for cardiovascular disorders, and that some individuals with a normal weight develop metabolic complications such as insulin resistance, gave rise to the idea that in obesity not only adipose tissue (AT) quantity matters but also AT function, with more relevance. It is known, that impaired AT function is caused by the interaction of genetic and environmental factors which lead to adipocyte hypertrophy, hypoxia and a variety of stresses, including inflammatory processes within the AT. Indeed, AT dysfunction translates into the imbalance between pro- and anti-inflammatory adipokines produced in the adipocyte and secreted into the systemic circulation. For instance, AT dysfunction has been characterized by decreased release of homeostatic protective factors (such as adiponectin, omentin or vaspin) and increased activation of stress-related pathways leading to pathological adipokine (leptin, resistin and visfatin) formation. Systemically, AT dysfunction promotes metabolic and vascular alterations, namely low-grade inflammation, hyperco-agulability, hypertension, dyslipidemia and insulin resistance. Thus, diagnosing AT dysfunction is of clinical relevance, serving as a tool for stratifying risk for cardiovascular disease or type 2 diabetes *mellitus*, and may guide preventive treatment with both medication and lifestyle interventions. It is believed that in the near future, a set of pro- and anti-inflammatory adipokines could be compiled, providing clinicians with an 'adipokine-score' indicative of the level of AT dysfunction. In this chapter, we

* Corresponding author Rosário Monteiro: Departamento de Biomedicina - Unidade de Bioquímica, Faculdade de Medicina, Universidade do Porto, Porto, Portugal; Tel/Fax: +351 225513624; E-mail: rosariom@med.up.pt

briefly discuss the current knowledge about the emerging biomarkers of dysfunctional AT and their potential impact on metabolic diseases associated with obesity.

Keywords: Adipocyte, Adipokine, Adiponectin, Adipose tissue dysfunction, Biomarker, Chemerin, Cytokine, Inflammation, Insulin resistance, Interleukin, Leptin, Lipocalin-2, Obesity, Omentin, Retinol-binding protein 4, Resistin, Serpin, Secreted frizzled-related protein 5, Tumor necrosis factor α, Vaspin, Visfatin.

INTRODUCTION

Obesity is a heterogeneous disorder characterized by multifactorial etiology being influenced by several factors including genetics and lifestyle habits, such as diet or physical activity [1]. Its incidence has been escalating for more than four decades causing a decline in life expectancy due to a set of comorbid associated conditions [2]. Although central obesity is broadly considered an important cardiometabolic risk factor for the development of type 2 diabetes *mellitus* (T2DM) and cardiovascular disease (CVD), empirical evidence has revealed that not all obese individuals develop these kind of disorders, potentially due to a preserved normal adipose tissue (AT) architecture and function [3]. Paradoxically, a subset of lean individuals is reported to have high risk for cardiometabolic complications, highlighting the notion that body mass index (BMI), waist circumference or intra-abdominal fat, although useful in clinical practice, are imperfect measures to estimate the contribution of adiposity to future disease risk and mortality [4]. These distinct subgroups of persons are referred to as metabolically healthy obese and metabolically unhealthy normal weight, respectively [5, 6]. Nowadays, it is already established that the amount of AT *per se* is not the causal factor in the occurrence of CVD or T2DM, but rather the metabolic consequences of obesity as a result of AT dysfunction [7].

The dysfunction of adipocytes seems to be the primary defect in obesity and may link obesity to several health problems. The excess of energy intake leads to an enlargement of adipocytes with the production of chemotactic adipokines that further attract macrophages and other emerging immune cells to AT [8]. Furthermore, a cascade of inflammatory events occurs on the AT with contribution of both adipose and non-adipose cells, including the release of large amounts of free fatty acids and proinflammatory adipokines such as tumor necrosis factor α (TNFα), leptin, chemerin, interleukins (IL) among others [9]. On the other hand, the production of anti-inflammatory adipokines, like adiponectin, is significantly reduced in hypertrophic adipocytes [10]. Consequently, an imbalanced production and release of pro- and anti-inflammatory adipokines occurs, favoring the secretion of a proinflammatory, atherogenic and diabetogenic adipokine pattern.

AT dysfunction rapidly evolves to general metabolic consequences namely systemic low-grade inflammation, elevated blood pressure, low high-density lipoprotein (HDL)-cholesterol, hypertriglyceridemia, atherosclerosis, fatty liver disease and even dementia, airway disease and some kinds of cancers [8], with many of its systemic metabolic consequences being clustered in the metabolic syndrome. AT dysfunction also contributes to the development of T2DM by causing insulin resistance due, among others, to the cytotoxic effects of proinflammatory adipokines and free fatty acids on pancreatic beta cells, decreasing insulin production [11]. Additionally, a hypercoagulability status and activation of renin-angiotensin-aldosterone system occurs as a result of plasminogen activator inhibitor-1 and angiotensinogen production by the AT [12]. So, diagnosing AT dysfunction may identify patients, independently of BMI, at high risk for the development of T2DM and CVD and may guide preventive measures in an early stage of disease, with greater chance of success.

ADIPOSE TISSUE AND ADIPOKINES

The AT consists of adipocytes and stromal vascular cells composed of preadipocytes, endothelial cells, macrophages, lymphocyte, haematopoietic progenitor cells, nerve endings and blood cells. As an endocrine organ, AT secretes several adipokines which have broad activities on carbohydrate and lipid metabolism and are implicated in the pathogenesis of insulin resistance, diabetes, metabolic syndrome and atherosclerosis [13]. Adipokines (*e.g.* leptin and adiponectin) derived almost exclusively from adipocytes are true adipokines compared with those also secreted by the non-adipocyte fraction of AT, such as TNFα and IL6. Most of these adipose-derived molecules reach the systemic circulation and can be measured in peripheral venous blood samples [14]. For instance, it is known that plasma concentrations of adipokines widely vary between patients and can be influenced by interventions such as weight loss and medications [15, 16]. It is also consensual that elevated levels of proinflammatory adipokines and decreased levels of anti-inflammatory adipokines exert a central role in AT dysfunction. In the next sections, we compile the more recent and relevant evidences concerning with this thematic.

Proinflammatory Adipokines

Leptin is an adipocyte-derived hormone and a subproduct of the ob-gene that regulates energy balance by its inhibitory effect on the sense of appetite. This hormone acts on receptors in the arcuate nucleus of the hypothalamus regulating appetite and energy homeostasis [17]. The leptin axis has functional interactions with elements of metabolism, such as insulin signaling and inflammation, including mediators of innate immunity, namely IL6. Moreover, leptin has a structural and functional relation to proinflammatory cytokines, such as IL6, reinforcing its classification as an adipokine [18]. The production of leptin by AT is stimulated by proinflammatory cytokines, such as TNFα, and by lipopolysaccharide [19, 20]. As a consequence, the brain may become desensitized for the inhibitory effects on food intake, a state called leptin resistance, creating a vicious circle of overeating, gaining weight and developing insulin resistance, despite high energy stores and high levels of leptin [21, 22]. It is well known that the level of leptin augments with the increase in weight gain, while adiponectin decreases. Measuring circulating levels of leptin and adiponectin as a screening tool may help recognize those individuals who do not only have obesity as a major risk factor toward developing cardiometabolic disease but also may have an unfavorable biomarker profile, putting them at the highest risk.

TNFα is a cell signaling protein involved in systemic inflammation and one of the cytokines that make up the acute phase reaction [23]. TNFα is produced chiefly by activated macrophages, although it can be also released from other cells, such as adipocytes, where it plays an important role in the development of insulin resistance by inducing apoptosis [24, 25] and interfering with intracellular insulin signaling pathway downstream from the insulin receptor [9]. Using murine models, it was demonstrated that TNFα gene deficiency can counteract obesity-induced insulin resistance [26]. Besides insulin resistance, increased levels of TNFα are also associated with hyperinsulinemia and elevated systolic blood pressure [27]. Furthermore, TNFα has many other distinct effects on AT including induction of leptin production, stimulation of lipolysis, suppression of lipogenesis, induction of adipocyte dedifferentiation and impairment of preadipocyte differentiation [24, 27, 28]. Currently, anti-TNFα agents are yet not associated with changes in insulin resistance or other kind of benefits concerning obesity and cardiometabolic disease in humans. However, the TNFα inhibiting pharmacotherapeutic strategy remains a promising approach.

IL6 is a pleiotropic proinflammatory cytokine involved in many biological functions. For instance, it regulates the immune response, haemopoiesis, the acute phase response and inflammation [29]. Although only small amounts, in the picogram range, can be detected in healthy humans, IL6 expression is highly and transiently upregulated in nearly all pathophysiological states [30]. Curiously, subcutaneous AT secretes about 30% of systemic IL6 and visceral AT appears to release more in human species [31]. It was demonstrated that IL6 inhibits insulin action in muscle, liver and adipocytes both *in vivo* and *in vitro* and contributes to the hepatic insulin resistance associated with obesity [32, 33]. Also, circulating levels of this cytokine correlates positively with fat mass and insulin resistance, and predicts the development of diabetes [34]. Additionally, IL6 is involved in the development of systemic inflammation, which alters lipid composition and causes atherogenesis, thus increasing cardiovascular risk [35, 36]. Therefore, the make use of IL6 as a biomarker of systemic inflammation and metabolic dysfunction has been consensual.

Apart from IL6, other adipokines are also augmented in obesity in relation with AT dysfunction. IL1 is secreted mainly by macrophages and adipocytes and is implicated in macrophages chemotaxis and thermogenesis. It is increased in obese mice and in human obesity and predictive of T2DM [37]. IL7, secreted mostly by stromal and vascular endothelial cells, is a homeostatic immune cytokine that regulates body weight, AT mass and function, and insulin signaling. It was found to be increased in morbidly obese subjects [37, 38]. IL8 is secreted by adipocytes (visceral white AT > subcutaneous white AT) and macrophages. Plasma IL8 concentration is augmented in obese subjects and related to fat mass and TNFα levels [39, 40]. Nowadays, the plasma level of these and other interleukins have been increasingly used as potential biomarkers of the function of AT.

Retinol-binding protein 4 (RBP4) is secreted by adipocytes and macrophages and serves to transport retinol from the liver to peripheral tissues [41, 42]. Elevated serum RBP4 was associated with components of the metabolic syndrome, including increased BMI, waist-to-hip ratio, serum triglyceride levels and systolic blood pressure as well as decreased HDL-cholesterol levels [43]. Reduced density of the membrane-type glucose transporter 4 (GLUT4) is considered as a direct cause for the stimulation of RBP4 release to the circulation by adipocytes. Circulating RBP4 inhibits the signaling pathways activated by insulin in skeletal muscle cells, resulting in the development of insulin resistance [44]. RBP4 is elevated in the serum before the development of diabetes and appears to identify insulin resistance and associated cardiovascular risk factors in subjects with various clinical presentations. These findings provide a rationale for antidiabetic therapies such as the thiazolidinediones stimulating peroxisome proliferator-activated receptor (PPAR) γ, that consequently inhibits the production of RBP4 by AT and increases tissues insulin sensitivity. Increased secretion of RBP4 stimulates the expression of adhesion molecules in the endothelial cells, promoting development of atherosclerosis and arterial hypertension [45]. Population studies demonstrated an association between serum RBP4 in the circulation and the severity of atherosclerosis and risk of the cardiovascular events and T2DM. It also appears that the rbp4 gene functional polymorphisms may influence the risk of metabolic complications of obesity, including vascular injury [45]. Therefore, the concentration of RBP4 in the circulation may be considered both as the causative factor and marker of chronic vascular injury.

Resistin has been initially postulated as a risk factor for insulin resistance, however, the subsequent available data have revealed contradictory findings both in rodents and humans. In rodents, resistin is primarily secreted from mature adipocytes and its expression can be upregulated by several factors, including insulin and glucose. The exposure of rodents, or their cells, to resistin results in decreased response to insulin. This is likely in part due to an upregulation of suppressor of cytokine signaling (SOCS) 3, which interferes with the activation of insulin receptor substrate (IRS) 1 [46]. In humans, resistin is derived mainly from macrophages and is involved in the regulation of inflammatory processes rather than in insulin sensitivity [47]. Indeed, it seems to be involved in the recruitment of immune cells and the secretion of proinflammatory factors, such as TNFα, through the activation of the nuclear factor-κB (NFκB) transcription factor [46]. Resistin also appears to mediate the pathogenesis of atherosclerosis by promoting endothelial dysfunction, vascular smooth muscle cell proliferation, arterial inflammation and the formation of foam cells [48]. Given the emerging interrelationship between inflammation and metabolic disease, and between adipocytes and macrophages, a conserved role of hyperesistinemia in the modulation of glucose metabolism and in the pathogenesis of insulin resistance is quite plausible [49]. Resistin may thus be a biomarker and, potentially, a mediator of metabolic and inflammatory disease that could be targeted by novel therapies aimed at stemming the tide of the epidemic of insulin resistance and its metabolic and cardiovascular complications.

Visfatin is not only synthesized and released by adipocytes but also by inflammatory cells, like activated macrophages [50]. It is also known as pre-B cell colony-enhancing factor (PBEF) and has been described as an adipokine with insulin-mimicking/-sensitizing effects due to its nicotinamide phosphoribosyltransferase (Nampt) activity. Despite the opposing effects of resistin and visfatin on the regulation of insulin sensitivity, both adipokines have proinflammatory properties [51]. Enhanced circulating visfatin/Nampt levels have been reported in metabolic diseases, such as obesity and T2DM [52, 53]. Concerning CVD, visfatin/Nampt was initially proposed as a clinical marker of atherosclerosis, endothelial dysfunction and vascular damage with a potential prognostic value. Nevertheless, beyond being a surrogate clinical marker, visfatin/Nampt is an active player in the promotion of vascular inflammation and atherosclerosis [54, 55]. Visfatin/Nampt effects on cytokine and chemokine secretion, macrophage survival, leukocyte recruitment by endothelial cells, vascular smooth muscle inflammation and plaque destabilization make of this adipokine a contributor to the development and progression of atherosclerosis [56]. More recently, in a cohort study, it was observed that the unstimulated whole saliva from T2DM subjects possessed significantly elevated levels of visfatin and resistin as compared to that from control subjects [57]. Elevated salivary visfatin and resistin in saliva have been shown to positively correlate with serum levels suggest that the two adipokines could represent potential noninvasive T2DM biomarkers [58, 59].

Lipocalin 2 (LCN2), also known as neutrophil gelatinase-associated lipocalin, is a secreted glycoprotein that belongs to a group of transporters of small lipophilic molecules in circulation. Although it is expressed in multiple tissues including uterus, liver, spleen, kidney, bone marrow, immune cells and chondrocytes, white AT is thought to be the main source [60]. LCN2 has been recently characterized as an adipose-derived cytokine involved in a variety of physiological processes, such as transport of fatty acids [61] and iron [62], and metabolic homeostasis [63]. Nevertheless, LCN2 have been linked to the pathogenesis of metabolic disorders through its association with inflammation. LCN2 expression and secretion have been shown to be strongly induced by TNFα in cultured murine and human adipocytes [64]. Interestingly, LCN2 promoter possesses the binding sites of two key transcription factors, NFkB and CCAAT/enhancer binding protein [65], suggesting that transcriptional activation of this gene in AT may not only be associated with inflammation and obesity but also have a function in AT remodeling. LCN2 has been also considered an inflammatory marker closely associated with obesity, insulin resistance and hyperglycemia in humans [66]. A study of Jang *et al* provides the first clinical evidence that serum concentration of LCN2 is related to obesity and its complications, chronic inflammation and metabolic dysfunction. Patients with metabolic syndrome showed higher levels of LCN2 than those without metabolic syndrome [67]. As an acute phase protein, LCN2 has become increasingly relevant in recent years as a potential biomarker in various clinical settings of obesity-related metabolic dysfunction and CVD. LCN2 levels in biological fluids are generally low, being upregulated in inflammatory states, which strongly indicates the potential of its use as a marker of disease onset and progression.

Chemerin stimulates chemotaxis of dendritic cells and macrophages towards inflammatory stimuli. In humans, chemerin mRNA is highly expressed in white AT, liver and lung, while its receptor, CMKLR1, is mostly expressed in immune cells as well as in adipocytes [68]. Moreover, chemerin levels show a significant correlation with body mass index, plasma triglyceride levels and blood pressure [69, 70]. Chemerin has been implicated in autocrine or paracrine signaling for adipocyte differentiation and lipolysis. Genetic knockdown of chemerin or its receptor impairs adipogenesis and reduces the expression of GLUT4 and adiponectin, while increasing expression of IL6 and insulin receptor. Furthermore, post-differentiation knockdown of chemerin diminished GLUT4, leptin, adiponectin expression and reduced lipolysis, suggesting that this adipokine plays a role in metabolic function of mature adipocytes [71]. Chemerin's role as a chemoattractant, along with the knowledge that macrophages are critical for adipose-associated inflammation, put this adipokine at the highlight when considering obesity-related insulin resistance and metabolic syndrome.

Anti-inflammatory Adipokines

Adiponectin, a protein synthesized and secreted mainly by adipocytes into the peripheral blood, is a cytokine that exerts insulin-sensitizing effects in the liver and skeletal muscle via adenosine monophosphate-activated protein kinase (AMPK) and PPARα activation [72]. Additionally, adiponectin can suppress atherosclerosis development in vascular wall possibly due to its anti-inflammatory and antioxidant properties [73]. Abdominal adiposity is an important negative predictor of plasma adiponectin with obese individuals presenting a higher subcutaneous/visceral AT ratio having higher adiponectin levels [74]. It has been observed that lower levels of adiponectin can substantially increase the risk of developing T2DM, metabolic syndrome and atherosclerosis in obese patients [75]. Although adiponectin has been recently proposed as a potential prognostic biomarker, it is not yet clear whether its levels have any clinical significance for risk stratification in CVD or if they simply reflect the activation of complex underlying mechanisms [73]. Further research on the potential clinical implications of adiponectin in the diagnosis and treatment of cardiometabolic diseases is needed.

Secreted frizzled-related protein 5 (Sfrp5) is a novel anti-inflammatory adipokine that sequesters Wnt5a in the extracellular space; the latter being an inflammatory protein that negatively regulates adipogenesis [76, 77]. Usually, higher levels of Wnt5a expression and increased Wnt5a/Sfrp5 ratio have been found in rodent models of obesity and T2DM. In Sfrp5-deficient mice, a high-calorie diet induced severe glucose intolerance, hepatic steatosis and an accumulation of activated macrophages in AT that was associated with the activation of c-Jun N-terminal kinase signaling pathway by Wnt5a protein. Conversely, the acute intravenous administration of Sfrp5 improved metabolic function and reduced AT inflammation [78]. It was also found that Sfrp5 is downregulated in obese individuals causing high levels of Wnt5a and leading to inflammation and insulin resistance [9]. Nevertheless, no studies have been performed yet towards the association between Sfrp5 and CVD or T2DM.

Omentin is an adipokine especially derived from visceral AT (mainly expressed in AT stromal vascular cells) positively related to adiponectin and HDL-cholesterol levels and negatively associated with BMI, waist circumference, insulin resistance, triglyceride and leptin levels [79]. Omentin-1, the major circulating isoform in human plasma, was significantly higher in lean subjects compared to obese and overweight subjects. Both omentin-1 and omentin-2 gene expression were decreased with obesity and were highly correlated with each other in visceral AT [80]. In another study, omentin circulating levels and its gene expression in visceral AT were both significantly lower in non-diabetic morbidly obese women than in controls [81]. It has been reported that lower plasma omentin-1 levels contribute to the pathogenesis of insulin resistance and T2DM in obese or overweight patients [82]. In addition to its insulin-sensitizing effects, omentin has anti-inflammatory and anti-atherogenic properties, causes vasodilatation and attenuates C-reactive protein-induced angiogenesis potentially via the NFκB signaling pathway, a potent proinflammatory signaling pathway [83]. The ability of omentin to reduce insulin resistance in conjunction with its anti-inflammatory and anti-atherogenic properties makes it a promising therapeutic target. Hence, omentin may have beneficial effects on the metabolic syndrome and could potentially be used as a biologic marker and/or pharmacologic agent in this respect.

Vaspin is a visceral AT-derived serine protease inhibitor that belongs to the serpin superfamily clade A (Serpina12). This adipokine has been implicated in counteracting insulin-resistance and inflammatory processes in obese mice [84]. Vaspin treatment or transgenic overexpression of vaspin in AT of obese and insulin resistant mice ameliorated expression of inflammatory genes *in vivo* [85]. It was found that IL1β-induced expression and secretion of proinflammatory cytokines, such as IL6, monocyte chemoattractant protein 1 (MCP1) and TNFα, was significantly blunted in vaspin expressing 3T3-L1 murine adipocytes. Additionally, treatment of 3T3-L1 cells with exogenous vaspin suppresses cytokine-induced inflammation via inhibition of NFκB pathway [86]. The same authors also found that endogenous vaspin positively affected insulin signaling by increasing insulin-stimulated phosphorylation of the key mediator protein kinase B (AKT). Based on these data, it has been assumed that vaspin serves as an insulin sensitizer with anti-inflammatory effects and might act as a compensatory mechanism that acts on the AT, which is activated in response to the decreased insulin sensitivity [87]. Therefore, it could be speculated that vaspin production antagonizes the effects of proteases which disrupt insulin action [88]. It is believed that vaspin could be regarded as a new biomarker in the field of obesity and related metabolic disorders, including glucose intolerance.

Lastly, anti-inflammatory IL10, is secreted by monocytes, macrophages, dendritic cells, and B and T cells. Unlike all other interleukins, IL10 improves insulin sensitivity and glucose transport and is attenuated in T2DM patients and increases with weight loss [37, 89]. In patients with obesity and T2DM, altered serum concentrations of IL10 seems to be dependent on the degree of insulin resistance and proinflammatory status [90].

The Adiponectin/Leptin Ratio

The evaluation of the adiponectin/leptin ratio has been a useful parameter for assessing insulin resistance in patients with and without diabetes. Indeed, it was reported that this ratio was more effective as a parameter of insulin resistance than was adiponectin or leptin alone and was a more sensitive and reliable marker of insulin resistance than was homeostasis model assessment (HOMA)-insulin resistance in subjects without hyperglycemia, as well as in T2DM patients [91 - 93]. Furthermore, Norata *et al* [94] reported that this ratio is a powerful independent predictor of intima-media thickness and other cardiometabolic parameters in healthy males. More recently, adiponectin/leptin ratio was also negatively correlated with markers of low-grade chronic inflammation [95]. Taken all this into account, it is not surprising consider this ratio as a predictive marker of AT dysfunction or obesity-associated cardiometabolic risk.

ARE ADIPOKINES IDEAL BIOMARKERS?

The concept that the AT plays an active role in energy balance and metabolic control came with the exploration of AT products, their effects and their possible interest as therapeutic targets. The more recent acknowledgment of the heterogeneous nature of obesity, with the debate on metabolically healthy/unhealthy obese/non-obese phenotypes, highlighted the need for sensitive and specific biomarkers to distinguish those with higher cardiometabolic risk, due to unhealthy AT accretion, independently of BMI. Having their source on the AT and being associated directly or indirectly with AT function, adipokines emerge as attractive candidates to assume this role. This chemically unrelated group of molecules is central to the dynamic regulation of energy metabolism, communicating the nutrient status of the organism with the tissues responsible for controlling both energy intake and expenditure as well as insulin sensitivity.

Unfortunately, their use in clinical practice has been limited. Ideal biomarkers should fulfill several criteria: i) easy measurement, ii) high diagnostic specificity and sensitivity, good reproducibility and precision and iii) good cost-effectiveness ratio [96]. Being present in systemic blood, adipokines represent an accessible means of determining AT function. However, so far, the inexistence of standard measurements protocols with impact on sensitivity and specificity, unavailability in routine laboratory measurements though automated methods, high cost and, most of all, lack of randomized controlled trials showing their association with metabolic outcomes and of recommended cut-off points for metabolic disorders, have limited their use in clinical practice. Although mounting evidence has been presented on their potential utility as translators of AT dysfunction, representing a group of informative biomarkers for the diagnosis of metabolic disorders and the prediction of outcome on a wide range of diseases, their actual use awaits their implementation into the routine laboratory menu.

CONCLUDING REMARKS

The list of molecules that suit the classification of "adipokines" is still growing and the evidence here presented is far from being complete. "Omics" approaches (proteomics and metabolomics) are currently popular and seem promising in identifying adipocyte products [96] related to higher or lower risk of metabolic complications in experimental or observational studies, but their application in the clinical setting is still questionable. Table **1** presents a summary of the characteristics of the main adipokines concerning their anti- or proinflammatory properties and, when known, their association with metabolic regulation, assumed as insulin sensitivity. Given the dimension of the obesity problem and the huge amount of research devoted to it, perhaps in the near future, either in isolation or integrated into indexes including other laboratory assessments (*e.g.* other cytokines/adipokines, glucose, triglycerides, HDL-cholesterol) or anthropometric measurements (*e.g.* waist circumference) they will indeed be useful in predicting metabolic outcomes and in guiding preventive or therapeutic interventions.

Table 1. Characteristics of the main adipokines concerning their anti- or proinflammatory properties and metabolic functions, adapted from Schrover *et al* [14].

Adipokine	Characteristics		
	Anti-inflammatory	Proinflammatory	Metabolic Function
Adiponectin	+	−	↑
Adipsin	+	−	↑
Apelin	−	−	↓
Adipolin	+	−	↑
Chemerin	−	−	−
Granulocyte colony stimulating factor	−	−	−
Hepatic growth factor (HGF)	−	−	−
Interleukin 1β (IL1β)	−	+	−
Interleukin 6 (IL6)	+	+	−
Interleukin 8 (IL8)	−	+	−
Interleukin 17β (IL17β)	−	+	−
Interleukin 21 (IL21)	−	+	−
Interferon gamma induced protein 10 (IP10)	−	+	−
Leptin	+	+	↓↑

(Table 1) cont.....

Adipokine	Characteristics		
	Anti-inflammatory	Proinflammatory	Metabolic Function
Monocyte chemoattractant protein 1 (MCP1)	+	−	−
Macrophage migration inhibitory factor (MIF)	−	+	−
Nerve growth factor (NGF)	−	−	−
Omentin	+	−	↑
Plasminogen activator inhibitor 1 (PAI1)	−	−	−
Retinol binding protein 4 (RBP4)	−	+	↓
Resistin	−	+	↓
Serpin	−	+	−
Serum amyloid A protein 1 (SAA1)	−	+	−
Secreted frizzled related protein (Sfrp5)	+	−	−
Tumor necrosis factor α (TNFα)	−	+	−
Thrombopoietin (TPO)	−	−	−
Transformation growth factor β (TGFβ)	+	−	−
Visfatin	−	−	↑
Vaspin	−	−	↑
Vascular cell adhesion molecule 1	−	+	−

(+) characteristic present, (−) characteristic absent, (↑) enhances metabolic function/insulin sensitivity, (↓) attenuates metabolic function/insulin sensitivity.

CONSENT FOR PUBLICATION

Not applicable.

CONFLICT OF INTEREST

The authors confirm that this chapter contents have no conflict of interest.

ACKNOWLEDGEMENTS

The authors would like to acknowledge financial support from by FEDER – Fundo Europeu de Desenvolvimento Regional, through NORTE 2020 Programa Operacional Regional do Norte- NORTE-01-0145-FEDER-000012 and Instituto de Investigação e Inovação em Saúde (Projeto Estratégico UID/BIM/04293/2013).

REFERENCES

[1]   González-Muniesa P, Mártinez-González M-A, Hu FB, *et al.* Obesity. Nat Rev Dis Primers 2017; 3: 17034.

[http://dx.doi.org/10.1038/nrdp.2017.34] [PMID: 28617414]

[2]   Gortmaker SL, Swinburn BA, Levy D, *et al.* Changing the future of obesity: science, policy, and action. Lancet 2011; 378(9793): 838-47.
[http://dx.doi.org/10.1016/S0140-6736(11)60815-5] [PMID: 21872752]

[3]   Han TS, Lean ME. A clinical perspective of obesity, metabolic syndrome and cardiovascular disease. JRSM Cardiovasc Dis 2016; 52048004016633371
[http://dx.doi.org/10.1177/2048004016633371] [PMID: 26998259]

[4]   Franssens BT, Westerink J, van der Graaf Y, Nathoe HM, Visseren FLJ. SMART study group. Metabolic consequences of adipose tissue dysfunction and not adiposity per se increase the risk of cardiovascular events and mortality in patients with type 2 diabetes. Int J Cardiol 2016; 222: 72-7.
[http://dx.doi.org/10.1016/j.ijcard.2016.07.081] [PMID: 27458826]

[5]   Mathew H, Farr OM, Mantzoros CS. Metabolic health and weight: Understanding metabolically unhealthy normal weight or metabolically healthy obese patients. Metabolism 2016; 65(1): 73-80.
[http://dx.doi.org/10.1016/j.metabol.2015.10.019] [PMID: 26683798]

[6]   Denis GV, Obin MS. 'Metabolically healthy obesity': origins and implications. Mol Aspects Med 2013; 34(1): 59-70.
[http://dx.doi.org/10.1016/j.mam.2012.10.004] [PMID: 23068072]

[7]   Choe SS, Huh JY, Hwang IJ, Kim JI, Kim JB. Adipose Tissue Remodeling: Its Role in Energy Metabolism and Metabolic Disorders. Front Endocrinol (Lausanne) 2016; 7: 30.
[http://dx.doi.org/10.3389/fendo.2016.00030] [PMID: 27148161]

[8]   Monteiro R, Azevedo I. Chronic inflammation in obesity and the metabolic syndrome. Mediators Inflamm 2010; 2010
[http://dx.doi.org/10.1155/2010/289645]

[9]   Ouchi N, Parker JL, Lugus JJ, Walsh K. Adipokines in inflammation and metabolic disease. Nat Rev Immunol 2011; 11(2): 85-97.
[http://dx.doi.org/10.1038/nri2921] [PMID: 21252989]

[10]   Slutsky N, Vatarescu M, Haim Y, *et al.* Decreased adiponectin links elevated adipose tissue autophagy with adipocyte endocrine dysfunction in obesity. Int J Obes 2016; 40(6): 912-20.
[http://dx.doi.org/10.1038/ijo.2016.5] [PMID: 26786352]

[11]   Gastaldelli A, Gaggini M, DeFronzo RA. Role of Adipose Tissue Insulin Resistance in the Natural History of Type 2 Diabetes: Results From the San Antonio Metabolism Study. Diabetes 2017; 66(4): 815-22.
[http://dx.doi.org/10.2337/db16-1167] [PMID: 28052966]

[12]   Jing F, Mogi M, Horiuchi M. Role of renin-angiotensin-aldosterone system in adipose tissue dysfunction. Mol Cell Endocrinol 2013; 378(1-2): 23-8.
[http://dx.doi.org/10.1016/j.mce.2012.03.005] [PMID: 22465098]

[13]   Galic S, Oakhill JS, Steinberg GR. Adipose tissue as an endocrine organ. Mol Cell Endocrinol 2010; 316(2): 129-39.
[http://dx.doi.org/10.1016/j.mce.2009.08.018] [PMID: 19723556]

[14]   Schrover IM, Spiering W, Leiner T, Visseren FL. Adipose Tissue Dysfunction: Clinical Relevance and Diagnostic Possibilities. Horm Metab Res 2016; 48(4): 213-25.
[http://dx.doi.org/10.1055/s-0042-103243] [PMID: 27065460]

[15]   Varady KA, Tussing L, Bhutani S, Braunschweig CL. Degree of weight loss required to improve adipokine concentrations and decrease fat cell size in severely obese women. Metabolism 2009; 58(8): 1096-101.
[http://dx.doi.org/10.1016/j.metabol.2009.04.010] [PMID: 19477470]

[16]   Tian F, Luo R, Zhao Z, Wu Y, Ban Dj. Blockade of the RAS increases plasma adiponectin in subjects with metabolic syndrome and enhances differentiation and adiponectin expression of human

preadipocytes. Exp Clin Endocrinol Diabetes 2010; 118(4): 258-65.
[http://dx.doi.org/10.1055/s-0029-1237706] [PMID: 19856251]

[17]   Brennan AM, Mantzoros CS. Drug Insight: the role of leptin in human physiology and pathophysiology--emerging clinical applications. Nat Clin Pract Endocrinol Metab 2006; 2(6): 318-27.
[http://dx.doi.org/10.1038/ncpendmet0196] [PMID: 16932309]

[18]   Tilg H, Moschen AR. Adipocytokines: mediators linking adipose tissue, inflammation and immunity. Nat Rev Immunol 2006; 6(10): 772-83.
[http://dx.doi.org/10.1038/nri1937] [PMID: 16998510]

[19]   Jéquier E. Leptin signaling, adiposity, and energy balance. Ann N Y Acad Sci 2002; 967: 379-88.
[http://dx.doi.org/10.1111/j.1749-6632.2002.tb04293.x] [PMID: 12079865]

[20]   van Dielen FM, van't Veer C, Schols AM, Soeters PB, Buurman WA, Greve JW. Increased leptin concentrations correlate with increased concentrations of inflammatory markers in morbidly obese individuals. Int J Obes Relat Metab Disord 2001; 25(12): 1759-66.
[http://dx.doi.org/10.1038/sj.ijo.0801825] [PMID: 11781755]

[21]   Pan H, Guo J, Su Z. Advances in understanding the interrelations between leptin resistance and obesity. Physiol Behav 2014; 130: 157-69.
[http://dx.doi.org/10.1016/j.physbeh.2014.04.003] [PMID: 24726399]

[22]   Engin A. Adiponectin-Resistance in Obesity. Adv Exp Med Biol 2017; 960: 415-41.
[http://dx.doi.org/10.1007/978-3-319-48382-5_18] [PMID: 28585210]

[23]   Streetz KL, Wüstefeld T, Klein C, Manns MP, Trautwein C. Mediators of inflammation and acute phase response in the liver. Cell Mol Biol 2001; 47(4): 661-73.
[PMID: 11502073]

[24]   Prins JB, Niesler CU, Winterford CM, *et al.* Tumor necrosis factor-alpha induces apoptosis of human adipose cells. Diabetes 1997; 46(12): 1939-44.
[http://dx.doi.org/10.2337/diab.46.12.1939] [PMID: 9392477]

[25]   Zhang Y, Huang C. Targeting adipocyte apoptosis: a novel strategy for obesity therapy. Biochem Biophys Res Commun 2012; 417(1): 1-4.
[http://dx.doi.org/10.1016/j.bbrc.2011.11.158] [PMID: 22172945]

[26]   Hotamisligil GS. Inflammation and metabolic disorders. Nature 2006; 444(7121): 860-7.
[http://dx.doi.org/10.1038/nature05485] [PMID: 17167474]

[27]   Hotamisligil GS. Inflammatory pathways and insulin action. Int J Obes Relat Metab Disord 2003; 27(S3) (Suppl. 3): S53-5.
[http://dx.doi.org/10.1038/sj.ijo.0802502] [PMID: 14704746]

[28]   Yu R, Kim C-S, Kang J-H. Inflammatory Components of Adipose Tissue as Target for Treatment of Metabolic Syndrome.Food Factors for Health Promotion Basel. KARGER 2009; pp. 95-103.
[http://dx.doi.org/10.1159/000212742]

[29]   Mihara M, Hashizume M, Yoshida H, Suzuki M, Shiina M. IL-6/IL-6 receptor system and its role in physiological and pathological conditions. Clin Sci (Lond) 2012; 122(4): 143-59.
[http://dx.doi.org/10.1042/CS20110340] [PMID: 22029668]

[30]   Wolf J, Rose-John S, Garbers C. Interleukin-6 and its receptors: a highly regulated and dynamic system. Cytokine 2014; 70(1): 11-20.
[http://dx.doi.org/10.1016/j.cyto.2014.05.024] [PMID: 24986424]

[31]   Klein J, Perwitz N, Kraus D, Fasshauer M. Adipose tissue as source and target for novel therapies. Trends Endocrinol Metab 2006; 17(1): 26-32.
[http://dx.doi.org/10.1016/j.tem.2005.11.008] [PMID: 16309918]

[32]   Klover PJ, Clementi AH, Mooney RA. Interleukin-6 depletion selectively improves hepatic insulin action in obesity. Endocrinology 2005; 146(8): 3417-27.

[http://dx.doi.org/10.1210/en.2004-1468] [PMID: 15845623]

[33] Kim H-J, Higashimori T, Park S-Y, *et al.* Differential effects of interleukin-6 and -10 on skeletal muscle and liver insulin action in vivo. Diabetes 2004; 53(4): 1060-7.
[http://dx.doi.org/10.2337/diabetes.53.4.1060] [PMID: 15047622]

[34] Fernández-Real JM, Ricart W. Insulin resistance and chronic cardiovascular inflammatory syndrome. Endocr Rev 2003; 24(3): 278-301.
[http://dx.doi.org/10.1210/er.2002-0010] [PMID: 12788800]

[35] Papanicolaou DA, Wilder RL, Manolagas SC, Chrousos GP. The pathophysiologic roles of interleukin-6 in human disease. Ann Intern Med 1998; 128(2): 127-37.
[http://dx.doi.org/10.7326/0003-4819-128-2-199801150-00009] [PMID: 9441573]

[36] Khovidhunkit W, Kim M-S, Memon RA, *et al.* Effects of infection and inflammation on lipid and lipoprotein metabolism: mechanisms and consequences to the host. J Lipid Res 2004; 45(7): 1169-96.
[http://dx.doi.org/10.1194/jlr.R300019-JLR200] [PMID: 15102878]

[37] Makki K, Froguel P, Wolowczuk I. Adipose tissue in obesity-related inflammation and insulin resistance: cells, cytokines, and chemokines. ISRN Inflamm 2013; 2013139239
[http://dx.doi.org/10.1155/2013/139239] [PMID: 24455420]

[38] Lucas S, Taront S, Magnan C, *et al.* Interleukin-7 regulates adipose tissue mass and insulin sensitivity in high-fat diet-fed mice through lymphocyte-dependent and independent mechanisms. 2012.
[http://dx.doi.org/10.1371/journal.pone.0040351]

[39] Bruun JM, Lihn AS, Madan AK, *et al.* Higher production of IL-8 in visceral vs. subcutaneous adipose tissue. Implication of nonadipose cells in adipose tissue. Am J Physiol Endocrinol Metab 2004; 286(1): E8-E13.
[http://dx.doi.org/10.1152/ajpendo.00269.2003] [PMID: 13129857]

[40] Straczkowski M, Dzienis-Straczkowska S, Stêpieñ A, Kowalska I, Szelachowska M, Kinalska I. Plasma interleukin-8 concentrations are increased in obese subjects and related to fat mass and tumor necrosis factor-alpha system. J Clin Endocrinol Metab 2002; 87(10): 4602-6.
[http://dx.doi.org/10.1210/jc.2002-020135] [PMID: 12364441]

[41] Broch M, Ramírez R, Auguet MT, *et al.* Macrophages are novel sites of expression and regulation of retinol binding protein-4 (RBP4). Physiol Res 2010; 59(2): 299-303.
[PMID: 19537932]

[42] Toloza FJK, Pérez-Matos MC, Ricardo-Silgado ML, *et al.* Comparison of plasma pigment epithelium-derived factor (PEDF), retinol binding protein 4 (RBP-4), chitinase-3-like protein 1 (YKL-40) and brain-derived neurotrophic factor (BDNF) for the identification of insulin resistance. J Diabetes Complications 2017; 31(9): 1423-9.
[http://dx.doi.org/10.1016/j.jdiacomp.2017.06.002] [PMID: 28648555]

[43] Graham TE, Yang Q, Blüher M, *et al.* Retinol-binding protein 4 and insulin resistance in lean, obese, and diabetic subjects. N Engl J Med 2006; 354(24): 2552-63.
[http://dx.doi.org/10.1056/NEJMoa054862] [PMID: 16775236]

[44] Wolf G. Serum retinol-binding protein: a link between obesity, insulin resistance, and type 2 diabetes. Nutr Rev 2007; 65(5): 251-6.
[http://dx.doi.org/10.1111/j.1753-4887.2007.tb00302.x] [PMID: 17566551]

[45] Majerczyk M, Olszanecka-Glinianowicz M, Puzianowska-Kuźnicka M, Chudek J. Retinol-binding protein 4 (RBP4) as the causative factor and marker of vascular injury related to insulin resistance. Postepy Hig Med Dosw 2016; 70(0): 1267-75.
[PMID: 28026829]

[46] Barnes KM, Miner JL. Role of resistin in insulin sensitivity in rodents and humans. Curr Protein Pept Sci 2009; 10(1): 96-107.
[http://dx.doi.org/10.2174/138920309787315239] [PMID: 19275676]

[47]   Haluzik M, Haluzikova D. The role of resistin in obesity-induced insulin resistance. Curr Opin Investig Drugs 2006; 7(4): 306-11.
[PMID: 16625816]

[48]   Park HK, Kwak MK, Kim HJ, Ahima RS. Linking resistin, inflammation, and cardiometabolic diseases. Korean J Intern Med (Korean Assoc Intern Med) 2017; 32(2): 239-47.
[http://dx.doi.org/10.3904/kjim.2016.229] [PMID: 28192887]

[49]   Lazar MA. Resistin- and Obesity-associated metabolic diseases. Horm Metab Res 2007; 39(10): 710-6.
[http://dx.doi.org/10.1055/s-2007-985897] [PMID: 17952831]

[50]   Curat CA, Wegner V, Sengenès C, et al. Macrophages in human visceral adipose tissue: increased accumulation in obesity and a source of resistin and visfatin. Diabetologia 2006; 49(4): 744-7.
[http://dx.doi.org/10.1007/s00125-006-0173-z] [PMID: 16496121]

[51]   Stofkova A. Resistin and visfatin: regulators of insulin sensitivity, inflammation and immunity. Endocr Regul 2010; 44(1): 25-36.
[http://dx.doi.org/10.4149/endo_2010_01_25] [PMID: 20151765]

[52]   Chen M-P, Chung F-M, Chang D-M, et al. Elevated plasma level of visfatin/pre-B cell colony-enhancing factor in patients with type 2 diabetes mellitus. J Clin Endocrinol Metab 2006; 91(1): 295-9.
[http://dx.doi.org/10.1210/jc.2005-1475] [PMID: 16234302]

[53]   Filippatos TD, Derdemezis CS, Gazi IF, et al. Increased plasma visfatin levels in subjects with the metabolic syndrome. Eur J Clin Invest 2008; 38(1): 71-2.
[http://dx.doi.org/10.1111/j.1365-2362.2007.01904.x] [PMID: 18173555]

[54]   Takebayashi K, Suetsugu M, Wakabayashi S, Aso Y, Inukai T. Association between plasma visfatin and vascular endothelial function in patients with type 2 diabetes mellitus. Metabolism 2007; 56(4): 451-8.
[http://dx.doi.org/10.1016/j.metabol.2006.12.001] [PMID: 17378999]

[55]   Vanhoutte PM. Endothelial dysfunction: the first step toward coronary arteriosclerosis. Circ J 2009; 73(4): 595-601.
[http://dx.doi.org/10.1253/circj.CJ-08-1169] [PMID: 19225203]

[56]   Romacho T, Sánchez-Ferrer CF, Peiró C. Visfatin/Nampt: an adipokine with cardiovascular impact. Mediators Inflamm 2013; 2013946427
[http://dx.doi.org/10.1155/2013/946427] [PMID: 23843684]

[57]   Srinivasan M, Meadows ML, Maxwell L. Assessment of salivary adipokines resistin, visfatin, and ghrelin as type 2 diabetes mellitus biomarkers. Biochem Res Int 2018; 20187463796
[http://dx.doi.org/10.1155/2018/7463796] [PMID: 29487749]

[58]   Desai GS, Mathews ST. Saliva as a non-invasive diagnostic tool for inflammation and insulin-resistance. World J Diabetes 2014; 5(6): 730-8.
[http://dx.doi.org/10.4239/wjd.v5.i6.730] [PMID: 25512775]

[59]   Mamali I, Roupas ND, Armeni AK, Theodoropoulou A, Markou KB, Georgopoulos NA. Measurement of salivary resistin, visfatin and adiponectin levels. Peptides 2012; 33(1): 120-4.
[http://dx.doi.org/10.1016/j.peptides.2011.11.007] [PMID: 22108712]

[60]   Abella V, Scotece M, Conde J, et al. The potential of lipocalin-2/NGAL as biomarker for inflammatory and metabolic diseases. Biomarkers 2015; 20(8): 565-71.
[http://dx.doi.org/10.3109/1354750X.2015.1123354] [PMID: 26671823]

[61]   Chu ST, Lin HJ, Huang HL, Chen YH. The hydrophobic pocket of 24p3 protein from mouse uterine luminal fluid: fatty acid and retinol binding activity and predicted structural similarity to lipocalins. J Pept Res 1998; 52(5): 390-7.
[http://dx.doi.org/10.1111/j.1399-3011.1998.tb00663.x] [PMID: 9894844]

[62]   Yang J, Goetz D, Li JY, *et al.* An iron delivery pathway mediated by a lipocalin. Mol Cell 2002; 10(5): 1045-56.
[http://dx.doi.org/10.1016/S1097-2765(02)00710-4] [PMID: 12453413]

[63]   Yan Q-W, Yang Q, Mody N, *et al.* The adipokine lipocalin 2 is regulated by obesity and promotes insulin resistance. Diabetes 2007; 56(10): 2533-40.
[http://dx.doi.org/10.2337/db07-0007] [PMID: 17639021]

[64]   Zhao P, Elks CM, Stephens JM. The induction of lipocalin-2 protein expression *in vivo* and *in vitro*. J Biol Chem 2014; 289(9): 5960-9.
[http://dx.doi.org/10.1074/jbc.M113.532234] [PMID: 24391115]

[65]   Shen F, Hu Z, Goswami J, Gaffen SL. Identification of common transcriptional regulatory elements in interleukin-17 target genes. J Biol Chem 2006; 281(34): 24138-48.
[http://dx.doi.org/10.1074/jbc.M604597200] [PMID: 16798734]

[66]   Wang Y, Lam KSL, Kraegen EW, *et al.* Lipocalin-2 is an inflammatory marker closely associated with obesity, insulin resistance, and hyperglycemia in humans. Clin Chem 2007; 53(1): 34-41.
[http://dx.doi.org/10.1373/clinchem.2006.075614] [PMID: 17040956]

[67]   Jang Y, Lee JH, Wang Y, Sweeney G. Emerging clinical and experimental evidence for the role of lipocalin-2 in metabolic syndrome. Clin Exp Pharmacol Physiol 2012; 39(2): 194-9.
[http://dx.doi.org/10.1111/j.1440-1681.2011.05557.x] [PMID: 21689137]

[68]   Bozaoglu K, Bolton K, McMillan J, *et al.* Chemerin is a novel adipokine associated with obesity and metabolic syndrome. Endocrinology 2007; 148(10): 4687-94.
[http://dx.doi.org/10.1210/en.2007-0175] [PMID: 17640997]

[69]   Roman AA, Parlee SD, Sinal CJ. Chemerin: a potential endocrine link between obesity and type 2 diabetes. Endocrine 2012; 42(2): 243-51.
[http://dx.doi.org/10.1007/s12020-012-9698-8] [PMID: 22610747]

[70]   Stojek M. The role of chemerin in human disease. Postepy Hig Med Dosw 2017; 71(0): 110-7.
[http://dx.doi.org/10.5604/01.3001.0010.3795] [PMID: 28258671]

[71]   Goralski KB, McCarthy TC, Hanniman EA, *et al.* Chemerin, a novel adipokine that regulates adipogenesis and adipocyte metabolism. J Biol Chem 2007; 282(38): 28175-88.
[http://dx.doi.org/10.1074/jbc.M700793200] [PMID: 17635925]

[72]   Matsuda M, Shimomura I. Roles of adiponectin and oxidative stress in obesity-associated metabolic and cardiovascular diseases. Rev Endocr Metab Disord 2014; 15(1): 1-10.
[http://dx.doi.org/10.1007/s11154-013-9271-7] [PMID: 24026768]

[73]   Katsiki N, Mantzoros C, Mikhailidis DP. Adiponectin, lipids and atherosclerosis. Curr Opin Lipidol 2017; 28(4): 347-54.
[http://dx.doi.org/10.1097/MOL.0000000000000431] [PMID: 28463859]

[74]   Guenther M, James R, Marks J, Zhao S, Szabo A, Kidambi S. Adiposity distribution influences circulating adiponectin levels. Transl Res 2014; 164(4): 270-7.
[http://dx.doi.org/10.1016/j.trsl.2014.04.008] [PMID: 24811003]

[75]   Lim S, Quon MJ, Koh KK. Modulation of adiponectin as a potential therapeutic strategy. Atherosclerosis 2014; 233(2): 721-8.
[http://dx.doi.org/10.1016/j.atherosclerosis.2014.01.051] [PMID: 24603219]

[76]   Bovolenta P, Esteve P, Ruiz JM, Cisneros E, Lopez-Rios J. Beyond Wnt inhibition: new functions of secreted Frizzled-related proteins in development and disease. J Cell Sci 2008; 121(Pt 6): 737-46.
[http://dx.doi.org/10.1242/jcs.026096] [PMID: 18322270]

[77]   Ross SE, Hemati N, Longo KA, *et al.* Inhibition of adipogenesis by Wnt signaling. Science 2000; 289(5481): 950-3.
[http://dx.doi.org/10.1126/science.289.5481.950] [PMID: 10937998]

[78]   Ouchi N, Higuchi A, Ohashi K, *et al.* Sfrp5 is an anti-inflammatory adipokine that modulates metabolic dysfunction in obesity. Science 2010; 329(5990): 454-7.
[http://dx.doi.org/10.1126/science.1188280] [PMID: 20558665]

[79]   Zhou J-Y, Chan L, Zhou S-W. Omentin: linking metabolic syndrome and cardiovascular disease. Curr Vasc Pharmacol 2014; 12(1): 136-43.
[http://dx.doi.org/10.2174/1570161112999140217095038] [PMID: 22724476]

[80]   de Souza Batista CM, Yang R-Z, Lee M-J, *et al.* Omentin plasma levels and gene expression are decreased in obesity. Diabetes 2007; 56(6): 1655-61.
[http://dx.doi.org/10.2337/db06-1506] [PMID: 17329619]

[81]   Auguet T, Quintero Y, Riesco D, *et al.* New adipokines vaspin and omentin. Circulating levels and gene expression in adipose tissue from morbidly obese women. BMC Med Genet 2011; 12(1): 60.
[http://dx.doi.org/10.1186/1471-2350-12-60] [PMID: 21526992]

[82]   Zhang Q, Zhu L, Zheng M, *et al.* Changes of serum omentin-1 levels in normal subjects, type 2 diabetes and type 2 diabetes with overweight and obesity in Chinese adults. Ann Endocrinol (Paris) 2014; 75(3): 171-5.
[http://dx.doi.org/10.1016/j.ando.2014.04.013] [PMID: 24997770]

[83]   Tan BK, Adya R, Randeva HS. Omentin: a novel link between inflammation, diabesity, and cardiovascular disease. Trends Cardiovasc Med 2010; 20(5): 143-8.
[http://dx.doi.org/10.1016/j.tcm.2010.12.002] [PMID: 21742269]

[84]   Heiker JT, Klöting N, Kovacs P, *et al.* Vaspin inhibits kallikrein 7 by serpin mechanism. Cell Mol Life Sci 2013; 70(14): 2569-83.
[http://dx.doi.org/10.1007/s00018-013-1258-8] [PMID: 23370777]

[85]   Nakatsuka A, Wada J, Iseda I, *et al.* Vaspin is an adipokine ameliorating ER stress in obesity as a ligand for cell-surface GRP78/MTJ-1 complex. Diabetes 2012; 61(11): 2823-32.
[http://dx.doi.org/10.2337/db12-0232] [PMID: 22837305]

[86]   Zieger K, Weiner J, Krause K, *et al.* Vaspin suppresses cytokine-induced inflammation in 3T3-L1 adipocytes via inhibition of NFκB pathway. Mol Cell Endocrinol 2018; 460: 181-8.
[http://dx.doi.org/10.1016/j.mce.2017.07.022] [PMID: 28756250]

[87]   Hida K, Wada J, Eguchi J, *et al.* Visceral adipose tissue-derived serine protease inhibitor: a unique insulin-sensitizing adipocytokine in obesity. Proc Natl Acad Sci USA 2005; 102(30): 10610-5.
[http://dx.doi.org/10.1073/pnas.0504703102] [PMID: 16030142]

[88]   Li Q, Chen R, Moriya J, *et al.* A novel adipocytokine, visceral adipose tissue-derived serine protease inhibitor (vaspin), and obesity. J Int Med Res 2008; 36(4): 625-9.
[http://dx.doi.org/10.1177/147323000803600402] [PMID: 18652756]

[89]   Jung SH, Park HS, Kim K-S, *et al.* Effect of weight loss on some serum cytokines in human obesity: increase in IL-10 after weight loss. J Nutr Biochem 2008; 19(6): 371-5.
[http://dx.doi.org/10.1016/j.jnutbio.2007.05.007] [PMID: 17614271]

[90]   Janowska J, Chudek J, Olszanecka-Glinianowicz M, Semik-Grabarczyk E, Zahorska-Markiewicz B. Interdependencies among Selected Pro-Inflammatory Markers of Endothelial Dysfunction, C-Peptide, Anti-Inflammatory Interleukin-10 and Glucose Metabolism Disturbance in Obese Women. Int J Med Sci 2016; 13(7): 490-9.
[http://dx.doi.org/10.7150/ijms.14110] [PMID: 27429585]

[91]   Inoue M, Yano M, Yamakado M, Maehata E, Suzuki S. Relationship between the adiponectin-leptin ratio and parameters of insulin resistance in subjects without hyperglycemia. Metabolism 2006; 55(9): 1248-54.
[http://dx.doi.org/10.1016/j.metabol.2006.05.010] [PMID: 16919546]

[92]   Inoue M, Maehata E, Yano M, Taniyama M, Suzuki S. Correlation between the adiponectin-leptin ratio and parameters of insulin resistance in patients with type 2 diabetes. Metabolism 2005; 54(3):

281-6.
[http://dx.doi.org/10.1016/j.metabol.2004.09.006] [PMID: 15736103]

[93] Zaletel J, Barlovic DP, Prezelj J. Adiponectin-leptin ratio: a useful estimate of insulin resistance in patients with Type 2 diabetes. J Endocrinol Invest 2010; 33(8): 514-8.
[http://dx.doi.org/10.1007/BF03346639] [PMID: 20142631]

[94] Norata GD, Raselli S, Grigore L, *et al.* Leptin:adiponectin ratio is an independent predictor of intima media thickness of the common carotid artery. Stroke 2007; 38(10): 2844-6.
[http://dx.doi.org/10.1161/STROKEAHA.107.485540] [PMID: 17823381]

[95] Frühbeck G, Catalán V, Rodríguez A, Gómez-Ambrosi J. Adiponectin-leptin ratio: A promising index to estimate adipose tissue dysfunction. Relation with obesity-associated cardiometabolic risk. Adipocyte 2018; 7(1): 57-62.
[http://dx.doi.org/10.1080/21623945.2017.1402151] [PMID: 29205099]

[96] Bergmann K, Sypniewska G. Diabetes as a complication of adipose tissue dysfunction. Is there a role for potential new biomarkers? Clin Chem Lab Med 2013; 51(1): 177-85.
[http://dx.doi.org/10.1515/cclm-2012-0490] [PMID: 23241684]

CHAPTER 5

Metabolic Inflammation at the Crossroads of Obesity Phenotypes

Inês Brandão[1,2], Célia Candeias[3] and Rosário Monteiro[1,2,3,*]

[1] *Department of Biomedicine, Biochemistry Unit, Faculty of Medicine, University of Porto, Porto, Portugal*

[2] *i3S - Instituto de Investigação e Inovação em Saúde, University of Porto, Porto, Portugal*

[3] *Unidade de Saúde Familiar Pedras Rubras, Agrupamento de Centros de Saúde Maia-Valongo, Maia, Portugal*

Abstract: The idea that there is heterogeneity among obese individuals in their risk for disease is not new, and may have begun with the acknowledgement that the distinct cardiovascular disease risk between males and females was influenced by their body pattern of adipose tissue accumulation (*i.e.* predominantly in the upper body *versus* in the lower body, respectively). Later came the debate on the pathophysiological meaning of adipose tissue accumulation in visceral as opposed to subcutaneous depots and even of distinct patterns of adipose tissue growth (hyperplasia *versus* hypertrophy). More recently, epidemiological evidence has shown that individuals with similar degrees of obesity may be at different ranges of metabolic abnormality and cardiometabolic risk spectrum. In addition, many subjects not fulfilling the criteria for obesity diagnosis share the same metabolic disturbances of some obese individuals. Although, it has been discussed that healthy obese people will sooner or later become unhealthy, the question on why some subjects attain a status of metabolic chaos earlier than others (for the same obesity levels or adipose tissue amount) is still matter of debate. In this chapter, we propose to discuss the contribution of obesity-related inflammation – metabolic inflammation – as cause or consequence of different obesity phenotypes, overviewing the main possible adipose tissue inflammation triggers.

Keywords: Adipocyte hypertrophy, Adipose tissue, Central obesity, Gut microbiota, Inflammasome, Metabolic inflammation, Metabolically healthy obese phenotype, Metabolically unhealthy normal-weight phenotype, Metabolically unhealthy obese phenotype, Obesity phenotypes, Peripheral obesity, Persistent organic pollutants, Sex hormones, Subcutaneous adipose tissue, Visceral adipose tissue.

** **Corresponding author Rosário Monteiro:** Departamento de Biomedicina - Unidade de Bioquímica, Faculdade de Medicina, Universidade do Porto, Porto, Portugal; Tel/Fax: +351 225513624; E-mail: rosariom@med.up.pt*

Rosário Monteiro and Maria João Martins (Eds.)

INTRODUCTION

Obesity, characterized by the World Health Organization as abnormal or excessive fat accumulation, poses a rising threat to the public health and welfare [1]. This medical condition has become epidemic in both developed and developing countries and is intimately associated with the prevalence of metabolic disorders associated with elevated risk of premature death such as type 2 diabetes, non-alcoholic fatty liver disease (NAFLD), cardiovascular diseases (CVD), dyslipidemia and certain types of cancer [2].

In recent years, it has come to light that there is heterogeneity among obese subjects in their cardiometabolic risk. While generally considered that obesity translates into metabolic disturbances leading to the metabolic syndrome and increased risk for developing CVD and type 2 diabetes, some subjects, despite being obese, are not affected by such metabolic abnormalities [3, 4]. A subset of non-obese subjects, on the other hand, may present those abnormalities, found commonly in the obese [5]. This has led to the distinction between obesity phenotypes, discussed in this chapter. Despite not being unanimous [6], this definition has practical consequences. Due to the enormous social and economic burden of obesity, rational allocation of resources for obesity treatment and prevention is warranted. Also, it is necessary to know which measures to apply and which individuals will profit the most from obesity treatment and prevention approaches.

The puzzling management of obesity and metabolic syndrome is correlated with their multifactorial nature where environmental, genetic and psychosocial factors interact through intricate networks [7]. Obesity is considered as a state of chronic low-grade inflammation initiated by metabolic surplus [8], thus considered by many as metabolic inflammation. Although adipose tissue (AT) is considered a central element in obesity-related inflammation, other organs and tissues also constitute important sources of inflammatory mediators in obesity. For instance, the liver, the pancreas and the muscle can simultaneously contribute to the inflammatory milieu and be affected by it [9, 10]. Adipose-originated metabolic inflammation is in close relationship with insulin resistance, being a determinant player for the observed metabolic alterations in metabolic syndrome, and has been under investigation for decades [10]. Inflammation and insulin resistance have been considered by many the main instigators of the metabolic syndrome [11, 12], being hallmarks of AT dysfunction. The list of triggers for AT inflammation is continuously growing and extends far beyond positive energy balance. This inflammatory signaling centered on the AT, which will be the main focus of this chapter, leads to a vicious cycle that perpetuates AT dysfunction, hinders metabolic adaptation [13, 14], and may be at the basis of unhealthy, opposed to heathy obesity.

THE HETEROGENEITY OF OBESITY

Despite the presence of metabolic disturbances in a vast majority of obese individuals, a considerable amount of people (10-25%) with a high body mass index (BMI) and excessive AT are not affected by such metabolic abnormalities although experiencing the same mechanical complications observed in other obesity phenotypes [3, 4]. These subjects have a lower risk of cardiovascular and liver diseases, presenting normal insulin sensitivity and glucose metabolism regardless of the excessive amount of body fat [15]. On the other hand, a subset of normal-weight individuals who are metabolically unhealthy has been identified in the 1980's by Ruderman *et al*, who suggested to characterize them by parameters such as hyperinsulinemia, insulin resistance, hypertriglyceridemia and coronary heart disease [5]. Obesity phenotypes that include metabolically unhealthy normal-weight (MUHNW), metabolically healthy obese (MHO) and metabolically unhealthy obese (MUO) have been widely reported within clinical and epidemiological studies (Table 1). Still, the phenotype categorization remains a matter of debate as it lacks standardized definitions such as the long-term outcomes of each phenotype [6].

The Metabolically Unhealthy Normal-weight Phenotype

The MUHNW phenotype is characterized by a normal BMI (18.5-25 kg/m^2) associated with increased levels of adiposity and ectopic fat distribution with augmented visceral AT (vAT), a distinctive feature of this category [16, 17]. MUHNW individuals tend to neglect prevention or clinical treatment, thus presenting an increased prevalence of clinical aspects often found in metabolic syndrome, such as low insulin sensitivity, low HDL-cholesterol and high levels of triglycerides and systemic inflammatory markers [18, 19]. In addition to the risk of developing metabolic syndrome, the MUHNW phenotype is characterized by increased risk of type 2 diabetes and CVD. Moreover, elderly people presenting this phenotype show a higher risk of all-cause and CVD-related mortality [20]. A standardized definition of MUHNW is still lacking, thus compromising an early diagnosis of this condition necessary for a suitable risk management [21]. During a prospective cohort study, Lee *et al* have proposed triglyceride-glucose index [ln (fasting triglycerides [mg/dL]×fasting plasma glucose [mg/dL]/2)] to be used as simple diagnostic criterion for MUHNW (above 8.82 for men and 8.73 for women) among normal weight people [20].

The Metabolically Healthy Obese Phenotype

Most articles suggest that individuals belonging to the MHO phenotype are obese with BMI over 30 kg/m^2 lacking metabolic anomalies, such as type 2 diabetes, dyslipidemia or hypertension [22 - 24]. The prevalence of MHO phenotype varies considerably among studies, ranging from 6% to 29% of the obese population [6, 25 - 27]. The disparity observed in these numbers results from the lack of consensus in the criteria used to define MHO [*e.g.* waist circumference, blood pressure, high density lipoprotein (HDL)-cholesterol, among others] [6].

Table 1. Obesity phenotypes, adapted from Cembrowska *et al* [16].

Phenotype	Metabolically unhealthy normal-weight (MUHNW)	Metabolically healthy obese (MHO)	Metabolically unhealthy obese (MUO)
BMI (kg/m^2)	18.5-25	>30	>30
Prevalence [1]	~10% - 37% of individuals with BMI <25 kg/m^2	~6% - 29% of obese individuals	Remaining obese individuals
Fat distribution	Low lean body mass, augmented adiposity. Ectopic fat Increased visceral and subcutaneous abdominal adipose tissue	Low visceral and ectopic fat Decreased hepatic steatosis	Ectopic fat Excessive visceral adipose tissue
Glucose metabolism	Low insulin sensitivity	Proper insulin sensitivity	Insulin resistance
Lipid profile	Improper lipid profile Low HDL-cholesterol levels High levels of triglycerides	Proper lipid profile	Improper lipid profile Low HDL-cholesterol levels High levels of triglycerides
Inflammatory profile	Elevated levels of systemic inflammatory markers, early inflammatory status	Low inflammatory degree, lower immune cell infiltration into adipose tissue	Permanent high inflammatory status
Clinical outcome	Type 2 diabetes risk Metabolic syndrome risk CVD risk Diminished muscle strength (lower physical activity)	Obesity complications. Possible deterioration of the metabolic risk profile	Metabolic syndrome progression, type 2 diabetes, CVD and higher mortality

[1]Prevalence depends on the ethnic population and the criteria used to define each phenotype. BMI, body mass index; CVD, cardiovascular disease; HDL, high density lipoprotein.

Several underlying factors have been proposed to explain the healthier profile in individuals with MHO (preserved metabolic health). Some of these factors comprise low vAT and ectopic fat accumulation (including decreased hepatic steatosis) observed in MHO, when compared to the more expandable subcutaneous fat depots [3]. Inflammatory status also appears to play a major role for the MHO phenotype as has it been linked to a low inflammatory degree, as further discussed ahead [28, 29].

Although the MHO group is associated with high insulin sensitivity, a favorable lipid profile (*e.g.* reduced levels of triglycerides), increased levels of adiponectin, absence of hypertension and reduced risk of developing type 2 diabetes and CVD, there is no evidence that these individuals will remain permanently protected from the risk of acquiring obesity-related comorbidities [16, 17, 21]. For instance, Marini *et al* have shown that a group of MHO women presented a less positive metabolic profile compared with non-obese women, with MHO having significantly increased blood pressure and carotid artery intima-media thickness and lower concentrations of HDL-cholesterol, which could represent early signs of atherosclerosis [30]. Oflaz *et al* further revealed that MHO women show signs of deteriorated endothelial function and atherosclerotic changes when compared with their healthy lean counterparts [31]. Additionally, a study from 2009 comprising 6011 men and women from the Third National Health and Nutrition Examination Survey (NHANES III), with public-access mortality data linkage, has shown that even in the absence of metabolic abnormalities, obesity is associated with augmented all-cause mortality risk [32].

Despite a multitude of studies focusing on MHO and its characteristics, there is still a large disparity both in the criteria used to define this phenotype and in the health outcomes analysed hence leading to a difficult comparison among published works [21, 25]. Also, variables that include lifestyle, physical fitness, ethnicity, gender or age account for the complexity in evaluating MHO [33].

The Metabolically Unhealthy Obese Phenotype

At last, the MUO phenotype is defined by a BMI over 30 kg/m^2 and high body fat percentage over 30% [34 - 36]. These patients typically reveal an ectopic fat distribution with excessive accumulation of vAT and are considered at risk to develop major health problems including metabolic syndrome progression, diabetes, CVD and higher mortality [15, 36, 37].

Given the dissimilarities observed in metabolic profiles among people within the same categories of BMI, several authors have considered that instead of the amount of AT other factors such as composition and distribution of body fat are determinants of metabolic function [38 - 40].

METABOLIC INFLAMMATION

Nowadays, although it is well established that inflammation is a major contributor for the development of obesity-related metabolic disorders (*e.g.* insulin resistance and type 2 diabetes), the underlying molecular mechanisms leading to the high inflammatory state in AT remain only partially understood [7, 41].

The first report establishing a link between inflammation and obesity revealed augmented levels of tumor necrosis factor α (TNFα) in AT of obese mice compared with lean controls [42]. Since then, a wealth of studies focusing on inflammation in obesity have revealed a growing list of proinflammatory cytokines produced by adipocytes and infiltrating macrophages that are increased in obese when compared to lean subjects, such as interleukin (IL) 6, IL1β, IL18, leptin, CC-chemokine ligand 2 (CCL2) and resistin [43 - 45].

In obesity, inflammatory responses present a chronic low-grade condition, distinct from the features observed in classical inflammation elicited by infection, cancer or injury [46]. The terms "meta-inflammation", signifying metabolically-triggered inflammation [46], or "para-inflammation" for an intermediate state between basal and inflammatory states [47], have been proposed to name the inflammatory state observed in obesity. Both metabolic and immune systems are highly interdependent, with common cellular machinery and sharing modulators and regulators, that include hormones, cytokines, signaling protein mediators, transcription factors and bioactive lipids [9, 48].

Besides functioning as energy reservoir, thermal regulator and mechanical protector for internal organs, AT is a central metabolically active endocrine organ. This tissue plays a role in energy homeostasis and insulin sensitivity through secretion of a wide range molecules, such as adipokines, cytokines, hormones and growth factors [49, 50].

Inflammatory processes in the AT, are now regarded as contributors to obesity-related metabolic disorders [9, 51]. The energy surplus in AT has been shown to not only induce proinflammatory responses but also to lead to endoplasmic reticulum stress, hypoxia, mitochondrial defects and ultimately, to systemic insulin resistance [51 - 53]. Augmenting lipid and carbohydrate substrates results in a higher demand on the mitochondrial electron transport chain. The increased demand for nutrient oxidation along with the augmented hypoxia, due to insufficient AT vascularization, generate abnormally high amounts of reactive oxygen species [7, 54]. Oxidative stress leads to activation of major inflammatory kinases such as c-Jun N-terminal kinase (JNK), p38 mitogen-activated protein kinases (MAPK), and inhibitor of kappa B kinase (IKK) that may directly interfere with insulin signaling or indirectly via induction of the nuclear factor kappa-light-chain-enhancer of activated B cells (NFκB) and increased proinflammatory cytokine and chemokine production [7, 55].

Understanding fully how metabolic homeostasis deteriorates and relates to inflammation and pinpointing triggering factors for inflammation in obesity still poses an extremely hard challenge.

ADIPOSE TISSUE INFLAMMATION AND PATHOGENESIS OF OBESITY

Adipose Tissue Cellularity, Remodelling and Inflammation

White AT (wAT) plays a key role in mediating the systemic inflammation observed in certain obesity phenotypes Fig. (**1**). Storage of nutrients in excess implicates hyperplasia (increase in adipocyte number) and adipocyte hypertrophy (increase in cell size) [41, 56]. Chronic nutrient overload results in excessive fat accumulation and adipocyte hypertrophy. Growing adipocyte size requires a constant remodeling in the extracellular matrix of the AT, ultimately leading to insufficient vascularization and innervation [27, 56].

Srdic *et al* have found that MUHNW subjects revealed higher adipocyte hypertrophy in vAT, when compared to healthy counterparts [27, 57, 58]. In the same line, MHO have been associated with smaller adipocytes relative to MUO controls [27, 58]. O´Connell *et al* reported a significant increase of the mean omental adipocyte size in MUO group when compared to MHO group. Adipocyte size strongly correlated with metabolic parameters such as insulin resistance, triglyceride levels and hepatic steatosis and fibrosis. The degree of steatosis measured was 43% in MUO phenotype and 3% in MHO. The size of adipocytes was suggested to be more relevant than the actual size of fat depot [59]. In fact, the importance of adipocyte size could potentially be explained by the overflow hypothesis that suggests adipocytes have a limit to store lipids. When this limit is reached, reminiscent fatty acids start to "overflow" to ectopic locations such as muscle or liver, leading to metabolic deterioration (*e.g.* hepatic insulin resistance) [59 - 61].

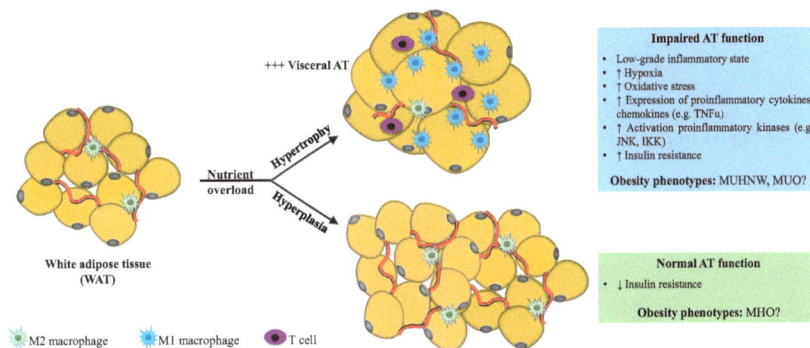

Fig. (1). Adipose tissue-centered inflammatory mechanisms that may underlie obesity phenotypes. IKK, inhibitor of kappa B kinase, JNK, c-Jun N-terminal kinase; MHO, metabolically healthy obese phenotype; MUHNW, metabolically unhealthy normal-weight phenotype; MUO, metabolically unhealthy obese phenotype; TNFα, tumor necrosis factor alpha.

Adipose Tissue Inflammatory Cells

Adipocyte hypertrophy, followed by augmented release of proinflammatory cytokines, promotes infiltration of immune cells and phenotypic changes in resident immune cells [27, 41]. Weisberg *et al* report an increase of AT proinflammatory macrophages in obese individuals, accompanied by overexpression of TNFα, IL6, inducible nitric oxide synthase, transforming growth factor β1, C-reactive protein (CRP), among others [53]. Also, Xu *et al* showed an upregulation of multiple inflammation and macrophage-specific genes in wAT of genetic and high-fat-induced obesity mouse models. The observed upregulation precedes a high increase in serum insulin levels. Furthermore, authors report a significant infiltration of macrophages in histological samples of wAT in obese mice and propose AT infiltrating macrophages and their inflammatory pathways to be major contributors to the pathogenesis of obesity-induced insulin resistance [52]. Diet-induced obesity has been shown to provoke a phenotypic switch in AT macrophage polarization into the proinflammatory M1-state, which relates to insulin resistance [62]. Interestingly, AT resident macrophages have been reported to be higher in vAT when compared to subcutaneous adipose tissue (sAT), which is in accordance with the worse metabolic risk profile observed in vAT [63]. Consistently, vAT adiposity has been reported to have a central role in the development of insulin resistance and inflammation [26, 27, 64].

MHO has been linked to a low inflammatory degree, with reduced white blood cell counts and low levels of TNFα, IL6 and CRP identified in the plasma [28, 29]. Opposing these findings, other studies have recently proposed an increase in circulating proinflammatory factors (*e.g.* CRP) in the MHO group [29, 65]. Also, a normal adipose function associated with a lower immune cell infiltration into adipose tissue and a normal adipokine secretion pattern has been reported in MHO individuals [66].

Patterns of Adipose Tissue Distribution

Vague firstly reported a distinct fat deposition between sexes, with a worse metabolic profile being related to the android (male) when compared to the gynoid (female) body type [67, 68]. These two terms are used to classify obesity in terms of fat distribution. In the android fat distribution, individuals present accumulation of AT mainly around the trunk and upper body (*e.g.* abdomen, chest). This central obesity pattern often named "apple-shaped" is more commonly found in men. In the gynoid fat pattern, AT is mainly deposited around the hips, thighs and lower trunk, leading to a "pear-shaped" shape more often found in women, also referred to as peripheral obesity [68, 69].

Even in the absence of obesity, accumulation of abdominal and central AT, has been related to metabolic and cardiovascular disease risk in healthy adults in multiple cohort studies [70 - 72]. Also, Fu *et al* have confirmed that central fat and central/peripheral fat ratio were significantly associated with increased metabolic risks in adult Chinese women [72]. Furthermore, in children aged 7 to 13-year-old, the central/peripheral ratio was closely linked to both insulin resistance and dyslipidemia. This ratio was suggested to be a good predictor for metabolic and CVD risk in normal weight, overweight and obese children [73].

The association of vAT with metabolic deterioration and cardiometabolic risk, regardless of BMI, has been at the basis of defining the MUHNW phenotype, characterized by a normal BMI with increased levels of adiposity and ectopic fat distribution with augmented vAT [16, 17] and an increased prevalence of metabolic syndrome features, such as low insulin sensitivity, increased blood pressure, low HDL-cholesterol and high levels of triglycerides and systemic inflammatory markers [18, 19, 30]. Indeed, multiple studies have shown that obesity phenotypes associated with poorer metabolic function (MUHNW and MUO) show increased vAT when compared to MHO individuals [27, 74, 75]. MUO patients typically reveal an ectopic fat distribution with excessive accumulation of vAT and are considered at risk to develop major health problems including metabolic syndrome progression, diabetes, CVD and higher mortality [15, 36, 37].

Distinct fat compartments within the abdominal adipose tissue also lead to different metabolic risk factors. Fox *et al* have shown that despite both vAT and sAT abdominal compartments are associated with metabolic risk factors, vAT seems to be more strongly correlated with cardiometabolic risk factors [76]. vAT depots show an increased secretion of proinflammatory cytokines (*e.g.* TNFα) and a reduced secretion of adiponectin, a hormone positively related with whole-body insulin sensitivity. Furthermore, abdominal vAT adipocytes, in comparison to abdominal sAT adipocytes, are more sensitive to catecholamine-induced lipolysis which translates into a greater release of free fatty acids (FFA) into the portal venous system and consequently, to increased lipotoxic effects, mainly in the liver and skeletal muscle. Also, vAT accumulation has been reported to be related with insulin resistance and hyperinsulinemia. Hence, vAT is nowadays considered as an independent risk factor for type 2 diabetes [77, 78]. Altogether, the vAT adipocyte profile could explain the deleterious effects observed in vAT accumulation [69, 79].

Noteworthy, peripheral fat appears to be concomitant with a lower metabolic risk, which could derive from the less inflammatory nature of the lower-body adipose tissue [72, 80, 81]. Interestingly, among the factors underlying the healthier profile found in individuals with MHO are a low vAT and ectopic fat accumulation (including decreased hepatic steatosis) and more expandable subcutaneous fat depot [3].

Interestingly, and demonstrating how much vAT contributes to determining obesity phenotypes, a novel mathematical model, the visceral adipose index (VAI), has been proposed to assess visceral adiposity based on anthropometric and lipid profiles. VAI calculation was assessed by equations comprising the waist circumference, the BMI and the levels of both low-density lipoprotein (LDL)-cholesterol and triglycerides. Kang *et al* have shown VAI to be a good predictive tool in determining the conversion of MHO to the more unfavorable MUO phenotype, in both genders [82].

Circulating Free Fatty Acids

The release of FFA into the circulation is augmented in most obese individuals due to over-expanding fat mass and has been linked to both peripheral insulin resistance and insufficient insulin production/release, two major factors for the etiology of type 2 diabetes [83]. Boden *et al* further show evidence for the role of augmented circulating FFAs in activating inflammatory processes in male rats, particularly by activating the proinflammatory IKK/IκB/NFκB pathway and by increasing expression of inflammatory cytokines in liver (IL1β and TNFα) and presence of monocyte chemoattractant protein-1 (MCP1) in the plasma [84]. A cohort study with 840 Chinese patients reveals high serum FFA levels correlate positively and significantly with metabolic syndrome parameters, inflammation indexes and hepatocellular damage. Furthermore, authors have shown that serum FFA can be used as a factor to predict advanced fibrosis in NAFLD patients [85]. Also, Ni *et al* have reported significantly elevated levels of circulating FFA in the MUO group when compared to both MHO and metabolically healthy lean groups. Authors advocate that FFA have a crucial role in the pathogenesis of metabolic syndrome [86]. We propose that circulating FFA may as well underlie the pathogenesis of obesity phenotypes.

Sex Hormones

Premenopausal women have been reported to present fewer metabolic disorders when compared to men [87 - 89]. However, in postmenopausal women presenting estrogen deficiency, the prevalence of these disorders raises dramatically along with the loss of subcutaneous fat and an increase in central fat [90, 91]. From these observations it was possible to hypothesize that estrogens may have a fundamental role in preventing the development of obesity and metabolic syndrome [9, 92]. Interestingly, according to an extensive analysis of multiple European cohort studies, MHO has been reported to be more frequent in women and to decrease with age in both sexes [33]. In accordance, very recently, a cohort study revealed that one-third of obese postmenopausal women within the MHO phenotype transitioned to the MUO phenotype, over a 6-year period, suggesting a link between excessive BMI and a predisposition toward metabolic deterioration [93], where the lack of estrogens may accelerate this transition.

Multiple studies have confirmed the link between estrogens and metabolic dysfunction ever since and it was shown that hormone replacement improves both insulin sensitivity and glycemic control [94, 95]. Stubbins *et al* have found estrogens could protect C57BL/6J female mice from adipocyte hypertrophy and from developing adipose tissue oxidative stress and inflammation when given high-fat diet. These mice appeared to be protected from developing liver steatosis and from becoming insulin resistant, when compared to ovariectomized female and male groups [96]. In the same line, Shen *et al* have shown that treatment of mice with estradiol, the major biologically active form of estrogen, could reverse both the recruitment of macrophages and the elevated macrophage infiltration observed in WAT of ovariectomized females fed with high-fat diet. Authors suggest this effect could result from a role of estrogens in suppressing inflammatory signaling in macrophages [16]. Indeed, the differences between pre- and postmenopausal women regarding adipose tissue distribution and inflammatory status, seem to mirror those that are observed among obesity phenotypes, and add evidence on the contribution of metabolic inflammation elicited by estrogen insufficiency in determining cardiometabolic risk.

Persistent Organic Pollutants

Other potential contributors to obesity and metabolic syndrome have been investigated. Among them, are persistent organic pollutants (POPs) that accumulate in AT. These heterogeneous compounds of both natural and anthropogenic origin are highly persistent and present endocrine-disrupting properties [97]. POPs have been studied for their adverse effects on human health. In 2014, Gauthier *et al* demonstrated the relationship of POPs with the variation in metabolic risk observed among obese individuals showing that the MHO phenotype is associated with lower plasma levels of POPs as compared with MUO subjects [98]. Although POP accumulation in AT may prevent the systemic effects of these compounds, this tissue can also be a target of their disruptive effects [98]. POP levels either in sAT and vAT have been shown to be higher in subjects with evidence of metabolic abnormalities. This pattern was especially evident for vAT, supported by higher vAT POP levels in patients with increased aggregation of metabolic syndrome components and higher 10-year cardiovascular risk based on the Framingham score [99].

Owing to this association, a paradigm shift of the view of POPs as mere obesogen compounds towards their acknowledgement as markers of dysmetabolic obesity was proposed [100]. Indeed, Teixeira *et al* have shown that the presence of xenoestrogens, such as hexachlorocyclohexane, in vAT and plasma in premenopausal women correlate positively with levels of the proinflammatory chemokine MCP1, thus contributing to a more proinflammatory status [101]. In accordance, xenostrogens have been shown to affect human peripheral blood-derived M1 and M2 macrophage migration, cytokine release, and estrogen-related signaling pathways. Effects were shown to be mediated by either estrogen receptor (ER) α or ERβ and were simultaneous to modulation of NFκB, activator protein-1, JNK, or extracellular signal-regulated kinase signaling pathways [102]. Also, Pestana *et al* have reported exposure to *p,p'*-dichlorodiphenyldichloro--thylene (*p,p'*-DDE) in male Wistar rats to be linked to impaired vAT normal function (*e.g.* decreased tissue development-related genes) and a reduction of the dynamic response to energy surplus, thus translating into exacerbated metabolic syndrome complications [103]. Smink *et al* have reported an association between prenatal exposure to hexachlorobenzene and increased BMI and weight in children aged 6.5 years in a study involving 482 children [104]. Finally, Lee *et al*, following a prospective cohort study with a group of diabetes-free individuals, have suggested low dose organochlorine pesticides and polychlorinated biphenyls may contribute to obesity, dyslipidemia, and insulin resistance [105].

Gut Microbiota and the Inflammasome

During the last decade, multiple studies have been appointing gut microbiota as another major environmental factor affecting host metabolic balance [106]. Studies comparing obese and lean human subjects have reported alterations on gut microbiota composition, such as a reduction of *Bacteroidetes* phylum and a related increase of *Firmicutes* [107, 108]. Changes in the normal gut microbial composition along with an augmented intestinal permeability, for example, as a result from a high-fat diet, been linked to a systemic low-grade elevation in bacterial derived endotoxin lipopolysaccharide (LPS), a condition termed metabolic endotoxemia [109 - 111]. Increased circulating LPS levels activate the pattern recognition receptor toll-like receptor 4 (TLR4) and trigger proinflammatory and oxidative cascades that can contribute to the development of metabolic imbalances observed in obesity [110]. For instance, Cani *et al* have shown metabolic endotoxemia can dysregulate the inflammatory tone and trigger body weight gain and diabetes in mice [112]. Creely *et al* have suggested LPS can activate an innate immune response in human adipose tissue in type 2 diabetes and obesity [113]. In the same line, a population-based cohort study comprising 7169 subjects has shown endotoxemia is tightly bound to increased risk of incident diabetes [114]. Finally, a 6-year follow-up study with 2529 middle-aged and older Chinese men and women has revealed elevated plasma LPS-binding protein (LBP) levels correlate significantly with an increased risk of developing metabolic syndrome [115]. Indeed, LPS binds LBP and activates the receptor protein CD14 located in the plasma membrane of macrophages which triggers the activation of proinflammatory pathways, such as NFκB [116, 117].

Apart from the distinction between lean and obese subjects, the gut microbiota is also now identified as a determining factor in the pathogenesis of the MUO phenotype and related comorbidities through increased endotoxemia, intestinal and systemic inflammation, as well as insulin resistance. In accordance, recent studies suggest that an healthy-like gut microbiota may contribute to the MHO phenotype [118].

The multiprotein signaling complex nucleotide-binding oligomerization domain-like receptor (NLRP) 3 inflammasome, which recognizes a wide range of microbial, stress and damage signals, leads to activation of caspase-1 and subsequent production of potent proinflammatory cytokines (IL1β and IL18). Noteworthy, NLRP3 inflammasome components as well as caspase-1 were found to be increased in adipose and liver tissues of obese mice and humans [119]. Vandanmagsar *et al* have reported a prominent role of NLRP3 inflammasome in inducing obesity and insulin resistance. NLRP3 inflammasome ablated mice did not show obesity-induced inflammasome activation in both fat depots and liver, and presented a better insulin signaling [119]. In spite of the potential role of the NLRP3 inflammasome in metabolic syndrome, activation of this pathway in fat occurs in a late phase of obesity, thus suggesting that NLRP3 inflammasome is actually not a primary etiologic factor in the disease [119, 120]. Yet, Esser *et al* have revealed that MUO phenotype appears to be related with an increased activation of the NLPR3 inflammasome in macrophages infiltrating vAT, and a less favorable inflammatory profile compared with the MHO phenotype [121]. In the opposite direction, NLRP1 inflammasome has been described to prevent obesity and metabolic syndrome through IL18 production. Murphy *et al* have found that mice lacking the NLRP1 inflammasome develop spontaneous obesity due to lipid accumulation. The same effect was observed in mice lacking IL18 [122].

TARGETING INFLAMMATION

Independently of its origin, the chronic low-grade inflammatory state observed in metabolic syndrome has, undoubtedly, a major role for the syndrome onset and its pathophysiological effects [7, 55].

In recent decades, extensive work has brought new insights to target metabolic inflammation involved in the pathogenesis of unhealthy obesity phenotypes. Two representative examples are presented ahead.

A diet rich in mixed fruits and fibres was shown to have no capacity to induce oxidative and inflammatory responses when compared to a high-fat diet presenting equal content of calories [123]. In the same line, Åsgård *et al* have suggested that fruit and vegetable intake may decrease oxidative stress and inflammation in type 2 diabetes patients [124]. Interestingly, mortality risk in MHO phenotype appears to be reduced by a Mediterranean dietary pattern, as proposed by a prospective cohort analysis in a representative obese USA population with a median follow-up of 18.5 years [125], underlining the role of dietary habits in preventing cardiometabolic risk, independently of BMI.

Another interesting example is the use of drugs that may impact on metabolism, inflammation or both. This is the case of the insulin-sensitizing thiazolidinediones (TZDs), released in the market during the 1990s, consisting of a class of drugs that activate the peroxisome proliferator-activated receptor-gamma (PPARγ), a receptor expressed in both adipocytes and macrophages in AT. Activation of PPARγ by TZDs reduces the inflammatory state both by promoting macrophage phenotype switching from proinflammatory M1 to anti-inflammatory M2 and by stimulating the enrichment of vAT with anti-inflammatory regulatory T (Treg) cells [126]. Esterson *et al* have reported significant decreases both in insulin resistance and adipose tissue inflammation in obese patients with type 2 diabetes upon treatment with pioglitazone [127]. Another anti-inflammatory drug, anakinra, an antagonist of human IL1 receptor, was shown to significantly diminish glycated hemoglobin, improve β-cell secretory function and lower systemic inflammatory markers in a trial involving 70 patients [126].

Thus, resolving the intricate network of triggering factors and inflammatory events involved in the metabolic syndrome development will pave the way for effective preventive and therapeutic treatments.

CONCLUDING REMARKS

Whatever the trigger for obesity-related inflammation, it is undisputable that it plays a central role in the pathogenesis of obesity comorbidities. We have presented evidence that the inflammatory status associated with adipocyte hypertrophy, proinflammatory AT macrophages, vAT, estrogen insufficiency, POPs present in the adipose tissue and metabolic endotoxemia elicited by an unfavourable gut microbiota may explain why a subset of obese subjects develop metabolic disturbances, while others on the opposite side of this spectrum, remain with relatively preserved metabolic function. However, one cannot ignore that the prognosis for the MHO phenotype remains a matter of intense debate and multiple prospective cohort studies provide evidence that MHO, when compared to their non-obese counterparts, are at higher risk to develop hypertension, type 2 diabetes and metabolic syndrome [18, 128]. Still, risk is lower when compared to MUO and MUHNW. Keeping in mind that inflammation may be at the crossroads between obesity phenotypes, interventions aiming to target metabolic inflammation may show promise in counteracting obesity metabolic comorbidities.

CONSENT FOR PUBLICATION

Not applicable.

CONFLICT OF INTEREST

The authors confirm that this chapter contents have no conflict of interest.

ACKNOWLEDGEMENTS

The authors would like to acknowledge financial support from by FEDER – Fundo Europeu de Desenvolvimento Regional, through NORTE 2020 Programa Operacional Regional do Norte- NORTE-01-0145-FEDER-000012 and Instituto de Investigação e Inovação em Saúde (Projeto Estratégico UID/BIM/04293/2013).

REFERENCES

[1]   World Health Organization Media Centre. Fact sheet Obesity and overweight WHO 2017 Available from: http://www.who.int/mediacentre/factsheets/fs311/en/

[2]   Mokdad AH, Ford ES, Bowman BA, *et al.* Prevalence of obesity, diabetes, and obesity-related health risk factors, 2001. JAMA 2003; 289(1): 76-9.
        [http://dx.doi.org/10.1001/jama.289.1.76] [PMID: 12503980]

[3]   Blüher M. The distinction of metabolically 'healthy' from 'unhealthy' obese individuals. Curr Opin Lipidol 2010; 21(1): 38-43.
        [http://dx.doi.org/10.1097/MOL.0b013e3283346ccc] [PMID: 19915462]

[4]   Karelis AD. To be obese--does it matter if you are metabolically healthy? Nat Rev Endocrinol 2011; 7(12): 699-700.
        [http://dx.doi.org/10.1038/nrendo.2011.181] [PMID: 22009160]

[5]   Ruderman NB, Schneider SH, Berchtold P. The "metabolically-obese," normal-weight individual. Am J Clin Nutr 1981; 34(8): 1617-21.
        [http://dx.doi.org/10.1093/ajcn/34.8.1617] [PMID: 7270486]

[6]   Jung CH, Lee WJ, Song K-H. Metabolically healthy obesity: a friend or foe? Korean J Intern Med (Korean Assoc Intern Med) 2017; 32(4): 611-21.
        [http://dx.doi.org/10.3904/kjim.2016.259] [PMID: 28602062]

[7]   Monteiro R, Azevedo I. Chronic inflammation in obesity and the metabolic syndrome. Mediators Inflamm 2010; 2010: 1-10.
        [http://dx.doi.org/10.1155/2010/289645] [PMID: 20706689]

[8]   Trayhurn P, Wood IS. Adipokines: inflammation and the pleiotropic role of white adipose tissue. Br J Nutr 2004; 92(3): 347-55.

[http://dx.doi.org/10.1079/BJN20041213] [PMID: 15469638]

[9]   Monteiro R, Teixeira D, Calhau C. Estrogen signaling in metabolic inflammation. Mediators Inflamm 2014; 2014615917
[http://dx.doi.org/10.1155/2014/615917] [PMID: 25400333]

[10]   Gregor MF, Hotamisligil GS. Inflammatory mechanisms in obesity. Annu Rev Immunol 2011; 29(1): 415-45.
[http://dx.doi.org/10.1146/annurev-immunol-031210-101322] [PMID: 21219177]

[11]   González AS, Guerrero DB, Soto MB, Díaz SP, Martinez-Olmos M, Vidal O. Metabolic syndrome, insulin resistance and the inflammation markers C-reactive protein and ferritin. Eur J Clin Nutr 2006; 60(6): 802-9.
[http://dx.doi.org/10.1038/sj.ejcn.1602384] [PMID: 16493453]

[12]   Wannamethee SG, Lowe GDO, Shaper AG, Rumley A, Lennon L, Whincup PH. The metabolic syndrome and insulin resistance: relationship to haemostatic and inflammatory markers in older non-diabetic men. Atherosclerosis 2005; 181(1): 101-8.
[http://dx.doi.org/10.1016/j.atherosclerosis.2004.12.031] [PMID: 15939060]

[13]   Goossens GH, Blaak EE. Adipose tissue dysfunction and impaired metabolic health in human obesity: a matter of oxygen? Front Endocrinol (Lausanne) 2015; 6: 55.
[http://dx.doi.org/10.3389/fendo.2015.00055] [PMID: 25964776]

[14]   Bremer AA, Jialal I. Adipose tissue dysfunction in nascent metabolic syndrome. J Obes 2013; 2013393192
[http://dx.doi.org/10.1155/2013/393192] [PMID: 23653857]

[15]   Dobson R, Burgess MI, Sprung VS, *et al.* Metabolically healthy and unhealthy obesity: differential effects on myocardial function according to metabolic syndrome, rather than obesity. Int J Obes 2016; 40(1): 153-61.
[http://dx.doi.org/10.1038/ijo.2015.151] [PMID: 26271188]

[16]   Cembrowska P, Stefańska A, Odrowąż-Sypniewska G. Obesity phenotypes: normal-weight individuals with metabolic disorders versus metabolically healthy obese. Med Res J 2017; 1(3): 95-9.
[http://dx.doi.org/10.5603/MRJ.2016.0016]

[17]   Mathew H, Farr OM, Mantzoros CS. Metabolic health and weight: Understanding metabolically unhealthy normal weight or metabolically healthy obese patients. Metabolism 2016; 65(1): 73-80.
[http://dx.doi.org/10.1016/j.metabol.2015.10.019] [PMID: 26683798]

[18]   Aung K, Lorenzo C, Hinojosa MA, Haffner SM. Risk of developing diabetes and cardiovascular disease in metabolically unhealthy normal-weight and metabolically healthy obese individuals. J Clin Endocrinol Metab 2014; 99(2): 462-8.
[http://dx.doi.org/10.1210/jc.2013-2832] [PMID: 24257907]

[19]   Dvorak RV, DeNino WF, Ades PA, Poehlman ET. Phenotypic characteristics associated with insulin resistance in metabolically obese but normal-weight young women. Diabetes 1999; 48(11): 2210-4.
[http://dx.doi.org/10.2337/diabetes.48.11.2210] [PMID: 10535456]

[20]   Lee S-H, Han K, Yang HK, *et al.* A novel criterion for identifying metabolically obese but normal weight individuals using the product of triglycerides and glucose. Nutr Diabetes 2015; 5(4)e149
[http://dx.doi.org/10.1038/nutd.2014.46] [PMID: 25915739]

[21]   Muñoz-Garach A, Cornejo-Pareja I, Tinahones FJ. Does Metabolically Healthy Obesity Exist? Nutrients 2016; 8(6)E320
[http://dx.doi.org/10.3390/nu8060320] [PMID: 27258304]

[22]   Sims EAH. Are there persons who are obese, but metabolically healthy? Metabolism 2001; 50(12): 1499-504.
[http://dx.doi.org/10.1053/meta.2001.27213] [PMID: 11735101]

[23]   Karelis AD. Metabolically healthy but obese individuals. Lancet 2008; 372(9646): 1281-3.

[http://dx.doi.org/10.1016/S0140-6736(08)61531-7] [PMID: 18929889]

[24] Stefan N, Kantartzis K, Machann J, *et al.* Identification and characterization of metabolically benign obesity in humans. Arch Intern Med 2008; 168(15): 1609-16.
[http://dx.doi.org/10.1001/archinte.168.15.1609] [PMID: 18695074]

[25] Phillips CM. Metabolically healthy obesity: definitions, determinants and clinical implications. Rev Endocr Metab Disord 2013; 14(3): 219-27.
[http://dx.doi.org/10.1007/s11154-013-9252-x] [PMID: 23928851]

[26] Goday A, Calvo E, Vázquez LA, *et al.* Prevalence and clinical characteristics of metabolically healthy obese individuals and other obese/non-obese metabolic phenotypes in a working population: results from the Icaria study. BMC Public Health 2016; 16: 248.
[http://dx.doi.org/10.1186/s12889-016-2921-4] [PMID: 27036105]

[27] Badoud F, Perreault M, Zulyniak MA, Mutch DM. Molecular insights into the role of white adipose tissue in metabolically unhealthy normal weight and metabolically healthy obese individuals.
[http://dx.doi.org/10.1096/fj.14-263913]

[28] Marques-Vidal P, Velho S, Waterworth D, Waeber G, von Känel R, Vollenweider P. The association between inflammatory biomarkers and metabolically healthy obesity depends of the definition used. Eur J Clin Nutr 2012; 66(4): 426-35.
[http://dx.doi.org/10.1038/ejcn.2011.170] [PMID: 21952696]

[29] Phillips CM, Perry IJ. Does inflammation determine metabolic health status in obese and nonobese adults? J Clin Endocrinol Metab 2013; 98(10): E1610-9.
[http://dx.doi.org/10.1210/jc.2013-2038] [PMID: 23979951]

[30] Marini MA, Succurro E, Frontoni S, *et al.* Metabolically healthy but obese women have an intermediate cardiovascular risk profile between healthy nonobese women and obese insulin-resistant women. Diabetes Care 2007; 30(8): 2145-7.
[http://dx.doi.org/10.2337/dc07-0419] [PMID: 17507694]

[31] Oflaz H, Ozbey N, Mantar F, *et al.* Determination of endothelial function and early atherosclerotic changes in healthy obese women. Diabetes Nutr Metab 2003; 16(3): 176-81.
[PMID: 14635735]

[32] Kuk JL, Ardern CI. Are metabolically normal but obese individuals at lower risk for all-cause mortality? Diabetes Care 2009; 32(12): 2297-9.
[http://dx.doi.org/10.2337/dc09-0574] [PMID: 19729521]

[33] van Vliet-Ostaptchouk JV, Nuotio M-L, Slagter SN, *et al.* The prevalence of metabolic syndrome and metabolically healthy obesity in Europe: a collaborative analysis of ten large cohort studies. BMC Endocr Disord 2014; 14(1): 9.
[http://dx.doi.org/10.1186/1472-6823-14-9] [PMID: 24484869]

[34] Alberti KGM, Zimmet P, Shaw J. IDF Epidemiology Task Force Consensus Group. The metabolic syndrome--a new worldwide definition. Lancet 2005; 366(9491): 1059-62.
[http://dx.doi.org/10.1016/S0140-6736(05)67402-8] [PMID: 16182882]

[35] Després J-P. Body fat distribution and risk of cardiovascular disease: an update. Circulation 2012; 126(10): 1301-13.
[http://dx.doi.org/10.1161/CIRCULATIONAHA.111.067264] [PMID: 22949540]

[36] De Lorenzo A, Soldati L, Sarlo F, Calvani M, Di Lorenzo N, Di Renzo L. New obesity classification criteria as a tool for bariatric surgery indication. World J Gastroenterol 2016; 22(2): 681-703.
[http://dx.doi.org/10.3748/wjg.v22.i2.681] [PMID: 26811617]

[37] Pajunen P, Kotronen A, Korpi-Hyövälti E, *et al.* Metabolically healthy and unhealthy obesity phenotypes in the general population: the FIN-D2D Survey. BMC Public Health 2011; 11(1): 754.
[http://dx.doi.org/10.1186/1471-2458-11-754] [PMID: 21962038]

[38] Björntorp P. Metabolic implications of body fat distribution. Diabetes Care 1991; 14(12): 1132-43.

[http://dx.doi.org/10.2337/diacare.14.12.1132] [PMID: 1773700]

[39]   Manolopoulos KN, Karpe F, Frayn KN. Gluteofemoral body fat as a determinant of metabolic health. Int J Obes 2010; 34(6): 949-59.
[http://dx.doi.org/10.1038/ijo.2009.286] [PMID: 20065965]

[40]   Jensen MD. Role of body fat distribution and the metabolic complications of obesity. J Clin Endocrinol Metab 2008; 93(11) (Suppl. 1): S57-63.
[http://dx.doi.org/10.1210/jc.2008-1585] [PMID: 18987271]

[41]   Makki K, Froguel P, Wolowczuk I. Adipose Tissue in Obesity-Related Inflammation and Insulin Resistance: Cells, Cytokines, and Chemokines. Int Sch Res Not 2013; 2013.

[42]   Hotamisligil GS, Arner P, Caro JF, Atkinson RL, Spiegelman BM. Increased adipose tissue expression of tumor necrosis factor-alpha in human obesity and insulin resistance. J Clin Invest 1995; 95(5): 2409-15.
[http://dx.doi.org/10.1172/JCI117936] [PMID: 7738205]

[43]   Ouchi N, Parker JL, Lugus JJ, Walsh K. Adipokines in inflammation and metabolic disease. Nat Rev Immunol 2011; 11(2): 85-97.
[http://dx.doi.org/10.1038/nri2921] [PMID: 21252989]

[44]   Schmidt FM, Weschenfelder J, Sander C, *et al.* Inflammatory cytokines in general and central obesity and modulating effects of physical activity. PLoS One 2015; 10(3)e0121971
[http://dx.doi.org/10.1371/journal.pone.0121971] [PMID: 25781614]

[45]   Makki K, Froguel P, Wolowczuk I. Adipose tissue in obesity-related inflammation and insulin resistance: cells, cytokines, and chemokines. ISRN Inflamm 2013; 2013139239
[http://dx.doi.org/10.1155/2013/139239] [PMID: 24455420]

[46]   Sun S, Ji Y, Kersten S, Qi L. Mechanisms of inflammatory responses in obese adipose tissue. Annu Rev Nutr 2012; 32: 261-86.
[http://dx.doi.org/10.1146/annurev-nutr-071811-150623] [PMID: 22404118]

[47]   Medzhitov R. Origin and physiological roles of inflammation. Nature 2008; 454(7203): 428-35.
[http://dx.doi.org/10.1038/nature07201] [PMID: 18650913]

[48]   Wellen KE, Hotamisligil GS. Inflammation, stress, and diabetes. J Clin Invest 2005; 115(5): 1111-9.
[http://dx.doi.org/10.1172/JCI25102] [PMID: 15864338]

[49]   Kershaw EE, Flier JS. Adipose tissue as an endocrine organ. J Clin Endocrinol Metab 2004; 89(6): 2548-56.
[http://dx.doi.org/10.1210/jc.2004-0395] [PMID: 15181022]

[50]   Prins JB. Adipose tissue as an endocrine organ. Best Pract Res Clin Endocrinol Metab 2002; 16(4): 639-51.
[http://dx.doi.org/10.1053/beem.2002.0222] [PMID: 12468412]

[51]   Kim JI, Huh JY, Sohn JH, *et al.* Lipid-overloaded enlarged adipocytes provoke insulin resistance independent of inflammation. Mol Cell Biol 2015; 35(10): 1686-99.
[http://dx.doi.org/10.1128/MCB.01321-14] [PMID: 25733684]

[52]   Xu H, Barnes GT, Yang Q, *et al.* Chronic inflammation in fat plays a crucial role in the development of obesity-related insulin resistance. J Clin Invest 2003; 112(12): 1821-30.
[http://dx.doi.org/10.1172/JCI200319451] [PMID: 14679177]

[53]   Weisberg SP, McCann D, Desai M, Rosenbaum M, Leibel RL, Ferrante AW Jr. Obesity is associated with macrophage accumulation in adipose tissue. J Clin Invest 2003; 112(12): 1796-808.
[http://dx.doi.org/10.1172/JCI200319246] [PMID: 14679176]

[54]   Rudich A, Kanety H, Bashan N. Adipose stress-sensing kinases: linking obesity to malfunction. Trends Endocrinol Metab 2007; 18(8): 291-9.
[http://dx.doi.org/10.1016/j.tem.2007.08.006] [PMID: 17855109]

[55] Qatanani M, Lazar MA. Mechanisms of obesity-associated insulin resistance: many choices on the menu. Genes Dev 2007; 21(12): 1443-55.
[http://dx.doi.org/10.1101/gad.1550907] [PMID: 17575046]

[56] Mulder P, Morrison MC, Verschuren L, *et al.* Reduction of obesity-associated white adipose tissue inflammation by rosiglitazone is associated with reduced non-alcoholic fatty liver disease in LDLr-deficient mice. Sci Rep 2016; 6(1): 31542.
[http://dx.doi.org/10.1038/srep31542] [PMID: 27545964]

[57] Srdić B, Stokić E, Korać A, Ukropina M, Veličković K, Breberina M. Morphological characteristics of abdominal adipose tissue in normal-weight and obese women of different metabolic profiles. Exp Clin Endocrinol Diabetes 2010; 118(10): 713-8.
[http://dx.doi.org/10.1055/s-0030-1254165] [PMID: 20533176]

[58] Stefan N, Häring H-U, Hu FB, Schulze MB. Metabolically healthy obesity: epidemiology, mechanisms, and clinical implications. Lancet Diabetes Endocrinol 2013; 1(2): 152-62.
[http://dx.doi.org/10.1016/S2213-8587(13)70062-7] [PMID: 24622321]

[59] O'Connell J, Lynch L, Cawood TJ, *et al.* The Relationship of Omental and Subcutaneous Adipocyte Size to Metabolic Disease in Severe Obesity.Sorensen TIA, editor PLoS One. 2010; 5: p. (4)e9997.
[http://dx.doi.org/10.1371/journal.pone.0009997]

[60] Unger RH. Lipid overload and overflow: metabolic trauma and the metabolic syndrome. Trends Endocrinol Metab 2003; 14(9): 398-403.
[http://dx.doi.org/10.1016/j.tem.2003.09.008] [PMID: 14580758]

[61] Sniderman AD, Bhopal R, Prabhakaran D, Sarrafzadegan N, Tchernof A. Why might South Asians be so susceptible to central obesity and its atherogenic consequences? The adipose tissue overflow hypothesis. Int J Epidemiol 2007; 36(1): 220-5.
[http://dx.doi.org/10.1093/ije/dyl245] [PMID: 17510078]

[62] Lumeng CN, Bodzin JL, Saltiel AR. Obesity induces a phenotypic switch in adipose tissue macrophage polarization. J Clin Invest 2007; 117(1): 175-84.
[http://dx.doi.org/10.1172/JCI29881] [PMID: 17200717]

[63] Cancello R, Tordjman J, Poitou C, *et al.* Increased infiltration of macrophages in omental adipose tissue is associated with marked hepatic lesions in morbid human obesity. Diabetes 2006; 55(6): 1554-61.
[http://dx.doi.org/10.2337/db06-0133] [PMID: 16731817]

[64] Bastien M, Poirier P, Lemieux I, Després J-P. Overview of epidemiology and contribution of obesity to cardiovascular disease. Prog Cardiovasc Dis 2014; 56(4): 369-81.
[http://dx.doi.org/10.1016/j.pcad.2013.10.016] [PMID: 24438728]

[65] Jung CH, Kang YM, Jang JE, *et al.* Fatty liver index is a risk determinant of incident type 2 diabetes in a metabolically healthy population with obesity. Obesity (Silver Spring) 2016; 24(6): 1373-9.
[http://dx.doi.org/10.1002/oby.21483] [PMID: 27112320]

[66] Goossens GH. The Metabolic Phenotype in Obesity: Fat Mass, Body Fat Distribution, and Adipose Tissue Function. Obes Facts 2017; 10(3): 207-15.
[http://dx.doi.org/10.1159/000471488] [PMID: 28564650]

[67] Vague J. Sexual differentiation. A determinant factor of the forms of obesity. 1947. Obes Res 1996; 4(2): 201-3.
[http://dx.doi.org/10.1002/j.1550-8528.1996.tb00535.x] [PMID: 8681056]

[68] Vague J. The degree of masculine differentiation of obesities: a factor determining predisposition to diabetes, atherosclerosis, gout, and uric calculous disease. Am J Clin Nutr 1956; 4(1): 20-34.
[http://dx.doi.org/10.1093/ajcn/4.1.20] [PMID: 13282851]

[69] Kyrou I, Randeva HS, Weickert MO. Clinical Problems Caused by ObesityEndotext MDTextcom, Inc 2000.

[70]   Okura T, Nakata Y, Yamabuki K, Tanaka K. Regional body composition changes exhibit opposing effects on coronary heart disease risk factors. Arterioscler Thromb Vasc Biol 2004; 24(5): 923-9. [http://dx.doi.org/10.1161/01.ATV.0000125702.26272.f6] [PMID: 15016639]

[71]   Kang SM, Yoon JW, Ahn HY, *et al.* Android fat depot is more closely associated with metabolic syndrome than abdominal visceral fat in elderly people. PLoS One 2011; 6(11)e27694 [http://dx.doi.org/10.1371/journal.pone.0027694] [PMID: 22096613]

[72]   Fu X, Song A, Zhou Y, *et al.* Association of regional body fat with metabolic risks in Chinese women. Public Health Nutr 2014; 17(10): 2316-24. [http://dx.doi.org/10.1017/S1368980013002668] [PMID: 24148901]

[73]   Samsell L, Regier M, Walton C, Cottrell L. Importance of android/gynoid fat ratio in predicting metabolic and cardiovascular disease risk in normal weight as well as overweight and obese children. J Obes 2014; 2014846578 [http://dx.doi.org/10.1155/2014/846578] [PMID: 25302115]

[74]   Messier V, Karelis AD, Robillard M-È, *et al.* Metabolically healthy but obese individuals: relationship with hepatic enzymes. Metabolism 2010; 59(1): 20-4. [http://dx.doi.org/10.1016/j.metabol.2009.06.020] [PMID: 19709695]

[75]   Brochu M, Tchernof A, Dionne IJ, *et al.* What are the physical characteristics associated with a normal metabolic profile despite a high level of obesity in postmenopausal women? J Clin Endocrinol Metab 2001; 86(3): 1020-5. [PMID: 11238480]

[76]   Fox CS, Massaro JM, Hoffmann U, *et al.* Abdominal visceral and subcutaneous adipose tissue compartments: association with metabolic risk factors in the Framingham Heart Study. Circulation 2007; 116(1): 39-48. [http://dx.doi.org/10.1161/CIRCULATIONAHA.106.675355] [PMID: 17576866]

[77]   Basat O, Ucak S, Ozkurt H, Basak M, Seber S, Altuntas Y. Visceral adipose tissue as an indicator of insulin resistance in nonobese patients with new onset type 2 diabetes mellitus. Exp Clin Endocrinol Diabetes 2006; 114(2): 58-62. [http://dx.doi.org/10.1055/s-2006-923886] [PMID: 16570234]

[78]   Sam S, Haffner S, Davidson MH, *et al.* Relationship of abdominal visceral and subcutaneous adipose tissue with lipoprotein particle number and size in type 2 diabetes. Diabetes 2008; 57(8): 2022-7. [http://dx.doi.org/10.2337/db08-0157] [PMID: 18469202]

[79]   Montague CT, O'Rahilly S. The perils of portliness: causes and consequences of visceral adiposity. Diabetes 2000; 49(6): 883-8. [http://dx.doi.org/10.2337/diabetes.49.6.883] [PMID: 10866038]

[80]   Snijder MB, Visser M, Dekker JM, *et al.* Health ABC Study. Low subcutaneous thigh fat is a risk factor for unfavourable glucose and lipid levels, independently of high abdominal fat. The Health ABC Study. Diabetologia 2005; 48(2): 301-8. [http://dx.doi.org/10.1007/s00125-004-1637-7] [PMID: 15660262]

[81]   Pinnick KE, Nicholson G, Manolopoulos KN, *et al.* MolPAGE Consortium. Distinct developmental profile of lower-body adipose tissue defines resistance against obesity-associated metabolic complications. Diabetes 2014; 63(11): 3785-97. [http://dx.doi.org/10.2337/db14-0385] [PMID: 24947352]

[82]   Kang YM, Jung CH, Cho YK, *et al.* Visceral adiposity index predicts the conversion of metabolically healthy obesity to an unhealthy phenotype.Fürnsinn C, editor PLoS One. 2017; 12: p. (6)e0179635.. [http://dx.doi.org/10.1371/journal.pone.0179635]

[83]   Arner P, Rydén M. Fatty Acids, Obesity and Insulin Resistance. Obes Facts 2015; 8(2): 147-55. [http://dx.doi.org/10.1159/000381224] [PMID: 25895754]

[84]   Boden G, She P, Mozzoli M, *et al.* Free fatty acids produce insulin resistance and activate the

proinflammatory nuclear factor-kappaB pathway in rat liver. Diabetes 2005; 54(12): 3458-65.
[http://dx.doi.org/10.2337/diabetes.54.12.3458] [PMID: 16306362]

[85]   Zhang J, Zhao Y, Xu C, *et al.* Association between serum free fatty acid levels and nonalcoholic fatty liver disease: a cross-sectional study. Sci Rep 2014; 4(1): 5832.
[http://dx.doi.org/10.1038/srep05832] [PMID: 25060337]

[86]   Ni Y, Zhao L, Yu H, *et al.* Circulating Unsaturated Fatty Acids Delineate the Metabolic Status of Obese Individuals. EBioMedicine 2015; 2(10): 1513-22.
[http://dx.doi.org/10.1016/j.ebiom.2015.09.004] [PMID: 26629547]

[87]   Krotkiewski M, Björntorp P, Sjöström L, Smith U. Impact of obesity on metabolism in men and women. Importance of regional adipose tissue distribution. J Clin Invest 1983; 72(3): 1150-62.
[http://dx.doi.org/10.1172/JCI111040] [PMID: 6350364]

[88]   Laws A, Hoen HM, Selby JV, Saad MF, Haffner SM, Howard BV. Insulin Resistance Atherosclerosis Study (IRAS) Investigators. Differences in insulin suppression of free fatty acid levels by gender and glucose tolerance status. Relation to plasma triglyceride and apolipoprotein B concentrations. Arterioscler Thromb Vasc Biol 1997; 17(1): 64-71.
[http://dx.doi.org/10.1161/01.ATV.17.1.64] [PMID: 9012639]

[89]   Frias JP, Macaraeg GB, Ofrecio J, Yu JG, Olefsky JM, Kruszynska YT. Decreased susceptibility to fatty acid-induced peripheral tissue insulin resistance in women. Diabetes 2001; 50(6): 1344-50.
[http://dx.doi.org/10.2337/diabetes.50.6.1344] [PMID: 11375335]

[90]   Ford ES. Prevalence of the metabolic syndrome defined by the International Diabetes Federation among adults in the U.S. Diabetes Care 2005; 28(11): 2745-9.
[http://dx.doi.org/10.2337/diacare.28.11.2745] [PMID: 16249550]

[91]   Toth MJ, Poehlman ET, Matthews DE, Tchernof A, MacCoss MJ. Effects of estradiol and progesterone on body composition, protein synthesis, and lipoprotein lipase in rats. Am J Physiol Endocrinol Metab 2001; 280(3): E496-501.
[http://dx.doi.org/10.1152/ajpendo.2001.280.3.E496] [PMID: 11171605]

[92]   Lizcano F, Guzmán G. Estrogen Deficiency and the Origin of Obesity during Menopause. BioMed Res Int 2014; 2014757461
[http://dx.doi.org/10.1155/2014/757461] [PMID: 24734243]

[93]   Kabat GC, Wu WY-Y, Bea JW, *et al.* Metabolic phenotypes of obesity: frequency, correlates and change over time in a cohort of postmenopausal women. Int J Obes 2017; 41(1): 170-7.
[http://dx.doi.org/10.1038/ijo.2016.179] [PMID: 27748744]

[94]   Salpeter SR, Walsh JME, Ormiston TM, Greyber E, Buckley NS, Salpeter EE. Meta-analysis: effect of hormone-replacement therapy on components of the metabolic syndrome in postmenopausal women. Diabetes Obes Metab 2006; 8(5): 538-54.
[http://dx.doi.org/10.1111/j.1463-1326.2005.00545.x] [PMID: 16918589]

[95]   Crespo CJ, Smit E, Snelling A, Sempos CT, Andersen RE. NHANES III. Hormone replacement therapy and its relationship to lipid and glucose metabolism in diabetic and nondiabetic postmenopausal women: results from the Third National Health and Nutrition Examination Survey (NHANES III). Diabetes Care 2002; 25(10): 1675-80.
[http://dx.doi.org/10.2337/diacare.25.10.1675] [PMID: 12351460]

[96]   Stubbins RE, Najjar K, Holcomb VB, Hong J, Núñez NP. Oestrogen alters adipocyte biology and protects female mice from adipocyte inflammation and insulin resistance. Diabetes Obes Metab 2012; 14(1): 58-66.
[http://dx.doi.org/10.1111/j.1463-1326.2011.01488.x] [PMID: 21834845]

[97]   Mouly TA, Toms LL. Breast cancer and persistent organic pollutants (excluding DDT): a systematic literature review. Environ Sci Pollut Res Int 2016; 23(22): 22385-407.
[http://dx.doi.org/10.1007/s11356-016-7577-1] [PMID: 27628920]

[98] Gauthier M-S, Rabasa-Lhoret R, Prud'homme D, *et al.* The metabolically healthy but obese phenotype is associated with lower plasma levels of persistent organic pollutants as compared to the metabolically abnormal obese phenotype. J Clin Endocrinol Metab 2014; 99(6): E1061-6.
[http://dx.doi.org/10.1210/jc.2013-3935] [PMID: 24606089]

[99] Pestana D, Faria G, Sá C, *et al.* Persistent organic pollutant levels in human visceral and subcutaneous adipose tissue in obese individuals--depot differences and dysmetabolism implications. Environ Res 2014; 133: 170-7.
[http://dx.doi.org/10.1016/j.envres.2014.05.026] [PMID: 24949816]

[100] Teixeira D, Pestana D, Calhau C, Monteiro R. Letter to the Editor. J Clin Endocrinol Metab 2014. Available from: http://press.endocrine.org/e-letters/10.1210/jc.2013-3935

[101] Teixeira D, Pestana D, Santos C, *et al.* Inflammatory and cardiometabolic risk on obesity: role of environmental xenoestrogens. J Clin Endocrinol Metab 2015; 100(5): 1792-801.
[http://dx.doi.org/10.1210/jc.2014-4136] [PMID: 25853792]

[102] Teixeira D, Marques C, Pestana D, *et al.* Effects of xenoestrogens in human M1 and M2 macrophage migration, cytokine release, and estrogen-related signaling pathways. Environ Toxicol 2016; 31(11): 1496-509.
[http://dx.doi.org/10.1002/tox.22154] [PMID: 26011183]

[103] Pestana D, Teixeira D, Meireles M, *et al.* Adipose tissue dysfunction as a central mechanism leading to dysmetabolic obesity triggered by chronic exposure to p,p'-DDE. Sci Rep 2017; 7(1): 2738.
[http://dx.doi.org/10.1038/s41598-017-02885-9] [PMID: 28572628]

[104] Smink A, Ribas-Fito N, Garcia R, *et al.* Exposure to hexachlorobenzene during pregnancy increases the risk of overweight in children aged 6 years. Acta Paediatr 2008; 97(10): 1465-9.
[http://dx.doi.org/10.1111/j.1651-2227.2008.00937.x] [PMID: 18665907]

[105] Lee D-H, Steffes MW, Sjödin A, *et al.* Low Dose Organochlorine Pesticides and Polychlorinated Biphenyls Predict Obesity, Dyslipidemia, and Insulin Resistance among People Free of Diabetes. Pan X, editor.PLoS One. 2011; 6: p. (1)e15977..

[106] Festi D, Schiumerini R, Eusebi LH, Marasco G, Taddia M, Colecchia A. Gut microbiota and metabolic syndrome. World J Gastroenterol 2014; 20(43): 16079-94.
[http://dx.doi.org/10.3748/wjg.v20.i43.16079] [PMID: 25473159]

[107] Ley RE, Turnbaugh PJ, Klein S, Gordon JI. Microbial ecology: human gut microbes associated with obesity. Nature 2006; 444(7122): 1022-3.
[http://dx.doi.org/10.1038/4441022a] [PMID: 17183309]

[108] Santacruz A, Collado MC, García-Valdés L, *et al.* Gut microbiota composition is associated with body weight, weight gain and biochemical parameters in pregnant women. Br J Nutr 2010; 104(1): 83-92.
[http://dx.doi.org/10.1017/S0007114510000176] [PMID: 20205964]

[109] Kim K-A, Gu W, Lee I-A, Joh E-H, Kim D-H. High Fat Diet-Induced Gut Microbiota Exacerbates Inflammation and Obesity in Mice via the TLR4 Signaling Pathway.Chamaillard M, editor PLoS One. 2012; 7: p. (10)e47713..
[http://dx.doi.org/10.1371/journal.pone.0047713]

[110] Boutagy NE, McMillan RP, Frisard MI, Hulver MW. Metabolic endotoxemia with obesity: Is it real and is it relevant? Biochimie 2016; 124: 11-20.
[http://dx.doi.org/10.1016/j.biochi.2015.06.020] [PMID: 26133659]

[111] Erridge C, Attina T, Spickett CM, Webb DJ. A high-fat meal induces low-grade endotoxemia: evidence of a novel mechanism of postprandial inflammation. Am J Clin Nutr 2007; 86(5): 1286-92.
[http://dx.doi.org/10.1093/ajcn/86.5.1286] [PMID: 17991637]

[112] Cani PD, Amar J, Iglesias MA, *et al.* Metabolic endotoxemia initiates obesity and insulin resistance. Diabetes 2007; 56(7): 1761-72.
[http://dx.doi.org/10.2337/db06-1491] [PMID: 17456850]

[113] Creely SJ, McTernan PG, Kusminski CM, *et al.* Lipopolysaccharide activates an innate immune system response in human adipose tissue in obesity and type 2 diabetes. Am J Physiol Endocrinol Metab 2007; 292(3): E740-7.
[http://dx.doi.org/10.1152/ajpendo.00302.2006] [PMID: 17090751]

[114] Pussinen PJ, Havulinna AS, Lehto M, Sundvall J, Salomaa V. Endotoxemia is associated with an increased risk of incident diabetes. Diabetes Care 2011; 34(2): 392-7.
[http://dx.doi.org/10.2337/dc10-1676] [PMID: 21270197]

[115] Liu X, Lu L, Yao P, *et al.* Lipopolysaccharide binding protein, obesity status and incidence of metabolic syndrome: a prospective study among middle-aged and older Chinese. Diabetologia 2014; 57(9): 1834-41.
[http://dx.doi.org/10.1007/s00125-014-3288-7] [PMID: 24906952]

[116] Neal MD, Leaphart C, Levy R, *et al.* Enterocyte TLR4 mediates phagocytosis and translocation of bacteria across the intestinal barrier. J Immunol 2006; 176(5): 3070-9.
[http://dx.doi.org/10.4049/jimmunol.176.5.3070] [PMID: 16493066]

[117] Boulangé CL, Neves AL, Chilloux J, Nicholson JK, Dumas M-E. Impact of the gut microbiota on inflammation, obesity, and metabolic disease. Genome Med 2016; 8(1): 42.
[http://dx.doi.org/10.1186/s13073-016-0303-2] [PMID: 27098727]

[118] Rial SA, Karelis AD, Bergeron KF, Mounier C. Gut microbiota and metabolic health: The potential beneficial effects of a medium chain triglyceride diet in obese individualsNutrients. Multidisciplinary Digital Publishing Institute (MDPI) 2016; 8.

[119] Vandanmagsar B, Youm Y-H, Ravussin A, *et al.* The NLRP3 inflammasome instigates obesity-induced inflammation and insulin resistance. Nat Med 2011; 17(2): 179-88.
[http://dx.doi.org/10.1038/nm.2279] [PMID: 21217695]

[120] Mori MA, Bezy O, Kahn CR. Metabolic syndrome: is Nlrp3 inflammasome a trigger or a target of insulin resistance? Circ Res 2011; 108(10): 1160-2.
[http://dx.doi.org/10.1161/RES.0b013e318220b57b] [PMID: 21566220]

[121] Esser N, L'homme L, De Roover A, *et al.* Obesity phenotype is related to NLRP3 inflammasome activity and immunological profile of visceral adipose tissue. Diabetologia 2013; 56(11): 2487-97.
[http://dx.doi.org/10.1007/s00125-013-3023-9] [PMID: 24013717]

[122] Murphy AJ, Kraakman MJ, Kammoun HL, *et al.* IL-18 Production from the NLRP1 Inflammasome Prevents Obesity and Metabolic Syndrome. Cell Metab 2016; 23(1): 155-64.
[http://dx.doi.org/10.1016/j.cmet.2015.09.024] [PMID: 26603191]

[123] Dandona P, Ghanim H, Chaudhuri A, Mohanty P. Macronutrient intake, insulin secretion, oxidative stress & inflammation: Clinico-pathological implications. Indian J Med Res 2016; 144(5): 645-9.
[http://dx.doi.org/10.4103/ijmr.IJMR_1807_16] [PMID: 28361814]

[124] Åsgård R, Rytter E, Basu S, *et al.* High intake of fruit and vegetables is related to low oxidative stress and inflammation in a group of patients with type 2 diabetes. Scand J Food Nutr 2007; 51(4): 149-58.
[http://dx.doi.org/10.1080/17482970701737285]

[125] Park Y-M, Steck SE, Fung TT, *et al.* Mediterranean diet and mortality risk in metabolically healthy obese and metabolically unhealthy obese phenotypes. Int J Obes 2016; 40(10): 1541-9.
[http://dx.doi.org/10.1038/ijo.2016.114] [PMID: 27339604]

[126] Larsen CM, Faulenbach M, Vaag A, *et al.* Interleukin-1-receptor antagonist in type 2 diabetes mellitus. N Engl J Med 2007; 356(15): 1517-26.
[http://dx.doi.org/10.1056/NEJMoa065213] [PMID: 17429083]

[127] Esterson YB, Zhang K, Koppaka S, *et al.* Insulin sensitizing and anti-inflammatory effects of thiazolidinediones are heightened in obese patients. J Investig Med 2013; 61(8): 1152-60.
[http://dx.doi.org/10.2310/JIM.0000000000000017] [PMID: 24141239]

[128] Bell JA, Kivimaki M, Hamer M. Metabolically healthy obesity and risk of incident type 2 diabetes: a meta-analysis of prospective cohort studies. Obes Rev 2014; 15(6): 504-15.
[http://dx.doi.org/10.1111/obr.12157] [PMID: 24661566]

CHAPTER 6

Environmental Chemical Obesogens

Diana Teixeira[1,2,3,4] and **Diogo Pestana**[1,4,*]

[1] *Nutrition and Metabolism, NOVA Medical School, Faculdade de Ciências Médicas, Universidade NOVA de Lisboa, Lisboa, Portugal*

[2] *Comprehensive Health Research Centre, Universidade NOVA de Lisboa, Lisboa, Portugal*

[3] *Unidade Universitária Lifestyle Medicine da José Mello Saúde by NOVA Medical School, Lisboa, Portugal*

[4] *CINTESIS - Center for Health Technology and Services Research, University of Porto, Porto, Portugal*

Abstract: Understanding the myriad of factors contributing to obesity is essential for curbing its decade-long expansion. Recently, despite the evidence of traditional contributing factors, the role of environmental chemicals with endocrine disrupting activity has also been highlighted. Undeniably, even very small concentrations of these endocrine disrupting chemicals (EDCs) have the capacity to induce severe health damages. The "environmental obesogen" hypothesis associates EDCs to the disruption of energy homeostasis, in particular because of their ability to modulate adipocyte biology. Further studies have revealed numerous potential mechanisms, including modulation of nuclear hormone receptor function and modification of the epigenome. More recently, their involvement in exacerbating metabolic dysfunction in an obesity context reinforces the hypothesis that EDCs have an important "environmental dysmetabolic" effect. Besides adulthood exposure, the perinatal effects are very important since they may allow a change in metabolic programming, encouraging the further development of obesity. Consequently, additional research directed at understanding the nature and action of EDCs will illuminate the connection between health and environment as well as the possible effects triggered by these compounds in respect to public health. Nutrition is being further substantiated as an important modulator of inflammatory and antioxidant pathways, especially associated with environmental insult; nutrition is also emerging as a tool to address exposure toxicity of ECDs as both a sensing and remediation platform. Ultimately, improving EDC exposure measurement, reducing confounding bias, identifying discrete periods of vulnerability and quantifying the effects of EDC mixtures will enhance inferences originated from epidemiological studies.

* **Corresponding author Diogo Pestana:** NOVA Medical School, Faculdade de Ciências Médicas, Universidade Nova de Lisboa. Campo dos Mártires da Pátria, 130, 1169-056 Lisboa, Portugal; Tel/Fax: +351 218803033; E-mail: diogopestana@nms.unl.pt

Rosário Monteiro and Maria João Martins (Eds.)

Keywords: Adipose tissue, Adipocytes, Cardiometabolic disease, Endocrine disrupting chemicals, Epigenetics, Inflammation, Metabolic syndrome, Metabolism-disrupting chemicals, Microbiota, Nutrition, Obesity, Obesity paradox, Obesogens, Type 2 diabetes.

INTRODUCTION

Obesity prevalence has been a global public health problem. What started being a concern of the wealthy nations, mainly due to their abundance-based society, soon began to spread worldwide reaching epidemic proportions [1 - 3]. Adding to this, child excessive weight and obesity are also rapidly increasing, an alarming perspective as it foretells them as obese adults [4]. Moreover, the rate at which the prevalence of obesity is increasing suggests that environmental and behavioural influences are "fuelling" the epidemic [1, 5].

In fact, the writings and insights on the ancient Greece are striking for the history of environmental health. Hippocrates, the father of medicine, highlighted the environment as an influence on the status of people's health in his work Airs, Waters and Places, suggesting that the environment (*e.g.*, quality of air, water and food) was influential in causing changes in human health. Despite the great increases in medical knowledge that have occurred since Hippocrates time, many of his principles remain plausible [6].

In 1970 Rachel Carson in "Silent Spring" underlined the potential dangers of pesticides. More recently, accumulating data suggest an important role for toxicology in obesity. In 2002, Baillie-Hamilton, in a provocative hypothesis to explain the global obesity epidemic, underscored the fact that the current exponential increase of obesity could not be justified merely by the alterations of food intake and a lack of physical activity [1].

ENDOCRINE DISRUPTING CHEMICALS - WHAT, WHY AND WHERE?

Endocrine disrupting chemicals (EDCs), are defined as "an exogenous chemical, or a mixture of chemicals, that interferes with any aspect of hormone action", according to the Endocrine Society [7], a simplified definition version of the originally proposed by the United States Environmental Protection Agency "EDCs are exogenous agents that interferes with the production, release, transport, metabolism, binding, action, or elimination of natural hormones in the body responsible for the maintenance of homeostasis and the regulation of developmental processes" [8]. Currently, the United Nations Environment Programme (UNEP) and the World Health Organization (WHO) definition of EDCs is "an exogenous substance or mixture that alters the function(s) of the endocrine system and consequently causes adverse health effects in an intact organism, or its progeny or (sub) populations" [9 - 11].

EDCs are an immense number of compounds, with distinct chemical structures, properties and applications, and until now approximately 1000 chemicals meet the criteria of an EDC [12, 13]. Some are plastics [*e.g.*, bisphenol A (BPA), phthalates], solvents [*e.g.*, polychlorinated biphenyls (PCBs), polybrominated biphenyls (PBBs), dioxins], pesticides and fungicides [*e.g.*, organotins, methoxychlor, chlorpyrifos, dichlorodiphenytrichloroethane (DDT), vinclozolin], personal care products (*e.g.*, triclosan), pharmaceutical agents (*e.g.*, thiazolidinediones, antihistamines, antidepressants) and synthetic hormones (*e.g.*, ethynilestradiol). Some natural compounds are also known as EDCs (*e.g.* phytoestrogens, including genistein and coumestrol) [14, 15]. Through the food-chain, these compounds can experience bioaccumulation and biomagnification, being persistent in the environment. In contrast, others are easily degraded but their continuous release into the environment still makes them cause of concern [16]. Several EDCs share a structural phenolic ring and other hydrophobic components Fig. (**1**), a characteristic of similarity with different nuclear receptor-activating compounds and steroid hormones. Additionally, they have potent lipophilic properties and long half-lives [17]. Finally, heavy metals, which may be involved in occupational or residential exposure, are another class of EDCs (*i.e.*, cadmium, mercury, and arsenic) [18, 19].

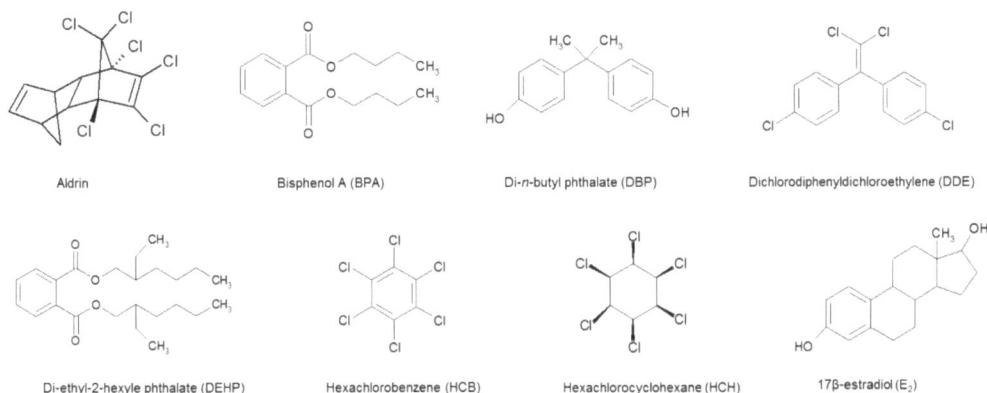

Fig. (1). Chemical structures of aldrin, bisphenol A (BPA), di-*n*-butyl phthalate (DBP), dichlorodiphenyldichloroethylene (DDE), di-ethyl-2-hexyle phthalate (DEHP), hexachlorobenzene (HCB), hexachlorocyclohexane (HCH) and 17β-estradiol (E_2).

Globally, the population is ubiquitously exposed to ECDs in daily life, which usually occurs through ingestion, inhalation or dermal absorption [20]. Thus, an individual should be contaminated with more than one compound, sometimes from different classes, enabling harmful effects potentially additive or synergistic [14].

Often occurring at very low levels, EDCs might induce tissue and time-dependent effects with non-monotonic responses (biphasic or U-shaped responses). For all of this, it is urgent that regulatory decisions on EDCs must be based on the principles of endocrinology and not only under a classical toxicological point of view [21, 22].

Given the lipophilic properties of EDCs, the adipose tissue (AT) has a main role on their kinetics. In fact, despite being constituted by different cell types, the EDCs storage in AT is believed to occur primarily in adipocytes [23]. Even more, AT is an endocrine and metabolic organ and could itself be a target of these pollutants Fig. (**2**) [24 - 26]. Several studies established that AT storage of EDCs has a central role in EDC toxicity [24, 27], however the complete knowledge of EDC distribution and dynamics in the body, mechanisms of action, and the molecular pathways involved in EDC toxicity remain unclear and constitute a hot topic of current research.

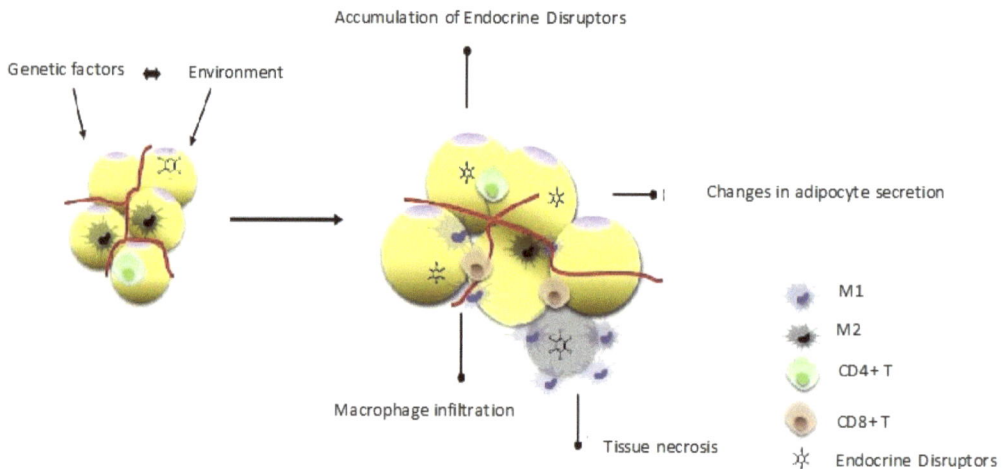

Fig. (2). Overview of the changes that occur during adipose tissue growth. Adapted from Myre *et al* [26].

EDCs action can be primarily mediated by two mechanisms: i) they can interfere in components of the endocrine system, or in the feedback loops in the brain, pituitary, gonads, thyroid, or others, temporarily or permanently, by mimicking hormone action and triggering their specific receptors, or ii) they block their action by binding to hormone receptors, antagonising its endocrine effect. EDCs may also interfere with the production, transport, and metabolism of endogenous hormones [28, 29]. Concerning their mechanism of action, there is still a paucity of data. In the light of current knowledge, it is known that they can interfere in pathways related to steroid biosynthesis and/or metabolism, and also act through nuclear receptors, nonnuclear steroid hormone receptors [such as membrane estrogen receptors (GPER) [30]], nonsteroid receptors (*e.g.,* neurotransmitter receptors) and orphan receptors [*e.g.,* aryl hydrocarbon receptor (AhR)] [31].

First of all, substances changing sex hormone signaling may be estrogenic, androgenic, antiestrogenic and antiandrogenic, which has been reported not only for individual compounds but also for complex mixtures of EDCs [32]. Furthermore, these chemical substances of anthropogenic origin may differ on agonistic/antagonistic potencies adding complexity to the study of their health effects [33]. EDCs, such as BPA, are known to act not only through classic nuclear estrogen receptors (ERs), but also via nonclassical estrogen-triggered pathways [34], leading to metabolic dysfunction and disruption of insulin signaling [35, 36]. By the inhibition of aromatase, these substances may also interfere with hormone synthesis [37]. Furthermore, circulating EDCs may deregulate the hypothalamus-pituitary-gonadal axis through the change on gonadotropin release [38], with consequences not only to reproductive function but also to metabolism, given the known roles of sex hormones in the regulation of energy balance. Upon exposure to EDCs with thyroid hormone-disrupting abilities [32], the regulation of key steps in organ development (brain, ear and bone) and in metabolism of carbohydrates, lipids and proteins that impact on the metabolic rate, may become impaired [39, 40].

Coordination the whole body's response to daily nutritional fluctuations is another target of action of EDCs. It is well known that hypothalamic-pituitary-adrenal (HPA) axis plays a critical role to regulate energy homeostasis. In peripheral tissues, glucocorticoid signaling can be influenced by EDCs, in addition to systemic adrenal production namely changes in 11β-hydroxysteroid dehydrogenase (11β-HSD) types 1 and 2 activities, the enzymes that mediate the interconversion between cortisone and cortisol, respectively [41].

A key integrator of detoxification and bioactivation of xenobiotics is the AhR, which has roles on the metabolism of endogenous (mainly hormones) and exogenous substances [42]. Moreover, AhR upon activation by dioxins, may affect cell proliferation, differentiation, apoptosis and intercellular communication [43, 44], being implicated in tumor promotion [43, 45, 46]. EDC interaction with AhR may compromise normal cell functions by activating oxidative stress-sensitive signaling and subsequent proinflammatory pathways. Environmental contaminants as PCBs, are AhR agonists, establishing a link between exposure and inflammation [47].

Peroxisome proliferator activated receptors (PPARs), liver X receptor (LXR), farnesoid X receptor (FXR), estrogen-related receptors (ERRs) and retinoid X receptors (RXRs), master transcriptional regulators critical to the regulation of metabolic pathways leading to obesity have also been demonstrated as possible EDC targets [48, 49]. The activation of nuclear receptors such as PPAR and LXR by EDCs interferes with the expression of an array of genes involved in lipid metabolism and inflammation [48, 50, 51]. EDC interference in the inflammatory processes may result from oxidative stress, mitochondrial dysfunction and epigenetic modifications [49, 52]. Given the largely demonstrated association between inflammation and metabolic dysfunction [53], inflammatory disruption is yet another mechanism exerted by EDCs likely to favor metabolic syndrome (MetS) development. Since estrogens affect the immune system and inflammatory processes [54 - 56], the ability of some EDCs to either interfere with estrogen signaling or metabolism may contribute to the dysfunction in these metabolic and inflammatory control homeostatic mechanisms [57, 58] and actions are exemplified by changes in cytokine, adipokine and autacoid synthesis with local and/or systemic effects [59 - 61].

Epigenetic processes are also involved in these endocrine disrupting effects, through modifications of factors that regulate gene expression independently of modifications to the DNA sequence. These effects include changes in DNA methyltransferases, histone acetyltransferases, histone deacetylases and histone methyltransferases, with possible significant and sustained effects on gene transcription [62, 63]. Indeed, epigenetic changes mediated by dietary and environmental factors, rather than genetic changes, are a more plausible explanation for the obesity epidemic in Western countries [64]. Showing the increased interest of the scientific community in this area, a recent paper points to the existence of epigenetic drivers of disease [65]. It demonstrates that nonalcoholic fatty liver disease has a specific DNA methylation signature that changes after bariatric surgery, thus providing a data set of epigenetic organ remodeling in humans [65].

In addition, an exciting aspect of epigenetics is the opportunity to integrate exposures as a type of 'exposome', leading to the expansion of environmental epigenetics field [66]. Although several EDCs have been shown to elicit modifications in DNA methylation or microRNA expression [67 - 69], knowledge regarding the epigenetic mechanisms and DNA methylation signatures related with disease progression and interaction with environmental exposures is still scarce, namely in relation to the obesogenic effect. Additionally, one of the ultimate goals is to define novel and potentially useful disease biomarkers, namely in the interaction with environmental exposures and disease progression.

ENDOCRINE DISRUPTING CHEMICALS AS OBESOGENS

In 2002 Baillie-Hamilton [1], presented evidence that confirmed earlier toxicologic studies published as far back as the 1970s in which low-dose chemical exposures were associated with weight gain in experimental animals.

Conceptually the "environmental obesogen" hypothesis postulates that chemicals are able to promote obesity by altering homeostatic metabolic set-points, disrupting appetite controls, perturbing lipid homeostasis to promote adipocyte hypertrophy, or stimulating adipogenic pathways that enhance adipocyte hyperplasia during development or in adulthood [70].

Epidemiological studies have shown that exposure to EDCs is near ubiquitous among humans. Wittassek *et al* [71] showed that 98% of urine samples in a German sample have detectable phthalate metabolites, indicating ubiquitous exposure through the last 20 years. In another study, Calafat *et al* [72] found that BPA was detected in 95% and 4-nonylphenol in 51% of the 394 adult urinary samples. Some studies have studied the distribution of EDCs among different fat depots. For example, Kim *et al* [73] recently found that visceral adipose tissue (vAT) contains higher levels of over 20 PCBs and p,p'-dichlorodiphenyldichloroethane (p,p'-DDD) but lower p,p'-DDT in a type 2 diabetes (T2D) case-control study of 50 hospitalized Korean patients. Pestana *et al* [74] also reported higher p,p'-DDD and p,p'-dichlorodiphenyldichloroethylene (p,p'-DDE) but lower hexachlorocyclohexane, aldrin, and dieldrin levels in vAT compared to those of subcutaneous adipose tissue (scAT) among obese portuguese subjects. Organochlorine pesticide (OCP) concentrations were also found in plasma and in abdominal and femoral scAT among men under a weight loss program [75, 76]. However, there is a scarcity of population-based epidemiologic studies evaluating associations between EDCs and obesity, and some controversy in existing data. In fact, Goncharov *et al* [77] in a Native American population, note that individuals with higher levels of PCBs tend to have higher levels of total serum lipids, showing a significant association among PCBs, lipids, age and BMI. Contrarily, Hue *et al* [78] reported no association in 53 individuals ranging from lean to obese. Even more, Pelletier *et al* [79] revealed that plasma OCPs concentrations are positively associated with higher BMI and fat mass in humans. Another study showed that serum BPA is higher in non-obese and obese women with polycystic ovary syndrome than in non-obese women without the syndrome [80]. In a population of the National Health and Nutrition Examination Survey (NHANES), an association between persistent organic pollutants (POPs; polychlorinated dibenzo-p-dioxins, and OCPs) and T2D was found among obese individuals [81]. Further investigations showed a decrease of non-dioxin PCBs levels with BMI and opposite association regarding to OCPs

[82, 83]. Taken together, these epidemiological reports suggest that environmental exposures to various EDCs play a role in overweight/obesity and comorbidities. Since there are so many diverse chemicals involved, they are most likely exerting their effects through multiple pathways.

Recently, the adipocyte has been proposed as a new target of EDCs. A newly emerging hypothesis is that exposure to environmental chemicals during development may play a role in the development of obesity later in life [84]. One example is a chemical widely used as surfactant, octylphenol, which may cause insulin-resistance and decrease adipocyte differentiation through upregulation of resistin, an adipocyte-specific hormone [1]. Other examples are a group of industrial chemicals produced in high quantities, highly lipophilic, the brominated flame retardants, that bioaccumulate in AT [85] as well as a high production volume chemical used in the manufacture of polycarbonate plastics, BPA, which can be used in baby and water bottles and epoxide resins that are used in food container linings [86]. Studies on the impact of BPA on AT yielded conflicting results, most likely due to the wide range of administered doses [87, 88]. The time of exposure is important too. When given to rats at high doses for 15 days, BPA causes reduction in body weight and in feeding efficiency [88] while others found that feeding BPA to rats for three months did not alter body weight, fat depots or triglyceride levels [89]. The role of BPA in AT development is provided by *in vitro* studies. BPA leads to an increase in 3T3-L1 differentiation and when in combination with insulin, accelerates adipocyte formation [89]. Recently, Hugo *et al* [90] reported that at low environmental-relevant doses, BPA inhibits adiponectin synthesis and stimulates the release of inflammatory adipokines, such as interleukin 6 (IL6) and tumor necrosis factor alpha (TNFα) from human AT, proposing an involvement of BPA in the inflammatory state associated with obesity.

An especially sensitive time frame for exposure to obesogens has been found to be either *in utero* or in the neonatal period [20].

Perinatal exposure is an important key factor, as the developing fetus is extremely sensitive to disturbance. Indeed, the epidemiological associations between poor fetal and infant growth and the subsequent development of metabolic diseases later in life result from the effects of poor nutrition in early life, which produces permanent changes in metabolism closes the 'thrifty-phenotype hypothesis' [91, 92]. In fact, the developing organism responds to cues of environmental quality by selecting an appropriate trajectory of growth in order to promote survival, leading to early-life metabolic adaptations and preparing the organism for its likely adult environment [93]. However, these established traits are misfits for the present obesogenic environment. An emerging additional view hypothesizes that perinatal exposure to EDCs at low environmentally-relevant doses might promote metabolic programming of obesity and metabolic risk [94 - 97]. Actually, it is now well known that perinatal exposure to these compounds may occur, influencing birth weight and later health outcomes [98 - 103]. The hormone-like activity of EDCs can disrupt the programming of endocrine signaling pathways that are established during perinatal differentiation, contributing to the development of obesity in adulthood. The specific pathways and mechanisms affected by perinatal exposure may be dependent upon the dose and the precise time of exposure, as well as other factors such as circulating endogenous hormone levels present during exposure [58].

To date, imprinting of obesity-related genes or changes in cell type and number (such as adipocytes) are pointed out as plausible molecular mechanisms [92, 104]. Epigenetic alterations appear to be the most likely mechanisms that could explain perinatal programming leading to later-life obesity and metabolic diseases [105], giving rise to the thrifty epigenotype hypothesis. Among the several environmental exposures, BPA exposure with influence in later disease risk is becoming increasingly well documented [106, 107]. Indeed, *in utero* exposure to environmentally relevant doses of BPA was shown to have a disruption impact on glucose homeostasis and gene expression of adult mice offspring, contributing to the development of metabolic disorders. Furthermore, the extensive harms of perinatal tobacco smoke exposure [108, 109], and its relationship with childhood overweight/obesity provide a proof-of-concept of how early-life exposure to EDCs can be a risk factor for obesity and MetS [109]. The mechanisms by which this perinatal exposure programs the AT and endocrine function are still under investigation, but it is already known that maternal tobacco smoke predisposes human and rat offspring to visceral obesity in early adulthood, possibly by programming AT dysfunction via alterations in the glucocorticoid pathway and development of leptin and insulin resistance [108, 110]. The increasing identification of genes with smoking-related methylation changes in newborns and adults reinforces epigenetic modifications, such as DNA methylation, as one of the main mechanisms by which smoking-related compounds (and other EDCs) might have long-lasting effects [111]. Furthermore, in animals, epigenetic effects, such as DNA methylation, can also be passed to successive generations, promoting a transgenerational inheritance of environmental obesogens [112, 113].

Evidently, these prenatal effects can initially occur through changes in the main organ involved in supplying nutrients to the fetus, the placenta, affecting feto-placental development and subsequent adulthood metabolic disease. In addition to changes in placenta size and morphology, changes in the epigenetic regulation of imprinting genes and transporter gene expression are also important to fetal programming [114].

Another mechanism of EDC action may the disturbance in neuroendocrine control, modifying the balance between energy intake and energy expenditure, especially by altering appetite and satiety regulation, as well as food preferences. Recently, in humans, BPA levels have been found to correlate with circulating levels of leptin and ghrelin. These adipokines act in opposing ways to regulate hunger, with leptin being inhibitory and ghrelin being stimulatory. Alterations in circulating levels of these hormones due to BPA exposure suggests that BPA may potentially be able interfere with hormonal control of hunger and satiety [115].

The gastrointestinal (GI) tract is exposed to high levels of pollutants, because the primary routes of exposure are through water and foods. Thus, interactions between EDCs and gut microbiota may disrupt homeostasis, leading to metabolic diseases such as obesity and diabetes.

Microbiota can directly metabolize a variety of environmental EDCs immediately after ingestion or subsequently to their conjugation by the liver. Reciprocally, EDCs can interfere with the composition and/or metabolic activity of the microbiota, with potentially deleterious consequences for the host [116 - 118].

Gut microbiota has the ability to perform diverse chemical transformations on drugs, including reduction, hydrolysis, the removal of a succinate group, dehydroxylation, acetylation, deacetylation, the cleavage of N-oxide bounds, proteolysis, denitration, deconjugation, thiazole ring opening, deglycosylation and demethylation [119].

The rate and extent of microbiota metabolism is influenced by the amounts of EDCs reaching the distal gut, where bacteria concentration is maximal. EDCs may be directly metabolized by the gut microbiota, since they may be poorly absorbed after ingestion, subsequently being swept to the distal small intestine and caecum by peristalsis. Several environmental chemicals have also been shown to inhibit gut microbiota growth or to induce dysbiosis *in vitro* and *in vivo* [119].

Furthermore, some EDCs might impact on GI microbiota physiology without inducing dysbiosis: exposure to EDCs during the perinatal period and early childhood may have a critical influence on the development of the gut microbiota and related microbiota-dependent host physiological functions, such as immune-system development [120]. It therefore seems plausible that chemical-induced disturbances of the composition of the GI microbiota may constitute an underestimated mechanism, which will compromise host physiology later in life.

EDCs (or their metabolites) may also be excreted in the bile. After being absorbed in the GI tract, most EDCs are transported by the portal blood to the liver for detoxification. The liver generally oxidizes EDCs and produces glucuronic acid, sulfate or glutathione conjugates and conjugates may be in most cases, eliminated in urine [119].

In adult male mice model, that either carried or lacked the AhR gene, Zang *et al* [121] confirm that 2,3,7,8-tetrachlorodibenzofuran (TCDF) (equivalent to approximately 3,000 ng/kg body weight in humans), in an AhR-dependent manner, increased gut inflammation, modulated the gut microbiota population (significantly shifting from *Firmicutes* toward *Bacteroidetes*), increased gut bacterial fermentation and had a profound impact on host metabolome.

The challenge of actual toxicology and EDC research are the mixture of multiple EDCs [122]. Thus, the analysis of complex mixtures and of the body burden in EDCs is currently a huge concern. In fact, an international effort to understand the true magnitude of human contamination being made. Nevertheless, despite this apparent commitment, many countries continue to disregard that hazard [123]. Thus, the development of easy and cost/effective procedures for EDC identification and quantification in the environment and biological samples and the clear demonstration of their effects on human health is a decisive step for the prosecution of biomonitoring programs and adds evidence for their wide recognition as health hazards.

YIN-YANG ROLE OF ADIPOSE TISSUE IN ENDOCRINE DISRUPTING CHEMICAL TOXICOLOGY

Attention was drawn to a specific group of EDCs, the POPs, that include numerous compounds with common features, such as dioxins, OCPs and PCBs [124]. Their lipophilic nature, allied with extreme resistance to chemical and biological degradation, are responsible for their persistence in environment and consequent harmful effects [125]. As lipophilic compounds, POPs are bioaccumulated in fatty tissues, and their levels increase along the trophic chain (biomagnification). In humans, the main exposure route is the ingestion of fat-containing food such as meat, fish and dairy products [125, 126]. Being at the top of the food chain, humans concentrate higher levels of POPs, that can be detected in several fluids and tissues, such as AT (the main reservoir), blood and breast milk [123, 127].

Indeed, it is now well recognized that AT is not a simple organ consisting of adipocytes (and other cell types), blood vessels and endogenous molecules, but can also be broadly contaminated with several man-made lipophilic chemicals [128]. Due to their continuous release into the environment, less lipophilic and resistant chemicals such as BPA, nonylphenol, polycyclic aromatic hydrocarbons and synthetic musk compounds have also been detected in AT [128 - 130].

Nonetheless, as a natural storage compartment for lipids and lipophilic molecules, AT is considered a relatively safe organ for EDC accumulation [24, 128]. However, as AT is also a highly active organ with important metabolic, endocrine and toxicological functions, the presence of these EDCs in AT goes beyond serving as their main accumulation site [24]. Despite seeming paradoxical, AT plays a central yin-yang role in EDC toxicology, acting as a protector/modulator and as a target of toxicity [24].

Upon exposure, the lipophilic EDCs are sequestered in AT, specifically within lipid droplets of adipocytes [23]. From a toxicokinetics and toxicodynamics perspective, this EDC accumulation in AT can be regarded as protective, as it can prevent free circulation of these toxic compounds and their systemic effects [1, 77, 131 - 133]. Experimental evidence supports that this accumulation can represent a protective function of AT, limiting the exposure of other critical organs and tissues to EDC toxicity [24], that could lead to metabolic dysfunction and T2D [127]. This yin role of AT may be determinant to sustain metabolic health. But although being protective to some extent under conditions of acute or subacute exposure, ultimately, it could also be a risk [24].

Indeed, if on one hand weight gain can somehow promote EDC "safe" accumulation in AT, it will also increase total body burden with expectable pressure upon AT efficacy [24]. Undeniably, due to the remodeling dynamics of AT biology, AT can also be a relevant source of circulating EDCs. They can be slowly released into circulation, turning AT into a chronic internal source of EDCs, resulting in a continuous low-grade systemic exposure with possible deleterious effects [24, 134]. Adding to the normal AT dynamic function, there are other situations that are associated with higher release of EDCs from AT, namely upon AT function impairment or major weight losses, such as those resulting from bariatric surgery or restrictive diets [135, 136]. Evidence collected from several studies proposes that EDCs may antagonize the positive effects of weight loss [80, 135 - 137].

Conversely, AT is a main organ for controlling energy homeostasis, insulin sensitivity and energy distribution to other tissues [138, 139]. In an insulin resistant individual, the loss of the function of insulin in AT can lead to elevated lipolysis and increased release of EDCs into the circulation [128, 140]. When in circulation, POPs can act in other organs, possibly leading to several disorders, including infertility and cancer [21, 22, 141 - 143].

However, the view of AT as an inert energy reservoir started to change when leptin was discovered and the role of AT as an endocrine organ was gradually recognized. The AT's complex and dynamic composition, mainly composed by adipocytes, but also with immunological and nervous system components [144], ensures an important association between the endocrine and inflammatory pathways [145, 146].

Since AT harbors the largest quantity of contaminants, it can function at the same time as a reservoir and a main target of EDC disruption effects, the yang role of AT in EDC toxicology, with putative local and systemic consequences [24].

Undoubtedly, it is not surprising that when accumulated in the AT, EDCs can also exert their endocrine disruption effects locally, interfering with adipocyte or AT biology and mediating part of their metabolic effects [24, 57, 58, 60]. Given the diversity of compounds, concentrations and mechanisms with distinct effects, the abilities of EDCs are still under intense discussion. Evidence is being gathered from different research groups showing that EDCs may trigger quantitative and qualitative alterations in AT, altering its functions, metabolism and adipocyte differentiation, as well as inducing a proinflammatory state in AT, that could lead to harmful metabolic effects [128, 147, 148].

ENDOCRINE DISRUPTING CHEMICALS AND ADIPOSE TISSUE DYSFUNCTION

AT is not just an energy storage or a repository for lipophilic chemicals. Adding to obesity's effects on AT structure and function, the interaction of ECDs with AT may lead to significant metabolic and endocrine dysfunction that could explain intriguing findings in obesity research. Indeed, notwithstanding all the efforts aiming to treat obesity, it is still intriguing why some individuals have more difficulty in losing weight than others or manifest different degrees of cardiometabolic complications, since metabolically healthy obese individuals correspond to 10 to 25% [149].

It remains uncertain how exactly obesity results in metabolic dysfunction, but there is the knowledge that pathologies resulting from abnormal or excessive fat accumulation are not responsibility of the mere increase in AT accumulation, but rather more dependent on location of AT accumulation, AT cellularity and adipocyte dysfunction [150]. In fact, we know today that AT dysfunction, especially visceral AT dysfunction, and inflammation have a fundamental part in unhealthy obesity, also known as dysmetabolic obesity [149, 151].

In a healthy white AT expansion, adipocytes undergo hyperplasia and AT mass increase should be accompanied by an increase in the vascularization to support the expansion (angiogenesis). An healthy AT should displays high insulin sensitivity and an anti-inflammatory state, characterized by high levels of M2 AT macrophages and regulatory T cells [150]. In normal conditions, if AT is able to accumulate more lipids, it undergoes AT remodeling, consisting in functional and morphological changes, in order to achieve a new equilibrium that confers defense from metabolic dysfunction and lipotoxicity [150, 152, 153]. This process depends on competent metabolic control cross-talk mechanisms resulting from signaling events between AT and the immune system and multiple tissues in the body (liver, brain, pancreas, heart, kidney, vascular endothelium and skeletal muscle) [150].

However, in an unhealthy white AT, the remodeling dynamics is disturbed and a state of inflammation is established, with an increase of natural killer (NK) cells and infiltrating proinflammatory M1 AT macrophages in comparison to anti-inflammatory M2 AT macrophages. In addition, the impairment of new vasculature formation to support AT growth and enhanced fibrosis and hypoxia, together with adipocyte hypertrophy and subsequent cellular stress, contribute to insulin resistance [150].

In a context of persistent positive caloric balance, the capacity of AT to safely store lipids and adequately expand gains vital importance. Evidence suggests that the risk of developing metabolic consequences of obesity may be related to how well AT can expand to accommodate the caloric excess, *i.e.*, from the inability to become more obese [154, 155]. Due to their abilities as disruptors of AT structure and function and obesogens, EDCs are considered as triggers of AT dysfunction, leading to the worsening of metabolic dysfunction and possibly functioning as environmental modifiers between obesity subphenotypes [24, 147].

Particularly at low doses, EDCs can modulate the development of AT, both through programming events, probably epigenetic mechanisms, taking place in early life but with impact on diseases in adulthood, or later in life with alteration of AT function and structure through metabolic disruption and inflammation [24]. In this regard, a recent study unravelled some of the mechanisms of vAT dysfunction and subsequent metabolic dysfunction caused by EDC exposure [147].

In fact, possibly due to its particular localization and unique metabolic characteristics [156], visceral obesity is considered determinant in the causal pathway of dysmetabolic obesity and MetS [149, 151]. In turn, data from obese individuals report that higher vAT POP levels, the main reservoir, are associated with metabolic abnormalities, inflammation and higher cardiovascular risk [74, 157].

Using an animal model, it was possible to show that *p,p'*-DDE exposure exacerbates the metabolic impact of a high-fat (HF) diet as a consequence of an impairment of the mesenteric vAT normal function and its growth ability [147].

The expected remodeling dynamic response to energy surplus was decreased by *p,p'*-DDE exposure and was characterized by an increase in inflammation and a reduction in competent metabolic control cross-talk mechanisms, resulting from a down-regulation of nervous system and tissue development-related genes, along with signaling and metabolism-related genes [147]. AT is innervated by the autonomic nervous system, especially by sympathetic nerves [158] and in response to higher energy influx and AT growth there is an increased sympathetic tone [159] that could be impaired by EDCs' ability, namely *p,p'*-DDE, as neurotoxicants and disruptors of neurotransmitter function [160, 161].

Altogether, these mechanisms could ultimately lead to AT dysfunction, disturbing its toxicological functions, namely of protection [24], and having local and systemic consequences [152, 162, 163], affecting the interplay with central (brain) and peripheral organs (gut, liver, muscle) [149, 151] and contributing to the dysfunction of other metabolically active organs [147, 164].

Since AT is the main reservoir of EDCs, their ability to promote AT dysfunction constitute a fundamental mechanism leading to dysmetabolic obesity and can help explain the interindividual variability of obesity effects [147]. Hence, EDCs stored in AT, in synergy with lifestyle factors, may be a key component in metabolic dysfunction pathologies [84, 162, 163] and possible markers of dysmetabolic obesity [147].

Early identification of AT and metabolic dysfunctions or prediction of responders to obesity treatment would help optimize the management of the disease and public health regulations. There has been an effort to associate plasma EDC levels with metabolic dysfunction and levels in AT [157]. However, we must take into consideration their more transient and irregular presence in blood, as a result of their toxicodynamics and of new exposures, making it difficult to truly reflect or infer their effects in AT. To surpass this issue, molecular tools (biomarkers) able to identify susceptible individuals, improve diagnosis and early detection of disease and predict major clinical outcomes in patients, can be used to overcome the challenge to identify weaker associations that require more accurate and sensitive tools [165].

CORNERSTONES OF THE METABOLISM-DISRUPTING CHEMICALS

Either acting in AT or systemically, EDCs add pressure onto metabolism homeostasis regulation. Undeniably, there is abundant evidence from epidemiological, *in vitro* and *in vivo* studies reporting a positive correlation of EDCs, both in plasma and AT, with the occurrence of obesity, insulin resistance, hypertension, MetS, and cardiovascular disease [7, 148, 163, 166, 167], as well as adipocyte dysfunction [162].

However, EDC effects in obesity and metabolism disruption are far more complex than the obesogenic effects of chemicals. Recently, Gauthier *et al* [168] confirmed the relationship between plasma POP levels and variation in metabolic risk amongst obese individuals by presenting an association of higher plasma POP levels with metabolically dysfunctional obesity.

Several other studies are aligned with these observations, demonstrating the potential role of EDCs in the development of metabolic dysfunction and cardiovascular risk in a context of obesity, and possibly also explaining the interindividual variability of obesity effects in metabolic dysfunction development, T2D pathogenesis and dissimilar susceptibility to successful weight loss [74, 147, 148, 157, 167]. Hence, the involvement of EDCs as markers of metabolic dysfunction in obesity and its reversibility shifts the view over their limited recognition as environmental obesogens [74, 147, 157, 169, 170]. On the other hand, EDCs also exert noteworthy effects even when not in an obesogenic context, as the induction of elevated fasting glucose, inflammation and hypertension [147].

Taken together, there is accumulating evidence to hypothesize that EDCs have an important metabolic dysregulation ability independent of their obesogenic effects. In 2015, the Parma Consensus Statement [169] proposed the expansion of the obesogen hypothesis, considering novel evidence of chemicals that increased susceptibility to liver lipid abnormalities, T2D and MetS; with these metabolic modifications probably playing a significant role in the global epidemics of obesity.

More recently, the term metabolism-disrupting chemicals (MDCs) was proposed [170] to refer to any EDC that modifies susceptibility to metabolic disorders and includes the term "obesogens", "diabesogens" and "diabetogens" [74, 157, 169 - 171]. Metabolic disorders such as cardiovascular diseases and T2D result from modifications of metabolic pathways in several organs, but despite the uttermost importance of obesity (particularly central obesity) [172, 173], EDC metabolism-disrupting effects can also be a result of their action in other metabolically-active organs or systems regardless of obesity [147, 170].

In fact, due to MDCs' complexity of targets and effects that often overlap, the comprehensive map of their mechanisms of action and targets is still relatively incomplete. An effort has been made by the scientific community to decipher this complexity, essential for the better understanding of the causal effects, and focus on preventing metabolic diseases instead on the current emphasis on interventions after the diseases are installed [170]. A recent publication by Heindel *et al* [170] reviewed the putative mechanisms of metabolic disruption that, with other recent contributions, are enabling the construction of a comprehensive roadmap of MDC actions [118, 174 - 178]. Briefly, we can highlight the effects on adipogenesis and adipokine production [170, 174, 179, 180], neuroendocrine control of metabolism and feeding [170, 175, 181, 182], energy homeostasis and T2D (through alteration of beta cell survival and function, insulin action and glucose disposal) [170, 174, 175, 183], as well as hepatic steatosis [170, 174, 177, 184], hyperlipidemia [170, 185] and gastrointestinal function and microbiota [118, 175].

Furthermore, one should not forget the importance of the timing of exposure, particularly as developmental exposures to MDCs are crucial for setting the sensitivity or susceptibility for metabolic disruption later in life [170, 174]. However, in some situations a "second hit" later in life, as an obesogenic environment, may be needed for the effects to become apparent as illness [170]. In addition, exposures to MDCs throughout life can also increase sensitivity to metabolic disturbance and lead to weight gain and metabolic diseases, either acting *per se* or by increasing the sensitivity or set point for disease [170].

CROSSROADS BETWEEN NUTRITION AND ENVIRONMENT - AN AVENUE FOR FUTURE INTERVENTIONS?

Over the past decade, great strides have been made to substantially reduce the amount of pollution generated; while total elimination is ideal, it is not a realistic or feasible goal in the immediate future. EDCs, and especially POPs, have been proven difficult to remove from contaminated sources due to their poor aqueous solubility and low volatility, even with the biological, chemical, physical and thermal remediation options available [186]. Strategies that modulate the effect of toxicants on pathophysiologic processes involved in disease etiology and progression will be of public health importance.

Recent findings implicate the importance of an individual's nutritional status and the use of protective bioactive food components to decrease the overall toxicity of environmental pollutants [187]. While complete remediation of a hazardous site may continue to be a crucial target for human exposure risk reduction, it is important to design and implement other biologically relevant ways to buffering toxicant exposure.

Importantly, there is increasing evidence of the protective tools of healthful nutrition, specifically regarding components of the Mediterranean diet (*i.e.*, polyphenols and omega-3 fatty acids), suggesting a means by which individuals may be able to control the development of pollutant-associated disease risks [188]. Concerning polyphenols, in mice exposed to 2,3,7,8-tetrachlorodibenzo-p-dioxin (TCDD) resveratrol (found abundantly in grapes, berries, and other plants) has been shown to attenuate hepatic steatosis and oxidative stress [189].

Furthermore, resveratrol may protect against the development of T2D associated with pollutant exposure since it can combat PCB-induced disruptions in adipocyte glucose homeostasis [190]. Additionally, it has been observed that individuals exhibit trends toward lower body burden of organochloride compounds after adopting vegetarian or vegan dietary patterns [191]. Due to the richness of these plant-based diets in polyphenols and antioxidant compounds, it is conceivable that specific bioactive and plant-derived compounds may be promoting greater excretion of pollutants [192].

Another intervention to reduce body burden and to enhance pollutant excretion, in addition to nutritional modulation, is the direct disruption or binding of these pollutants via the enterohepatic circulation [128].

Recent evidence advocated that a possible intervention is to block the enterohepatic recirculation of EDCs. Accordingly dietary fibre, olestra a nonabsorbable lipid, or cholestyramine a bile acid resin, have the capability to adsorb EDCs in the bile and increase their excretion in feces [128]. Moreover, green tea consumption lowers plasma levels and enhances fecal excretion of lipids and lipid-soluble compounds, including lipophilic EDCs [193, 194]. In fact, during enterohepatic recirculation pollutants become exposed to the intestinal environment, thus providing an avenue for potential dietary intervention.

Regarding health behaviors to increase the elimination of EDCs, time-restricted feeding combined with intermittent fasting and exercise/physical activity are important strategies. Therefore chronic physical activity substantially increased the hepatobiliary clearance of endogenous and exogenous chemicals, in animal experiments [128]. However, these associations need to be further explored to determine if this is indeed the case. There is a great need to explore this lifestyle paradigm in environmental toxicology and to improve our understanding of the relationship between nutrition and exercise/physical activity, exposure to environmental toxicants and disease [195].

Finally, avoiding EDC-contaminated animal fat, including fish, is another important dietary intervention that can reduce EDC exposure. Although fish is generally recommended as the best source of omega-3 fatty acids, it is also a significant source of EDCs. In line with this, recent contradictory epidemiological findings regarding the health effects of fish consumption can also be explained by the mixed effects of the beneficial nutrients and harmful chemicals contained in fish [196 - 199].

Notwithstanding, it has been established that certain unhealthy dietary practices can worsen the toxicity of ECDs exposure. The overconsumption of processed and refined foods contributes to diets high in *trans* and saturate fatty acids and free sugars, which exacerbate not only diet-induced metabolic complications, but also pollutant-associated inflammatory processes, which could be due to the fact that the mechanisms of pollutant-induced toxicity and dietary-induced inflammatory responses are similar [147].

CONCLUDING REMARKS

Public health risk assessment can no longer be based on the assumption that obesity and metabolic disorders are just the result of personal choices, but rather a combination of complex events that may be contributing to this metabolic dysfunction epidemic, namely factors such as the exposure to EDCs. Indeed, the EDCs' concept has received increasing attention and is now a focus of debate and concern among scientists, physicians, regulators, and the public [200].

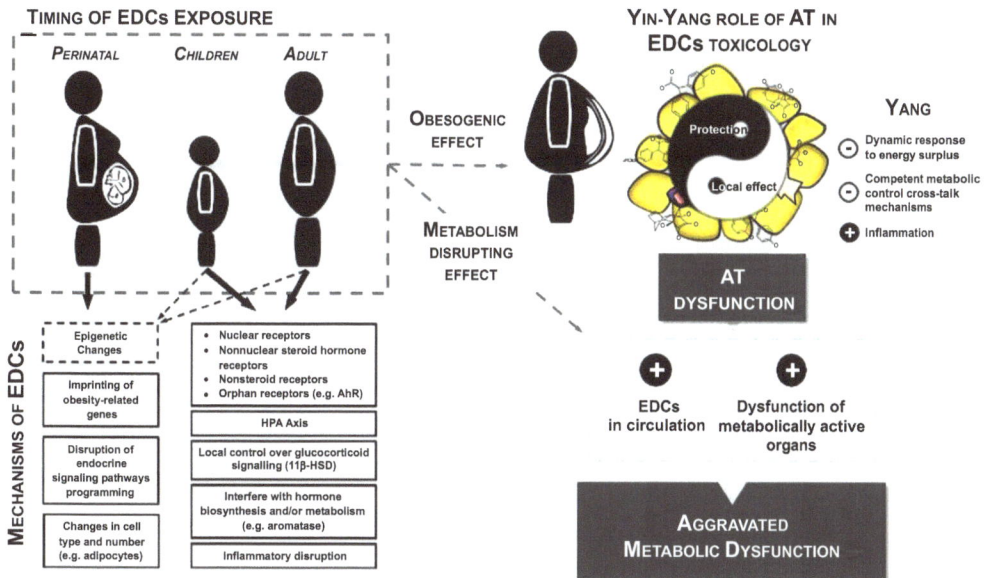

Fig. (3). Schematic representation of the proposed mechanisms for the obesogenic and metabolism disruption effects of endocrine disrupting chemicals (EDCs). 11β-HSD, 11β-hydroxysteroid dehydrogenase; AT, adipose tissue; AhR, aryl hydrocarbon receptor; HPA, hypothalamic-pituitary-adrenal axis.

Recent research provides accumulating evidence to state that EDCs have an important obesogenic and metabolism disruption ability that, to some extent, can also explain the obesity subphenotypes and the aggravation of metabolic disorders, even without being in a context of obesity Fig. (**3**). AT yin-yang role in EDC toxicology can play an important part in their disruption effect, acting both as a modulator/protector and as a target of toxicity, that could ultimately lead to the AT dysfunction with metabolic consequences.

As a complex field, researchers continue to wrestle with important issues, such as low-dose effects, non-monotonic dose responses, effects of mixtures and the importance of windows of susceptibility, especially early life exposures, which require a thorough evaluation to assemble a comprehensive roadmap of EDC actions. To this end, there is a need to biomonitor and evaluate all the exposures across the lifespan and how they interact with our own unique characteristics, the 'exposome'. Then, new avenues of intervention and prevention can appear, such as nutrition, an emerging tool to address ECD exposure toxicity.

CONSENT FOR PUBLICATION

Not applicable.

CONFLICT OF INTEREST

The authors confirm that this chapter contents have no conflict of interest.

ACKNOWLEDGEMENTS

Declared none.

REFERENCES

[1]   Baillie-Hamilton PF. Chemical toxins: a hypothesis to explain the global obesity epidemic. J Altern Complement Med 2002; 8(2): 185-92.
[http://dx.doi.org/10.1089/107555302317371479] [PMID: 12006126]

[2]   Bundred P, Kitchiner D, Buchan I. Prevalence of overweight and obese children between 1989 and 1998: population based series of cross sectional studies. BMJ 2001; 322(7282): 326-8.
[http://dx.doi.org/10.1136/bmj.322.7282.326] [PMID: 11159654]

[3]   Flegal KM, Carroll MD, Kuczmarski RJ, Johnson CL. Overweight and obesity in the United States: prevalence and trends, 1960-1994. Int J Obes Relat Metab Disord 1998; 22(1): 39-47.
[http://dx.doi.org/10.1038/sj.ijo.0800541] [PMID: 9481598]

[4]   Sardinha LB, Santos R, Vale S, *et al.* Prevalence of overweight and obesity among Portuguese youth: a study in a representative sample of 10-18-year-old children and adolescents International journal of pediatric obesity : IJPO : an official journal of the International Association for the Study of Obesity 2011; 6(2-2): e124-8.

[5]   Heindel JJ, Newbold R, Schug TT. Endocrine disruptors and obesity. Nat Rev Endocrinol 2015; 11(11): 653-61.
[http://dx.doi.org/10.1038/nrendo.2015.163] [PMID: 26391979]

[6]   Tountas Y. The historical origins of the basic concepts of health promotion and education: the role of ancient Greek philosophy and medicine. Health Promot Int 2009; 24(2): 185-92.
[http://dx.doi.org/10.1093/heapro/dap006] [PMID: 19304737]

[7]   Gore AC, Chappell VA, Fenton SE, *et al.* EDC-2: The Endocrine Society's Second Scientific Statement on Endocrine-Disrupting Chemicals. Endocr Rev 2015; 36(6): E1-E150.
[http://dx.doi.org/10.1210/er.2015-1010] [PMID: 26544531]

[8]   Kavlock RJ, Daston GP, DeRosa C, *et al.* Research needs for the risk assessment of health and environmental effects of endocrine disruptors: a report of the U.S. EPA-sponsored workshop. Environ

Health Perspect 1996; 104(4) (Suppl. 4): 715-40.
[PMID: 8880000]

[9]   Bergman Å, Andersson AM, Becher G, *et al.* Science and policy on endocrine disrupters must not be mixed: a reply to a "common sense" intervention by toxicology journal editors. Environ Health 2013; 12: 69.
[http://dx.doi.org/10.1186/1476-069X-12-69] [PMID: 23981490]

[10]   IPCS. Global assessment of the state-of-the-science of endocrine disruptors. Geneva: International Programme on Chemical Safety, World Health Organization and United Nations Environment Programme 2002.

[11]   WHO/UNEP. State of the science of Endocrine Disrupting Chemicals 2012. Geneva: United Nations Environment Programme and World Health Organization 2013.

[12]   Trasande L, Zoeller RT, Hass U, *et al.* Estimating burden and disease costs of exposure to endocrine-disrupting chemicals in the European union. J Clin Endocrinol Metab 2015; 100(4): 1245-55.
[http://dx.doi.org/10.1210/jc.2014-4324] [PMID: 25742516]

[13]   Li Y, Luh CJ, Burns KA, *et al.* Endocrine-Disrupting Chemicals (EDCs): In Vitro Mechanism of Estrogenic Activation and Differential Effects on ER Target Genes. Environ Health Perspect 2013; 121(4): 459-66.
[http://dx.doi.org/10.1289/ehp.1205951] [PMID: 23384675]

[14]   Diamanti-Kandarakis E, Bourguignon JP, Giudice LC, *et al.* Endocrine-disrupting chemicals: an Endocrine Society scientific statement. Endocr Rev 2009; 30(4): 293-342.
[http://dx.doi.org/10.1210/er.2009-0002] [PMID: 19502515]

[15]   Kuiper GG, Lemmen JG, Carlsson B, *et al.* Interaction of estrogenic chemicals and phytoestrogens with estrogen receptor beta. Endocrinology 1998; 139(10): 4252-63.
[http://dx.doi.org/10.1210/endo.139.10.6216] [PMID: 9751507]

[16]   Gregoraszczuk EL, Kovacevic R. The impact of endocrine disruptors on endocrine targets. Int J Endocrinol 2013; 2013340453
[http://dx.doi.org/10.1155/2013/340453] [PMID: 23935618]

[17]   Kojima H, Sata F, Takeuchi S, Sueyoshi T, Nagai T. Comparative study of human and mouse pregnane X receptor agonistic activity in 200 pesticides using in vitro reporter gene assays. Toxicology 2011; 280(3): 77-87.
[http://dx.doi.org/10.1016/j.tox.2010.11.008] [PMID: 21115097]

[18]   Tchounwou PB, Yedjou CG, Patlolla AK, Sutton DJ. Heavy metal toxicity and the environment. Exp Suppl 2012; 101: 133-64.
[PMID: 22945569]

[19]   La Merrill M, Birnbaum LS. Childhood obesity and environmental chemicals. Mt Sinai J Med 2011; 78(1): 22-48.
[http://dx.doi.org/10.1002/msj.20229] [PMID: 21259261]

[20]   Darbre PD. Endocrine Disruptors and Obesity. Curr Obes Rep 2017; 6(1): 18-27.
[http://dx.doi.org/10.1007/s13679-017-0240-4] [PMID: 28205155]

[21]   Vandenberg LN, Colborn T, Hayes TB, *et al.* Regulatory decisions on endocrine disrupting chemicals should be based on the principles of endocrinology. Reprod Toxicol 2013; 38: 1-15.
[http://dx.doi.org/10.1016/j.reprotox.2013.02.002] [PMID: 23411111]

[22]   Vandenberg LN, Colborn T, Hayes TB, *et al.* Hormones and endocrine-disrupting chemicals: low-dose effects and nonmonotonic dose responses. Endocr Rev 2012; 33(3): 378-455.
[http://dx.doi.org/10.1210/er.2011-1050] [PMID: 22419778]

[23]   Bourez S, Le Lay S, Van den Daelen C, *et al.* Accumulation of polychlorinated biphenyls in adipocytes: selective targeting to lipid droplets and role of caveolin-1. PLoS One 2012; 7(2)e31834
[http://dx.doi.org/10.1371/journal.pone.0031834] [PMID: 22363745]

[24]   La Merrill M, Emond C, Kim MJ, *et al*. Toxicological function of adipose tissue: focus on persistent organic pollutants. Environ Health Perspect 2013; 121(2): 162-9.
[http://dx.doi.org/10.1289/ehp.1205485] [PMID: 23221922]

[25]   Lee DH, Porta M, Jacobs DR Jr, Vandenberg LN. Chlorinated persistent organic pollutants, obesity, and type 2 diabetes. Endocr Rev 2014; 35(4): 557-601.
[http://dx.doi.org/10.1210/er.2013-1084] [PMID: 24483949]

[26]   Myre M, Imbeault P. Persistent organic pollutants meet adipose tissue hypoxia: does cross-talk contribute to inflammation during obesity? Obes Rev 2014; 15(1): 19-28.
[http://dx.doi.org/10.1111/obr.12086] [PMID: 23998203]

[27]   Arrebola JP, Fernández MF, Martín-Olmedo P, *et al*. Adipose tissue concentrations of persistent organic pollutants and total cancer risk in an adult cohort from Southern Spain: preliminary data from year 9 of the follow-up. Sci Total Environ 2014; 500-501: 243-9.
[http://dx.doi.org/10.1016/j.scitotenv.2014.08.043] [PMID: 25217999]

[28]   Gutendorf B, Westendorf J. Comparison of an array of in vitro assays for the assessment of the estrogenic potential of natural and synthetic estrogens, phytoestrogens and xenoestrogens. Toxicology 2001; 166(1-2): 79-89.
[http://dx.doi.org/10.1016/S0300-483X(01)00437-1] [PMID: 11518614]

[29]   Swedenborg E, Rüegg J, Mäkelä S, Pongratz I. Endocrine disruptive chemicals: mechanisms of action and involvement in metabolic disorders. J Mol Endocrinol 2009; 43(1): 1-10.
[http://dx.doi.org/10.1677/JME-08-0132] [PMID: 19211731]

[30]   Prossnitz ER, Barton M. Estrogen biology: new insights into GPER function and clinical opportunities. Mol Cell Endocrinol 2014; 389(1-2): 71-83.
[http://dx.doi.org/10.1016/j.mce.2014.02.002] [PMID: 24530924]

[31]   Sanderson JT. The steroid hormone biosynthesis pathway as a target for endocrine-disrupting chemicals. Toxicol Sci 2006; 94(1): 3-21.
[http://dx.doi.org/10.1093/toxsci/kfl051] [PMID: 16807284]

[32]   De Coster S, van Larebeke N. Endocrine-disrupting chemicals: associated disorders and mechanisms of action. J Environ Public Health 2012; 2012713696
[http://dx.doi.org/10.1155/2012/713696] [PMID: 22991565]

[33]   Degen GH, Bolt HM. Endocrine disruptors: update on xenoestrogens. Int Arch Occup Environ Health 2000; 73(7): 433-41.
[http://dx.doi.org/10.1007/s004200000163] [PMID: 11057411]

[34]   Alonso-Magdalena P, Ropero AB, Soriano S, *et al*. Bisphenol-A acts as a potent estrogen via non-classical estrogen triggered pathways. Mol Cell Endocrinol 2012; 355(2): 201-7.
[http://dx.doi.org/10.1016/j.mce.2011.12.012] [PMID: 22227557]

[35]   Soriano S, Alonso-Magdalena P, García-Arévalo M, *et al*. Rapid insulinotropic action of low doses of bisphenol-A on mouse and human islets of Langerhans: role of estrogen receptor β. PLoS One 2012; 7(2)e31109
[http://dx.doi.org/10.1371/journal.pone.0031109] [PMID: 22347437]

[36]   Batista TM, Alonso-Magdalena P, Vieira E, *et al*. Short-term treatment with bisphenol-A leads to metabolic abnormalities in adult male mice. PLoS One 2012; 7(3)e33814
[http://dx.doi.org/10.1371/journal.pone.0033814] [PMID: 22470480]

[37]   Whitehead SA, Rice S. Endocrine-disrupting chemicals as modulators of sex steroid synthesis. Best Pract Res Clin Endocrinol Metab 2006; 20(1): 45-61.
[http://dx.doi.org/10.1016/j.beem.2005.09.003] [PMID: 16522519]

[38]   Raven G, de Jong FH, Kaufman JM, de Ronde W. In men, peripheral estradiol levels directly reflect the action of estrogens at the hypothalamo-pituitary level to inhibit gonadotropin secretion. J Clin Endocrinol Metab 2006; 91(9): 3324-8.

[http://dx.doi.org/10.1210/jc.2006-0462] [PMID: 16787981]

[39]   Köhrle J. Environment and endocrinology: the case of thyroidology. Ann Endocrinol (Paris) 2008; 69(2): 116-22.
[http://dx.doi.org/10.1016/j.ando.2008.02.008] [PMID: 18440490]

[40]   Hofmann PJ, Schomburg L, Köhrle J. Interference of endocrine disrupters with thyroid hormone receptor-dependent transactivation. Toxicol Sci 2009; 110(1): 125-37.
[http://dx.doi.org/10.1093/toxsci/kfp086] [PMID: 19403856]

[41]   Grün F, Blumberg B. Perturbed nuclear receptor signaling by environmental obesogens as emerging factors in the obesity crisis. Rev Endocr Metab Disord 2007; 8(2): 161-71.
[http://dx.doi.org/10.1007/s11154-007-9049-x] [PMID: 17657605]

[42]   Werck-Reichhart D, Feyereisen R. Cytochromes P450: a success story. Genome Biol 2000; 1(6): reviews3003.1-.

[43]   Dietrich C, Kaina B. The aryl hydrocarbon receptor (AhR) in the regulation of cell-cell contact and tumor growth. Carcinogenesis 2010; 31(8): 1319-28.
[http://dx.doi.org/10.1093/carcin/bgq028] [PMID: 20106901]

[44]   Puga A, Ma C, Marlowe JL. The aryl hydrocarbon receptor cross-talks with multiple signal transduction pathways. Biochem Pharmacol 2009; 77(4): 713-22.
[http://dx.doi.org/10.1016/j.bcp.2008.08.031] [PMID: 18817753]

[45]   Huff JE, Salmon AG, Hooper NK, Zeise L. Long-term carcinogenesis studies on 2,3,7,8-tetrachlorodibenzo-p-dioxin and hexachlorodibenzo-p-dioxins. Cell Biol Toxicol 1991; 7(1): 67-94.
[http://dx.doi.org/10.1007/BF00121331] [PMID: 2054688]

[46]   Sjögren M, Ehrenberg L, Rannug U. Relevance of different biological assays in assessing initiating and promoting properties of polycyclic aromatic hydrocarbons with respect to carcinogenic potency. Mutat Res 1996; 358(1): 97-112.
[http://dx.doi.org/10.1016/0027-5107(96)00175-3] [PMID: 8921980]

[47]   Hennig B, Meerarani P, Slim R, *et al.* Proinflammatory properties of coplanar PCBs: in vitro and in vivo evidence. Toxicol Appl Pharmacol 2002; 181(3): 174-83.
[http://dx.doi.org/10.1006/taap.2002.9408] [PMID: 12079426]

[48]   Casals-Casas C, Feige JN, Desvergne B. Interference of pollutants with PPARs: endocrine disruption meets metabolism. Int J Obes 2008; 32(6) (Suppl. 6): S53-61.
[http://dx.doi.org/10.1038/ijo.2008.207] [PMID: 19079281]

[49]   Grün F, Blumberg B. Environmental obesogens: organotins and endocrine disruption via nuclear receptor signaling. Endocrinology 2006; 147(6) (Suppl.): S50-5.
[http://dx.doi.org/10.1210/en.2005-1129] [PMID: 16690801]

[50]   Hong C, Tontonoz P. Coordination of inflammation and metabolism by PPAR and LXR nuclear receptors. Curr Opin Genet Dev 2008; 18(5): 461-7.
[http://dx.doi.org/10.1016/j.gde.2008.07.016] [PMID: 18782619]

[51]   Arzuaga X, Reiterer G, Majkova Z, Kilgore MW, Toborek M, Hennig B. PPARalpha ligands reduce PCB-induced endothelial activation: possible interactions in inflammation and atherosclerosis. Cardiovasc Toxicol 2007; 7(4): 264-72.
[http://dx.doi.org/10.1007/s12012-007-9005-8] [PMID: 17955387]

[52]   Lee DH, Steffes MW, Jacobs DR Jr. Can persistent organic pollutants explain the association between serum gamma-glutamyltransferase and type 2 diabetes? Diabetologia 2008; 51(3): 402-7.
[http://dx.doi.org/10.1007/s00125-007-0896-5] [PMID: 18071669]

[53]   Monteiro R, Azevedo I. Chronic inflammation in obesity and the metabolic syndrome. Mediators Inflamm 2010; 2010
[http://dx.doi.org/10.1155/2010/289645]

[54]   Straub RH. The complex role of estrogens in inflammation. Endocr Rev 2007; 28(5): 521-74.
        [http://dx.doi.org/10.1210/er.2007-0001] [PMID: 17640948]

[55]   Nilsson BO. Modulation of the inflammatory response by estrogens with focus on the endothelium and
        its interactions with leukocytes. Inflamm Res 2007; 56(7): 269-73.
        [http://dx.doi.org/10.1007/s00011-007-6198-z] [PMID: 17659431]

[56]   De Bosscher K, Vanden Berghe W, Haegeman G. Cross-talk between nuclear receptors and nuclear
        factor kappaB. Oncogene 2006; 25(51): 6868-86.
        [http://dx.doi.org/10.1038/sj.onc.1209935] [PMID: 17072333]

[57]   Newbold RR, Padilla-Banks E, Jefferson WN, Heindel JJ. Effects of endocrine disruptors on obesity.
        Int J Androl 2008; 31(2): 201-8.
        [http://dx.doi.org/10.1111/j.1365-2605.2007.00858.x] [PMID: 18315718]

[58]   Newbold RR, Padilla-Banks E, Snyder RJ, Jefferson WN. Perinatal exposure to environmental
        estrogens and the development of obesity. Mol Nutr Food Res 2007; 51(7): 912-7.
        [http://dx.doi.org/10.1002/mnfr.200600259] [PMID: 17604389]

[59]   Ben-Jonathan N, Hugo ER, Brandebourg TD. Effects of bisphenol A on adipokine release from human
        adipose tissue: Implications for the metabolic syndrome. Mol Cell Endocrinol 2009; 304(1-2): 49-54.
        [http://dx.doi.org/10.1016/j.mce.2009.02.022] [PMID: 19433247]

[60]   Wada K, Sakamoto H, Nishikawa K, *et al.* Life style-related diseases of the digestive system:
        endocrine disruptors stimulate lipid accumulation in target cells related to metabolic syndrome. J
        Pharmacol Sci 2007; 105(2): 133-7.
        [http://dx.doi.org/10.1254/jphs.FM0070034] [PMID: 17928741]

[61]   Han EH, Kim JY, Kim HK, Hwang YP, Jeong HG. o,p′-DDT induces cyclooxygenase-2 gene
        expression in murine macrophages: Role of AP-1 and CRE promoter elements and PI3-
        kinase/Akt/MAPK signaling pathways. Toxicol Appl Pharmacol 2008; 233(2): 333-42.
        [http://dx.doi.org/10.1016/j.taap.2008.09.003] [PMID: 18840457]

[62]   Tabb MM, Blumberg B. New modes of action for endocrine-disrupting chemicals. Mol Endocrinol
        2006; 20(3): 475-82.
        [http://dx.doi.org/10.1210/me.2004-0513] [PMID: 16037129]

[63]   Janesick A, Blumberg B. Endocrine disrupting chemicals and the developmental programming of
        adipogenesis and obesity. Birth Defects Res C Embryo Today 2011; 93(1): 34-50.
        [http://dx.doi.org/10.1002/bdrc.20197] [PMID: 21425440]

[64]   Udali S, Guarini P, Moruzzi S, Choi SW, Friso S. Cardiovascular epigenetics: from DNA methylation
        to microRNAs. Mol Aspects Med 2013; 34(4): 883-901.
        [http://dx.doi.org/10.1016/j.mam.2012.08.001] [PMID: 22981780]

[65]   Ahrens M, Ammerpohl O, von Schönfels W, *et al.* DNA methylation analysis in nonalcoholic fatty
        liver disease suggests distinct disease-specific and remodeling signatures after bariatric surgery. Cell
        Metab 2013; 18(2): 296-302.
        [http://dx.doi.org/10.1016/j.cmet.2013.07.004] [PMID: 23931760]

[66]   Burris HH, Baccarelli AA. Environmental epigenetics: from novelty to scientific discipline. J Appl
        Toxicol 2014; 34(2): 113-6.
        [http://dx.doi.org/10.1002/jat.2904] [PMID: 23836446]

[67]   Baccarelli A, Wright RO, Bollati V, *et al.* Rapid DNA methylation changes after exposure to traffic
        particles. Am J Respir Crit Care Med 2009; 179(7): 572-8.
        [http://dx.doi.org/10.1164/rccm.200807-1097OC] [PMID: 19136372]

[68]   Manikkam M, Guerrero-Bosagna C, Tracey R, Haque MM, Skinner MK. Transgenerational actions of
        environmental compounds on reproductive disease and identification of epigenetic biomarkers of
        ancestral exposures. PLoS One 2012; 7(2)e31901
        [http://dx.doi.org/10.1371/journal.pone.0031901] [PMID: 22389676]

[69]   McClure EA, North CM, Kaminski NE, Goodman JI. Changes in DNA methylation and gene expression during 2,3,7,8-tetrachlorodibenzo-p-dioxin-induced suppression of the lipopolysaccharide-stimulated IgM response in splenocytes Toxicological sciences : an official journal of the Society of Toxicology 2011; 120(2): 339-48.

[70]   Obesogens GF. Curr Opin Endocrinol Diabetes Obes 2010; 17(5): 453-9.
[http://dx.doi.org/10.1097/MED.0b013e32833ddea0] [PMID: 20689419]

[71]   Thomas P, Dong J. Binding and activation of the seven-transmembrane estrogen receptor GPR30 by environmental estrogens: a potential novel mechanism of endocrine disruption. J Steroid Biochem Mol Biol 2006; 102(1-5): 175-9.
[http://dx.doi.org/10.1016/j.jsbmb.2006.09.017] [PMID: 17088055]

[72]   Wittassek M, Wiesmüller GA, Koch HM, *et al.* Internal phthalate exposure over the last two decades--a retrospective human biomonitoring study. Int J Hyg Environ Health 2007; 210(3-4): 319-33.
[http://dx.doi.org/10.1016/j.ijheh.2007.01.037] [PMID: 17400024]

[73]   Kim KS, Lee YM, Kim SG, *et al.* Associations of organochlorine pesticides and polychlorinated biphenyls in visceral vs. subcutaneous adipose tissue with type 2 diabetes and insulin resistance. Chemosphere 2014; 94: 151-7.
[http://dx.doi.org/10.1016/j.chemosphere.2013.09.066] [PMID: 24161582]

[74]   Pestana D, Faria G, Sá C, *et al.* Persistent organic pollutant levels in human visceral and subcutaneous adipose tissue in obese individuals--depot differences and dysmetabolism implications. Environ Res 2014; 133: 170-7.
[http://dx.doi.org/10.1016/j.envres.2014.05.026] [PMID: 24949816]

[75]   Calafat AM, Kuklenyik Z, Reidy JA, Caudill SP, Ekong J, Needham LL. Urinary concentrations of bisphenol A and 4-nonylphenol in a human reference population. Environ Health Perspect 2005; 113(4): 391-5.
[http://dx.doi.org/10.1289/ehp.7534] [PMID: 15811827]

[76]   Pelletier C, Doucet E, Imbeault P, Tremblay A. Associations between weight loss-induced changes in plasma organochlorine concentrations, serum T(3) concentration, and resting metabolic rate. Toxicol Sci 2002; 67(1): 46-51.
[http://dx.doi.org/10.1093/toxsci/67.1.46] [PMID: 11961215]

[77]   Chevrier J, Dewailly E, Ayotte P, Mauriège P, Després JP, Tremblay A. Body weight loss increases plasma and adipose tissue concentrations of potentially toxic pollutants in obese individuals. Int J Obes Relat Metab Disord 2000; 24(10): 1272-8.
[http://dx.doi.org/10.1038/sj.ijo.0801380] [PMID: 11093288]

[78]   Hue O, Marcotte J, Berrigan F, *et al.* Plasma concentration of organochlorine compounds is associated with age and not obesity. Chemosphere 2007; 67(7): 1463-7.
[http://dx.doi.org/10.1016/j.chemosphere.2006.10.033] [PMID: 17126879]

[79]   Goncharov A, Haase RF, Santiago-Rivera A, *et al.* Akwesasne Task Force on the Environment. High serum PCBs are associated with elevation of serum lipids and cardiovascular disease in a Native American population. Environ Res 2008; 106(2): 226-39.
[http://dx.doi.org/10.1016/j.envres.2007.10.006] [PMID: 18054906]

[80]   Pelletier C, Després JP, Tremblay A. Plasma organochlorine concentrations in endurance athletes and obese individuals. Med Sci Sports Exerc 2002; 34(12): 1971-5.
[http://dx.doi.org/10.1097/00005768-200212000-00017] [PMID: 12471304]

[81]   Takeuchi T, Tsutsumi O, Ikezuki Y, Takai Y, Taketani Y. Positive relationship between androgen and the endocrine disruptor, bisphenol A, in normal women and women with ovarian dysfunction. Endocr J 2004; 51(2): 165-9.
[http://dx.doi.org/10.1507/endocrj.51.165] [PMID: 15118266]

[82]   Lee DH, Lee IK, Song K, *et al.* A strong dose-response relation between serum concentrations of

persistent organic pollutants and diabetes: results from the National Health and Examination Survey 1999-2002. Diabetes Care 2006; 29(7): 1638-44.
[http://dx.doi.org/10.2337/dc06-0543] [PMID: 16801591]

[83] Glynn AW, Granath F, Aune M, *et al.* Organochlorines in Swedish women: determinants of serum concentrations. Environ Health Perspect 2003; 111(3): 349-55.
[http://dx.doi.org/10.1289/ehp.5456] [PMID: 12611665]

[84] Lee DH, Lee IK, Porta M, Steffes M, Jacobs DR Jr. Relationship between serum concentrations of persistent organic pollutants and the prevalence of metabolic syndrome among non-diabetic adults: results from the National Health and Nutrition Examination Survey 1999-2002. Diabetologia 2007; 50(9): 1841-51.
[http://dx.doi.org/10.1007/s00125-007-0755-4] [PMID: 17624515]

[85] Lee MJ, Lin H, Liu CW, *et al.* Octylphenol stimulates resistin gene expression in 3T3-L1 adipocytes via the estrogen receptor and extracellular signal-regulated kinase pathways. Am J Physiol Cell Physiol 2008; 294(6): C1542-51.
[http://dx.doi.org/10.1152/ajpcell.00403.2007] [PMID: 18417718]

[86] Vandenberg LN, Hauser R, Marcus M, Olea N, Welshons WV. Human exposure to bisphenol A (BPA). Reprod Toxicol 2007; 24(2): 139-77.
[http://dx.doi.org/10.1016/j.reprotox.2007.07.010] [PMID: 17825522]

[87] Shin BS, Kim CH, Jun YS, *et al.* Physiologically based pharmacokinetics of bisphenol A. J Toxicol Environ Health A 2004; 67(23-24): 1971-85.
[http://dx.doi.org/10.1080/15287390490514615] [PMID: 15513896]

[88] Nunez AA, Kannan K, Giesy JP, Fang J, Clemens LG. Effects of bisphenol A on energy balance and accumulation in brown adipose tissue in rats. Chemosphere 2001; 42(8): 917-22.
[http://dx.doi.org/10.1016/S0045-6535(00)00196-X] [PMID: 11272914]

[89] Seidlová-Wuttke D, Jarry H, Christoffel J, Rimoldi G, Wuttke W. Effects of bisphenol-A (BPA), dibutylphtalate (DBP), benzophenone-2 (BP2), procymidone (Proc), and linurone (Lin) on fat tissue, a variety of hormones and metabolic parameters: a 3 months comparison with effects of estradiol (E2) in ovariectomized (ovx) rats. Toxicology 2005; 213(1-2): 13-24.
[http://dx.doi.org/10.1016/j.tox.2005.05.001] [PMID: 15951094]

[90] Sakurai K, Kawazuma M, Adachi T, *et al.* Bisphenol A affects glucose transport in mouse 3T3-F442A adipocytes. Br J Pharmacol 2004; 141(2): 209-14.
[http://dx.doi.org/10.1038/sj.bjp.0705520] [PMID: 14707028]

[91] Hales CN, Barker DJ. The thrifty phenotype hypothesis. Br Med Bull 2001; 60: 5-20.
[http://dx.doi.org/10.1093/bmb/60.1.5] [PMID: 11809615]

[92] Ozanne SE, Constância M. Mechanisms of disease: the developmental origins of disease and the role of the epigenotype. Nat Clin Pract Endocrinol Metab 2007; 3(7): 539-46.
[http://dx.doi.org/10.1038/ncpendmet0531] [PMID: 17581623]

[93] Wells JC. The thrifty phenotype as an adaptive maternal effect. Biol Rev Camb Philos Soc 2007; 82(1): 143-72.
[http://dx.doi.org/10.1111/j.1469-185X.2006.00007.x] [PMID: 17313527]

[94] Mendez MA, Garcia-Esteban R, Guxens M, *et al.* Prenatal organochlorine compound exposure, rapid weight gain, and overweight in infancy. Environ Health Perspect 2011; 119(2): 272-8.
[http://dx.doi.org/10.1289/ehp.1002169] [PMID: 20923745]

[95] Naville D, Pinteur C, Vega N, *et al.* Low-dose food contaminants trigger sex-specific, hepatic metabolic changes in the progeny of obese mice. FASEB J 2013; 27(9): 3860-70.
[http://dx.doi.org/10.1096/fj.13-231670] [PMID: 23756648]

[96] Chamorro-García R, Sahu M, Abbey RJ, Laude J, Pham N, Blumberg B. Transgenerational inheritance of increased fat depot size, stem cell reprogramming, and hepatic steatosis elicited by

prenatal exposure to the obesogen tributyltin in mice. Environ Health Perspect 2013; 121(3): 359-66.
[http://dx.doi.org/10.1289/ehp.1205701] [PMID: 23322813]

[97]   Newbold RR. Prenatal exposure to diethylstilbestrol (DES). Fertil Steril 2008; 89(2) (Suppl.): e55-6.
[http://dx.doi.org/10.1016/j.fertnstert.2008.01.062] [PMID: 18308064]

[98]   Schoeters GE, Den Hond E, Koppen G, *et al.* Biomonitoring and biomarkers to unravel the risks from
prenatal environmental exposures for later health outcomes. Am J Clin Nutr 2011; 94(6) (Suppl.):
1964S-9S.
[http://dx.doi.org/10.3945/ajcn.110.001545] [PMID: 21543535]

[99]   Govarts E, Nieuwenhuijsen M, Schoeters G, *et al.* Birth weight and prenatal exposure to
polychlorinated biphenyls (PCBs) and dichlorodiphenyldichloroethylene (DDE): a meta-analysis
within 12 European Birth Cohorts. Environ Health Perspect 2012; 120(2): 162-70.
[http://dx.doi.org/10.1289/ehp.1103767] [PMID: 21997443]

[100]   Kezios KL, Liu X, Cirillo PM, *et al.* Dichlorodiphenyltrichloroethane (DDT), DDT metabolites and
pregnancy outcomes. Reprod Toxicol 2013; 35: 156-64.
[http://dx.doi.org/10.1016/j.reprotox.2012.10.013] [PMID: 23142753]

[101]   Li LX, Chen L, Meng XZ, *et al.* Exposure levels of environmental endocrine disruptors in mother-
newborn pairs in China and their placental transfer characteristics. PLoS One 2013; 8(5)e62526
[http://dx.doi.org/10.1371/journal.pone.0062526] [PMID: 23667484]

[102]   Dewan P, Jain V, Gupta P, Banerjee BD. Organochlorine pesticide residues in maternal blood, cord
blood, placenta, and breastmilk and their relation to birth size. Chemosphere 2013; 90(5): 1704-10.
[http://dx.doi.org/10.1016/j.chemosphere.2012.09.083] [PMID: 23141556]

[103]   Al-Saleh I, Al-Doush I, Alsabbaheen A, Mohamed GelD, Rabbah A. Levels of DDT and its
metabolites in placenta, maternal and cord blood and their potential influence on neonatal
anthropometric measures. Sci Total Environ 2012; 416: 62-74.
[http://dx.doi.org/10.1016/j.scitotenv.2011.11.020] [PMID: 22192892]

[104]   Martin-Gronert MS, Ozanne SE. Mechanisms underlying the developmental origins of disease. Rev
Endocr Metab Disord 2012; 13(2): 85-92.
[http://dx.doi.org/10.1007/s11154-012-9210-z] [PMID: 22430227]

[105]   Barouki R, Gluckman PD, Grandjean P, Hanson M, Heindel JJ. Developmental origins of non-
communicable disease: implications for research and public health. Environmental health : a global
access science source 2012; 11: 42.
[http://dx.doi.org/10.1186/1476-069X-11-42]

[106]   García-Arevalo M, Alonso-Magdalena P, Rebelo Dos Santos J, Quesada I, Carneiro EM, Nadal A.
Exposure to bisphenol-A during pregnancy partially mimics the effects of a high-fat diet altering
glucose homeostasis and gene expression in adult male mice. PLoS One 2014; 9(6)e100214
[http://dx.doi.org/10.1371/journal.pone.0100214] [PMID: 24959901]

[107]   Alonso-Magdalena P, Vieira E, Soriano S, *et al.* Bisphenol A exposure during pregnancy disrupts
glucose homeostasis in mothers and adult male offspring. Environ Health Perspect 2010; 118(9):
1243-50.
[http://dx.doi.org/10.1289/ehp.1001993] [PMID: 20488778]

[108]   Lisboa PC, de Oliveira E, de Moura EG. Obesity and endocrine dysfunction programmed by maternal
smoking in pregnancy and lactation. Front Physiol 2012; 3: 437.
[http://dx.doi.org/10.3389/fphys.2012.00437] [PMID: 23181022]

[109]   Behl M, Rao D, Aagaard K, *et al.* Evaluation of the association between maternal smoking, childhood
obesity, and metabolic disorders: a national toxicology program workshop review. Environ Health
Perspect 2013; 121(2): 170-80.
[http://dx.doi.org/10.1289/ehp.1205404] [PMID: 23232494]

[110]   Zinkhan EK, Lang BY, Yu B, *et al.* Maternal tobacco smoke increased visceral adiposity and serum

corticosterone levels in adult male rat offspring. Pediatr Res 2014; 76(1): 17-23.
[http://dx.doi.org/10.1038/pr.2014.58] [PMID: 24727947]

[111] Markunas CA, Xu Z, Harlid S, *et al.* Identification of DNA methylation changes in newborns related to maternal smoking during pregnancy. Environ Health Perspect 2014; 122(10): 1147-53.
[http://dx.doi.org/10.1289/ehp.1307892] [PMID: 24906187]

[112] Hanson MA, Gluckman PD. Developmental origins of health and disease: new insights. Basic Clin Pharmacol Toxicol 2008; 102(2): 90-3.
[http://dx.doi.org/10.1111/j.1742-7843.2007.00186.x] [PMID: 18226060]

[113] Farber HJ. Harm of in utero tobacco smoke exposure: a heritable trait? Chest 2014; 145(6): 1182-4.
[http://dx.doi.org/10.1378/chest.13-2868] [PMID: 24889426]

[114] Sandovici I, Hoelle K, Angiolini E, Constância M. Placental adaptations to the maternal-fetal environment: implications for fetal growth and developmental programming. Reprod Biomed Online 2012; 25(1): 68-89.
[http://dx.doi.org/10.1016/j.rbmo.2012.03.017] [PMID: 22560117]

[115] Rönn M, Lind L, Örberg J, *et al.* Bisphenol A is related to circulating levels of adiponectin, leptin and ghrelin, but not to fat mass or fat distribution in humans. Chemosphere 2014; 112: 42-8.
[http://dx.doi.org/10.1016/j.chemosphere.2014.03.042] [PMID: 25048886]

[116] Greenblum S, Turnbaugh PJ, Borenstein E. Metagenomic systems biology of the human gut microbiome reveals topological shifts associated with obesity and inflammatory bowel disease. Proc Natl Acad Sci USA 2012; 109(2): 594-9.
[http://dx.doi.org/10.1073/pnas.1116053109] [PMID: 22184244]

[117] Snedeker SM, Hay AG. Do interactions between gut ecology and environmental chemicals contribute to obesity and diabetes? Environ Health Perspect 2012; 120(3): 332-9.
[http://dx.doi.org/10.1289/ehp.1104204] [PMID: 22042266]

[118] Velmurugan G, Ramprasath T, Gilles M, Swaminathan K, Ramasamy S. Gut Microbiota, Endocrine-Disrupting Chemicals, and the Diabetes Epidemic. Trends Endocrinol Metab 2017; 28(8): 612-25.
[http://dx.doi.org/10.1016/j.tem.2017.05.001] [PMID: 28571659]

[119] Claus SP, Guillou H, Ellero-Simatos S. The gut microbiota: a major player in the toxicity of environmental pollutants? NPJ Biofilms Microbiomes 2016; 2: 16003.
[http://dx.doi.org/10.1038/npjbiofilms.2016.3] [PMID: 28721242]

[120] Ménard S, Guzylack-Piriou L, Lencina C, *et al.* Perinatal exposure to a low dose of bisphenol A impaired systemic cellular immune response and predisposes young rats to intestinal parasitic infection. PLoS One 2014; 9(11)e112752
[http://dx.doi.org/10.1371/journal.pone.0112752] [PMID: 25415191]

[121] Zhang L, Nichols RG, Correll J, *et al.* Persistent Organic Pollutants Modify Gut Microbiota-Host Metabolic Homeostasis in Mice Through Aryl Hydrocarbon Receptor Activation. Environ Health Perspect 2015; 123(7): 679-88.
[http://dx.doi.org/10.1289/ehp.1409055] [PMID: 25768209]

[122] Sosa-Ferrera Z, Mahugo-Santana C, Santana-Rodríguez JJ. Analytical methodologies for the determination of endocrine disrupting compounds in biological and environmental samples. BioMed Res Int 2013; 2013674838
[http://dx.doi.org/10.1155/2013/674838] [PMID: 23738329]

[123] Porta M, Puigdomènech E, Ballester F, *et al.* Monitoring concentrations of persistent organic pollutants in the general population: the international experience. Environ Int 2008; 34(4): 546-61.
[http://dx.doi.org/10.1016/j.envint.2007.10.004] [PMID: 18054079]

[124] WHO/UNEP. Ridding the world of POPs: a guide to the Stockholm convention on persistent organic pollutants. Geneva 2005.

[125] Li QQ, Loganath A, Chong YS, Tan J, Obbard JP. Persistent organic pollutants and adverse health

effects in humans. J Toxicol Environ Health A 2006; 69(21): 1987-2005.
[http://dx.doi.org/10.1080/15287390600751447] [PMID: 16982537]

[126]   Lee SA, Dai Q, Zheng W, *et al.* Association of serum concentration of organochlorine pesticides with dietary intake and other lifestyle factors among urban Chinese women. Environ Int 2007; 33(2): 157-63.
[http://dx.doi.org/10.1016/j.envint.2006.08.010] [PMID: 17055057]

[127]   Porta M. Persistent organic pollutants and the burden of diabetes. Lancet 2006; 368(9535): 558-9.
[http://dx.doi.org/10.1016/S0140-6736(06)69174-5] [PMID: 16905002]

[128]   Lee YM, Kim KS, Jacobs DR Jr, Lee DH. Persistent organic pollutants in adipose tissue should be considered in obesity research. Obes Rev 2017; 18(2): 129-39.
[http://dx.doi.org/10.1111/obr.12481] [PMID: 27911986]

[129]   Moon HB, Lee DH, Lee YS, Kannan K. Occurrence and accumulation patterns of polycyclic aromatic hydrocarbons and synthetic musk compounds in adipose tissues of Korean females. Chemosphere 2012; 86(5): 485-90.
[http://dx.doi.org/10.1016/j.chemosphere.2011.10.008] [PMID: 22055311]

[130]   Geens T, Neels H, Covaci A. Distribution of bisphenol-A, triclosan and n-nonylphenol in human adipose tissue, liver and brain. Chemosphere 2012; 87(7): 796-802.
[http://dx.doi.org/10.1016/j.chemosphere.2012.01.002] [PMID: 22277880]

[131]   Kamel F, Hoppin JA. Association of pesticide exposure with neurologic dysfunction and disease. Environ Health Perspect 2004; 112(9): 950-8.
[http://dx.doi.org/10.1289/ehp.7135] [PMID: 15198914]

[132]   Demers A, Ayotte P, Brisson J, Dodin S, Robert J, Dewailly E. Plasma concentrations of polychlorinated biphenyls and the risk of breast cancer: a congener-specific analysis. Am J Epidemiol 2002; 155(7): 629-35.
[http://dx.doi.org/10.1093/aje/155.7.629] [PMID: 11914190]

[133]   Svensson BG, Hallberg T, Nilsson A, Schütz A, Hagmar L. Parameters of immunological competence in subjects with high consumption of fish contaminated with persistent organochlorine compounds. Int Arch Occup Environ Health 1994; 65(6): 351-8.
[http://dx.doi.org/10.1007/BF00383243] [PMID: 8034358]

[134]   Needham LL, Burse VW, Head SL, *et al.* Adipose tissue/serum partitioning of chlorinated hydrocarbon pesticides in humans. Chemosphere 1990; 20(7): 975-80.
[http://dx.doi.org/10.1016/0045-6535(90)90208-B]

[135]   Kim MJ, Marchand P, Henegar C, *et al.* Fate and complex pathogenic effects of dioxins and polychlorinated biphenyls in obese subjects before and after drastic weight loss. Environ Health Perspect 2011; 119(3): 377-83.
[http://dx.doi.org/10.1289/ehp.1002848] [PMID: 21156398]

[136]   Imbeault P, Tremblay A, Simoneau JA, Joanisse DR. Weight loss-induced rise in plasma pollutant is associated with reduced skeletal muscle oxidative capacity. Am J Physiol Endocrinol Metab 2002; 282(3): E574-9.
[http://dx.doi.org/10.1152/ajpendo.00394.2001] [PMID: 11832359]

[137]   Tremblay A, Chaput JP. Adaptive reduction in thermogenesis and resistance to lose fat in obese men. Br J Nutr 2009; 102(4): 488-92.
[http://dx.doi.org/10.1017/S0007114508207245] [PMID: 19660148]

[138]   Kershaw EE, Flier JS. Adipose tissue as an endocrine organ. J Clin Endocrinol Metab 2004; 89(6): 2548-56.
[http://dx.doi.org/10.1210/jc.2004-0395] [PMID: 15181022]

[139]   Lafontan M. Fat cells: afferent and efferent messages define new approaches to treat obesity. Annu Rev Pharmacol Toxicol 2005; 45: 119-46.

[http://dx.doi.org/10.1146/annurev.pharmtox.45.120403.095843] [PMID: 15822173]

[140] Irigaray P, Newby JA, Lacomme S, Belpomme D. Overweight/obesity and cancer genesis: more than a biological link. Biomed Pharmacother 2007; 61(10): 665-78.
[http://dx.doi.org/10.1016/j.biopha.2007.10.008] [PMID: 18035514]

[141] Valera B, Jørgensen ME, Jeppesen C, Bjerregaard P. Exposure to persistent organic pollutants and risk of hypertension among Inuit from Greenland. Environ Res 2013; 122: 65-73.
[http://dx.doi.org/10.1016/j.envres.2012.12.006] [PMID: 23375553]

[142] Sjöberg Lind Y, Lind PM, Salihovic S, van Bavel B, Lind L. Circulating levels of persistent organic pollutants (POPs) are associated with left ventricular systolic and diastolic dysfunction in the elderly. Environ Res 2013; 123: 39-45.
[http://dx.doi.org/10.1016/j.envres.2013.02.007] [PMID: 23562393]

[143] Wolff MS, Toniolo PG, Lee EW, Rivera M, Dubin N. Blood levels of organochlorine residues and risk of breast cancer. J Natl Cancer Inst 1993; 85(8): 648-52.
[http://dx.doi.org/10.1093/jnci/85.8.648] [PMID: 8468722]

[144] Cinti S. The adipose organ: morphological perspectives of adipose tissues. Proc Nutr Soc 2001; 60(3): 319-28.
[http://dx.doi.org/10.1079/PNS200192] [PMID: 11681806]

[145] Caspar-Bauguil S, Cousin B, Galinier A, *et al.* Adipose tissues as an ancestral immune organ: site-specific change in obesity. FEBS Lett 2005; 579(17): 3487-92.
[http://dx.doi.org/10.1016/j.febslet.2005.05.031] [PMID: 15953605]

[146] Bays HE, González-Campoy JM, Bray GA, *et al.* Pathogenic potential of adipose tissue and metabolic consequences of adipocyte hypertrophy and increased visceral adiposity. Expert Rev Cardiovasc Ther 2008; 6(3): 343-68.
[http://dx.doi.org/10.1586/14779072.6.3.343] [PMID: 18327995]

[147] Pestana D, Teixeira D, Meireles M, *et al.* Adipose tissue dysfunction as a central mechanism leading to dysmetabolic obesity triggered by chronic exposure to p,p′-DDE. Sci Rep 2017; 7(1): 2738.
[http://dx.doi.org/10.1038/s41598-017-02885-9] [PMID: 28572628]

[148] Ibrahim MM, Fjære E, Lock EJ, *et al.* Chronic consumption of farmed salmon containing persistent organic pollutants causes insulin resistance and obesity in mice. PLoS One 2011; 6(9)e25170
[http://dx.doi.org/10.1371/journal.pone.0025170] [PMID: 21966444]

[149] Blüher M. The distinction of metabolically 'healthy' from 'unhealthy' obese individuals. Curr Opin Lipidol 2010; 21(1): 38-43.
[http://dx.doi.org/10.1097/MOL.0b013e3283346ccc] [PMID: 19915462]

[150] Kusminski CM, Bickel PE, Scherer PE. Targeting adipose tissue in the treatment of obesity-associated diabetes. Nat Rev Drug Discov 2016; 15(9): 639-60.
[http://dx.doi.org/10.1038/nrd.2016.75] [PMID: 27256476]

[151] Wernstedt Asterholm I, Tao C, Morley TS, *et al.* Adipocyte inflammation is essential for healthy adipose tissue expansion and remodeling. Cell Metab 2014; 20(1): 103-18.
[http://dx.doi.org/10.1016/j.cmet.2014.05.005] [PMID: 24930973]

[152] Ukropec J, Ukropcova B, Kurdiova T, Gasperikova D, Klimes I. Adipose tissue and skeletal muscle plasticity modulates metabolic health. Arch Physiol Biochem 2008; 114(5): 357-68.
[http://dx.doi.org/10.1080/13813450802535812] [PMID: 19016045]

[153] Reilly SM, Saltiel AR. Adapting to obesity with adipose tissue inflammation. Nat Rev Endocrinol 2017; 13(11): 633-43.
[http://dx.doi.org/10.1038/nrendo.2017.90] [PMID: 28799554]

[154] Virtue S, Vidal-Puig A. Adipose tissue expandability, lipotoxicity and the Metabolic Syndrome--an allostatic perspective. Biochim Biophys Acta 2010; 1801(3): 338-49.
[http://dx.doi.org/10.1016/j.bbalip.2009.12.006] [PMID: 20056169]

[155] Tan CY, Vidal-Puig A. Adipose tissue expandability: the metabolic problems of obesity may arise from the inability to become more obese. Biochem Soc Trans 2008; 36(Pt 5): 935-40.
[http://dx.doi.org/10.1042/BST0360935] [PMID: 18793164]

[156] Palaniappan L, Carnethon MR, Wang Y, *et al.* Insulin Resistance Atherosclerosis Study. Predictors of the incident metabolic syndrome in adults: the Insulin Resistance Atherosclerosis Study. Diabetes Care 2004; 27(3): 788-93.
[http://dx.doi.org/10.2337/diacare.27.3.788] [PMID: 14988303]

[157] Teixeira D, Pestana D, Santos C, *et al.* Inflammatory and cardiometabolic risk on obesity: role of environmental xenoestrogens. J Clin Endocrinol Metab 2015; 100(5): 1792-801.
[http://dx.doi.org/10.1210/jc.2014-4136] [PMID: 25853792]

[158] Das UN. Obesity: genes, brain, gut, and environment. Nutrition 2010; 26(5): 459-73.
[http://dx.doi.org/10.1016/j.nut.2009.09.020] [PMID: 20022465]

[159] Schwartz JH, Young JB, Landsberg L. Effect of dietary fat on sympathetic nervous system activity in the rat. J Clin Invest 1983; 72(1): 361-70.
[http://dx.doi.org/10.1172/JCI110976] [PMID: 6874952]

[160] Tshala-Katumbay D, Mwanza JC, Rohlman DS, Maestre G, Oriá RB. A global perspective on the influence of environmental exposures on the nervous system. Nature 2015; 527(7578): S187-92.
[http://dx.doi.org/10.1038/nature16034] [PMID: 26580326]

[161] Fonnum F, Mariussen E. Mechanisms involved in the neurotoxic effects of environmental toxicants such as polychlorinated biphenyls and brominated flame retardants. J Neurochem 2009; 111(6): 1327-47.
[http://dx.doi.org/10.1111/j.1471-4159.2009.06427.x] [PMID: 19818104]

[162] Regnier SM, Sargis RM. Adipocytes under assault: environmental disruption of adipose physiology. Biochim Biophys Acta 2014; 1842(3): 520-33.
[http://dx.doi.org/10.1016/j.bbadis.2013.05.028] [PMID: 23735214]

[163] Sargis RM. The hijacking of cellular signaling and the diabetes epidemic: mechanisms of environmental disruption of insulin action and glucose homeostasis. Diabetes Metab J 2014; 38(1): 13-24.
[http://dx.doi.org/10.4093/dmj.2014.38.1.13] [PMID: 24627823]

[164] Rodríguez-Alcalá LM, Sá C, Pimentel LL, *et al.* Endocrine Disruptor DDE Associated with a High-Fat Diet Enhances the Impairment of Liver Fatty Acid Composition in Rats. J Agric Food Chem 2015; 63(42): 9341-8.
[http://dx.doi.org/10.1021/acs.jafc.5b03274] [PMID: 26449595]

[165] Gallo V, Egger M, McCormack V, *et al.* STROBE Statement. STrengthening the Reporting of OBservational studies in Epidemiology--Molecular Epidemiology (STROBE-ME): an extension of the STROBE Statement. PLoS Med 2011; 8(10)e1001117
[http://dx.doi.org/10.1371/journal.pmed.1001117] [PMID: 22039356]

[166] Kirkley AG, Sargis RM. Environmental endocrine disruption of energy metabolism and cardiovascular risk. Curr Diab Rep 2014; 14(6): 494.
[http://dx.doi.org/10.1007/s11892-014-0494-0] [PMID: 24756343]

[167] Ruzzin J, Petersen R, Meugnier E, *et al.* Persistent organic pollutant exposure leads to insulin resistance syndrome. Environ Health Perspect 2010; 118(4): 465-71.
[http://dx.doi.org/10.1289/ehp.0901321] [PMID: 20064776]

[168] Gauthier MS, Rabasa-Lhoret R, Prud'homme D, *et al.* The metabolically healthy but obese phenotype is associated with lower plasma levels of persistent organic pollutants as compared to the metabolically abnormal obese phenotype. J Clin Endocrinol Metab 2014; 99(6): E1061-6.
[http://dx.doi.org/10.1210/jc.2013-3935] [PMID: 24606089]

[169] Heindel JJ, Vom Saal FS, Blumberg B, *et al.* Parma consensus statement on metabolic disruptors.

Environ Health 2015; 14: 54.
[http://dx.doi.org/10.1186/s12940-015-0042-7] [PMID: 26092037]

[170]   Heindel JJ, Blumberg B, Cave M, *et al.* Metabolism disrupting chemicals and metabolic disorders. Reprod Toxicol 2017; 68: 3-33.
[http://dx.doi.org/10.1016/j.reprotox.2016.10.001] [PMID: 27760374]

[171]   Pestana D, Teixeira D, Sá C, *et al.* The Role of Endocrine Disruptors on Metabolic Dysfunction. Open Biotechnology Journal 2016; 10(1,M9): 108-21.
[http://dx.doi.org/10.2174/1874070701610010108]

[172]   Eckel RH, Grundy SM, Zimmet PZ. The metabolic syndrome. Lancet 2005; 365(9468): 1415-28.
[http://dx.doi.org/10.1016/S0140-6736(05)66378-7] [PMID: 15836891]

[173]   Alberti KG, Eckel RH, Grundy SM, *et al.* Harmonizing the metabolic syndrome: a joint interim statement of the International Diabetes Federation Task Force on Epidemiology and Prevention; National Heart, Lung, and Blood Institute; American Heart Association; World Heart Federation; International Atherosclerosis Society; and International Association for the Study of Obesity. Circulation 2009; 120(16): 1640-5.
[http://dx.doi.org/10.1161/CIRCULATIONAHA.109.192644] [PMID: 19805654]

[174]   Mimoto MS, Nadal A, Sargis RM. Polluted Pathways: Mechanisms of Metabolic Disruption by Endocrine Disrupting Chemicals. Curr Environ Health Rep 2017; 4(2): 208-22.
[http://dx.doi.org/10.1007/s40572-017-0137-0] [PMID: 28432637]

[175]   Nadal A, Quesada I, Tudurí E, Nogueiras R, Alonso-Magdalena P. Endocrine-disrupting chemicals and the regulation of energy balance. Nat Rev Endocrinol 2017; 13(9): 536-46.
[http://dx.doi.org/10.1038/nrendo.2017.51] [PMID: 28524168]

[176]   Deierlein AL, Rock S, Park S. Persistent Endocrine-Disrupting Chemicals and Fatty Liver Disease. Curr Environ Health Rep 2017; 4(4): 439-49.
[http://dx.doi.org/10.1007/s40572-017-0166-8] [PMID: 28980219]

[177]   Foulds CE, Treviño LS, York B, Walker CL. Endocrine-disrupting chemicals and fatty liver disease. Nat Rev Endocrinol 2017; 13(8): 445-57.
[http://dx.doi.org/10.1038/nrendo.2017.42] [PMID: 28524171]

[178]   Park SH, Lim JE, Park H, Jee SH. Body burden of persistent organic pollutants on hypertension: a meta-analysis. Environ Sci Pollut Res Int 2016; 23(14): 14284-93.
[http://dx.doi.org/10.1007/s11356-016-6568-6] [PMID: 27055888]

[179]   Howell GE III, Meek E, Kilic J, Mohns M, Mulligan C, Chambers JE. Exposure to p,p′-dichlorodiphenyldichloroethylene (DDE) induces fasting hyperglycemia without insulin resistance in male C57BL/6H mice. Toxicology 2014; 320: 6-14.
[http://dx.doi.org/10.1016/j.tox.2014.02.004] [PMID: 24582731]

[180]   Arsenescu V, Arsenescu RI, King V, Swanson H, Cassis LA. Polychlorinated biphenyl-77 induces adipocyte differentiation and proinflammatory adipokines and promotes obesity and atherosclerosis. Environ Health Perspect 2008; 116(6): 761-8.
[http://dx.doi.org/10.1289/ehp.10554] [PMID: 18560532]

[181]   Bo E, Farinetti A, Marraudino M, *et al.* Adult exposure to tributyltin affects hypothalamic neuropeptide Y, Y1 receptor distribution, and circulating leptin in mice. Andrology 2016; 4(4): 723-34.
[http://dx.doi.org/10.1111/andr.12222] [PMID: 27310180]

[182]   Giatti S, Foglio B, Romano S, *et al.* Effects of Subchronic Finasteride Treatment and Withdrawal on Neuroactive Steroid Levels and Their Receptors in the Male Rat Brain. Neuroendocrinology 2016; 103(6): 746-57.
[http://dx.doi.org/10.1159/000442982] [PMID: 26646518]

[183]   Alonso-Magdalena P, Quesada I, Nadal A. Endocrine disruptors in the etiology of type 2 diabetes

mellitus. Nat Rev Endocrinol 2011; 7(6): 346-53.
[http://dx.doi.org/10.1038/nrendo.2011.56] [PMID: 21467970]

[184] Wahlang B, Beier JI, Clair HB, *et al.* Toxicant-associated steatohepatitis. Toxicol Pathol 2013; 41(2): 343-60.
[http://dx.doi.org/10.1177/0192623312468517] [PMID: 23262638]

[185] Penell J, Lind L, Salihovic S, van Bavel B, Lind PM. Persistent organic pollutants are related to the change in circulating lipid levels during a 5 year follow-up. Environ Res 2014; 134: 190-7.
[http://dx.doi.org/10.1016/j.envres.2014.08.005] [PMID: 25173051]

[186] Gomes HI, Dias-Ferreira C, Ribeiro AB. Overview of in situ and ex situ remediation technologies for PCB-contaminated soils and sediments and obstacles for full-scale application. Sci Total Environ 2013; 445-446: 237-60.
[http://dx.doi.org/10.1016/j.scitotenv.2012.11.098] [PMID: 23334318]

[187] Petriello MC, Newsome B, Hennig B. Influence of nutrition in PCB-induced vascular inflammation. Environ Sci Pollut Res Int 2014; 21(10): 6410-8.
[http://dx.doi.org/10.1007/s11356-013-1549-5] [PMID: 23417440]

[188] Hennig B, Ettinger AS, Jandacek RJ, *et al.* Using nutrition for intervention and prevention against environmental chemical toxicity and associated diseases. Environ Health Perspect 2007; 115(4): 493-5.
[http://dx.doi.org/10.1289/ehp.9549] [PMID: 17450213]

[189] Ishida T, Takeda T, Koga T, *et al.* Attenuation of 2,3,7,8-tetrachlorodibenzo-p-dioxin toxicity by resveratrol: a comparative study with different routes of administration. Biol Pharm Bull 2009; 32(5): 876-81.
[http://dx.doi.org/10.1248/bpb.32.876] [PMID: 19420757]

[190] Baker NA, English V, Sunkara M, Morris AJ, Pearson KJ, Cassis LA. Resveratrol protects against polychlorinated biphenyl-mediated impairment of glucose homeostasis in adipocytes. J Nutr Biochem 2013; 24(12): 2168-74.
[http://dx.doi.org/10.1016/j.jnutbio.2013.08.009] [PMID: 24231106]

[191] Arguin H, Sánchez M, Bray GA, *et al.* Impact of adopting a vegan diet or an olestra supplementation on plasma organochlorine concentrations: results from two pilot studies. Br J Nutr 2010; 103(10): 1433-41.
[http://dx.doi.org/10.1017/S000711450999331X] [PMID: 20030906]

[192] Hoffman JB, Hennig B. Protective influence of healthful nutrition on mechanisms of environmental pollutant toxicity and disease risks. Ann N Y Acad Sci 2017; 1398(1): 99-107.
[http://dx.doi.org/10.1111/nyas.13365] [PMID: 28574588]

[193] Yang TT, Koo MW. Chinese green tea lowers cholesterol level through an increase in fecal lipid excretion. Life Sci 2000; 66(5): 411-23.
[http://dx.doi.org/10.1016/S0024-3205(99)00607-4] [PMID: 10670829]

[194] Morita K, Matsueda T, Iida T. [Effect of green tea (matcha) on gastrointestinal tract absorption of polychlorinated biphenyls, polychlorinated dibenzofurans and polychlorinated dibenzo-p-dioxins in rats]. Fukuoka Igaku Zasshi 1997; 88(5): 162-8. [Effect of green tea (matcha) on gastrointestinal tract absorption of polychlorinated biphenyls, polychlorinated dibenzofurans and polychlorinated dibenzo-p-dioxins in rats].
[PMID: 9194336]

[195] Hennig B, Toborek M, Bachas LG, Suk WA. Emerging issues: nutritional awareness in environmental toxicology. J Nutr Biochem 2004; 15(4): 194-5.
[http://dx.doi.org/10.1016/j.jnutbio.2004.01.002] [PMID: 15068811]

[196] Assmuth T. Policy and science implications of the framing and qualities of uncertainty in risks: toxic and beneficial fish from the Baltic Sea. Ambio 2011; 40(2): 158-69.
[http://dx.doi.org/10.1007/s13280-010-0127-z] [PMID: 21446394]

[197] Foran JA, Good DH, Carpenter DO, Hamilton MC, Knuth BA, Schwager SJ. Quantitative analysis of the benefits and risks of consuming farmed and wild salmon. J Nutr 2005; 135(11): 2639-43.
[http://dx.doi.org/10.1093/jn/135.11.2639] [PMID: 16251623]

[198] Ruzzin J, Jacobs DR. The secret story of fish: decreasing nutritional value due to pollution? Br J Nutr 2012; 108(3): 397-9.
[http://dx.doi.org/10.1017/S0007114512002048] [PMID: 22621708]

[199] Hong MY, Lumibao J, Mistry P, Saleh R, Hoh E. Fish Oil Contaminated with Persistent Organic Pollutants Reduces Antioxidant Capacity and Induces Oxidative Stress without Affecting Its Capacity to Lower Lipid Concentrations and Systemic Inflammation in Rats. J Nutr 2015; 145(5): 939-44.
[http://dx.doi.org/10.3945/jn.114.206607] [PMID: 25788582]

[200] Schug TT, Johnson AF, Birnbaum LS, *et al.* Minireview: Endocrine Disruptors: Past Lessons and Future Directions. Mol Endocrinol 2016; 30(8): 833-47.
[http://dx.doi.org/10.1210/me.2016-1096] [PMID: 27477640]

CHAPTER 7

Medical Management of the Obese Patient

Paula Freitas[1,2,3,*], **Vanessa Guerreiro**[1,2] and **Davide Carvalho**[1,2,3]

[1] *Department of Endocrinology, Diabetes, and Metabolism, Centro Hospitalar S. João, Porto, Portugal*

[2] *Department of Endocrinology, Diabetes, and Metabolism, Faculty of Medicine, Universidade do Porto, Porto, Portugal*

[3] *i3S - Instituto de Investigação e Inovação em Saúde, Universidade do Porto, Porto, Portugal*

Abstract: Obesity is a common, chronic, complex, and multifactorial disorder and its management requires a multidisciplinary approach, including diet, exercise, behavior modifications, and drugs, all of which are key components of the treatment. Antiobesity drugs often have to be prescribed, despite adherence to appropriate lifestyle modifications. The goal of pharmacological management of obesity is not only to induce weight loss, but also to improve comorbidities associated with obesity, namely the components of metabolic syndrome, sleep apnoea, *etc.*, and also to help patients maintain compliance, maintain body weight loss, prevent weight regain, as well as to improve their quality of life. The efficacy of the treatment should be evaluated after the first three months, and the drug should be withdrawal in non-responders, or - if possible - an alternative therapy may be tried. There are marked differences regarding drug availability in the world, however the long-term use of approved antiobesity drugs is limited to five drugs (orlistat, phentermine/topiramate, lorcaserin, naltrexone/bupropion, and liraglutide), all of which must be used in conjunction with lifestyle intervention. We will review currently approved antiobesity medications, focussing mainly on clinical aspects, and we will also discuss some of the new drugs that are in the pipeline.

Keywords: Antiobesity drugs, Bupropion, Liraglutide, Lorcaserin, Medical treatment, Naltrexone, Obesity, Obesity pharmacotherapy, Orlistat, Phentermine, Topiramate.

INTRODUCTION

Obesity is a common, chronic and complex disease of multifactorial origin, associated with internal and external factors, such as biological, psychological and social/situational susceptibility conditions, among many others [1]. Obesity mana-

* **Corresponding author Paula Freitas:** Department of Endocrinology, Diabetes, and Metabolism, Centro Hospitalar S. João, Al. Prof. Hernâni Monteiro, 4200-319 Porto, Portugal; Tel: +351 225513600; Fax: +351 225513601; E-mail: paula_freitas@sapo.pt

gement requires a multidisciplinary team with a global approach of the factors that contribute to obesity and excess weight preservation. Lifestyle intervention, like diet, exercise, and behavior modification are key components of treatment [2].

American College of Endocrinology, American Association of Clinical Endocrinologists (2016), and American Heart Association/American College of Cardiology/The Obesity Society (2016) published guidelines for managing overweight and obesity in adults considering using weight loss medication in those who do not respond to lifestyle modification and have a body mass index (BMI) of $\geq$30kg/m^2, or $\geq$27kg/m^2 with related comorbidities, namely diabetes, hypertension, sleep apnea, *etc* [3].

The goals of pharmacological treatment of obesity are to reduce weight, to control the metabolic syndrome components and improve or prevent atherosclerotic heart disease [2]. Pharmacological interventions should be considered as part of a comprehensive strategy of obesity management [4]. Yet, administering pharmacotherapy in conjunction with lifestyle modifications can improve compliance, comorbidities, and quality of life [1]. Weight loss goals should be realistic, individualised, and aimed at the long-term. Most of the times losing 5-10% over six months is achievable, maintainable, and has proven health benefits [1, 5].

After the first three months of pharmacotherapy responders should be identified. If >5% weight loss in patients without diabetes and >3% in patients with diabetes has occurred treatment may be continued. Also, an improvement in body composition and/or waist circumference may be alternative and realistic indicators of success of the treatment. In non-responders drug therapy should be discontinued or switched to an alternative drug if possible [1, 6].

The treatment of current comorbidities, the prevention of new comorbidities and maintenance of weight loss constitute the three main criteria for success. Given the chronic character of obesity, continued care is required to monitor and treat comorbidities, and avoid weight regain [1, 7].

Currently, the approved antiobesity drugs are extremely limited and the options for obesity pharmacotherapy worldwide vary between Europe and United States of America. There are currently two groups of licensed obesity drugs: those that inhibit pancreatic lipase and those that act centrally to suppress appetite. Those drugs that acted by increasing energy expenditure were withdrawn, due to adverse health effects [8]. By the end of the year 2000, only orlistat was approved for long-term use in North America and Europe. The effectiveness versus safety binomial is of utmost importance. Concerns about the safety of drugs, in many cases, were highlighted only after they were brought to the market [9].

The Food and Drug Administration (FDA), defines therapy effectiveness based on mean efficacy or categorical efficacy after one-year of treatment, and for this case, mean efficacy is a weight reduction of 5% (after subtracting the effect of placebo). Categorical efficacy related to the proportion of subjects (at least 35%) treated that maintained 5% weight loss compared with placebo-receiving controls. Until current days, orlistat, phentermine/topiramate (PHEN/TPM), lorcaserin, naltrexone/bupropion (NB) and liraglutide are approved for long-term use and all are to be combined with dietary measures [10]. This chapter will a) review the currently approved antiobesity medications, focusing mainly on clinical aspects, and b) discuss some of the new drugs that are in the pipeline.

CURRENTLY APPROVED ANTIOBESITY MEDICATIONS

Orlistat

Orlistat acts in the gastrointestinal tract to inhibit pancreatic and gastric lipases, limiting the digestion of triglycerides containing long-chain fatty acids [11].

It is a derivative of lipstatin, a naturally-occurring lipase inhibitor produced by *Streptomyces toxytricini*. Orlistat acts in the intestinal lumen binding covalentelly to gastric and pancreatic lipases that become inactivated being unable to hydrolyse triglycerides into absorbable free fatty acids and monoglycerides. This produces caloric deficit and a positive effect on weight control [11]. Approximately only 1% of orlistat is absorbed being unlikely to produce systemic lipase inhibition. A few cases of hypersensitivity (rash, urticaria and angioedema) have been reported [11]. Two metabolites have been identified, both of which have extremely weak lipase inhibitory activity and are considered to be pharmacologically inactive [12, 13]. The orlistat effect is dose-dependent, so daily doses greater so that daily doses greater than 360 mg provide little additional benefit - the recommended dose is 120 mg, three times a day (*tid*) [11] taken immediately before, during, or up to one hour after a main meal [11]. Capsules containing 60 mg of orlistat are also as an over-the-counter drug [14].

The most frequent side-effects of orlistat are gastrointestinal and may increase when meals have a high content in fat (30% total daily calories from fat). In patients consuming less than 30% of calories from fat, orlistat effect on weight loss attenuated. Elder patients may be treated with similar doses but all patients should take a multivitamin supplement once a day (*od;* at least 2 hours before, or after the administration of orlistat, or at bedtime) during orlistat treatment as it decreases fat-soluble vitamin absorption [11]. Orlistat may interfere with acyclovir absorption [14]. Orlistat has been used to treat patients with uncomplicated obesity and patients with obesity and diabetes in long-term clinical trials [14].

A 4-year, double-blind, randomised, placebo-controlled trial with lifestyle changes, as well as the prescription of either orlistat 120 mg, or a placebo, *tid* was carried out in 3305 patients. Participants had a BMI $\geq 30 kg/m^2$, and normal (79%), or impaired (21%) glucose tolerance. Primary endpoints were changes in body weight and time to onset of type 2 diabetes. After 4 years, the cumulative incidence of type 2 diabetes was 9.0% with a placebo, and 6.2% with orlistat, corresponding to a reduction of 37.3% (p=0.0032). Mean weight loss after 4 years was significantly greater with orlistat (5.8 *vs.* 3.0 kg with a placebo; p<0.001) and was similar between orlistat-recipients with impaired (5.7 kg) or normal glucose tolerance (5.8 kg) at baseline. Treatment with orlistat in addition to lifestyle changes resulted in early and significant improvements in cardiovascular risk factors, including high waist circumference, high blood pressure and dyslipidemia. Total and LDL cholesterol, as well as LDL-to-HDL cholesterol ratio decreased significantly more with orlistat than with a placebo, at both 1 and 4 years. The authors concluded that orlistat plus lifestyle changes resulted in a greater reduction in the incidence of type 2 diabetes and produced greater weight loss in a clinically-representative obese population compared with lifestyle changes alone, over 4 years [15].

The use of orlistat has also been studied in children. In a study of 539 adolescents receiving 120 mg of orlistat or a placebo, *tid,* BMI decreased on average by 0.55 kg/m^2 in the orlistat-treated group, compared to a mean increase of 0.31 kg/m^2 in the placebo group [16].

Another clinically important issue is regaining weight. In a study by Karhunen *et al*, of the initial 96 obese subjects who participated in the weight reduction programme, 72 subjects with the complete set of data for 2 years were included for the study. After a 4-week lead period, the subjects were randomised to either orlistat 120 mg, or a placebo (both *tid*), in addition to a mildly hypoenergetic balanced diet for one year. This was followed by a 1 year double-blind period with the subjects within each treatment group being reassigned to receive orlistat 120 mg, or a placebo (both *tid*), in conjunction with a weight maintenance diet. During the first year, the orlistat-treated group had greater reduction of body weight and fat mass, but not of fat-free mass or resting energy expenditure (REE), when compared to the placebo group. During the second year, orlistat treatment was associated with smaller regain of body weight and fat mass, with no significant differences in the changes of fat-free mass or REE, when compared to placebo treatment. In addition to higher weight loss and the maintenance of reduced weight, orlistat treatment is associated with beneficial changes in body composition, although with no excess decrease in REE, when compared to that achieved with the placebo with a dietary therapy alone [17]. In a meta-analysis of trials with orlistat, the weighted mean weight loss of those treated with orlistat was -5.70±7.28 kg and in the placebo group was -2.40±6.99 kg, for a net effect of -2.87 [95% confidence interval (CI): -3.21 to -2.53] [18].

Lorcaserin

Lorcaserin selectively activates the central serotonin $(5HT)_{2C}$ receptor, and has a much greater affinity for this receptor compared with $5HT_{2A}$ and $5HT_{2B}$ receptors. Lorcaserin reduces appetite by binding to $5HT_{2C}$ receptors on anorexigenic proopiomelanocortin (POMC) neurons in the hypothalamus and has been designed to avoid cardiac valvular effects mediated through the $5HT_{2B}$ receptor [2] Fig. (**1**). Lorcaserin is commercialised under the brand name of Belviq® (Arena Pharmaceuticals and Eisai Pharmaceuticals, San Diego, California, USA) [14]. There has been no evidence of an increased risk of valvulopathy with lorcaserin over 2 years [19]. The recommended treatment dose of lorcaserin is 10 mg *bid*. There is also a recently approved 20 mg *od* extended release (ER) tablet. Treatment should be discontinued if ≥5% weight loss is not achieved after 12 weeks like for all other drugs for the obesity management [2].

The BLOSSOM trial is a randomised, placebo-controlled, double-blind, parallel arm trial carried out in 97 US research centres, that included 4008 patients, aged 18-65 years, with a BMI between 30 and 45 kg/m^2, or between 27 and 29.9 kg/m^2, with an obesity-related comorbid condition. Patients were randomly assigned at a 2:1:2 ratio to receive lorcaserin 10 mg *bid*, lorcaserin 10 mg *od*, or a placebo. All patients received diet and exercise counselling. Significantly more patients that had been treated with lorcaserin 10 mg *bid* and *od* lost at least 5% of baseline body weight (47.2 and 40.2%, respectively), when compared with a placebo (25%, p<0.001 *vs.* lorcaserin *bid*). Weight loss of at least 10% was achieved in 22.6 and 17.4% of patients receiving lorcaserin 10 mg *bid* or *od*, respectively, and 9.7% of patients in the placebo group (p<0.001 *vs.* lorcaserin *bid*). Authors concluded that lorcaserin administered in conjunction with a lifestyle modification programme is associated with dose-dependent weight loss that was significantly greater than in the placebo group [20].

Early response to weight loss interventions is a key motivator for continuing therapy and maintaining weight loss [21]. However, individuals respond differently to weight loss regimens. In order to maximize the therapeutic benefits of lorcaserin, while minimizing unnecessary drug exposure and cost, week 12 response to lorcaserin could be utilised as a predictor of long-term weight loss outcomes and, therefore, of cardiometabolic risk factor improvement. This emphasizes that pharmacological treatment must be continued in the early responders but as with any drug, benefits must be weighed against risks. Smith *et al* showed that early weight loss while on lorcaserin, in patients with or without type 2 diabetes, is a predictor of long-term weight loss outcomes at 1 year. Furthermore, sustained benefits with regard to cardiometabolic risk factor reductions were found, and they considered that these results should be used to guide the patient-physician conversation around initiation and continuation of lorcaserin treatment for chronic weight management [22].

In another double-blind clinical trial, 3182 randomised obese or overweight adults were assigned to receive lorcaserin at a dose of 10 mg, or a placebo, *bid* for 52 weeks. Additionally, all patients underwent lifestyle modifications (diet and exercise counselling). At week 52, patients in the placebo group continued to receive a placebo, but patients in the lorcaserin group were randomly reassigned to receive either a placebo or lorcaserin. Primary outcomes were weight loss at one year, and maintenance of weight loss at 2 years. At 1 year, 47.5% of patients in the lorcaserin group and 20.3% in the placebo group had lost 5% or more of their body weight (p<0.001), corresponding to an average loss of 5.8±0.2 kg with lorcaserin and 2.2±0.1 kg with a placebo during year 1 (p<0.001). Among those patients who received lorcaserin during year 1, and who had lost 5% or more of their baseline weight at 1 year, the loss was maintained in more patients who continued to receive lorcaserin during year 2 (67.9%) than in patients who received a placebo during year 2 (50.3%; p<0.001). The authors concluded that, in conjunction with lifestyle modification, lorcaserin was associated with significant weight loss and improved maintenance of weight loss, when compared with a placebo [19].

In the BLOOM-DM study, in patients with type 2 diabetes in a year-long study, randomised, placebo-controlled trial with 604 patients, lorcaserin was associated with significant weight loss and improvement in glycemic control [23].

The most common side-effects of lorcaserin include headache, dizziness, fatigue, nausea, dry mouth and constipation, which were mild and resolved quickly [14]. There is a theoretical interaction with other serotonergic drugs, such as serotonin reuptake inhibitors (SSRIs). Although no incidents were reported in phase 3 studies, coadministration can lead to development of serotonin syndrome [2]. There was also some concern regarding the use of monoamine oxidase inhibitors (MAOIs), because of the risk of serotonin syndrome [14]. Ideal candidates for the use of lorcaserin are often patients who manifest inadequate meal satiety.

Recently, the CAMELLIA-TIMI 61 trial demonstrated that lorcaserin was effective at promoting weight loss without an increase in adverse cardiovascular events, in overweight and obese patients with a mean age of 64 years and cardiovascular disease or multiple cardiovascular risk factors. The mean follow-up was 3.3 years [24].

At the beginning of February, the FDA requested the voluntary withdrawal of the weight loss drug lorcaserin from the market, stating that the drug's potential risk for cancer outweighs its benefits. This action follows the agency's January announcement that it was reviewing data from a post-marketing safety trial, which found higher cancer rates — specifically, cancers of the colorectum, lung, and pancreas — in lorcaserin users. Over 5 years, 7.7% of lorcaserin users and 7.1% of placebo recipients were diagnosed with cancer. Special cancer screening for lorcaserin users is not recommended.

Topiramate and Phentermine/Topiramate Combination

The combination PHEN/TPM as an ER medication is the first new drug combination that has been approved for chronic weight management in overweight and subjects with obesity in more than a decade. It is commercialised under the brand name of Qsymia® (by Vivus Inc., Mountain View, California, USA) [14]. This drug combination was designed to suppress appetite and to enhance satiety Fig. (1); however, it has not been approved in Europe. In 2012 and 2013 the Committee for Medicinal Products for Human Use of the European Medicines Agency voted against the approval of this PHEN/TPM combination on the basis "that the long-term safety of this combination, particularly in the cardiovascular and psychiatric areas, had not been completely defined" [1]. The combination uses lower doses of phentermine (3.75 mg in the starting dose, 7.5 mg in the recommended dose, and 15 mg in the full dose) than are usually prescribed when phentermine is used as a single agent [14]. Topiramate acts through an appetite-reducing mechanism that is not thoroughly understood - although it may be through its effect on γ-aminobutyric acid (GABA) receptors - and phentermine acts to reduce appetite through increasing norepinephrine in the hypothalamus [14].

Topiramate exists in an ER formulation and the dose in the combination with phentermine (23 mg in the starting dose, 46 mg in the recommended dose, and 92 mg in the full dose) is lower than when topiramate is used for migraine prophylaxis or to control seizures [14]. Topiramate is a sulfamate-substituted monosaccharide, which is currently approved in more than 75 countries worldwide for the treatment of selective seizures disorders [25]. In clinical trials of topiramate for seizures disorders, weight loss has been noted and, additionally, weight loss associated with topiramate (normal formulation) has also been observed in several rodent models of obesity [25, 26].

Topiramate (normal formulation) in low doses (96, 192 and 256 mg/day) promotes clinically relevant weight loss in the long-term treatment of obese subjects as well as an improvement in glucose tolerance and blood pressure. Weight loss has been shown ongoing until week 60, with maintenance of body weight for the longest follow-up at 76 weeks [25]. The most frequently-observed common adverse events in the topiramate-treated patients occur mostly during the titration phase and are related to the central or peripheral nervous system (including paresthesia, difficulty with concentration/attention, difficulty with memory, nervousness and psychomotor slowing, language problems and depression [25].

The EQUIP study, a 56-week randomised, controlled trial with the controlled-release (CR) combination of PHEN/TPM, for two doses (3.75/23 mg or 15/92 mg), in conjunction with lifestyle modification, was performed in patients with class II and III obesity, which and produced statistically significant weight loss when compared with a placebo. The largest dose provided weight loss and concomitant improvement in comorbidities that exceeds weight losses reported at 1 year for other currently available pharmaceutical treatments. PHEN/TPM CR demonstrated dose-dependent beneficial effects on weight and metabolic parameters without serious adverse events induced by treatment [27].

In the CONQUER study, a 56-week phase 3 trial, patients, who were overweight or obese with 2 or more comorbidities (abdominal obesity, hypertension, dyslipidemia, diabetes or prediabetes), were randomised to a placebo or phentermine 7.5 mg plus topiramate 46.0 mg (CR) *od* or phentermine 15.0 mg plus topiramate 92.0 mg (CR) *od*, in 93 centres in the USA. At week 56, changes in body weight were -1.4 kg (least-squares mean -1.2%, 95% CI -1.8 to -0.7), -8.1 kg (-7.8%, -8.5 to -7.1), and -10.2 kg (-9.8%, -10.4 to -9.3) in the patients placebo-treated, phentermine 7.5 mg plus topiramate 46.0 mg or phentermine 15.0 mg plus topiramate 92.0 mg, respectively. The weight loss with PHEN/TPM CR was associated by improvements in most risk factors, namely, lowered blood pressure, improved glycemic control, increased HDL-cholesterol and lowered triglycerides [28].

Furthermore, in the SEQUEL study, a placebo-controlled, double-blind, 52-weeks extension study of the long-term efficacy and safety of PHEN/TPM CR was performed in overweight and obese subjects with cardiometabolic disease. PHEN/TPM CR used in conjunction with lifestyle intervention was well tolerated and produced significant, dose-related weight loss that was maintained during a 108-week period. PHENT/TPM CR was also associated with sustained improvements in the clinical manifestations of weight-related cardiometabolic disease, including hyperglycemia, dyslipidemia, and elevated blood pressure, despite reduced use of concomitant medications. and led to a reduction in the rate of progression to type 2 diabetes [29].

The most common adverse events of PHEN/TPM CR are paresthesias, dizziness dysgeusia, dry mouth, constipation and insomnia [14, 27]. Phentermine, as a sympathomimetic agent, causes insomnia and dry mouth, usually at the beginning of treatment and then resolves. Topiramate, which is a carbonic anhydrase inhibitor, is associated with altered taste for carbonated beverages and tingling of fingers, toes, and perioral areas and mild metabolic acidosis. Topiramate if used during pregnancy is associated with oral clefts. If a patient becomes pregnant, treatment should be immediately terminated. A rare side-effect of topiramate is acute glaucoma and it is contraindicated in the case of glaucoma. PHEN/TPM ER is also contraindicated in hyperthyroidism and within 14 days of treatment with MAOIs. Other potential issues, though rare, include a risk of kidney stones (associated with topiramate) and increased heart rate in patients susceptible to sympathomimetic drugs (associated with phentermine) [14]. Due to the phentermine component, this drug should not be prescribed to patients with a history of cardiovascular disease or other conditions that could be exacerbated by a stimulant. Patients who have weight gain partially attributable to antidepressants, specifically SSRIs or serotonin-norepinephrine reuptake inhibitors, are reasonable candidates for PHEN/TPM ER, as the EQUIP, CONQUER and SEQUEL trials all included patients with histories of depression who were on these medications [2]. The ideal patient to prescribe PHEN/TPM ER to is someone who could benefit from the appetite-suppressant effects of the agent [2].

Naltrexone/Bupropion Combination

Bupropion is a dopamine and norepinephrine reuptake inhibitor that is FDA-approved as an antidepressant and to assist with stopping smoking. By inhibiting the reuptake of dopamine and norepinephrine it modulates the central reward pathways at the hypothalamus level which are triggered by food, and consequently reduces food intake Fig. (**1**) [2, 14].

Naltrexone is an opioid antagonist that is FDA-approved for the treatment of alcohol and opioid dependence and antagonises an inhibitory feedback loop that would otherwise limit bupropion's anorectic properties [2, 14]. Bupropion *per se* has minimal effect on weight loss [14]. The rationale for combining naltrexone with bupropion (NB) is that naltrexone might block the inhibitory influences of opioid receptors activated by β-endorphin that is released in the hypothalamus and stimulates feeding, while allowing the activity of alpha melanocyte-stimulating hormone (αMSH), which inhibits food intake [2, 30]. Each commercial tablet of

NB (Contrave®, Orexigen Therapeutics, Inc., La Jolla, California, USA) contains 8 mg naltrexone and 90 mg bupropion ER. Initial prescription should be for one tablet a day in the morning, with instructions to increase by one tablet a week to a maximum dose of two tablets *bid* (32/360 mg). The medication should be discontinued if a patient has achieved ≤5% weight loss at 16 weeks (after 12 weeks at the maintenance dose), as already mentioned for other antiobesity drugs [2].

The COR-I study, a randomised, double-blind, placebo-controlled, phase 3 trial undertaken at 34 sites in the USA, evaluated the effect of combination treatment with NB sustained release (SR) on men and women aged 18-65 years who had a BMI of 30-45 kg/m² and uncomplicated obesity or BMI 27-45 kg/m² with dyslipidaemia or hypertension. Participants were prescribed mild hypocaloric diet and exercise and were randomly assigned in a 1:1:1 ratio to receive naltrexone SR 32 mg *per day* plus bupropion SR 360 mg *per day*, combined in fixed-dose tablets (NB32), or naltrexone SR 16 mg per day plus bupropion SR 360 mg *per day*, combined in fixed-dose tablets (NB16), or a matching placebo *bid*, given orally for 56 weeks. Mean change in bodyweight was -1.3% (standard error: 0.3) in the placebo group, -6.1% (standard error: 0.3) in the NB32 group (p<0.0001 *vs.* the placebo) and -5.0% (standard error: 0.3) in the NB16 group (p<0.0001 *vs.* the placebo) [31].

In the placebo-controlled, double-blind COR-II study, for up to 56 weeks, 1496 obese or overweight patients with dyslipidemia and/or hypertension were randomised 2:1 to combined naltrexone SR 32 mg per day plus bupropion SR 360 mg per day, or a placebo. Patients on NB demonstrated greater improvements in weight and various cardiometabolic risk markers as well as weight-related quality of life, and control of eating [32].

The COR-BMOD study was a 56-week, randomised, placebo-controlled trial that examined the efficacy and safety of naltrexone plus bupropion in conjunction with intensive behavior modification (BMOD). The study showed that NB used in the study produced significantly greater mean weight loss than BMOD alone and helped a significantly greater percentage of participants to lose ≥5%, ≥10% and ≥15% or more of initial weight [33].

The COR-Diab was a 56-week study designed to assess the efficacy and safety of naltrexone SR 32 mg plus bupropion SR 360 mg in overweight/obese individuals with type 2 diabetes, with or without background oral antidiabetic drugs. NB therapy in these overweight/obese patients with type 2 diabetes, when compared with a placebo, induced significantly greater weight reduction and proportion of patients achieving ≥5% weight loss, as well as significantly greater HbA1c reduction and percentage of patients achieving HbA1c <7% and an improvement in triglycerides and HDL-cholesterol. NB therapy was associated with improvements in glycemic control and specific cardiovascular risk factors. Additionally, it was generally well-tolerated, with a safety profile similar to that of patients without diabetes [34].

The most common adverse event with NB was nausea (which was generally mild to moderate and transient), constipation, headache, dizziness, insomnia and dry mouth [2, 32]. Medication interactions include MAOIs and opioids. NB should be avoided in patients with uncontrolled hypertension, uncontrolled pain, a history of seizures, or any condition that predisposes to a seizure, such as anorexia or bulimia nervosa, and in whom the abrupt discontinuation of alcohol, benzodiazepines, barbiturates or antiepileptic drugs occurred [2]. NB was not associated with an increase in the number of cases of depression or suicidality *vs* placebo [32]. Ideal candidates for NB may include patients that have concomitant depression, patients who are trying to quit smoking or to reduce alcohol intake and patients who describe cravings for food and/or addictive behaviours related to food [2].

Liraglutide

Liraglutide 3.0 mg (Saxenda®, Novo Nordisk Inc., Plainsboro, New Jersey, USA) was approved by the FDA for the treatment of obesity in 2014, and was also previously FDA-approved for the treatment of type 2 diabetes in doses of up to 1.8 mg, under the brand name Victoza® (Novo Nordisk Inc., Plainsboro, New Jersey, USA) [2]. Liraglutide is an analogue to receptor 1 (GLP1R) and is 97% similar to that of the human endogenous GLP1, but it has a much longer half-life (13 hours *vs* 2 minutes, respectively) [35]. Peripheral administration of liraglutide results in an uptake in brain regions regulating appetite, including the hypothalamus Fig. (**1**) [2]. A study involving individuals with obesity and without diabetes demonstrated that liraglutide administered at 3.0 mg *od* decreased food intake, as well as subjective hunger, and delayed gastric emptying [36].

Astrup *et al* carried out a double-blind, placebo-controlled, 20-week trial, with an open-label orlistat comparator in 19 sites in Europe, with 564 patients with obesity, randomly assigned to 1 of 4 liraglutide doses (1.2 mg, 1.8 mg, 2.4 mg or 3.0 mg), or to a placebo administrated *od* subcutaneously, or orlistat *tid* orally. All individuals had a 500 kcal per day energy-deficit diet and increased their physical activity throughout the trial. Liraglutide treatment over 20 weeks was well-tolerated and induced more weight loss, in a dose-dependent manner, than a placebo or orlistat. More individuals lost more than 5% weight with liraglutide 3.0 mg than with a placebo or orlistat. Liraglutide treatment not only reduced blood pressure at all doses but also the prevalence of prediabetes at 1.8-3.0 mg [37]. After having demonstrated short-term weight loss with liraglutide in obese adults, Astrup *et al* demonstrated that liraglutide was well-tolerated and that it promoted sustained weight loss over 2 years, and improved blood pressure and lipid profile, and it also decreased the prevalence of prediabetes and metabolic syndrome [38]. Liraglutide monotherapy for a period of 2 years provided significant and sustained improvements in glycemic control, and sustained improvements in glycemic control and body weight, when compared with glimepiride monotherapy, with a lower risk of hypoglycemia in type 2 diabetes patients [39].

In the SCALE study, a 56-week, double-blind trial involved 3731 patients [without type 2 diabetes and who were obese or overweight (if treated or untreated dyslipidemia or hypertension occurred in the latter BMI category)] that were randomly assigned in a 2:1 ratio to receive *od* subcutaneous injections of liraglutide at a dose of 3.0 mg or a placebo. At week 56, patients in the liraglutide group had lost a mean of 8.4 kg of body weight, and those in the placebo group had lost a mean of 2.8 kg weight. A total of 63.2% of the patients in the liraglutide group lost at least 5% of their body weight (p<0.001), when compared with 27.1% in the placebo group, and 33.1% and 10.6%, respectively, lost more than 10% of their body weight (p<0.001). In this study, 3.0 mg *od* subcutaneous liraglutide was administered, in conjunction with lifestyle modifications (diet and exercise) and was associated with clinically meaningful weight loss, reductions in glycemic variables and multiple cardiometabolic risk factors, and improvements in health-related quality of life in overweight or obese patients [40].

In the SCALE diabetes study, the objective was to investigate the efficacy and safety of liraglutide *vs.* a placebo for weight management in adults who were overweight or obese, with type 2 diabetes. A 56-week, randomised (2:1:1), double-blind, placebo-controlled parallel-group trial was performed, with a 12-week 'off-drugs' observational follow-up period. Subcutaneous liraglutide 3.0 mg, liraglutide 1.8 mg or a placebo *od* were administered in conjunction with a 500 kcal/day deficit and increased physical activity. Weight loss was 6.0% with liraglutide 3.0 mg, 4.7% with liraglutide 1.8 mg, and 2.0% with a placebo. Weight loss of 5% or greater occurred in 54.3% of cases with liraglutide 3.0 mg and in 40.4% with liraglutide 1.8 mg, *vs.* 21.4% with a placebo. Weight loss greater than 10% occurred in 25.2% of cases with liraglutide 3.0 mg and in 15.9% with liraglutide 1.8 mg *vs.* 6.7% with a placebo. The authors concluded that the use of subcutaneous liraglutide 3.0 mg daily among overweight and obese participants with type 2 diabetes, compared with a placebo, resulted in weight loss over 56 weeks [41].

The SCALE Maintenance study was a 45 weeks, randomised phase 3 trial that assessed the efficacy of liraglutide in maintaining weight loss achieved with a low-calorie diet in patients with obesity or who were overweight with comorbidities, who lost ≥5% of initial weight during a low calorie-diet run-in, that were randomly assigned to subcutaneous administration of liraglutide 3.0 mg *od* or a placebo. Participants lost a mean 6.0% of screening weight during the run-in. From randomisation to week 56, weight decreased an additional mean 6.2% with liraglutide and 0.2% with a placebo. More participants receiving liraglutide (81.4%) maintained the ≥5% run-in weight loss compared with those receiving a placebo. Liraglutide produces small, but statistically significant improvements in waist circumference, fasting plasma glucose, systolic blood pressure and high sensitivity C-reactive protein when compared with a placebo. The authors conclude that liraglutide, prescribed at 3.0 mg *od*, shows promise for improving the maintenance of lost weight [42].

In the SCALE Sleep apnoea trial [43], the objective was to investigate whether liraglutide 3.0 mg reduces obstructive sleep apnoea (OSA), compared with a placebo. This was a randomised, double-blind trial, where non-diabetic participants with obesity, who had moderate OSA [apnea-hypopnea index (AHI) 15-29.9 events per hour] or severe OSA (AHI ≥30 events per hour) and who were unwilling/unable to use continuous positive airway pressure therapy, were randomised for 32 weeks to liraglutide 3.0 mg, or a placebo, both in conjunction with diet and exercise. After 32 weeks, the mean reduction in AHI as well as the mean percentage weight loss were greater with liraglutide than with a placebo. A statistically significant association between the degree of weight loss and improvement in OSA end points was demonstrated *post-hoc*, and greater reductions in HbA1C and systolic blood pressure were seen with liraglutide *vs.* a placebo. In conclusion, the study confirmed that greater weight loss led to greater improvements in AHI and other sleep-related endpoints, and it suggested that liraglutide 3.0 mg, in conjunction with a diet and exercise regimen, may be useful as a weight management component of a comprehensive therapeutic approach for OSA management. Furthermore, given its range of beneficial pharmacodynamic effects, liraglutide 3.0 mg may also be a useful tool for individuals who are already undergoing continuous positive airway pressure treatment [43].

The most common side-effects of liraglutide include nausea, vomiting, gastrointestinal distress (abdominal pain, dyspepsia, diarrhea and constipation), hypoglycaemia, appetite reduction and headache [35, 44]. A mild increase in heart rate with the use of liraglutide can occur [44]. Although liraglutide was related to an association with medullary thyroid cancer only in rodents, and the relevance to humans has not yet been determined, liraglutide is contraindicated in patients who have had medullary thyroid cancer, or who have a family history of multiple endocrine neoplasia type 2 [2]. The risk of hypoglycaemia increases with the concomitant use of liraglutide with insulin, or insulin secretagogues [2]. The drug should be discontinued if a patient has not achieved 4% weight loss after 16 weeks. Ideal patients for the administration of liraglutide include patients who are overweight or obese, who report inadequate meal satiety and/or have type 2 diabetes, prediabetes or impaired glucose tolerance. Unlike the other antiobesity medications, liraglutide does not appear to alter the neurotransmitters involved in mood regulation. In this regard, it is a good choice in patients who have to use concomitant psychiatric medications [2]. Dose titration is recommended to minimize the side-effect of nausea. The initial dose is a 0.6 mg subcutaneous *od* injection, which should be increased by increments of 0.6 mg subcutaneous every week until a maximum dose of 3.0 mg is reached. If patients develop nausea during the process of dose escalation, then the dose should not be further increased until the present dose is better tolerated [35, 45].

Other Considerations

In a recent systematic review and a network meta-analysis carried out by Khera *et al*, including 28 randomised clinical trials with 29018 patients (median age, 46 years; 74% women; median baseline body weight: 100.5 kg; median baseline BMI: 36.1 kg/m^2), the authors compared the effectiveness and safety of five US FDA-approved medications for long-term weight loss (orlistat, lorcaserin, NB, PHEN/TPM and liraglutide), for at least 1 year, compared to another active agent or a placebo. A median 23% of placebo participants had at least 5% weight loss, *vs*. 75% of participants taking PHEN/TPM, 63% taking liraglutide, 55% taking NB, 49% taking lorcaserin and 44% taking orlistat. All active agents were associated with significant excess weight loss, when compared with a placebo at 1 year: PHEN/TPM, 8.8 kg; liraglutide, 5.3 kg; NB, 5.0 kg; lorcaserin, 3.2 kg; and orlistat, 2.6 kg. The authors concluded that among overweight or obese adults, orlistat, lorcaserin, NB, PHEN/TPM and liraglutide, compared with a placebo, were each associated with achieving at least 5% weight loss at 52 weeks, PHEN/TPM and liraglutide being associated with the highest odds of achieving at least 5% weight loss [46]. When choosing a drug for obesity, several factors need to be considered, such as comorbidities, medications interactions and risk of potential adverse effects [47]. Moreover, beyond interactions, contraindications, side effects risk, average efficacy, additional benefits (beyond weight loss), should also be considered patient preferences (dosing, mode of administration) and cost to patient of the drug.

There are several potential combination therapies approaches that can be beneficial. However, additional long-term studies are needed, especially for centrally-acting antiobesity drugs, in order to evaluate the potential neuropsychiatric adverse effects and the benefit-to-risk ratio. Future studies focussing not only on central, but also on peripheral targets governing energy expenditure may offer novel treatment strategies [48]. The mechanisms of action of centrally-acting approved antiobesity medications is summarised in Fig. (**1**).

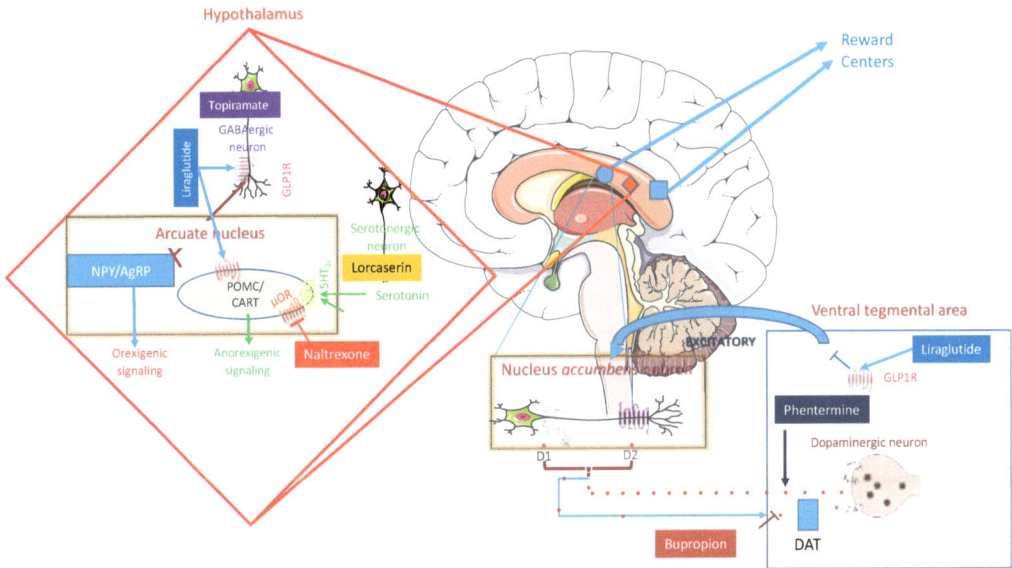

Fig. (1). Most currently available antiobesity pharmacotherapies act on the central nervous system, in the hypothalamus and reward centers. Lorcaserin selectively activates the central serotonin (5HT)$_{2C}$ receptors on anorexigenic proopiomelanocortin (POMC)/cocaine- and amphetamine-regulated transcript (CART) neurons in the hypothalamus. Topiramate acts through an appetite-reducing mechanism that is not thoroughly understood and may involve γ-aminobutyric acid (GABA) receptors. Phentermine primarily acts as a releasing agent of norepinephrine in neurons, although, to a lesser extent, it releases dopamine and serotonin into synapses. It seems to reduce appetite through increasing norepinephrine signalling in the hypothalamus. Bupropion is a dopamine and norepinephrine reuptake inhibitor, namely antagonising the dopamine active transporter (DAT), that increases monoamine concentration at synapses increasing signalling at central reward pathways and other hypothalamic areas [*e.g.* in dopamine receptors types 1 (D1) and 2 (D2)], increasing food-associated rewards and reducing food intake. Naltrexone antagonises *mu* opioid receptor (μOR) preventing an inhibitory feedback loop that would otherwise limit bupropion's anorectic properties (not shown). Liraglutide is an analogue of glucagon-like peptide 1 (GLP1A) that acting on central GLP1R receptors (GLP1RA) stimulates anorexigenic pathways (*e.g.* POMC/CART pathways) and decreases orexigenic pathways [e.g. neuropeptide Y (NPY)/agouti-related peptide (AgRP) signalling].

Semaglutide

Semaglutide shares 94% homology with native GLP-1 and was developed from liraglutide in an attempt to increase the half-life while maintaining the physiological effects of liraglutide [49]. An amino acid substitution protects semaglutide from dipeptidyl-peptidase-4 degradation, the acylation has been modified and a more flexible linker has been used [49]. These changes have increased the affinity of semaglutide to the GLP-1 receptor threefold compared with liraglutide and increased its half-life to 165 h in humans [49]. Semaglutide trials have shown dose-dependent weight loss and adverse events [50, 51]. In a randomized, double-blind, placebo controlled, compared with liraglutide 3mg, phase 2 study, 83% of participants in the semaglutide arm, 66% in the liraglutide arm, and 23% in the placebo arm lost at least 5% of baseline body weight at 52 weeks of intervention. At 52 weeks, mean weight reductions for the semaglutide arm ranged from 6.0% (0.05 mg) to 13.8% (0.4 mg) of baseline weight, patients receiving a fast-escalation dose (every 2 weeks) of semaglutide ranged from 11.4% (0.3 mg) to 16.3% (0.4 mg), the liraglutide arm had a 7.8% reduction in baseline weight, and the placebo arm had a 2.3% reduction. Thirty-five percent of participants in the semaglutide arm, 6% in the liraglutide arm, and 2% in the placebo arm lost 20% or more over the 52 weeks [50]. The most common adverse events were gastrointestinal disorders, which were largely mild to moderate (range 15-38% with placebo, 38-82% with semaglutide). In Marso et al. [44], Sorli et al. [52] and O'Neil et al. [50], most adverse event-related withdrawals were due to gastrointestinal events, commonly reported as nausea, vomiting, and constipation or diarrhoea, with nausea the most common. No unexpected safety concerns were identified in any of the trials [44, 50, 52, 53]. Four phase III studies (STEP 1-4) are set for completion in 2020 and a cardiovascular trial that is estimated for completion in 2023 (SELECT [Semaglutide Effects on Cardiovascular Outcomes in People with Overweight or Obesity]). In conclusion, semaglutide is a potential viable low-risk option to aid in weight loss through appetite suppression and enhanced satiety. It is available in the subcutaneous formulation once a week. Trials on the oral formulation are being performed.

NEW DRUGS IN THE PIPELINE AND NEW STRATEGIES

The new perspectives in the complex central/peripheral relationship that underlies the balance between energy intake and expenditure and a better understanding of energy homeostasis have shown capable of providing more effective molecular targets for obesity. The traditional pathways were revisited with new drugs, and new strategies are also being developed. New promising drugs direct to different targets are currently being evaluated, such as leptin analogs (metreleptin) and sensitizers (amylin analogs - pramlintide, davalintide), GLP1R agonists (TTP-054) and multiple agonists (glucagon-like peptide 1 receptor, GLP1RA; gastric inhibitory polypeptide receptor, GIPR; glucagon receptor, GcgR), melanocortin 4 receptor (MC4R) agonists (RM-493), neuropeptide Y (NPY) antagonists (velneperit), cannabinoid receptor type 1 (CB1) blockers (AM-6545), methionine aminopeptidase 2 (MetAP2) inhibitors (beloranib), lipase inhibitors (cetilistat), and antiobesity vaccines (ghrelin; somatostatin; adenovirus-36, Ad36). These medicines are aggregated in clusters: "satiety signals" drugs, "orexigenic signals" antagonists, "fat utilisation" promoters and "absorption of fats" inhibitors. As these drugs act through different pathways, it makes sense to use 2 or more classes acting in complementary targets and opens numerous therapeutic avenues. Indeed, like in many other multifactorial diseases, the monotherapy approach is condemned to the unsuccess. We have a large story of combination therapies that were able to circumvent such challenges, namely for the treatment of diabetes, hypertension, dyslipidaemia or tuberculosis. Hence, the dream of the personalised medicine is on the way of the obesity management.

From Leptin Analogs to Leptin Sensitizers

Leptin and leptin analogs directly stimulate the anorexigenic POMC neurons and inhibit the orexigenic NPY neurons in the hypothalamic arcuate nucleus (ARC), therefore promoting satiety and weight reduction. Since weight loss causes leptin reduction, normalization of leptin to pre-weight loss levels, through the human hormone leptin analogue metreleptin supplementation, reduces weight loss induced counter-regulation [54]. Recently, pramlintide, an injectable synthetic amylin analogue demonstrated to have leptin-sensitising effects. The antiobesity properties of the pramlintide and metreleptin (pramlintide/metreleptin) combined treatment were evaluated. The amount of weight loss was dose and baseline BMI-dependent. Participants with a baseline BMI of less than 35 kg/m^2 obtained the best weight loss efficacy from the combination. The 52-week blinded, placebo-controlled phase 2 extension study of pramlintide/metreleptin results were presented later. The combined treatment results showed marked and maintained weight loss through; again, the most robust efficacy was seen in patients with a BMI of less than 35 kg/m^2 [55]. Despite these promising results, the pramlintide/metreleptin combination drug development was stopped in 2011. A new amylinomimetic has been tested, and it appears to be more potent in reducing food energy ingestion and body weight [56]. Davalintide is a high affinity agonist of amylin, calcitonin and calcitonin gene-related peptide receptors [56]. Recent studies indicated that dual amylin and calcitonin receptor agonists (DACRAs) are very potent with an efficacy far beyond classical amylin agonists, such as pramlintide, although the reason for this remains to be clarified. A new DACRA (KBP-088) with prolonged receptor activation, is superior to davalintide in terms of efficacy, inducing a significant weight loss that could be explained by an anorectic effect, which led to a reduced amount of body fat, and in addition, improved both insulin action and glucose tolerance [57].

From New Glucagon-like Peptide 1 Analogs to Multiligand Therapies

Currently prescribed GLP1 receptors agonists induce significant, yet not sufficient body weight reductions in most obese patients, primarily through both anorectic (central) or satiation (peripheral) actions Fig. (**1**). New, second generation, oral, GLP1R analogs are under evaluation for body weight reduction, such as TTP

054-021 [58]; TTP273 was presented at the American Diabetes Association annual meeting of 2017 [59]. No further studies are on way. Recently, several authors have tried to develop multiple agonists. They tried to combine drugs that induce satiety, such as GLP1RA, with other drugs with a different mechanism of action. Glucagon, a pancreatic hormone, in chronic use increases thermogenesis and lipolysis [60, 61]. The problem is that glucagon is diabetogenic [62]. Combination of GLP1RA agonism with glucagon will be a mean to counterbalance the glucose increase risk of glucagon effect, but will also provide additional efficacy by a different mechanism of action. The body weight reduction is almost entirely due to fat mass decrease and there was no sign of glucose intolerance until the GLP1R activity was reduced to a level lower than glucagon action. Unexpectedly, these GcgR/GLP1 dual agonists decrease hepatic steatosis and hyperinsulinemia and improve glucose tolerance. Oxyntomodulin (OXM), a gut hormone involved in metabolic control, could be taken as an endogenous GLP1R/glucagon co-agonist; however, OXM is a not very strong, imbalanced agonist of both receptors [63]. Interestingly, glucagon is a fibroblast growth factor 21 (FGF21) secretagogue, an endogenous peptide with action at the central nervous system, hepatic, and fat tissues that induces weight reductions and improves dyslipidemia, which also seems to have demonstrated benefits as an antiobesity therapy [64, 65].

Other GLP1R/gastric inhibitory polypeptide (GIP) co-agonists were also developed [66]. These chimeric peptides bind and activate both the GLP1R and GIP receptors with higher efficacy in humans when compared to equimolar monoagonists. The intracellular mode of action that guide the synergistic effect on weight loss are being investigated, although enhanced anorectic actions and hormonal sensitivity appear to mediate the weight loss. These mixed dual agonists - GcgR/GLP1RA and GIPR/GLP1RA co-agonists - were developed to bind to either one or the other receptor with equally-balanced preference, leading to equal relative levels of occupancy for each receptor. They were not designed to simultaneously bind two different similar nature receptors at the same target cell. A few months ago, new data of a novel compound tirzepatide (LY3298176) were published [67].Tirzepatide induces weight loss from -0.9 kg to -11.3 kg. At the end of study, 14 - 71% of the participants achieved at least 5% body weight reduction and 6-39% get at least 10%. Waist circumference reductions could be of 10.2 cm. There was also improvement in lipids and glycemic control, because the trial was performed in type 2 diabetic persons. No trials in obese are on the way.

More recently triple agonists - GLP1R, glucagon and GIP - were developed with efficacy for body weight reduction [68]. When compared to the previously described dual incretin co-agonists, these novel triple agonists were superior in correcting the excess of fat mass. A new compound results were presented in the

ADA 2018 meeting with promise results in weight reductions in animal models [69].

These perceived benefits need to be demonstrated in human clinical trials across broad populations.

Oxyntomodulin Analogs

After food ingestion, hormones such as GLP1R, Oxyntomodulin (OXM), peptide YY and cholecystokinin, are released from gut L-cells. These hormones play a critical role in satiety signalling and possibly an essential function in energy homeostasis and long-term body weight maintenance [70]. OXM and GLP1R are derived from the *preproglucagon* gene. Preproglucagon is expressed in the pancreas, gut L-cells and in the *nucleus tractus solitarius* of the brainstem. OXM is a naturally occurring 37-amino acid peptide hormone produced and released from the endocrine L-cells of the gut after enzymatic processing by the precursor prohormone convertase [71]. OXM is a dual agonist of GLP1R receptor and GcgR receptor. In normal-weight human subjects, OXM infusion is anoretic, inducing a 19.3 reduction in caloric intake with a long lasting post-infusion effect for 12 hours. This effect was partly explained by ghrelin levels decrease. It was also demonstrated to be a weak incretin and induces a slight increase in the insulin plasma levels [72]. In a 4 weeks study of overweight and obese subjects, subcutaneous administration of OXM *tid* resulted in 2.3 kg weight reduction, compared with 0.5 kg in the placebo group [73]. Furthermore, OXM is able to in induce energy expenditure [74].

To circumvent the inactivation by dipeptidyl peptidase-4 (DPP4) enzyme, amino acid substitutions were performed to produce OXM analogs (glucagon-37). Covalent linking of lipid moieties is used to prolong half-life. The new compounds have a longer *in vivo* half-life, in comparison with the native OXM. The analogs induce weight loss through food intake reduction, increase energy expenditure, improve glucose tolerance and mediate glucose-dependent pancreatic insulin secretion. Therefore, they seem to be promising tools for obesity and other metabolic related comorbidities management. Other process of prolong the plasma half-life of a drug is covalent and non-covalent attachment or amalgamation of polyethylene glycol (PEG) to molecules (PEGylation), apart from improving other pharmacokinetic parameters [75]. PEGylated OXM (PEGOXM) analogs, injected subcutaneously for two weeks, every other day during the light cycle, were tested in lean and diet-induced obese mice. The 40 kDa PEG conjugate was the most efficacious on day 1, with the longest duration of action. It was also shown to significantly inhibit ingestion, improve dysglycemia and reduce adiposity and body weight in mice. Studies in monkeys indicate that PEGOXM could have the potential for once a week use in humans. Therefore, this seems to be a promising therapy for diabetes and obesity [76].

Antagonism of the Neuropeptide Y Y5 Receptor

Velneperit (S-2367) is a novel drug developed by the Japanese pharmaceutic company Shionogi, which acts as a potent antagonist for the NPY Y5 receptor. It has anorectic effects and was developed as a possible treatment for obesity. In a programme of multicentric trials including 1566 randomised subjects, an oral dose of velneperit 800 mg *od*, combined with a hypocaloric diet, showed a significant weight reduction (5% from the baseline weight or greater in 35% of patients as compared to 12% of patients on placebo) and decreased waist circumference [77]. Regarding the velneperit safety profile, it was well tolerated, with nasopharyngitis, upper respiratory infections, sinusitis, and headache being the most frequent adverse effects. Recently hepatic safety problems were raised [78]. Although the difference in weight regain between placebo- and MK-0557 (another NPY Y5 receptor antagonist)-treated patients was statistically significant, the magnitude of the effect was small and without clinical meaning. Antagonism of the NPY Y5 receptor do not seems to be an efficient treatment strategy for reducing weight regain after very low calorie diets [78]. Targeting the NPY Y5 receptor in future drug development programmes need to be associated with other compounds to induce significant therapeutic efficacy.

Antiobesity Vaccines

Vaccines against appetite-stimulating hormones might be a new target for the treatment of obesity. Ghrelin, the hunger hormone, is the only known circulating hormone that increases body weight by simultaneously stimulating food ingestion and decreasing energy expenditure. It is principally synthesised in endocrine cells of the gastric fundus, termed X/A-like or ghrelin cells from a precursor, preproghrelin. Vaccination could be a promising alternative for the obesity management due to its prolonged therapeutic effect. A vaccine against ghrelin entered phase 2a trials as an antiobesity therapy in 2006 [79]. It acts *via* ARC NPY/agouti-related peptide (AgRP) neurons, almost all of which express the growth hormone secretagogue receptor 1a (GHSR1a). In a recent study, a chemical conjugate of active ghrelin was tested at a dose of 75 μg intraperitoneally in adult male mice with normal weight and with diet-induced obesity (DIO). It resulted in an acute decrease in food intake, higher energy expenditure and decrease of NPY gene expression in the basal hypothalamus, thereby reflecting a decrease in central orexigenic signals in vaccinated DIO mice [80]. A new nasal vaccine was recently evaluated with promising results [81]. Recently, interest for somatostatin vaccination as a tool to treat obesity has increased. Somatostatin is a hypothalamic peptide hormone also present in digestive system. Somatostatin to inhibits GH release from the anterior pituitary. Using DIO male mice, immunization with 2 somatostatin vaccines, JH17 and JH18, was evaluated. A 10% reduction in body weight of vaccinated mice was found 4 days after the first injection of modified somatostatin. At the end of 6 weeks the control mice exhibited a 15% increase in their body weight compared with baseline, and mice vaccinated with JH17 and JH18 exhibited 4% and 7% decrease in their body weight, respectively, despite similar food intake between the groups. Hence, the somatostatin vaccines seems to be effective in reducing weight gain [82].

Several other vaccines are in development to fight obesity. Ad36, is a human adenovirus, that induces TNFα and MCP1 mRNA in adipose tissue, but improves glycemic control in mice. Ad36 is associated, in several studies, with adult and childhood obesity [83, 84]. Wistar rats were inoculated with live Ad36, UV-irradiated Ad36, or the medium alone. A 23% increase in epidydimal fat pad weight in just 4 days post-Ad36 infection was noted. No change in the fat pad weight of the UV-inactivated group further supports the role of an active virus in increasing the adipose tissue [85]. In a recent study it was demonstrated that when a vaccine candidate from purified Ad36 and UV-inactivated virus was injected into mice, the serum levels of proinflammatory cytokines and infiltrated immune cells decreased in fat tissue [86]. It appears that the Ad36 vaccination can be used prophylactically to protect against virus-induced weight gain.

Antagonists of the Cannabinoid Receptor Type 1

The endocannabinoid system remains as a potential target for treating obesity. AM6545 is a peripheral acting neutral CB1 antagonist. It is less lipophilic than rimonabant (the CB1 antagonist/inverse agonist SR141716 formerly introduced in Europe in 2006 and withdrawn in 2008 due to side effects) but maintains high affinity and selectivity for CB1. AM6545 is several folds more CB1/CB2 selective, and remarkably improved the metabolic parameters in rodents, without leading to central side effects like low body temperature or behavioural modifications [87]. AM6545 administered intraperitoneally at 4.0, 8.0 and 16.0 mg/kg also inhibited diminished the appetite and induces weight loss in rodents and, at these doses, it did not appear to induce adverse events [88]. Peripheral CB1 antagonists appear to be a good way to reduce obesity.

The Melonocortin System - from Melanin-Concentrating Hormone Receptor 1 Antagonists to Melanocortin 4 Receptor Agonists and Multitarget Drugs

αMSH, which is a cleavage product of ProOpioMelanoCortin (POMC), plays an essential role in the regulation of food ingestion and energy expenditure. In the adipose tissue-leptin-melanocortin signalling pathway, αMSH transmits the anorexigenic action of leptin through the Melanocortin 4 Receptor [89]. Melanin-concentrating hormone (MCH) is a cyclic 19-aminoacid orexigenic hypothalamic peptide originally isolated from the pituitary. Is predominantly expressed in the lateral hypothalamus and *zona incerta*, and had projections to different central areas [90]. MCH acts *via* MCH Receptors 1 (MCHR1) and 2 (MCHR2), two G-protein-coupled receptors [91]. These receptors are present in humans and several other species, although MCHR2 is not expressed in rodents [92]. MCHR1 is widely distributed in the brain [93] including areas associated with feeding behavior, mood, sleep-wake cycle and energy balance, such as the ARC, ventromedial and dorsomedial nuclei in the hypothalamus [94]. Acute intra-cerebro-ventricular (ICV) injection of MCH stimulated water and food ingestion in rats [95]. Chronic ICV infusion of MCH in rats [96] and diet induced obesity mice [97] promoted increased food intake and obesity, especially on a high-fat diet. On contrary, mice lacking MCH presented hypophagia and were lean compared to wild-type mice [98]. Genetic ablation of the *MCHR1* gene resulted in a lean phenotype accompanied by decrease food intake and increased energy expenditure [99]. Acute or chronic ICV administration of agonists of MCHR1 resulted in the similar effect observed with MCH treatment [100], whereas central and peripheral administration of a MCHR1 antagonist led to reduced food intake and body weight [101]. In addition to energy balance actions, despite controversial it seems that MCH has also some role in glucose regulation. MCHR1 knockout mice are more insulin sensitive, presenting insulin levels lower than wild-type mice [99]. Is necessary that MCHR1 antagonists are able to penetrate central nervous system to induce hypophagia and weight loss [102]. New small antagonists for MCHR1 have been designed regarding obesity management. However, the antiobesity mechanisms of these compounds are not yet very clear. Compared with pair-fed matched, rats treated with one of those compounds lost significantly more weight [103]. A highly selective and potent MCHR1 antagonist with good oral bioavailability and high CNS penetration when acutely administered, increased metabolic rate in obese mice [104]. The central effects of these compounds were also demonstrated because, when chronically treated, mice exhibited a significantly higher body temperature compared to pair-fed controls. GW803430 is a new potent and selective non-peptide MCHR1 antagonist with anorectic and anxiolytic actions [105]. Recently GW803430, produced a persistent antiobesity effect due to both a hypophagia and an increase in physical activity and through this, increased energy expenditure, without any significant effect on glucose metabolism [106]. AMG 076, also a potent selective MCHR1 antagonist, demonstrated significant benefits in animal models [107].

Setmelanotide, an 8-AA cyclic peptide also known as RM-493, is a MC4R agonist [108]. Previous MC4R agonists were found to induce considerable adverse events, such as high blood pressure and penile erections [109 - 112]. Setmelanotide has been used in the treatment of two obese patients with POMC deficiency; reductions of 20 and 51 kg after 12 and 42 weeks, respectively, without significant side effects, were observed [113].

The efficacy of double agonists of GLP1RA and MC4R for the management of increased body weight and diabetes was also evaluated in rodents. Obese mice were chronically treated with either the long-acting GLP1RA agonist liraglutide, the MC4R agonist setmelanotide, or a combination of both. The combination treatment with MC4R agonist and GLP1RA agonist induces weight reduction and improves glucose homeostasis and controls dyslipidaemia beyond that which can be achieved with each drug per se. The better metabolic action of the combined therapy is attributed to the anorectic and glycemic control actions of both drugs, along with the ability of setmelatonide to increase energy expenditure. Compared to mice treated with liraglutide alone, hypothalamic GLP1RA expression was higher in mice treated with the combination therapy after both acute and chronic treatment. The same seems to happen with setmelanotide enhancing hypothalamic MC4R expression. In conclusion, dual therapy with MC4R and GLP1R agonists increases the expression of each receptor, minimizes desensitisation, and increased metabolic efficacy. Together, these findings suggest new perspectives for employing combination treatments that comprise parallel MC4R and GLP1R agonism for the treatment of obesity and diabetes [114].

Methionine Aminopeptidase 2 Inhibition

MetAP2, a member of the dimetallohydrolase family, is a cytosolic metalloenzyme encoded by the *METAP2* gene in humans (106). Initially studied as anticancer agents, MetAP2 inhibitors are potent antiangiogenic agents that prevent tumour vascularisation and metastasis [115]. Inhibitors of MetAP2 induce important maintained weight loss. Low dose MetAP2 inhibitors had antiobesity effects either in obese animals or in humans without anti-angiogenic effects [116, 117].

MetAP2 inhibitors demonstrated to suppress extracellular signal-regulated kinases (ERK) 1 and 2, leading to the sterol regulatory element-binding protein (SREBP) activity suppression, and consequently to decreased biosynthesis of lipid and cholesterol. New human studies with an MetAP2 inhibitor, beloranib, demonstrated an increase in the levels of key catabolic hormones, adiponectin and FGF21. These catabolic effects were associated with the increased production of beta-hydroxybutyrate, suggesting that these drugs stimulates fat burning and lipid excretion and increased energy expenditure. The negative energy balance, induces a decrease in adipose tissue and consequently a decrease in leptin levels [118].

Beloranib phase 2 trials were successfully completed [109]. Belonarib demonstrates that it cannot only reduce body weight but also improve cardiovascular disease risk factors. Beloranib induced a significant decreased in weight in patients with Prader-Willi syndrome and hypothalamic obesity, in a phase 2, double-blinded, randomised controlled trial. Other metabolic improvements namely in dyslipidaemia, and in abdominal circumference, were observed. Since side effects, gastrointestinal and sleep disturbances, are dose related, lower doses were generally well-tolerated [119]. Unfortunately in a phase 3 trial in Prader-Willi patients, an increase in venous thrombotic events (2 fatal pulmonary embolism and 2 deep vein thrombosis events) was registered and the drug studies were stopped. However, MetAP2 inhibition seems to be a promising tool for increased body weight [120].

Double Sodium-Dependent Glucose Transporter 1 and 2 Inhibitors

Inhibition of sodium-dependent glucose transporter (SGLT) 1 and 2 leads to diminished renal glucose reabsorption and increased glucose excretion [121]. Glucose excretion with canagliflozin is dose-dependent, so canagliflozin induces a net caloric loss in patients with and without diabetes [122]. The effects of various doses of canagliflozin compared with placebo on body weight in overweight and obese subjects without diabetes were evaluated in a 12-week phase 2b study. Canagliflozin induced a significant weight reduction without marked adverse events [123]. More recently combination therapy of canagliflozina with phentermine (CAN/PHEN) showed promising results: at week 26 CAN/PHEN therapy induces a 6.9% weight reduction in comparison with placebo ($p<0.001$), associated with a blood pressure reduction, and with good tolerance [124]. Theoretically, SGLT2 inhibition should induce a urinary loss of 160 g of glucose per day, but in clinical terms we only are able to count 50% of the predicted glucose excretion. We admit that results of compensatory increased reabsorption by the SGLT1 expressed distal to SGLT2. So, what could be expect from more potent inhibitors of both co-transporters? New dual drug could be also an obesity breakthrough [125].

In summary, the novel targets include agents which function as "satiety signs (amylin analogs, leptin analogs, GLP1R agonists, MCR4 agonists, OXM analogs and ghrelin vaccines), drugs that inhibit orexigenic signals (NPY antagonists and CB1blockers), agents which increase fat utilisation (MetAP2 inhibitors and somatostatin vaccines), drugs which decrease absorption of fats (lipase inhibitors) and others that protect against adenoviral infections (Ad36 vaccine).

CONCLUDING REMARKS

Obesity is a serious public health problem. Prevention is a long-term solution. As a chronic disease with multifactorial origin requires multiple interventions. Medications for chronic weight loss management should always be considered for obesity treatment in conjunction with a combination of caloric intake restriction, exercise, and lifelong lifestyle modifications. The advance in the knowledge of the mechanisms underlying of appetite, hunger, satiety and energy homeostasis has led to the design of novel drugs and the recent approval of new obesity medications. Drugs are useful for the treatment of patients with obesity, as they can induce appetite control but also if they are able to reinforce behavioral intentions that lead to lifestyle changes. Some medications that we described above are now available, having been approved by the EMA and FDA for long-term obesity management. These medications have the potential to reduce obesity burden and the complications and risk factors associated with obesity, and they could help achieve and maintain weight loss. Tailoring treatment to patients' behaviors, clinical history, preferences, and comorbidities is necessary for successful pharmacotherapy. However, personalised treatment requires the adherence to treatment-termination rules according to the initial response. Not losing at least 5% of initial weight in 3-6 months indicates that an alternative strategy should be initiated. Despite the advent of these novel medications, we still need new drugs to be able to treat this chronic disorder, especially in the case of non-responders.

Another problem in many countries is that, despite the availability of new compounds to treat obesity, the percentage of patients receiving pharmacotherapy for their problem is still small, due to the dearth of obesity specialists, the social problems of obese persons that in general are low-income populations, and the poor level of insurance coverage for the new medications [126].

CONSENT FOR PUBLICATION

Not applicable.

CONFLICT OF INTEREST

The authors confirm that this chapter contents have no conflict of interest.

ACKNOWLEDGEMENTS

Declared none.

REFERENCES

[1]   Toplak H, Woodward E, Yumuk V, *et al.* 2014 EASO Position Statement on the Use of Anti-Obesity Drugs. Obes Facts 2015; 8(3): 166-74.
[http://dx.doi.org/10.1159/000430801] [PMID: 25968960]

[2]   Igel LI, Kumar RB, Saunders KH, Aronne LJ. Practical Use of Pharmacotherapy for Obesity. Gastroenterology 2017; 152(7): 1765-79.
[http://dx.doi.org/10.1053/j.gastro.2016.12.049] [PMID: 28192104]

[3]   Jensen MD, Ryan DH, Apovian CM, *et al.* 2013 AHA/ACC/TOS guideline for the management of overweight and obesity in adults: a report of the American College of Cardiology/American Heart Association Task Force on Practice Guidelines and The Obesity Society. Circulation 2014; 129(25) (Suppl. 2): S102-38.
[http://dx.doi.org/10.1161/01.cir.0000437739.71477.ee] [PMID: 24222017]

[4]   Hainer V, Toplak H, Mitrakou A. Treatment modalities of obesity: what fits whom? Diabetes Care 2008; 31 (Suppl. 2): S269-77.
[http://dx.doi.org/10.2337/dc08-s265] [PMID: 18227496]

[5]   Frühbeck G, Toplak H, Woodward E, Yumuk V, Maislos M, Oppert JM. Obesity: the gateway to ill health - an EASO position statement on a rising public health, clinical and scientific challenge in Europe. Obes Facts 2013; 6(2): 117-20.
[http://dx.doi.org/10.1159/000350627] [PMID: 23548858]

[6]   Yumuk V, Frühbeck G, Oppert JM, Woodward E, Toplak H. An EASO position statement on multidisciplinary obesity management in adults. Obes Facts 2014; 7(2): 96-101.
[http://dx.doi.org/10.1159/000362191] [PMID: 24685592]

[7]   Tsigos C, Hainer V, Basdevant A, *et al.* Management of obesity in adults: European clinical practice guidelines. Obes Facts 2008; 1(2): 106-16.
[http://dx.doi.org/10.1159/000126822] [PMID: 20054170]

[8]   Chen Y. Regulation of food intake and the development of anti-obesity drugs. Drug Discov Ther 2016; 10(2): 62-73.
[http://dx.doi.org/10.5582/ddt.2016.01014] [PMID: 27063550]

[9]   Jones BJ, Bloom SR. The New Era of Drug Therapy for Obesity: The Evidence and the Expectations. Drugs 2015; 75(9): 935-45.
[http://dx.doi.org/10.1007/s40265-015-0410-1] [PMID: 25985865]

[10]   Gotthardt JD, Bello NT. Can we win the war on obesity with pharmacotherapy? Expert Rev Clin Pharmacol 2016; 9(10): 1289-97.
[http://dx.doi.org/10.1080/17512433.2016.1232164] [PMID: 27590007]

[11]   Ballinger A, Peikin SR. Orlistat: its current status as an anti-obesity drug. Eur J Pharmacol 2002; 440(2-3): 109-17.
[http://dx.doi.org/10.1016/S0014-2999(02)01422-X] [PMID: 12007529]

[12]   Zhi J, Melia AT, Funk C, *et al.* Metabolic profiles of minimally absorbed orlistat in obese/overweight volunteers. J Clin Pharmacol 1996; 36(11): 1006-11.
[http://dx.doi.org/10.1177/009127009603601104] [PMID: 8973989]

[13]   Zhi J, Mulligan TE, Hauptman JB. Long-term systemic exposure of orlistat, a lipase inhibitor, and its metabolites in obese patients. J Clin Pharmacol 1999; 39(1): 41-6.
[http://dx.doi.org/10.1177/00912709922007543] [PMID: 9987699]

[14]   Bray GA, Ryan DH. Update on obesity pharmacotherapy. Ann N Y Acad Sci 2014; 1311: 1-13.
[http://dx.doi.org/10.1111/nyas.12328] [PMID: 24641701]

[15]   Torgerson JS, Hauptman J, Boldrin MN, Sjöström L. XENical in the prevention of diabetes in obese subjects (XENDOS) study: a randomized study of orlistat as an adjunct to lifestyle changes for the prevention of type 2 diabetes in obese patients. Diabetes Care 2004; 27(1): 155-61.
[http://dx.doi.org/10.2337/diacare.27.1.155] [PMID: 14693982]

[16]   Chanoine JP, Hampl S, Jensen C, Boldrin M, Hauptman J. Effect of orlistat on weight and body composition in obese adolescents: a randomized controlled trial. JAMA 2005; 293(23): 2873-83.
[http://dx.doi.org/10.1001/jama.293.23.2873] [PMID: 15956632]

[17] Karhunen L, Franssila-Kallunki A, Rissanen P, *et al.* Effect of orlistat treatment on body composition and resting energy expenditure during a two-year weight-reduction programme in obese Finns. Int J Obes Relat Metab Disord 2000; 24(12): 1567-72.
[http://dx.doi.org/10.1038/sj.ijo.0801443] [PMID: 11126207]

[18] Rucker D, Padwal R, Li SK, Curioni C, Lau DC. Long term pharmacotherapy for obesity and overweight: updated meta-analysis. BMJ 2007; 335(7631): 1194-9.
[http://dx.doi.org/10.1136/bmj.39385.413113.25] [PMID: 18006966]

[19] Smith SR, Weissman NJ, Anderson CM, *et al.* Multicenter, placebo-controlled trial of lorcaserin for weight management. N Engl J Med 2010; 363(3): 245-56.
[http://dx.doi.org/10.1056/NEJMoa0909809] [PMID: 20647200]

[20] Fidler MC, Sanchez M, Raether B, *et al.* A one-year randomized trial of lorcaserin for weight loss in obese and overweight adults: the BLOSSOM trial. J Clin Endocrinol Metab 2011; 96(10): 3067-77.
[http://dx.doi.org/10.1210/jc.2011-1256] [PMID: 21795446]

[21] Elfhag K, Rössner S. Who succeeds in maintaining weight loss? A conceptual review of factors associated with weight loss maintenance and weight regain. Obes Rev 2005; 6(1): 67-85.
[http://dx.doi.org/10.1111/j.1467-789X.2005.00170.x] [PMID: 15655039]

[22] Smith SR, O'Neil PM, Astrup A, *et al.* Early weight loss while on lorcaserin, diet and exercise as a predictor of week 52 weight-loss outcomes. Obesity (Silver Spring) 2014; 22(10): 2137-46.
[http://dx.doi.org/10.1002/oby.20841] [PMID: 25044799]

[23] O'Neil PM, Smith SR, Weissman NJ, *et al.* Randomized placebo-controlled clinical trial of lorcaserin for weight loss in type 2 diabetes mellitus: the BLOOM-DM study. Obesity (Silver Spring) 2012; 20(7): 1426-36.
[http://dx.doi.org/10.1038/oby.2012.66] [PMID: 22421927]

[24] Bohula EA, Wiviott SD, McGuire DK, *et al.* Cardiovascular Safety of Lorcaserin in Overweight or Obese Patients. N Engl J Med 2018; 379(12): 1107-17.
[http://dx.doi.org/10.1056/NEJMoa1808721] [PMID: 30145941]

[25] Wilding J, Van Gaal L, Rissanen A, Vercruysse F, Fitchet M. A randomized double-blind placebo-controlled study of the long-term efficacy and safety of topiramate in the treatment of obese subjects. Int J Obes Relat Metab Disord 2004; 28(11): 1399-410.
[http://dx.doi.org/10.1038/sj.ijo.0802783] [PMID: 15486569]

[26] Richard D, Ferland J, Lalonde J, Samson P, Deshaies Y. Influence of topiramate in the regulation of energy balance. Nutrition 2000; 16(10): 961-6.
[http://dx.doi.org/10.1016/S0899-9007(00)00452-4] [PMID: 11054602]

[27] Allison DB, Gadde KM, Garvey WT, *et al.* Controlled-release phentermine/topiramate in severely obese adults: a randomized controlled trial (EQUIP). Obesity (Silver Spring) 2012; 20(2): 330-42.
[http://dx.doi.org/10.1038/oby.2011.330] [PMID: 22051941]

[28] Gadde KM, Allison DB, Ryan DH, *et al.* Effects of low-dose, controlled-release, phentermine plus topiramate combination on weight and associated comorbidities in overweight and obese adults (CONQUER): a randomised, placebo-controlled, phase 3 trial. Lancet 2011; 377(9774): 1341-52.
[http://dx.doi.org/10.1016/S0140-6736(11)60205-5] [PMID: 21481449]

[29] Garvey WT, Ryan DH, Look M, *et al.* Two-year sustained weight loss and metabolic benefits with controlled-release phentermine/topiramate in obese and overweight adults (SEQUEL): a randomized, placebo-controlled, phase 3 extension study. Am J Clin Nutr 2012; 95(2): 297-308.
[http://dx.doi.org/10.3945/ajcn.111.024927] [PMID: 22158731]

[30] Greenway FL, Dunayevich E, Tollefson G, *et al.* Comparison of combined bupropion and naltrexone therapy for obesity with monotherapy and placebo. J Clin Endocrinol Metab 2009; 94(12): 4898-906.
[http://dx.doi.org/10.1210/jc.2009-1350] [PMID: 19846734]

[31] Greenway FL, Fujioka K, Plodkowski RA, *et al.* Effect of naltrexone plus bupropion on weight loss in

overweight and obese adults (COR-I): a multicentre, randomised, double-blind, placebo-controlled, phase 3 trial. Lancet 2010; 376(9741): 595-605.
[http://dx.doi.org/10.1016/S0140-6736(10)60888-4] [PMID: 20673995]

[32]   Apovian CM, Aronne L, Rubino D, *et al.* A randomized, phase 3 trial of naltrexone SR/bupropion SR on weight and obesity-related risk factors (COR-II). Obesity (Silver Spring) 2013; 21(5): 935-43.
[http://dx.doi.org/10.1002/oby.20309] [PMID: 23408728]

[33]   Wadden TA, Foreyt JP, Foster GD, *et al.* Weight loss with naltrexone SR/bupropion SR combination therapy as an adjunct to behavior modification: the COR-BMOD trial. Obesity (Silver Spring) 2011; 19(1): 110-20.
[http://dx.doi.org/10.1038/oby.2010.147] [PMID: 20559296]

[34]   Hollander P, Gupta AK, Plodkowski R, *et al.* Effects of naltrexone sustained-release/bupropion sustained-release combination therapy on body weight and glycemic parameters in overweight and obese patients with type 2 diabetes. Diabetes Care 2013; 36(12): 4022-9.
[http://dx.doi.org/10.2337/dc13-0234] [PMID: 24144653]

[35]   Velazquez A, Apovian CM. Pharmacological management of obesity. Minerva Endocrinol 2017.
[PMID: 28462579]

[36]   van Can J, Sloth B, Jensen CB, Flint A, Blaak EE, Saris WH. Effects of the once-daily GLP-1 analog liraglutide on gastric emptying, glycemic parameters, appetite and energy metabolism in obese, non-diabetic adults. Int J Obes 2014; 38(6): 784-93.
[http://dx.doi.org/10.1038/ijo.2013.162] [PMID: 23999198]

[37]   Astrup A, Rössner S, Van Gaal L, *et al.* Effects of liraglutide in the treatment of obesity: a randomised, double-blind, placebo-controlled study. Lancet 2009; 374(9701): 1606-16.
[http://dx.doi.org/10.1016/S0140-6736(09)61375-1] [PMID: 19853906]

[38]   Astrup A, Carraro R, Finer N, *et al.* Safety, tolerability and sustained weight loss over 2 years with the once-daily human GLP-1 analog, liraglutide. Int J Obes 2012; 36(6): 843-54.
[http://dx.doi.org/10.1038/ijo.2011.158] [PMID: 21844879]

[39]   Garber A, Henry RR, Ratner R, Hale P, Chang CT, Bode B. Liraglutide, a once-daily human glucagon-like peptide 1 analogue, provides sustained improvements in glycaemic control and weight for 2 years as monotherapy compared with glimepiride in patients with type 2 diabetes. Diabetes Obes Metab 2011; 13(4): 348-56.
[http://dx.doi.org/10.1111/j.1463-1326.2010.01356.x] [PMID: 21205128]

[40]   Pi-Sunyer X, Astrup A, Fujioka K, *et al.* A Randomized, Controlled Trial of 3.0 mg of Liraglutide in Weight Management. N Engl J Med 2015; 373(1): 11-22.
[http://dx.doi.org/10.1056/NEJMoa1411892] [PMID: 26132939]

[41]   Davies MJ, Bergenstal R, Bode B, *et al.* Efficacy of Liraglutide for Weight Loss Among Patients With Type 2 Diabetes: The SCALE Diabetes Randomized Clinical Trial. JAMA 2015; 314(7): 687-99.
[http://dx.doi.org/10.1001/jama.2015.9676] [PMID: 26284720]

[42]   Wadden TA, Hollander P, Klein S, *et al.* Weight maintenance and additional weight loss with liraglutide after low-calorie-diet-induced weight loss: the SCALE Maintenance randomized study. Int J Obes 2013; 37(11): 1443-51.
[http://dx.doi.org/10.1038/ijo.2013.120] [PMID: 23812094]

[43]   Blackman A, Foster GD, Zammit G, *et al.* Effect of liraglutide 3.0 mg in individuals with obesity and moderate or severe obstructive sleep apnea: the SCALE Sleep Apnea randomized clinical trial. Int J Obes 2016; 40(8): 1310-9.
[http://dx.doi.org/10.1038/ijo.2016.52] [PMID: 27005405]

[44]   Marso SP, Bain SC, Consoli A, *et al.* Semaglutide and Cardiovascular Outcomes in Patients with Type 2 Diabetes. N Engl J Med 2016; 375(19): 1834-44.
[http://dx.doi.org/10.1056/NEJMoa1607141] [PMID: 27633186]

[45]   Apovian CM, Aronne LJ, Bessesen DH, *et al.* Pharmacological management of obesity: an endocrine Society clinical practice guideline. J Clin Endocrinol Metab 2015; 100(2): 342-62.
[http://dx.doi.org/10.1210/jc.2014-3415] [PMID: 25590212]

[46]   Khera R, Murad MH, Chandar AK, *et al.* Association of Pharmacological Treatments for Obesity With Weight Loss and Adverse Events: A Systematic Review and Meta-analysis. JAMA 2016; 315(22): 2424-34.
[http://dx.doi.org/10.1001/jama.2016.7602] [PMID: 27299618]

[47]   Kumar RB, Aronne LJ. Efficacy comparison of medications approved for chronic weight management. Obesity (Silver Spring) 2015; 23 (Suppl. 1): S4-7.
[http://dx.doi.org/10.1002/oby.21093] [PMID: 25900871]

[48]   Narayanaswami V, Dwoskin LP. Obesity: Current and potential pharmacotherapeutics and targets. Pharmacol Ther 2017; 170: 116-47.
[http://dx.doi.org/10.1016/j.pharmthera.2016.10.015] [PMID: 27773782]

[49]   Lau J, Bloch P, Schäffer L, *et al.* Discovery of the Once-Weekly Glucagon-Like Peptide-1 (GLP-1) Analogue Semaglutide. J Med Chem 2015; 58(18): 7370-80.
[http://dx.doi.org/10.1021/acs.jmedchem.5b00726] [PMID: 26308095]

[50]   O'Neil PM, Birkenfeld AL, McGowan B, *et al.* Efficacy and safety of semaglutide compared with liraglutide and placebo for weight loss in patients with obesity: a randomised, double-blind, placebo and active controlled, dose-ranging, phase 2 trial. Lancet 2018; 392(10148): 637-49.
[http://dx.doi.org/10.1016/S0140-6736(18)31773-2] [PMID: 30122305]

[51]   Nauck MA, Petrie JR, Sesti G, *et al.* A Phase 2, Randomized, Dose-Finding Study of the Novel Once-Weekly Human GLP-1 Analog, Semaglutide, Compared With Placebo and Open-Label Liraglutide in Patients With Type 2 Diabetes. Diabetes Care 2016; 39(2): 231-41.
[PMID: 26358288]

[52]   Sorli C, Harashima SI, Tsoukas GM, *et al.* Efficacy and safety of once-weekly semaglutide monotherapy versus placebo in patients with type 2 diabetes (SUSTAIN 1): a double-blind, randomised, placebo-controlled, parallel-group, multinational, multicentre phase 3a trial. Lancet Diabetes Endocrinol 2017; 5(4): 251-60.
[http://dx.doi.org/10.1016/S2213-8587(17)30013-X] [PMID: 28110911]

[53]   Davies M, Pieber TR, Hartoft-Nielsen ML, Hansen OKH, Jabbour S, Rosenstock J. Effect of Oral Semaglutide Compared With Placebo and Subcutaneous Semaglutide on Glycemic Control in Patients With Type 2 Diabetes: A Randomized Clinical Trial. JAMA 2017; 318(15): 1460-70.
[http://dx.doi.org/10.1001/jama.2017.14752] [PMID: 29049653]

[54]   Kissileff HR, Thornton JC, Torres MI, *et al.* Leptin reverses declines in satiation in weight-reduced obese humans. Am J Clin Nutr 2012; 95(2): 309-17.
[http://dx.doi.org/10.3945/ajcn.111.012385] [PMID: 22237063]

[55]   Roth JD, Roland BL, Cole RL, *et al.* Leptin responsiveness restored by amylin agonism in diet-induced obesity: evidence from nonclinical and clinical studies. Proc Natl Acad Sci USA 2008; 105(20): 7257-62.
[http://dx.doi.org/10.1073/pnas.0706473105] [PMID: 18458326]

[56]   Mack CM, Soares CJ, Wilson JK, *et al.* Davalintide (AC2307), a novel amylin-mimetic peptide: enhanced pharmacological properties over native amylin to reduce food intake and body weight. Int J Obes 2010; 34(2): 385-95.
[http://dx.doi.org/10.1038/ijo.2009.238] [PMID: 19935749]

[57]   Gydesen S, Andreassen KV, Hjuler ST, Christensen JM, Karsdal MA, Henriksen K. KBP-088, a novel DACRA with prolonged receptor activation, is superior to davalintide in terms of efficacy on body weight. Am J Physiol Endocrinol Metab 2016; 310(10): E821-7.
[http://dx.doi.org/10.1152/ajpendo.00514.2015] [PMID: 26908506]

[58] Gustavson S, Grimes I, Valcarce C, Burstein A, Mjalli A, Eds. TTP054, a Novel, Orally-Available Glucagon-like Peptide-1 (GLP-1) Agonist, Lowers HbA1c in Subjects with Type 2 Diabetes Mellitus (T2DM). DIABETES; 2014: AMER DIABETES ASSOC 1701 N BEAUREGARD ST, ALEXANDRIA, VAUSA 2014; pp. 22311-1717.

[59] Freeman J, Dvergsten C, Dunn I, Valcarce C, Eds. TTP273, Oral (Nonpeptide) GLP-1R Agonist: Improved Glycemic Control without Nausea and Vomiting in Phase 2. DIABETES; 2017: AMER DIABETES ASSOC 1701 N BEAUREGARD ST, ALEXANDRIA, VAUSA 2017; pp. 22311-1717.

[60] Joel CD. Stimulation of metabolism of rat brown adipose tissue by addition of lipolytic hormones in vitro. J Biol Chem 1966; 241(4): 814-21.
[PMID: 4285845]

[61] Kuroshima A, Yahata T. Thermogenic responses of brown adipocytes to noradrenaline and glucagon in heat-acclimated and cold-acclimated rats. Jpn J Physiol 1979; 29(6): 683-90.
[http://dx.doi.org/10.2170/jjphysiol.29.683] [PMID: 541897]

[62] Müller WA, Faloona GR, Aguilar-Parada E, Unger RH. Abnormal alpha-cell function in diabetes. Response to carbohydrate and protein ingestion. N Engl J Med 1970; 283(3): 109-15.
[http://dx.doi.org/10.1056/NEJM197007162830301] [PMID: 4912452]

[63] Dakin CL, Gunn I, Small CJ, *et al*. Oxyntomodulin inhibits food intake in the rat. Endocrinology 2001; 142(10): 4244-50.
[http://dx.doi.org/10.1210/endo.142.10.8430] [PMID: 11564680]

[64] Habegger KM, Stemmer K, Cheng C, *et al*. Fibroblast growth factor 21 mediates specific glucagon actions. Diabetes 2013; 62(5): 1453-63.
[http://dx.doi.org/10.2337/db12-1116] [PMID: 23305646]

[65] Talukdar S, Zhou Y, Li D, *et al*. A Long-Acting FGF21 Molecule, PF-05231023, Decreases Body Weight and Improves Lipid Profile in Non-human Primates and Type 2 Diabetic Subjects. Cell Metab 2016; 23(3): 427-40.
[http://dx.doi.org/10.1016/j.cmet.2016.02.001] [PMID: 26959184]

[66] Finan B, Ma T, Ottaway N, *et al*. Unimolecular dual incretins maximize metabolic benefits in rodents, monkeys, and humans. Sci Transl Med 2013; 5(209)209ra151
[http://dx.doi.org/10.1126/scitranslmed.3007218] [PMID: 24174327]

[67] Frias JP, Nauck MA, Van J, *et al*. Efficacy and safety of LY3298176, a novel dual GIP and GLP-1 receptor agonist, in patients with type 2 diabetes: a randomised, placebo-controlled and active comparator-controlled phase 2 trial. Lancet 2018; 392(10160): 2180-93.
[http://dx.doi.org/10.1016/S0140-6736(18)32260-8] [PMID: 30293770]

[68] Finan B, Yang B, Ottaway N, *et al*. A rationally designed monomeric peptide triagonist corrects obesity and diabetes in rodents. Nat Med 2015; 21(1): 27-36.
[http://dx.doi.org/10.1038/nm.3761] [PMID: 25485909]

[69] Kim J, Lee J, Choi J, *et al*. Novel Combination of a Long-Acting GLP-1/GIP/Glucagon Triple Agonist (HM15211) and Once-Weekly Basal Insulin (HM12460a) Offers Improved Glucose Lowering and Weight Loss in a Diabetic Animal Model. Diabetes 2018; 67 (Suppl. 1): 719.
[http://dx.doi.org/10.2337/db18-77-OR]

[70] Wren AM, Bloom SR. Gut hormones and appetite control. Gastroenterology 2007; 132(6): 2116-30.
[http://dx.doi.org/10.1053/j.gastro.2007.03.048] [PMID: 17498507]

[71] Holst JJ. On the physiology of GIP and GLP-1. Horm Metab Res 2004; 36(11-12): 747-54.
[http://dx.doi.org/10.1055/s-2004-826158] [PMID: 15655703]

[72] Cohen MA, Ellis SM, Le Roux CW, *et al*. Oxyntomodulin suppresses appetite and reduces food intake in humans. J Clin Endocrinol Metab 2003; 88(10): 4696-701.
[http://dx.doi.org/10.1210/jc.2003-030421] [PMID: 14557443]

[73] Wynne K, Park AJ, Small CJ, *et al.* Subcutaneous oxyntomodulin reduces body weight in overweight and obese subjects: a double-blind, randomized, controlled trial. Diabetes 2005; 54(8): 2390-5.
[http://dx.doi.org/10.2337/diabetes.54.8.2390] [PMID: 16046306]

[74] Wynne K, Park AJ, Small CJ, *et al.* Oxyntomodulin increases energy expenditure in addition to decreasing energy intake in overweight and obese humans: a randomised controlled trial. Int J Obes 2006; 30(12): 1729-36.
[http://dx.doi.org/10.1038/sj.ijo.0803344] [PMID: 16619056]

[75] Harris JM, Chess RB. Effect of pegylation on pharmaceuticals. Nat Rev Drug Discov 2003; 2(3): 214-21.
[http://dx.doi.org/10.1038/nrd1033] [PMID: 12612647]

[76] Bianchi E, Carrington PE, Ingallinella P, *et al.* A PEGylated analog of the gut hormone oxyntomodulin with long-lasting antihyperglycemic, insulinotropic and anorexigenic activity. Bioorg Med Chem 2013; 21(22): 7064-73.
[http://dx.doi.org/10.1016/j.bmc.2013.09.016] [PMID: 24094437]

[77] Agaku IT, Singh T, Jones SE, *et al.* Combustible and Smokeless Tobacco Use Among High School Athletes - United States, 2001-2013. MMWR Morb Mortal Wkly Rep 2015; 64(34): 935-9.
[http://dx.doi.org/10.15585/mmwr.mm6434a2] [PMID: 26334565]

[78] Wong D, Sullivan K, Heap G. The pharmaceutical market for obesity therapies. Nat Rev Drug Discov 2012; 11(9): 669-70.
[http://dx.doi.org/10.1038/nrd3830] [PMID: 22935797]

[79] Melnikova I, Wages D. Anti-obesity therapies. Nat Rev Drug Discov 2006; 5(5): 369-70.
[http://dx.doi.org/10.1038/nrd2037] [PMID: 16802443]

[80] Andrade S, Pinho F, Ribeiro AM, *et al.* Immunization against active ghrelin using virus-like particles for obesity treatment. Curr Pharm Des 2013; 19(36): 6551-8.
[http://dx.doi.org/10.2174/13816128113199990506] [PMID: 23859551]

[81] Azegami T, Yuki Y, Sawada S, *et al.* Nanogel-based nasal ghrelin vaccine prevents obesity. Mucosal Immunol 2017; 10(5): 1351-60.
[http://dx.doi.org/10.1038/mi.2016.137] [PMID: 28120848]

[82] Haffer KN. Effects of novel vaccines on weight loss in diet-induced-obese (DIO) mice. J Anim Sci Biotechnol 2012; 3(1): 21.
[http://dx.doi.org/10.1186/2049-1891-3-21] [PMID: 22958753]

[83] Na HN, Hong YM, Kim J, Kim HK, Jo I, Nam JH. Association between human adenovirus-36 and lipid disorders in Korean schoolchildren. Int J Obes 2010; 34(1): 89-93.
[http://dx.doi.org/10.1038/ijo.2009.207] [PMID: 19823186]

[84] Almgren M, Atkinson R, He J, *et al.* Adenovirus-36 is associated with obesity in children and adults in Sweden as determined by rapid ELISA. PLoS One 2012; 7(7)e41652
[http://dx.doi.org/10.1371/journal.pone.0041652] [PMID: 22848557]

[85] Pasarica M, Loiler S, Dhurandhar NV. Acute effect of infection by adipogenic human adenovirus Ad36. Arch Virol 2008; 153(11): 2097-102.
[http://dx.doi.org/10.1007/s00705-008-0219-2] [PMID: 18830560]

[86] Na HN, Nam JH. Proof-of-concept for a virus-induced obesity vaccine; vaccination against the obesity agent adenovirus 36. Int J Obes 2014; 38(11): 1470-4.
[http://dx.doi.org/10.1038/ijo.2014.41] [PMID: 24614097]

[87] Cluny NL, Vemuri VK, Chambers AP, *et al.* A novel peripherally restricted cannabinoid receptor antagonist, AM6545, reduces food intake and body weight, but does not cause malaise, in rodents. Br J Pharmacol 2010; 161(3): 629-42.
[http://dx.doi.org/10.1111/j.1476-5381.2010.00908.x] [PMID: 20880401]

[88]   Randall PA, Vemuri VK, Segovia KN, *et al.* The novel cannabinoid CB1 antagonist AM6545 suppresses food intake and food-reinforced behavior. Pharmacol Biochem Behav 2010; 97(1): 179-84.
[http://dx.doi.org/10.1016/j.pbb.2010.07.021] [PMID: 20713079]

[89]   Farooqi IS, O'Rahilly S. Mutations in ligands and receptors of the leptin-melanocortin pathway that lead to obesity. Nat Clin Pract Endocrinol Metab 2008; 4(10): 569-77.
[http://dx.doi.org/10.1038/ncpendmet0966] [PMID: 18779842]

[90]   Bittencourt JC, Presse F, Arias C, *et al.* The melanin-concentrating hormone system of the rat brain: an immuno- and hybridization histochemical characterization. J Comp Neurol 1992; 319(2): 218-45.
[http://dx.doi.org/10.1002/cne.903190204] [PMID: 1522246]

[91]   Tan CP, Sano H, Iwaasa H, *et al.* Melanin-concentrating hormone receptor subtypes 1 and 2: species-specific gene expression. Genomics 2002; 79(6): 785-92.
[http://dx.doi.org/10.1006/geno.2002.6771] [PMID: 12036292]

[92]   Hill J, Duckworth M, Murdock P, *et al.* Molecular cloning and functional characterization of MCH2, a novel human MCH receptor. J Biol Chem 2001; 276(23): 20125-9.
[http://dx.doi.org/10.1074/jbc.M102068200] [PMID: 11274220]

[93]   Kokkotou EG, Tritos NA, Mastaitis JW, Slieker L, Maratos-Flier E. Melanin-concentrating hormone receptor is a target of leptin action in the mouse brain. Endocrinology 2001; 142(2): 680-6.
[http://dx.doi.org/10.1210/endo.142.2.7981] [PMID: 11159839]

[94]   Saito Y, Cheng M, Leslie FM, Civelli O. Expression of the melanin-concentrating hormone (MCH) receptor mRNA in the rat brain. J Comp Neurol 2001; 435(1): 26-40.
[http://dx.doi.org/10.1002/cne.1191] [PMID: 11370009]

[95]   Qu D, Ludwig DS, Gammeltoft S, *et al.* A role for melanin-concentrating hormone in the central regulation of feeding behaviour. Nature 1996; 380(6571): 243-7.
[http://dx.doi.org/10.1038/380243a0] [PMID: 8637571]

[96]   Rossi M, Beak SA, Choi SJ, *et al.* Investigation of the feeding effects of melanin concentrating hormone on food intake--action independent of galanin and the melanocortin receptors. Brain Res 1999; 846(2): 164-70.
[http://dx.doi.org/10.1016/S0006-8993(99)02005-3] [PMID: 10556632]

[97]   Gomori A, Ishihara A, Ito M, *et al.* Chronic intracerebroventricular infusion of MCH causes obesity in mice. Melanin-concentrating hormone. Am J Physiol Endocrinol Metab 2003; 284(3): E583-8.
[http://dx.doi.org/10.1152/ajpendo.00350.2002] [PMID: 12453827]

[98]   Shimada M, Tritos NA, Lowell BB, Flier JS, Maratos-Flier E. Mice lacking melanin-concentrating hormone are hypophagic and lean. Nature 1998; 396(6712): 670-4.
[http://dx.doi.org/10.1038/25341] [PMID: 9872314]

[99]   Marsh DJ, Weingarth DT, Novi DE, *et al.* Melanin-concentrating hormone 1 receptor-deficient mice are lean, hyperactive, and hyperphagic and have altered metabolism. Proc Natl Acad Sci USA 2002; 99(5): 3240-5.
[http://dx.doi.org/10.1073/pnas.052706899] [PMID: 11867747]

[100] Shearman LP, Camacho RE, Sloan Stribling D, *et al.* Chronic MCH-1 receptor modulation alters appetite, body weight and adiposity in rats. Eur J Pharmacol 2003; 475(1-3): 37-47.
[http://dx.doi.org/10.1016/S0014-2999(03)02146-0] [PMID: 12954357]

[101] Borowsky B, Durkin MM, Ogozalek K, *et al.* Antidepressant, anxiolytic and anorectic effects of a melanin-concentrating hormone-1 receptor antagonist. Nat Med 2002; 8(8): 825-30.
[http://dx.doi.org/10.1038/nm741] [PMID: 12118247]

[102] Eric Hu X, Wos JA, Dowty ME, *et al.* Small-molecule melanin-concentrating hormone-1 receptor antagonists require brain penetration for inhibition of food intake and reduction in body weight. J Pharmacol Exp Ther 2008; 324(1): 206-13.
[http://dx.doi.org/10.1124/jpet.107.130435] [PMID: 17932246]

[103] Huang H, Acuna-Goycolea C, Li Y, Cheng HM, Obrietan K, van den Pol AN. Cannabinoids excite hypothalamic melanin-concentrating hormone but inhibit hypocretin/orexin neurons: implications for cannabinoid actions on food intake and cognitive arousal. J Neurosci 2007; 27(18): 4870-81.
[http://dx.doi.org/10.1523/JNEUROSCI.0732-07.2007] [PMID: 17475795]

[104] Ito M, Ishihara A, Gomori A, *et al.* Mechanism of the anti-obesity effects induced by a novel melanin-concentrating hormone 1-receptor antagonist in mice. Br J Pharmacol 2010; 159(2): 374-83.
[http://dx.doi.org/10.1111/j.1476-5381.2009.00536.x] [PMID: 20015294]

[105] Gehlert DR, Rasmussen K, Shaw J, *et al.* Preclinical evaluation of melanin-concentrating hormone receptor 1 antagonism for the treatment of obesity and depression. J Pharmacol Exp Ther 2009; 329(2): 429-38.
[http://dx.doi.org/10.1124/jpet.108.143362] [PMID: 19182070]

[106] Zhang LN, Sinclair R, Selman C, *et al.* Effects of a specific MCHR1 antagonist (GW803430) on energy budget and glucose metabolism in diet-induced obese mice. Obesity (Silver Spring) 2014; 22(3): 681-90.
[http://dx.doi.org/10.1002/oby.20418] [PMID: 23512845]

[107] Motani AS, Luo J, Liang L, *et al.* Evaluation of AMG 076, a potent and selective MCHR1 antagonist, in rodent and primate obesity models. Pharmacol Res Perspect 2013; 1(1)e00003
[http://dx.doi.org/10.1002/prp2.3] [PMID: 25505557]

[108] Chen KY, Muniyappa R, Abel BS, *et al.* RM-493, a melanocortin-4 receptor (MC4R) agonist, increases resting energy expenditure in obese individuals. J Clin Endocrinol Metab 2015; 100(4): 1639-45.
[http://dx.doi.org/10.1210/jc.2014-4024] [PMID: 25675384]

[109] Greenfield JR, Miller JW, Keogh JM, *et al.* Modulation of blood pressure by central melanocortinergic pathways. N Engl J Med 2009; 360(1): 44-52.
[http://dx.doi.org/10.1056/NEJMoa0803085] [PMID: 19092146]

[110] Kuo JJ, da Silva AA, Tallam LS, Hall JE. Role of adrenergic activity in pressor responses to chronic melanocortin receptor activation. Hypertension 2004; 43(2): 370-5.
[http://dx.doi.org/10.1161/01.HYP.0000111836.54204.93] [PMID: 14707160]

[111] Ni XP, Butler AA, Cone RD, Humphreys MH. Central receptors mediating the cardiovascular actions of melanocyte stimulating hormones. J Hypertens 2006; 24(11): 2239-46.
[http://dx.doi.org/10.1097/01.hjh.0000249702.49854.fa] [PMID: 17053546]

[112] Molinoff PB, Shadiack AM, Earle D, Diamond LE, Quon CY. PT-141: a melanocortin agonist for the treatment of sexual dysfunction. Ann N Y Acad Sci 2003; 994: 96-102.
[http://dx.doi.org/10.1111/j.1749-6632.2003.tb03167.x] [PMID: 12851303]

[113] Kühnen P, Clément K, Wiegand S, *et al.* Proopiomelanocortin Deficiency Treated with a Melanocortin-4 Receptor Agonist. N Engl J Med 2016; 375(3): 240-6.
[http://dx.doi.org/10.1056/NEJMoa1512693] [PMID: 27468060]

[114] Clemmensen C, Finan B, Fischer K, *et al.* Dual melanocortin-4 receptor and GLP-1 receptor agonism amplifies metabolic benefits in diet-induced obese mice. EMBO Mol Med 2015; 7(3): 288-98.
[http://dx.doi.org/10.15252/emmm.201404508] [PMID: 25652173]

[115] Yeh JJ, Ju R, Brdlik CM, *et al.* Targeted gene disruption of methionine aminopeptidase 2 results in an embryonic gastrulation defect and endothelial cell growth arrest. Proc Natl Acad Sci USA 2006; 103(27): 10379-84.
[http://dx.doi.org/10.1073/pnas.0511313103] [PMID: 16790550]

[116] White HM, Acton AJ, Considine RV. The angiogenic inhibitor TNP-470 decreases caloric intake and weight gain in high-fat fed mice. Obesity (Silver Spring) 2012; 20(10): 2003-9.
[http://dx.doi.org/10.1038/oby.2012.87] [PMID: 22510957]

[117] Hughes TE, Kim DD, Marjason J, Proietto J, Whitehead JP, Vath JE. Ascending dose-controlled trial

of beloranib, a novel obesity treatment for safety, tolerability, and weight loss in obese women. Obesity (Silver Spring) 2013; 21(9): 1782-8.
[http://dx.doi.org/10.1002/oby.20356] [PMID: 23512440]

[118] Baratta R, Amato S, Degano C, *et al.* Adiponectin relationship with lipid metabolism is independent of body fat mass: evidence from both cross-sectional and intervention studies. J Clin Endocrinol Metab 2004; 89(6): 2665-71.
[http://dx.doi.org/10.1210/jc.2003-031777] [PMID: 15181039]

[119] Kim DD, Krishnarajah J, Lillioja S, *et al.* Efficacy and safety of beloranib for weight loss in obese adults: a randomized controlled trial. Diabetes Obes Metab 2015; 17(6): 566-72.
[http://dx.doi.org/10.1111/dom.12457] [PMID: 25732625]

[120] McCandless SE, Yanovski JA, Miller J, *et al.* Effects of MetAP2 inhibition on hyperphagia and body weight in Prader-Willi syndrome: A randomized, double-blind, placebo-controlled trial. Diabetes Obes Metab 2017; 19(12): 1751-61.
[http://dx.doi.org/10.1111/dom.13021] [PMID: 28556449]

[121] Bays H. From victim to ally: the kidney as an emerging target for the treatment of diabetes mellitus. Curr Med Res Opin 2009; 25(3): 671-81.
[http://dx.doi.org/10.1185/03007990802710422] [PMID: 19232040]

[122] Liang Y, Arakawa K, Ueta K, *et al.* Effect of canagliflozin on renal threshold for glucose, glycemia, and body weight in normal and diabetic animal models. PLoS One 2012; 7(2)e30555
[http://dx.doi.org/10.1371/journal.pone.0030555] [PMID: 22355316]

[123] Bays HE, Weinstein R, Law G, Canovatchel W. Canagliflozin: effects in overweight and obese subjects without diabetes mellitus. Obesity (Silver Spring) 2014; 22(4): 1042-9.
[http://dx.doi.org/10.1002/oby.20663] [PMID: 24227660]

[124] Hollander P, Bays HE, Rosenstock J, *et al.* Coadministration of Canagliflozin and Phentermine for Weight Management in Overweight and Obese Individuals Without Diabetes: A Randomized Clinical Trial. Diabetes Care 2017; 40(5): 632-9.
[http://dx.doi.org/10.2337/dc16-2427] [PMID: 28289041]

[125] Sands AT, Zambrowicz BP, Rosenstock J, *et al.* Sotagliflozin, a Dual SGLT1 and SGLT2 Inhibitor, as Adjunct Therapy to Insulin in Type 1 Diabetes. Diabetes Care 2015; 38(7): 1181-8.
[http://dx.doi.org/10.2337/dc14-2806] [PMID: 26049551]

[126] Saunders KH, Kumar RB, Igel LI, Aronne LJ. Pharmacologic Approaches to Weight Management: Recent Gains and Shortfalls in Combating Obesity. Curr Atheroscler Rep 2016; 18(7): 36.
[http://dx.doi.org/10.1007/s11883-016-0589-y] [PMID: 27181165]

CHAPTER 8

Current Pharmacological Approaches in Obesity Treatment

Nuno Borges[1,2,*] and **Alejandro Santos**[1,3]

[1] *Faculty of Nutrition and Food Sciences, University of Porto, Porto, Portugal*

[2] *CINTESIS - Center for Health Technology and Services Research, University of Porto, Porto, Portugal*

[3] *i3S - Instituto de Investigação e Inovação em Saúde, University of Porto, Porto, Portugal*

Abstract: The recognition of obesity as a chronic disease and its relentless expansion throughout the world in the last few decades has driven the need for more efficient treatments. Pharmacological approaches have been attempted since the twentieth century, but most of the drugs failed to demonstrate an adequate balance between weight loss and side effects. In the last few years, new, less stringent criteria from the Food and Drug Administration allowed the introduction of new compounds or combinations of old ones. The single new compounds are lorcaserin, an agonist of central $5HT2_C$ receptors and liraglutide, an agonist of glucagon-like peptide 1 receptors. New, fixed-dose combination drugs are naltrexone-bupropion (an opioid antagonist and an antidepressant, respectively) and phentermine-topiramate (a central noradrenaline release stimulant and an antiepileptic, respectively). Orlistat, an inhibitor of gastrointestinal lipases, has also been available for some years. Weight loss effect after one year found in double blind, placebo controlled clinical trials ranges from *circa* 3 kg for orlistat and lorcaserin to 9 kg for the phentermine-topiramate combination. Drugs with higher weight reductions generally present a higher probability of adverse effects. The relatively modest effect of all the drugs approved for obesity treatment clearly shows that pharmacotherapy cannot be the sole solution for the overwhelming obesity epidemic. Nevertheless, a more personalized use of the existing compounds and the possibility of new drugs based on different mechanisms may certainly help to circumvent the powerful energy-conserving mechanisms that make sustained weight loss extremely difficult to achieve.

Keywords: Appetite, Bupropion, Cardiovascular effects, Clinical trials, Diabetes *mellitus*, Drug combination, Efficacy, Liraglutide, Lorcaserin, Monotherapy, Naltrexone, Obesity, Orlistat, Overweight, Pharmacotherapy, Phentermine, Safety, Side-effects, Topiramate, Weight loss.

* **Corresponding author Nuno Borges:** Faculty of Nutrition and Food Sciences, University of Porto, Porto Portugal; Tel: +351 225074320; Fax: +351 225074329; E-mail:nunoborges@fcna.up.pt

Rosário Monteiro and Maria João Martins (Eds.)

INTRODUCTION - HISTORY OF DRUG TREATMENT IN OBESITY

The recognition of obesity as a disease is, historically, quite recent. The American Medical Association only classified it as such in 2013, when its worldwide epidemic was already well established [1]. Yet, attempts to treat it with drugs have been made with increasing intensity since the middle of the twentieth century [2]. The first compounds to be used were dinitrophenol and amphetamine and both produced significant weight loss within a short-time period [2]. Dinitrophenol, a mitochondrial oxidative phosphorylation uncoupling agent, induced a higher energy expenditure, therefore leading to weight loss, but it was soon verified that its side effects were frequent and severe: liver and renal toxicity and hyperthermia were often observed [3]. Amphetamine and some of its derivatives, like methamphetamine or dexamphetamine, were also used as appetite inhibitors. These compounds, that enhanced noradrenaline release in brain areas related to appetite control, such as the lateral hypothalamus, led to a subsequent weight loss. Again, the short-time action upon appetite and weight was noticeable, but side effects compromised their use in the treatment of obesity: their potential of abuse, dependency and cardiovascular effects were some of the most important [2].

Subsequent research tried to develop compounds that kept this appetite inhibitor action of amphetamine, but lacked the above mentioned central and peripheral effects. From this effort, some drugs, such as phentermine, phenylpropanolamine or diethylpropion, were introduced in the market, with mixed results. Phentermine is still available as an appetite suppressant for short-term use in the USA and its fixed dose combination with topiramate has recently been approved (see below). Diethylpropion shares most properties with phentermine and is also available in the USA, but phenylpropanolamine was withdrawn due to an association with increased stroke incidence [2]. Fenfluramine and its isomer, dexfenfluramine, were both approved and used in obese patients. Both stimulated the release and inhibited the reuptake of serotonin, reducing appetite and body weight. The combination of fenfluramine with phentermine, popularly known as fen-phen, achieved a considerable success in the USA, but fenfluramine and dexfenfluramine were withdrawn from the market worldwide in 2004, due to an increase in the risk of pulmonary hypertension and cardiac valvulopathy [4].

In 1997, a new drug, sibutramine, was introduced. This compound inhibited serotonin and noradrenaline neuronal reuptake and produced appetite inhibition and weight loss. Sibutramine was available in many countries for almost a decade but again, long-term studies of cardiovascular safety (namely the SCOUT study) [5] revealed significant side-effects, namely increases in non-fatal myocardial infarction and stroke. Therefore, sibutramine was withdrawn from the market in 2011.

A drug with a new mechanism of action, rimonabant, was developed and reached the market in 2006. Rimonabant, a cannabinoid CB1 receptor inverse agonist, explored the role of endogenous cannabinoids on appetite control [6] and displayed significant reductions in body weight and improvements in some cardiometabolic parameters, thus providing an alternative for obesity management and control through a previously unexplored mechanism [2, 7]. Nevertheless, this drug was also withdrawn from the market in 2008, after reports of increased suicidal ideation in treated patients.

Although not extensive, the previous list of anti-obesity drugs clearly shows the difficulty of achieving a balanced combination of efficacy and safety when weight loss is the therapeutic goal. Energy balance, a crucial element in survival, is under the control of several mechanisms, involving brain centers but also peripheral organs such as the gastrointestinal tract or the adipose tissue. The redundancy of these control systems and their capacity to hamper humans to maintain a sustained energy deficit is certainly one of the factors contributing to the failure of single-action drugs, especially in the long-term.

ORLISTAT

Orlistat is an inhibitor of pancreatic and gastric lipases, chemically derived from lipstatin, a compound produced by *Streptomyces toxytricini*. By inhibiting *circa* 30% of triglyceride cleavage into absorbable glycerol and free fatty acids, orlistat reduces fat absorption, thereby reducing energy availability from diet sources. The unabsorbed triglycerides are excreted in the feces [8]. Orlistat itself has a very low absorption in the gastrointestinal tract and its blood concentrations are considered negligible [9]. The actions of orlistat are, thus, confined to the gastrointestinal tract.

Orlistat was approved for weight reduction and weight maintenance in 1999 and has been available in many countries across the world ever since. It was and still is the sole drug approved for obesity in several countries and it is also approved for adolescents [10]. It has originally been marketed as a prescription drug, with a dose of 120 mg, given three times daily, before the main meals. Later, in 2007, a second posology (60 mg) was marketed as an over-the-counter, also with the same therapeutic scheme, three times daily, before meals [11, 12].

Weight loss achieved with orlistat has been studied in several clinical trials, most using the 3x120 mg dosage. According to a recent meta-analysis, average weight difference compared to placebo is -2.63 kg with 95% confidence limits (CL) -2.94, -2.32 [13]. Other reviews, with different inclusion criteria, point to a weight loss of 3.4 kg [14], 3.05 kg [15] or 2.87 kg [16] after one year.

Orlistat effects upon other parameters have also been studied, namely on blood lipids, blood pressure and glycemia. A recent meta-analysis [17] reviewed the published results on plasma total cholesterol, low-density lipoprotein (LDL), high-density lipoprotein (HDL), triglycerides and lipoprotein(a). The conclusions point to a statistically significant reducing effect of orlistat on total cholesterol (-0.30 mmol/L), LDL (-0.27 mmol/L), HDL (-0.034 mmol/L) and triglycerides (-0.09 mmol/L), with no significant effect on lipoprotein(a). These results were more consistent in patients that experienced higher body weight loss; no evidence of any additional mechanism of orlistat upon blood lipids was found.

The meta-analysis of Zhou *et al* [18] reported an overall significant reduction of blood pressure with orlistat. Results show -1.85 mmHg in systolic and -1.49 mmHg in diastolic blood pressure. The review by Siebenhofer *et al* reported a reduction in systolic blood pressure of 2.46 mmHg [19]. This effect is most probably linked to weight loss alone, highlighting the importance of even small reductions in body weight in lowering the cardiovascular risk factor impact in obesity.

Blood glucose control is often impaired in the obese, leading to an increased risk of type 2 diabetes *mellitus* (T2DM) in these patients [20]. A 4-year clinical trial analysed the cumulative incidence of impaired glucose tolerance and T2DM in overweight or obese patients undergoing orlistat 3x120mg treatment [21]. Results show that, despite the relatively modest weight loss, treatment could reduce the number of T2DM patients after 4 years by 37.3% and 45.0% in the whole group or in the group with impaired glucose tolerance at baseline, respectively. This effect of orlistat on the group of patients with impaired glucose tolerance at baseline explains the global effect in all patients and allowed the authors to extrapolate that treating 10 obese patients with impaired glucose tolerance for 4 years will avoid one case of T2DM. The meta-analysis of Zhou *et al* [18] revealed an overall significant reduction of fasting blood glucose of 0.12 mmol/L.

All these effects of orlistat on metabolic parameters are in line with the well-known benefits of weight loss and reinforce the usefulness of even small reductions.

Due to its mechanism of action and lack of systemic absorption, orlistat side effects are relatively scarce and confined to its intestinal actions. The most prevalent of these side effects results from the presence of unabsorbed fat in distal portions of the gut, which often lead to fecal incontinence, flatus with discharge, oily fecal spotting, fecal urgency, oily evacuation and soft stools [16]. These effects appear in a significant number of treated patients, reports ranging from 15-30% [16] to 7% for fecal incontinence [16]. Treatment discontinuation due to side effects occurred in 12%, a value which is significantly higher than in the placebo group [16]. A recent meta-analysis found an odds ratio for discontinuation of orlistat therapy *vs.* placebo of 1.84 (1.55 to 2.18) [13]. Another issue found in orlistat-treated patients is the reduction of plasma levels of fat soluble vitamins A, D, E and K, another direct consequence of reduced fat absorption. The XENDOS study found that after 4 years of treatment, there were reductions in all the 4 vitamins that were significantly higher than in the placebo group, albeit small. Despite these reductions, fat soluble vitamin levels were found to never fall below the respective normal ranges during the whole study [21]. However, a vitamin supplement is now recommended for all patients taking orlistat [16]. A few rare cases of liver failure in orlistat-treated patients raised concern about the putative role of the drug in this serious effect. The Food and Drug Administration (FDA), in the USA, issued a warning for a possible relation between orlistat treatment and liver injury. This analysis was made from 32 cases reported between 1999 and 2008 [22]. A study from 2013, using a self-controlled case series study design, reported no causal relationship between orlistat treatment and acute liver injury in 94695 treated patients [23].

In conclusion, orlistat produces significant, yet modest, weight loss. This effect is often accompanied by improvements in metabolic parameters such as blood lipids, blood pressure and glycemia. Overall safety is good, but gastrointestinal side effects are frequent and may induce withdrawal of treatment due to discomfort.

LORCASERIN

Lorcaserin is a 5-hydroxytryptamine (5-HT, serotonin) receptor agonist. It has a high selectivity for the $5-HT_{2C}$ subtype, being 15 and 100 times more selective than for the $5-HT_{2A}$ and the $5HT_{2B}$ subtypes, respectively [24]. The $5-HT_{2C}$ subtype is thought to be responsible for the appetite inhibition induced by serotonin through the opiomelanocortin neuronal network in the brain [25]. This drug was approved by the FDA and has been in the US market since 2013. Three randomized, double-blind, placebo controlled clinical trials using lorcaserin were the basis for determining both the weight-loss and the side-effects of lorcaserin [26 - 28]. A subsequent meta-analysis [29] shows an overall weight difference of -3.23 kg (-3.75, -2.70, 95% CL) after one year of treatment. The meta-analysis of Khera *et al* [13] reports that 49% and 25% of patients achieved > 5% and > 10% initial weight loss, compared with only 29% and 9% patients in the placebo group, respectively. Other metabolic parameters have been studied in lorcaserin clinical trials, namely blood lipids, blood pressure and glycemia. Results point to statistically significant, albeit small, decreases in: systolic and diastolic pressure (0.61 mmHg and 0.49 mmHg, respectively), total cholesterol (1.06%), LDL

(1.29%) and triglycerides (4.7%). No significant differences were observed for HDL cholesterol. The BLOOM-DM study [28], aimed at studying lorcaserin effects on body weight and glycemic control in T2DM patients, showed statistically significant reductions in glycated hemoglobin (HbA1C) (1.0% *vs.* 0.5% in the placebo group) and in fasting blood glucose (27.4 mg/dL *vs.* 11.9 mg/dL for placebo) using the 10 mg twice daily dosage.

The choice of developing a selective 5-HT$_{2C}$ agonist for weight loss is related to the fact that other drugs, such as fenfluramine or dexfenfluramine, which non-selectively activate all 5-HT$_2$ receptors, presented an increased risk of cardiac valvular disease. In fact, this was one of the problems that led to withdrawal of these drugs and is related to the activation of the 5-HT$_{2B}$ subtype [30]. The selectivity of lorcaserin for the 5-HT$_{2C}$ subtype reduces the probability of such effects. Available data show no significant difference in valvular problems between lorcaserin and placebo treated groups [31]. The most common side-effects associated with lorcaserin use are headache, nausea, dizziness, fatigue, urinary tract infection, constipation, dry mouth and diarrhea [29]. According to a recent meta-analysis by Khera *et al* [13], lorcaserin presents the lowest probability of discontinuation of therapy among the drugs approved for obesity treatment (orlistat, naltrexone-bupropion, phentermine-topiramate and liraglutide). It also showed the highest probability of having fewer side effects using surface under the cumulative ranking (SUCRA) probabilities. Nevertheless, lorcaserin has not been approved in Europe, due to the application withdrawal from the company (Arena Pharmaceuticals). Concerns from the European Medicines Agency Committee for Medicinal Products for Human Use (CHMP) about potential risk of tumors in the long-term use (based on laboratory data), psychiatric disorders (like depression) and cardiac valvulopathy could not be addressed by the company within the timetable for the application [32].

In conclusion, lorcaserin shows a significant weight loss effect, and this effect is accompanied with some favorable changes in the metabolic profile of obese patients. These effects are, however, modest in size. Safety seems to be adequate, but some concerns remain especially in the long-term use of this drug.

PHENTERMINE/TOPIRAMATE COMBINATION

Phentermine is an atypical amphetamine derivative that stimulates norepinephrine release in the central nervous system (CNS), presenting limited effects on dopamine and serotonin. This CNS-acting drug was approved for short-term treatment of obesity in 1959 [33]. The results of a quantitative analysis of 6 trials, published in 2002, estimated that treating patients with the typical daily dose of 30 mg yields an average weight loss of 3.6 kg compared to placebo after 8 to 24 weeks [34]. A meta-analysis performed in 2005 suggests that phentermine as monotherapy results in modest weight loss for up to 6 months [35]. Patients' tolerance to phentermine is good, the most common side-effects are insomnia, dry mouth and constipation [36]. Exposure to phentermine monotherapy can cause modest increases in heart rate and blood pressure, the isolated use of the drug has not been linked to a higher risk of valvular heart disease [37].

Topiramate is a sulphamate-substituted monosaccharide that is widely available as an anti-convulsant, with weight loss properties. Multiple mechanisms of action have been described for this drug including blockade of sodium and L-type calcium channels, antagonism of glutamate AMPA/Kainate receptors, facilitation of GABA-mediated chloride fluxes and inhibition of carbonic anhydrase activity. However, the precise mechanisms of action of topiramate for weight loss remain unclear [38]. Dose-ranging studies have observed significant weight loss at 60 weeks with 96, 192 and 256 mg/day (7, 9.1 and 9.7%, respectively) [39]. In 1996, it was marketed as an antiepileptic drug and in 2004 for migraine prophylaxis. Weight loss was observed in topiramate epilepsy trials, particularly among patients with higher BMI [40]. Consequently, several long-term randomized clinical trials tested the weight loss effectiveness of topiramate in doses up to 384 mg/day in overweight and obese adults, some trials including patients with comorbidities like T2DM and hypertension revealed improvement in glycemic control in topiramate treated patients [39, 41 - 43]. Topiramate treatment-associated weight loss was shown in a 2011 meta-analysis of 10 randomized clinical trials, although 2 of these trials did not have weight loss as a primary outcome. The average weight loss observed in overweight and obese adults was 5.3 kg. Nonetheless, topiramate tolerability as a monotherapy is questionable considering that twice the number of patients withdraw the therapy *vs.* placebo because of adverse events [44].

The fixed dose combination of phentermine immediate release and topiramate extended release was approved by the FDA for weight management on July 2012, under the commercial designation Qsymia®. The drug combination was approved for weight management in obese (BMI > 30 kg/m^2) and overweight (BMI 27-29.9 kg/m^2) patients presenting at least one weight-related comorbidity. The initial dosage proposed is: phentermine/topiramate extended-release (3.75/23 mg); the maintenance dosage proposed is: phentermine/topiramate extended-release (7.5/46 mg) [45]. In Europe, the marketing authorization of this combination, under the commercial name Qsiva®, was refused by the European Medicines Agency (EMA) in 2012 and again in 2013 [46]. Phentermine is presently approved separately for short-term obesity management and topiramate is used in the treatment of epilepsy and migraine prevention. The combination of phentermine with topiramate as a pharmacotherapy for obesity is based on the concept that combining lower doses of each drug will minimize undesired cardiovascular effects while having a synergistic effect on weight loss [47].

As a combination therapy phentermine and topiramate controlled release (CR) were initially tested in a 24-week randomized controlled trial, 200 obese adults were allocated to four groups (50 subjects each) for daily treatment with placebo, phentermine (15 mg), topiramate CR (100 mg) or phentermine/topiramate CR (15/100 mg). The observed weight loss was greater with the combination therapy (10.7%) *vs.* all other groups: placebo (2.1%), phentermine (4.6%) and topiramate CR (6.3%) [48].

The safety and efficacy of phentermine-topiramate CR combination in the treatment of obesity has been evaluated in phase III randomized, placebo-controlled clinical trials. The 56-week EQUIP trial assessed 1267 obese patients with BMI > 35 kg/m^2. Study participants were assigned to 3 treatment groups: placebo, phentermine/topiramate CR (3.75/23 mg) and phentermine/topiramate CR (15/92 mg). The mean weight loss observed in the highest dosage group was 14.4%, whereas 67% patients reduced their body weight by at least 5% and 47% patients showed at least 10% body weight reduction [47]. The 56-week CONQUER trial assessed the safety and efficacy of this combination on 2487 patients with BMI ≥ 27 and ≤ 45 kg/m^2. Patients received placebo or phentermine/topiramate CR (either 7.5/46 mg or 15/92 mg). Mean weight loss from baseline in the maximum dosage group was 12.4%, while 70% patients lost at least 5% body weight, and 48% lost at least 10% body weight [49]. The SEQUEL study was a double-blind, placebo-controlled, 52-week extension of the CONQUER study. This study concludes that fentermine/topiramate CR when used in addition to lifestyle intervention for the treatment of obesity was well tolerated resulting in significant, dose-dependent weight loss that was sustained during a 108-week period. Fentermine/topiramate CR treatment was associated with continued improvements of weight-related cardiometabolic disease manifestations, including hypertension, hyperglycemia and dyslipidemia, regardless of the reduced use of concomitant medications. The effects of this combination therapy ended in a reduction in the rate of progression to T2DM, the biggest benefits were seen in patients receiving phentermine/topiramate CR (15/92 mg) [50]. Paresthesia, dry mouth, upper respiratory tract infection constipation, insomnia, dizziness, and dysgeusia were the most frequent adverse effects of fentermine/topiramate CR in phase 3 trials [49, 50]. Fentermine/topiramate CR use was associated with more frequent cognitive adverse events (language difficulties, memory impairment, attention deficit and psychomotor slowing). In one-year trials, psychiatric disorders, as a class, were twice as common with fentermine/topiramate CR full-dose (23%) than with placebo (11%) [51]. Because of increased risk of cleft lip with or without cleft palate among babies born to mothers who were exposed to topiramate during first trimester of pregnancy, the combination is contraindicated during pregnancy due to its teratogenic potential [52].

Treatment with fentermine/topiramate CR follows a complex dosing protocol: it starts at 3.75/23 mg once daily and increases to 7.5/46 mg after 2 weeks. After 3 months of treatment, if weight loss is < 3% with the 7.5/46 mg dose, the recommended options are to discontinue the drug or rise the dosage to 15/92 mg. When rising from 7.5/46 to 15/92 mg, there is a middle dosage of 11.25/69 mg for a period of 2 weeks. If after 3 months on the 15/92 mg dosage the measured weight loss is < 5% treatment discontinuation is recommended [45].

NALTREXONE/BUPROPION COMBINATION

Bupropion is an aminoketone used as an antidepressant and also as an aid to smoking cessation, it is a norepinephrine and dopamine reuptake inhibitor. Naltrexone is used in the treatment of alcohol and opioid dependence. Anorectic effects have been described for both drugs and the combination has been proven effective in stimulating weight loss [53 - 55].

The FDA approved naltrexone sustained release (SR)/bupropion SR in September 2014, withdrawing the FDA's initial rejection of the combination in 2011 [56]. Naltrexone/buproprion was approved in Europe in April 2015. For the first time, the EMA introduced a stopping rule in its recent approval of naltrexone/buproprion, indicating that treatment must be discontinued if a weight reduction of at least 5% is not attained after 16 weeks [57].

Bupropion can reduce energy intake and increase energy expenditure, one of the underlying mechanisms involves the stimulation of hypothalamic pro-opiomelanocortin (POMC) producing neurons with the subsequent release of α-melanocyte stimulating hormone (α-MSH), which then binds to melanocortin-4 receptor (MC4R) [58]. However, when POMC neurons release α-MSH they also release β-endorphin, which, as an agonist of the μ-opioid receptors on POMC neurons, retroinhibits α-MSH release. Naltrexone administration can block this negative feedback loop, resulting in a stronger and durable activation of POMC neurons explaining the cooperative action of both drugs in weight loss [59]. Additionally, there is evidence that both drugs affect the mesolimbic dopaminergic reward pathway, which is normally involved in behavior reinforcement, namely feeding. Therefore, this drug combination may cause a reduction in reward-driven food intake [60, 61].

The naltrexone/bupropion prolonged release combination has been tested in 4 phase 3, placebo controlled, double-blind, randomized clinical trials. The combination was well tolerated and significant weight loss was observed in all those trials (around 4 to 5% additional weight loss compared with patients on placebo and similar lifestyle modification programs) [62 - 65]. One of these trials showed improvements in glycemic control and in some cardiovascular risk factors in patients with T2DM treated with naltrexone/bupropion [64]. A more recent open label trial studied the use of this combination simultaneously with the use of a commercially available comprehensive lifestyle intervention program or usual care given by their physician. It was concluded that treatment with naltrexone/bupropion prolonged release combination, together with comprehensive lifestyle intervention, significantly enhanced weight loss over usual care alone (8.52% difference). This weight loss was sustained for 78 weeks and was considered safe and well tolerated [66]. In the first 8 weeks of treatment, naltrexone/bupropion increased mean heart rate (2.4 bpm) compared to placebo; increases in systolic and diastolic blood pressure were also observed in the first 8 weeks with a mean increase of 2.4 and 2.0 mmHg, respectively. Heart rate and blood pressure remained increased after 56 weeks, although by lower levels. The FDA initially rejected the approval of this combination requiring a pre-approval cardiovascular outcomes trial. The marketing approval of this combination by the FDA was given after review of provisional data from an at the time ongoing cardiovascular outcomes trial [56].

The presence of bupropion in this combination led to the inclusion of a warning to alert patients and prescribers to the higher risk of suicidal thoughts and behaviors related to antidepressant drugs. Reports of neuropsychiatric events in patients using bupropion for smoking cessation were included in the warning. The naltrexone/bupropion combination most commonly reported adverse effects are nervous system related (seizures, headache, dizziness, insomnia and anxiety) and gastrointestinal (dry mouth, nausea, vomiting and constipation). This combination should not be prescribed to patients with uncontrolled hypertension, seizure disorders and eating disorders, like anorexia nervosa or bulimia. Also, it should not be used in patients receiving chronic opioid treatment and in those that suddenly stop taking alcohol, benzodiazepines, barbiturates or antiepileptic drugs. Naltrexone/bupropion is presented as fixed-dose tablets containing naltrexone/bupropion (8/90 mg) prolonged release tablets. Treatment with naltrexone/bupropion follows a complex protocol, dosage should be escalated as follows: first week, start with 1 tablet each morning; second week, 1 tablet twice daily; third week, 2 tablets in the morning and 1 in the evening; fourth week onward, 2 tablets twice daily. According to the FDA, treatment should be discontinued if weight loss is inferior to 5% after 12 weeks of treatment with maintenance dosage or 16 weeks according to the EMA [67].

LIRAGLUTIDE

When the Glucagon-Like Peptides drug class was originally approved for the treatment of T2DM, it was noted that patients lost weight with continued use, leading to the testing of their weight loss effects [68]. After food intake, glucagon-like peptide 1 (GLP1) is secreted from the L cells in the ileum; this incretin hormone decreases gastric emptying and glucagon secretion [69, 70]. GLP1 has also been shown to act in hypothalamic regions involved in the regulation of appetite and satiety resulting in decreased food intake. It is also known to modulate CNS pathways regulating energy homeostasis, therefore GLP1 acts not only as an incretin but also as a neuropeptide [69, 71]. The observed weight loss may be in part attributed to the gastrointestinal side effects of this class of drugs: nausea, constipation and, in some patients, diarrhea. In patients with diabetes a decrease in glycemia may occur, therefore patients with insulin therapy should avoid liraglutide [71].

Liraglutide is a GLP1 receptor agonist marketed under the commercial name Saxenda® with a 97% homology with endogenous GLP1. The endogenous peptide suffers fast degradation by the enzyme dipeptidyl peptidase IV (DPPIV); on the contrary liraglutide has long lasting effects with a half-life of 10 to 14 hours. Liraglutide was initially approved in 2010 for the treatment of T2DM with a maximum daily dosage of 1.8 mg administered via subcutaneous injections. More recently, both the FDA (2014) and the EMA (2015) approved the drug at the 3.0 mg injectable dose as an adjunct therapy to a reduced-energy diet and increased physical activity for long-term weight management in adults with obesity, or to those who are overweight (BMI > 27 kg/m^2) with comorbidities such as hypertension, T2DM, dyslipidemia or sleep apnea [72, 73].

The development of liraglutide as an obesity treatment started with a phase 2 trial that randomized obese subjects to a double-blind, 20-week daily treatment with placebo or one of 4 doses of liraglutide or orlistat 120 mg, 3 times daily for 20 weeks; each treatment group included 90 to 98 subjects [74]. Liraglutide treatment reduced mean weight in a dose-dependent manner: 1.2, 1.8, 2.4 and 3.0 mg resulted in -4.8, -5.5, -6.3 and -7.2 kg weight change, respectively. Treatment with placebo or orlistat mean weight loss was 2.8 kg and 4.1 kg, respectively. The efficacy and safety of liraglutide 3.0 mg daily injections for weight loss in overweight or obese patients was studied in 4 phase 3 randomized clinical trials; one of these trials also included the lower dosage of 1.8 mg [73]. The SCALE trials (SCALE - Diabetes, SCALE - Obesity and prediabetes and SCALE - maintenance) assessed the clinical safety and efficacy of liraglutide in the treatment of obesity and diabetes [75 - 77]. The SCALE - Obesity and Prediabetes trial enrolled 3731 overweight or obese participants in a 56-week, double-blind, randomized controlled trial, 2487 participants received 3.0 mg of liraglutide and 1244 participants were allocated in the placebo group, all participants received lifestyle modification counseling. By the end of week 56, a 5% body weight loss was observed in 63% of participants in the treated group *vs.* 27% with placebo. A 10% body weight loss was observed in 33% of participants *vs.* 11% in those taking placebo. Treated patient average weight loss was 8.4 ± 7.3 kg, the placebo group lost 2.8 ± 6.5 kg. In the treated group, the observed net weight loss from baseline body weight was 8% *vs.* 3% in the placebo group. Comparable results were observed across trials as well as further improvements in cardiovascular and metabolic risk factors [75]. In the treated group mean systolic blood pressure decreased from baseline 6 to 9 mmHg, no significant changes to diastolic blood pressure were observed and heart rate slightly increased. Liraglutide treatment also reduced the prevalence of prediabetes and metabolic syndrome by 52% and 59% in that order. Liraglutide-treated patients with lifestyle changes (diet and exercise) preserved weight loss achieved through dietary energy restriction and obtained additional weight loss during the 56-week trial period [77]. In patients with moderate/severe obstructive sleep apnea, liraglutide treatment improved the apnea-hypopnea index [78]. At doses up to 3.0 mg, the safety profile and tolerability in adolescents is identical as in adults; however the use of liraglutide for weight loss in this age group is yet to be approved by the FDA and the EMA [79]. The use of liraglutide in patients with T2DM that underwent bariatric surgery was proved safe, induced additional weight loss and reductions in HbA1C [80].

The most common side-effects with liraglutide (which may affect more than 1 in 10 people) are nausea (feeling sick), vomiting, diarrhea and constipation [72, 73]. Liraglutide is contraindicated in patients with a personal or family history of medullary thyroid cancer or with multiple endocrine neoplasia syndrome type 2. Liraglutide use must be discontinued if pancreatitis is suspected. The treatment protocol for weight management with liraglutide recommends a maximum dosage of 3 mg daily. The initial dosage is 0.6 mg, increasing by 0.6 mg weekly until the maximum dosage of 3 mg is reached. The drug is administered through subcutaneous injection in the abdomen, thigh, or upper arm. According to the FDA and the EMA treatment should be discontinued if weight loss is inferior to 5% after 12 weeks of treatment with the maximum dosage [81].

CONCLUDING REMARKS

Obesity remains a major public health problem and its worldwide incidence and prevalence are still increasing. It is recognized that preventing excessive weight gain, especially among children, is probably the best way to invert this tendency, but efforts, which involve social, economic and public health measures, still seem insufficient at this point. Among the therapeutic options for obesity treatment, pharmacotherapy remains at a relatively modest position, although several efforts have been made recently, with the approval of new single or combination drugs. Because some of these were recently introduced in the market, there is still a lack of long-term information on the delicate balance between efficacy and safety, a crucial issue regarding the chronic nature of obesity.

Several new pharmacological mechanisms of action are currently being studied, exploring the diversity of mediators involved in energy homeostasis. The redundancy of these mechanisms and its overwhelming efficacy in preserving fat stores is surely a formidable barrier to transpose by these putative anti-obesity drugs.

CONSENT FOR PUBLICATION

Not applicable.

CONFLICT OF INTEREST

The authors confirm that this chapter contents have no conflict of interest.

ACKNOWLEDGEMENTS

Declared none.

REFERENCES

[1]   Pollack AAMA. Recognizes Obesity as a Disease. New York Times 2013; 2013.

[2]   Bray GA. Medical treatment of obesity: the past, the present and the future. Best Pract Res Clin Gastroenterol 2014; 28(4): 665-84.
        [http://dx.doi.org/10.1016/j.bpg.2014.07.015] [PMID: 25194183]

[3]   Grundlingh J, Dargan PI, El-Zanfaly M, Wood DM. 2,4-dinitrophenol (DNP): a weight loss agent with significant acute toxicity and risk of death. J Med Toxicol 2011; 7(3): 205-12.
        [http://dx.doi.org/10.1007/s13181-011-0162-6] [PMID: 21739343]

[4]   Connolly HM, Crary JL, McGoon MD, *et al.* Valvular heart disease associated with fenfluramine-phentermine. N Engl J Med 1997; 337(9): 581-8.
        [http://dx.doi.org/10.1056/NEJM199708283370901] [PMID: 9271479]

[5]   James WPT, Caterson ID, Coutinho W, *et al.* SCOUT Investigators. Effect of sibutramine on cardiovascular outcomes in overweight and obese subjects. N Engl J Med 2010; 363(10): 905-17.
        [http://dx.doi.org/10.1056/NEJMoa1003114] [PMID: 20818901]

[6]   Freund TF, Katona I, Piomelli D. Role of endogenous cannabinoids in synaptic signaling. Physiol Rev 2003; 83(3): 1017-66.
        [http://dx.doi.org/10.1152/physrev.00004.2003] [PMID: 12843414]

[7]   Després J-P, Golay A, Sjöström L. Rimonabant in Obesity-Lipids Study Group. Effects of rimonabant on metabolic risk factors in overweight patients with dyslipidemia. N Engl J Med 2005; 353(20): 2121-34.
        [http://dx.doi.org/10.1056/NEJMoa044537] [PMID: 16291982]

[8]   Hogan S, Fleury A, Hadvary P, *et al.* Studies on the antiobesity activity of tetrahydrolipstatin, a potent and selective inhibitor of pancreatic lipase. Int J Obes 1987; 11 (Suppl. 3): 35-42.
[PMID: 3440690]

[9]   Zhi J, Melia AT, Eggers H, Joly R, Patel IH. Review of limited systemic absorption of orlistat, a lipase inhibitor, in healthy human volunteers. J Clin Pharmacol 1995; 35(11): 1103-8.
[http://dx.doi.org/10.1002/j.1552-4604.1995.tb04034.x] [PMID: 8626884]

[10]   Chanoine J-P, Hampl S, Jensen C, Boldrin M, Hauptman J. Effect of orlistat on weight and body composition in obese adolescents: a randomized controlled trial. JAMA 2005; 293(23): 2873-83.
[http://dx.doi.org/10.1001/jama.293.23.2873] [PMID: 15956632]

[11]   Hauptman J, Lucas C, Boldrin MN, Collins H, Segal KR. Orlistat in the long-term treatment of obesity in primary care settings. Arch Fam Med 2000; 9(2): 160-7.
[http://dx.doi.org/10.1001/archfami.9.2.160] [PMID: 10693734]

[12]   Rössner S, Sjöström L, Noack R, Meinders AE, Noseda G. European Orlistat Obesity Study Group. Weight loss, weight maintenance, and improved cardiovascular risk factors after 2 years treatment with orlistat for obesity. Obes Res 2000; 8(1): 49-61.
[http://dx.doi.org/10.1038/oby.2000.8] [PMID: 10678259]

[13]   Khera R, Murad MH, Chandar AK, *et al.* Association of Pharmacological Treatments for Obesity With Weight Loss and Adverse Events: A Systematic Review and Meta-analysis. JAMA 2016; 315(22): 2424-34.
[http://dx.doi.org/10.1001/jama.2016.7602] [PMID: 27299618]

[14]   Yanovski SZ, Yanovski JA. Long-term drug treatment for obesity: a systematic and clinical review. JAMA 2014; 311(1): 74-86.
[http://dx.doi.org/10.1001/jama.2013.281361] [PMID: 24231879]

[15]   Peirson L, Douketis J, Ciliska D, Fitzpatrick-Lewis D, Ali MU, Raina P. Treatment for overweight and obesity in adult populations: a systematic review and meta-analysis. CMAJ Open 2014; 2(4): E306-17.
[http://dx.doi.org/10.9778/cmajo.20140012] [PMID: 25485258]

[16]   Rucker D, Padwal R, Li SK, Curioni C, Lau DCW. Long term pharmacotherapy for obesity and overweight: updated meta-analysis. BMJ 2007; 335(7631): 1194-9.
[http://dx.doi.org/10.1136/bmj.39385.413113.25] [PMID: 18006966]

[17]   Sahebkar A, Simental-Mendía LE, Reiner Ž, *et al.* Effect of orlistat on plasma lipids and body weight: A systematic review and meta-analysis of 33 randomized controlled trials. Pharmacol Res 2017; 122: 53-65.
[http://dx.doi.org/10.1016/j.phrs.2017.05.022] [PMID: 28559211]

[18]   Zhou Y-H, Ma X-Q, Wu C, *et al.* Effect of anti-obesity drug on cardiovascular risk factors: a systematic review and meta-analysis of randomized controlled trials. PLoS One 2012; 7(6)e39062
[http://dx.doi.org/10.1371/journal.pone.0039062] [PMID: 22745703]

[19]   Siebenhofer A, Jeitler K, Horvath K, Berghold A, Siering U, Semlitsch T. Long-term effects of weight-reducing drugs in hypertensive patients. Cochrane Database Syst Rev 2013; (3): CD007654
[http://dx.doi.org/10.1002/14651858.CD007654.pub3] [PMID: 23543553]

[20]   Dale CE, Fatemifar G, Palmer TM, *et al.* UCLEB Consortium; METASTROKE Consortium. Causal Associations of Adiposity and Body Fat Distribution With Coronary Heart Disease, Stroke Subtypes, and Type 2 Diabetes Mellitus: A Mendelian Randomization Analysis. Circulation 2017; 135(24): 2373-88.
[http://dx.doi.org/10.1161/CIRCULATIONAHA.116.026560] [PMID: 28500271]

[21]   Torgerson JS, Hauptman J, Boldrin MN, Sjöström L. XENical in the prevention of diabetes in obese subjects (XENDOS) study: a randomized study of orlistat as an adjunct to lifestyle changes for the prevention of type 2 diabetes in obese patients. Diabetes Care 2004; 27(1): 155-61.
[http://dx.doi.org/10.2337/diacare.27.1.155] [PMID: 14693982]

[22] FDA Drug Safety Communication: Completed safety review of Xenical/Alli (orlistat) and severe liver injury 2010 [Available from:. https://www.fda.gov/Drugs/DrugSafety/PostmarketDrugSafetyInformationforPatientsandProviders/ucm213038.htm

[23] Douglas IJ, Langham J, Bhaskaran K, Brauer R, Smeeth L. Orlistat and the risk of acute liver injury: self controlled case series study in UK Clinical Practice Research Datalink. BMJ 2013; 346: f1936. [http://dx.doi.org/10.1136/bmj.f1936] [PMID: 23585064]

[24] Smith BM, Smith JM, Tsai JH, *et al.* Discovery and structure-activity relationship of (1R)-8-chloro-2,3,4,5-tetrahydro-1-methyl-1H-3-benzazepine (Lorcaserin), a selective serotonin 5-HT2C receptor agonist for the treatment of obesity. J Med Chem 2008; 51(2): 305-13. [http://dx.doi.org/10.1021/jm0709034] [PMID: 18095642]

[25] Lam DD, Przydzial MJ, Ridley SH, *et al.* Serotonin 5-HT2C receptor agonist promotes hypophagia via downstream activation of melanocortin 4 receptors. Endocrinology 2008; 149(3): 1323-8. [http://dx.doi.org/10.1210/en.2007-1321] [PMID: 18039773]

[26] Smith SR, Weissman NJ, Anderson CM, *et al.* Behavioral Modification and Lorcaserin for Overweight and Obesity Management (BLOOM) Study Group. Multicenter, placebo-controlled trial of lorcaserin for weight management. N Engl J Med 2010; 363(3): 245-56. [http://dx.doi.org/10.1056/NEJMoa0909809] [PMID: 20647200]

[27] Fidler MC, Sanchez M, Raether B, *et al.* BLOSSOM Clinical Trial Group. A one-year randomized trial of lorcaserin for weight loss in obese and overweight adults: the BLOSSOM trial. J Clin Endocrinol Metab 2011; 96(10): 3067-77. [http://dx.doi.org/10.1210/jc.2011-1256] [PMID: 21795446]

[28] O'Neil PM, Smith SR, Weissman NJ, *et al.* Randomized placebo-controlled clinical trial of lorcaserin for weight loss in type 2 diabetes mellitus: the BLOOM-DM study. Obesity (Silver Spring) 2012; 20(7): 1426-36. [http://dx.doi.org/10.1038/oby.2012.66] [PMID: 22421927]

[29] Chan EW, He Y, Chui CSL, Wong AYS, Lau WCY, Wong ICK. Efficacy and safety of lorcaserin in obese adults: a meta-analysis of 1-year randomized controlled trials (RCTs) and narrative review on short-term RCTs. Obes Rev 2013; 14(5): 383-92. [http://dx.doi.org/10.1111/obr.12015] [PMID: 23331711]

[30] Rothman RB, Baumann MH, Savage JE, *et al.* Evidence for possible involvement of 5-HT(2B) receptors in the cardiac valvulopathy associated with fenfluramine and other serotonergic medications. Circulation 2000; 102(23): 2836-41. [http://dx.doi.org/10.1161/01.CIR.102.23.2836] [PMID: 11104741]

[31] Weissman NJ, Sanchez M, Koch GG, Smith SR, Shanahan WR, Anderson CM. Echocardiographic assessment of cardiac valvular regurgitation with lorcaserin from analysis of 3 phase 3 clinical trials. Circ Cardiovasc Imaging 2013; 6(4): 560-7. [http://dx.doi.org/10.1161/CIRCIMAGING.112.000128] [PMID: 23661689]

[32] Withdrawal of the marketing authorisation application for Belviq (lorcaserin): European Medicines Agency; 2013 [Available from:. http://www.ema.europa.eu/docs/en_GB/document_library/Medicine_QA/2013/05/WC500143811.pdf

[33] Rothman RB, Baumann MH, Dersch CM, *et al.* Amphetamine-type central nervous system stimulants release norepinephrine more potently than they release dopamine and serotonin. Synapse 2001; 39(1): 32-41. [http://dx.doi.org/10.1002/1098-2396(20010101)39:1<32::AID-SYN5>3.0.CO;2-3] [PMID: 11071707]

[34] Haddock CK, Poston WS, Dill PL, Foreyt JP, Ericsson M. Pharmacotherapy for obesity: a quantitative analysis of four decades of published randomized clinical trials. Int J Obes Relat Metab Disord 2002; 26(2): 262-73.

[http://dx.doi.org/10.1038/sj.ijo.0801889] [PMID: 11850760]

[35]   Li Z, Maglione M, Tu W, *et al.* Meta-analysis: pharmacologic treatment of obesity. Ann Intern Med 2005; 142(7): 532-46.
[http://dx.doi.org/10.7326/0003-4819-142-7-200504050-00012] [PMID: 15809465]

[36]   Silverstone T. Appetite suppressants. A review. Drugs 1992; 43(6): 820-36.
[http://dx.doi.org/10.2165/00003495-199243060-00003] [PMID: 1379155]

[37]   Jick H, Vasilakis C, Weinrauch LA, Meier CR, Jick SS, Derby LE. A population-based study of appetite-suppressant drugs and the risk of cardiac-valve regurgitation. N Engl J Med 1998; 339(11): 719-24.
[http://dx.doi.org/10.1056/NEJM199809103391102] [PMID: 9731087]

[38]   Rosenfeld WE. Topiramate: a review of preclinical, pharmacokinetic, and clinical data. Clin Ther 1997; 19(6): 1294-308.
[http://dx.doi.org/10.1016/S0149-2918(97)80006-9] [PMID: 9444441]

[39]   Wilding J, Van Gaal L, Rissanen A, Vercruysse F, Fitchet M. OBES-002 Study Group. A randomized double-blind placebo-controlled study of the long-term efficacy and safety of topiramate in the treatment of obese subjects. Int J Obes Relat Metab Disord 2004; 28(11): 1399-410.
[http://dx.doi.org/10.1038/sj.ijo.0802783] [PMID: 15486569]

[40]   Verrotti A, Scaparrotta A, Agostinelli S, Di Pillo S, Chiarelli F, Grosso S. Topiramate-induced weight loss: a review. Epilepsy Res 2011; 95(3): 189-99.
[http://dx.doi.org/10.1016/j.eplepsyres.2011.05.014] [PMID: 21684121]

[41]   Tonstad S, Tykarski A, Weissgarten J, *et al.* Efficacy and safety of topiramate in the treatment of obese subjects with essential hypertension. Am J Cardiol 2005; 96(2): 243-51.
[http://dx.doi.org/10.1016/j.amjcard.2005.03.053] [PMID: 16018851]

[42]   Eliasson B, Gudbjornsdottir S, Cederholm J, Liang Y, Vercruysse F, Smith U. Weight loss and metabolic effects of topiramate in overweight and obese type 2 diabetic patients: randomized double-blind placebo-controlled trial. Int J Obes (2005) 2007; 31(7): 1140-7.
[http://dx.doi.org/10.1038/sj.ijo.0803548]

[43]   Rosenstock J, Hollander P, Gadde KM, Sun X, Strauss R, Leung A. OBD-202 Study Group. A randomized, double-blind, placebo-controlled, multicenter study to assess the efficacy and safety of topiramate controlled release in the treatment of obese type 2 diabetic patients. Diabetes Care 2007; 30(6): 1480-6.
[http://dx.doi.org/10.2337/dc06-2001] [PMID: 17363756]

[44]   Kramer CK, Leitão CB, Pinto LC, Canani LH, Azevedo MJ, Gross JL. Efficacy and safety of topiramate on weight loss: a meta-analysis of randomized controlled trials. Obes Rev 2011; 12(5): e338-47.
[http://dx.doi.org/10.1111/j.1467-789X.2010.00846.x] [PMID: 21438989]

[45]   Drug Approval Package - Qsymia. US Food and Drug Administration 2012.https://www.accessdata.fda.gov/drugsatfda_docs/nda/2012/022580orig1s000_qsymia_toc.cfm

[46]   Human medicines - Qsiva: European Medicines Agency; 2013 [Available from:.
http://www.ema.europa.eu/ema/index.jsp?curl=pages/medicines/human/medicines/002350/smops/Negative/human_smop_000435.jsp&mid=WC0b01ac058001d127

[47]   Allison DB, Gadde KM, Garvey WT, *et al.* Controlled-release phentermine/topiramate in severely obese adults: a randomized controlled trial (EQUIP). Obesity (Silver Spring) 2012; 20(2): 330-42.
[http://dx.doi.org/10.1038/oby.2011.330] [PMID: 22051941]

[48]   Gadde KMYG, Foust MS, Tam PY, Najarian T. A 24-week randomized controlled trial of VI-0521, a combination weight loss therapy, in obese adults. Obesity (Silver Spring) 2006; 14 (Suppl.): A17-8.

[49]   Gadde KM, Allison DB, Ryan DH, *et al.* Effects of low-dose, controlled-release, phentermine plus topiramate combination on weight and associated comorbidities in overweight and obese adults

(CONQUER): a randomised, placebo-controlled, phase 3 trial. Lancet 2011; 377(9774): 1341-52.
[http://dx.doi.org/10.1016/S0140-6736(11)60205-5] [PMID: 21481449]

[50] Garvey WT, Ryan DH, Look M, *et al.* Two-year sustained weight loss and metabolic benefits with controlled-release phentermine/topiramate in obese and overweight adults (SEQUEL): a randomized, placebo-controlled, phase 3 extension study. Am J Clin Nutr 2012; 95(2): 297-308.
[http://dx.doi.org/10.3945/ajcn.111.024927] [PMID: 22158731]

[51] Shin JH, Gadde KM. Clinical utility of phentermine/topiramate (Qsymia™) combination for the treatment of obesity. Diabetes Metab Syndr Obes 2013; 6: 131-9.
[PMID: 23630428]

[52] Mines D, Tennis P, Curkendall SM, *et al.* Topiramate use in pregnancy and the birth prevalence of oral clefts. Pharmacoepidemiol Drug Saf 2014; 23(10): 1017-25.
[http://dx.doi.org/10.1002/pds.3612] [PMID: 24692316]

[53] Gadde KM, Allison DB. Combination therapy for obesity and metabolic disease. Curr Opin Endocrinol Diabetes Obes 2009; 16(5): 353-8.
[http://dx.doi.org/10.1097/MED.0b013e3283304f90] [PMID: 19625958]

[54] Gadde KM, Parker CB, Maner LG, *et al.* Bupropion for weight loss: an investigation of efficacy and tolerability in overweight and obese women. Obes Res 2001; 9(9): 544-51.
[http://dx.doi.org/10.1038/oby.2001.71] [PMID: 11557835]

[55] Greig SL, Keating GM. Naltrexone ER/Bupropion ER: A Review in Obesity Management. Drugs 2015; 75(11): 1269-80.
[http://dx.doi.org/10.1007/s40265-015-0427-5] [PMID: 26105116]

[56] Drug Approval Package - Contrave: U.S. Food and Drug Administration; 2014 [Available from:. https://www.accessdata.fda.gov/drugsatfda_docs/nda/2014/200063Orig1s000TOC.cfm

[57] Human Medicines - Mysimba: European Medicines Agency; 2015 [Available from:. http://www.ema.europa.eu/ema/index.jsp?curl=pages/medicines/human/medicines/003687/human_me d_001845.jsp&mid=WC0b01ac058001d124

[58] Mercer SL. ACS chemical neuroscience molecule spotlight on contrave. ACS Chem Neurosci 2011; 2(9): 484-6.
[http://dx.doi.org/10.1021/cn200076y] [PMID: 22860172]

[59] Yanovski SZ, Yanovski JA. Naltrexone extended-release plus bupropion extended-release for treatment of obesity. JAMA 2015; 313(12): 1213-4.
[http://dx.doi.org/10.1001/jama.2015.1617] [PMID: 25803343]

[60] Morton GJ, Cummings DE, Baskin DG, Barsh GS, Schwartz MW. Central nervous system control of food intake and body weight. Nature 2006; 443(7109): 289-95.
[http://dx.doi.org/10.1038/nature05026] [PMID: 16988703]

[61] Billes SK, Sinnayah P, Cowley MA. Naltrexone/bupropion for obesity: an investigational combination pharmacotherapy for weight loss. Pharmacol Res 2014; 84: 1-11.
[http://dx.doi.org/10.1016/j.phrs.2014.04.004] [PMID: 24754973]

[62] Apovian CM, Aronne L, Rubino D, *et al.* COR-II Study Group. A randomized, phase 3 trial of naltrexone SR/bupropion SR on weight and obesity-related risk factors (COR-II). Obesity (Silver Spring) 2013; 21(5): 935-43.
[http://dx.doi.org/10.1002/oby.20309] [PMID: 23408728]

[63] Greenway FL, Fujioka K, Plodkowski RA, *et al.* COR-I Study Group. Effect of naltrexone plus bupropion on weight loss in overweight and obese adults (COR-I): a multicentre, randomised, double-blind, placebo-controlled, phase 3 trial. Lancet 2010; 376(9741): 595-605.
[http://dx.doi.org/10.1016/S0140-6736(10)60888-4] [PMID: 20673995]

[64] Hollander P, Gupta AK, Plodkowski R, *et al.* COR-Diabetes Study Group. Effects of naltrexone sustained-release/bupropion sustained-release combination therapy on body weight and glycemic

parameters in overweight and obese patients with type 2 diabetes. Diabetes Care 2013; 36(12): 4022-9.
[http://dx.doi.org/10.2337/dc13-0234] [PMID: 24144653]

[65] Wadden TA, Foreyt JP, Foster GD, *et al.* Weight loss with naltrexone SR/bupropion SR combination therapy as an adjunct to behavior modification: the COR-BMOD trial. Obesity (Silver Spring) 2011; 19(1): 110-20.
[http://dx.doi.org/10.1038/oby.2010.147] [PMID: 20559296]

[66] Halseth A, Shan K, Walsh B, Gilder K, Fujioka K. Method-of-use study of naltrexone sustained release (SR)/bupropion SR on body weight in individuals with obesity. Obesity (Silver Spring) 2017; 25(2): 338-45.
[http://dx.doi.org/10.1002/oby.21726] [PMID: 28026920]

[67] Krentz AJ, Fujioka K, Hompesch M. Evolution of pharmacological obesity treatments: focus on adverse side-effect profiles. Diabetes Obes Metab 2016; 18(6): 558-70.
[http://dx.doi.org/10.1111/dom.12657] [PMID: 26936802]

[68] Shyangdan DS, Royle P, Clar C, Sharma P, Waugh N, Snaith A. Glucagon-like peptide analogues for type 2 diabetes mellitus. Cochrane Database Syst Rev 2011; (10): CD006423
[http://dx.doi.org/10.1002/14651858.CD006423.pub2] [PMID: 21975753]

[69] van Can J, Sloth B, Jensen CB, Flint A, Blaak EE, Saris WH. Effects of the once-daily GLP-1 analog liraglutide on gastric emptying, glycemic parameters, appetite and energy metabolism in obese, non-diabetic adults. Int J Obes (2005) 2014; 38(6): 784-93.

[70] Hansen L, Deacon CF, Orskov C, Holst JJ. Glucagon-like peptide-1-(7-36)amide is transformed to glucagon-like peptide-1-(9-36)amide by dipeptidyl peptidase IV in the capillaries supplying the L cells of the porcine intestine. Endocrinology 1999; 140(11): 5356-63.
[http://dx.doi.org/10.1210/endo.140.11.7143] [PMID: 10537167]

[71] Turton MD, O'Shea D, Gunn I, *et al.* A role for glucagon-like peptide-1 in the central regulation of feeding. Nature 1996; 379(6560): 69-72.
[http://dx.doi.org/10.1038/379069a0] [PMID: 8538742]

[72] Drug Approval Package - Saxenda: U.S. Food and Drug Administration; 2014 [Available from:. https://www.accessdata.fda.gov/scripts/cder/daf/index.cfm?event=overview.process&ApplNo=206321

[73] Human Medicines - Saxenda: EMA; 2015 [Available from:. http://www.ema.europa.eu/ema/index.jsp?curl=pages/medicines/human/medicines/003780/human_me d_001855.jsp&mid=WC0b01ac058001d124

[74] Astrup A, Rössner S, Van Gaal L, *et al.* NN8022-1807 Study Group. Effects of liraglutide in the treatment of obesity: a randomised, double-blind, placebo-controlled study. Lancet 2009; 374(9701): 1606-16.
[http://dx.doi.org/10.1016/S0140-6736(09)61375-1] [PMID: 19853906]

[75] Pi-Sunyer X, Astrup A, Fujioka K, *et al.* SCALE Obesity and Prediabetes NN8022-1839 Study Group. A Randomized, Controlled Trial of 3.0 mg of Liraglutide in Weight Management. N Engl J Med 2015; 373(1): 11-22.
[http://dx.doi.org/10.1056/NEJMoa1411892] [PMID: 26132939]

[76] Davies MJ, Bergenstal R, Bode B, *et al.* NN8022-1922 Study Group. Efficacy of Liraglutide for Weight Loss Among Patients With Type 2 Diabetes: The SCALE Diabetes Randomized Clinical Trial. JAMA 2015; 314(7): 687-99.
[http://dx.doi.org/10.1001/jama.2015.9676] [PMID: 26284720]

[77] Wadden TA, Hollander P, Klein S, *et al.* Weight maintenance and additional weight loss with liraglutide after low-calorie-diet-induced weight loss: the SCALE Maintenance randomized study. Int J Obes (2005) 2013; 37(11): 1443-51.

[78] Blackman A, Foster GD, Zammit G, *et al.* Effect of liraglutide 3.0 mg in individuals with obesity and moderate or severe obstructive sleep apnea: the SCALE Sleep Apnea randomized clinical trial Int J

Obes (2005) 2016; 40(8): 1310-9.

[79]   Danne T, Biester T, Kapitzke K, *et al.* Liraglutide in an Adolescent Population with Obesity: A Randomized, Double-Blind, Placebo-Controlled 5-Week Trial to Assess Safety, Tolerability, and Pharmacokinetics of Liraglutide in Adolescents Aged 12-17 Years. J Pediatr 2017; 181: 146-153.e3.
[http://dx.doi.org/10.1016/j.jpeds.2016.10.076] [PMID: 27979579]

[80]   Gorgojo-Martínez JJ, Feo-Ortega G, Serrano-Moreno C. Effectiveness and tolerability of liraglutide in patients with type 2 diabetes mellitus and obesity after bariatric surgery. Surg Obes Relat Dis 2016; 12(10): 1856-63.
[http://dx.doi.org/10.1016/j.soard.2016.02.013] [PMID: 27256860]

[81]   Gadde KM, Pritham Raj Y. Pharmacotherapy of Obesity: Clinical Trials to Clinical Practice. Curr Diab Rep 2017; 17(5): 34.
[http://dx.doi.org/10.1007/s11892-017-0859-2] [PMID: 28378293]

Recent Advances in Obesity Research, 2020, Vol. 1, 211-235

CHAPTER 9

Managing Obesity with Bariatric Surgery

Gil Faria[1,2,*]

[1] *ULS Matosinhos/Hospital de Pedro Hispano, Serviço de Cirurgia Geral, Matosinhos, Portugal*

[2] *CINTESIS - Center for Health Technology and Services Research, Faculty of Medicine, University of Porto, Porto, Portugal*

Abstract: Obesity is associated with several comorbidities, especially cardiovascular and metabolic diseases. Bariatric surgery is the most effective treatment for obesity, leading to long-term weight loss, reversal of the associated diseases and reduction in long-term mortality. The relative effectiveness of each type of surgery is not yet fully clear, but all the surgeries lead to a significant improvement in metabolic diseases. Resistance to insulin is associated to obesity and is an essential step in the pathophysiology of diabetes. The metabolic effects of surgery (most studied are the effects of gastric bypass) lead to an early improvement of insulin resistance even before significant weight loss has occurred. Metabolic syndrome clusters several cardiovascular risk factors and is increased in obese patients. Surgery leads to remission of metabolic syndrome in up to 80% of patients. The remission of type 2 diabetes after surgery is significantly greater after surgery than with the best medical management, varying between 50-80%. Severity and control of type 2 diabetes are related to the resolution rates after surgery. Coronary artery disease, atherosclerosis, gastro-esophageal reflux disease, obstructive sleep apnea, cardiac failure, renal failure, non-alcoholic hepatic steatosis and other obesity-associated diseases are significantly improved after bariatric surgery. Patients with higher body mass indexes and lower disease burden seem to be those that improve the most, achieving higher remission rates of obesity-associated diseases. Even in the most severe forms of uncontrolled metabolic disease, bariatric surgery leads to a significant improvement of comorbidities.

Keywords: Bariatric surgery, Body mass index, Cardiovascular risk factor, Chronic kidney disease, Dislypidemia, Gastro-esophageal reflux disease, Glycemic control, High blood pressure, Metabolic surgery, Metabolic syndrome, Mortality, Non-alcoholic fatty liver disease, Obstructive sleep apnea, Predictors, Quality of life, Remission, Resistance to insulin, Roux-en-Y gastric bypass, Sleeve gastrectomy, Type 2 diabetes *mellitus*, Weight loss.

---

* **Corresponding author Gil Faria:** CINTESIS - Center for Health Technology and Services Research, Faculty of Medicine, University of Porto, Porto, Portugal; Tel: +351225513600; Fax: +351 225513601; E-mail: gilrfaria@gmail.com

Rosário Monteiro and Maria João Martins (Eds.)

INTRODUCTION

Cardiovascular and metabolic diseases [especially type 2 diabetes *mellitus* (T2DM), high blood pressure (HBP) and dyslipidemia (DLP)] are highly prevalent worldwide and obesity is one of the major risk factors. It is estimated that T2DM affects 8.5% of the human populations and HBP and DLP affect up to 40% [1 - 3].

Before bariatric surgery, the main tools available for managing obesity and metabolic disease were lifestyle modification and medical therapy with dismal results [4 - 7]. Bariatric surgery is the most effective treatment and the only allowing significant and durable weight loss, reversal of the metabolic syndrome and reduction in cardiovascular events and long-term mortality [4, 5, 8 - 14].

However, the evaluation of outcomes in bariatric surgery, although difficult, is of utmost importance. There are several different risks at stake (including death) and different outcomes to be achieved: quality of life (QoL), weight loss and the resolution of associated diseases.

Also, due to the technical nature of the procedures, small variations in the technique (such as pouch size, anastomoses diameter or limb lengths) or different techniques - Roux-en-Y gastric bypass (RYGB), gastric band (GB), sleeve gastrectomy (SG), etc. - make it more difficult to analyse the results and compare data. Patient follow-up and reporting are usually sub-optimal and the parameters used to measure improvement or resolution of comorbidities have not been standardized [15]. So, despite the more than 350000 surgeries performed worldwide each year, we are still lacking consensus on which is the most appropriate surgery for each patient and what outcomes can be expected [16].

Although the operative mortality rates for bariatric surgery range between 0.1% and 2%, the most recent data report mortality rates of 0.15%, making bariatric surgery one of the safest surgical procedures, on par with childbirth [17]. Some of the factors associated with higher mortality are visceral obesity, male sex, BMI > 50 kg/m², T2DM, sleep apnea, older age and low volume centres [17 - 19].

Weight loss is commonly represented as the percentage of excess weight loss (%EWL) and represents the lost weight relative to the weight in excess. Although the %EWL is not the most important outcome of surgery, it is highly correlated with the risk factors and patient satisfaction [15]. Several reports concluded that among groups of patients on medical therapy, net weight change (usually at 2 years) ranged from +0.5% to -21.6%, while in the surgical groups it decreased between 36% and 87% [20 - 23]. The 2009 Cochrane Database Report concludes that "bariatric surgery is a more effective intervention for weight loss than nonsurgical options" [24]. Buchwald's meta-analysis concluded that the mean %EWL was 47.5% after GB and 61.6% after RYGB [25]. The most recent data from International Federation for the Surgery of Obesity (IFSO) concludes that the %EWL is directly related with the initial weight and varies from 106.7% for patients with BMI 30-35 kg/m^2 and 57.8% for patients with BMI ≥ 65 kg/m^2 for RYGB [26]. Furthermore, the SOS study has concluded that this weight loss is sustained up to 15 years after surgery [20].

Although GB, SG, RYGB and biliopancreatic diversion (BPD) are all superior to non-surgical management, the relative effectiveness of these procedures is still not completely established. This is due to studies reporting different follow-up periods and rates, differences in the metric used for reports and variations in the surgical techniques and perioperative protocols [15]. Despite the evolution in the safety and perioperative protocols of the surgeries and the now residual place for GB, a summary of the characteristics of each surgery, as reported in 2011, might be useful (Table **1**).

Table 1. Comparison of surgical procedures (gastric band, sleeve gastrectomy and gastric bypass). Adapted from Dumon *et al* [15].

	Gastric band	Sleeve Gastrectomy	Gastric Bypass
Operative time (min)	77.5	100.4	64.8
Hospital stay (days)	1.7	4.4	4.2
%EWL 1 year	37.8	59.8	62.8
%EWL 3 years	55.0	66.0	66.0
Diabetes resolution (%)	47.8	77.2	83.8
Hypertension resolution (%)	38.4	71.7	75.4
Dyslipidemia improved (%)	71.1	61.0	93.6
Overall Complications (%)	9	11.2	23
Major Complications (%)	0.2	4.7	2
Mortality (%)	0.05	0.5	0.3

%EWL: percentage of excess weight loss (the lost weight relative to the weight in excess).

Despite the perioperative mortality, surgical patients have a lower 5-year mortality than nonsurgical patients (0.68% *vs.* 6.17%) [27]. The reduced mortality is caused by decreases in cardiovascular mortality, diabetes and cancer-related deaths [5, 12, 20, 27].

Obesity is associated with reduced QoL and, in general, QoL improves after bariatric surgery [28, 29]. The differential effect of each surgery on QoL is not yet fully understood, but it seems that RYGB is associated with better measures and greatest improvement in QoL [15, 29 - 31].

SURGERY, WEIGHT LOSS AND INSULIN METABOLISM

Insulin resistance is thought to be a fundamental step in the genesis and development of T2DM. Obesity has long been thought to produce insulin resistance; however, some authors suggest that it might just be another manifestation of insulin resistance. For overt T2DM to establish, both insulin resistance and β-cell dysfunction are required [32 - 34].

Several reports concluded that there is a hyperinsulinemic state associated with obesity [35]. This hyperinsulinism is thought to arise from increased insulin production to compensate for insulin resistance. According to some authors, besides its effects on glucose and lipid metabolism, this hyperinsulinemic state is also related to intracellular mechanisms that lead to cancer development, hence the need to reverse this pathological condition known as insulin resistance [36].

The remission rate of T2DM after bariatric surgery is variable and the underlying mechanisms of this improvement are not yet known. Some studies point out that this improvement occurs early on after surgery, much before any significant weight loss has occurred [33, 37, 38].

After RYGB, patients have been reported to experience a rapid improvement in insulin resistance and T2DM remission as early as 3 days after surgery [33, 37, 39]. A meta-analysis concluded that insulin resistance was significantly improved 2 weeks after RYGB and BPD, but not after SG or GB [40].

Lima *et al* [41] reported an improved insulin resistance 1 month after RYGB and according to Rubino *et al* [42] there was a significant decrease in glucose and insulin levels 3 weeks after RYGB. A meta-analysis concluded that Homeostasis Model Assessment of Insulin Resistance (HOMA-IR) improved by 33% at 1-2 weeks and by 59% at 6 months after RYGB [40]. As early as 3 days after surgery, a decrease in insulin levels and insulin resistance has been documented, both in patients with clinical insulin resistance or with normal glucose tolerance test [39]. Furthermore, these improvements were unchanged up to 12 months after surgery, despite a continuing weight loss [33, 39]. This early improvement in insulin resistance is clinically significant as up to 30% of diabetic patients who undergo RYGB surgery might be discharged with no anti-diabetic medication [43].

Prolonged starvation and calorie restriction have been proposed as tentative hypotheses for the early improvement in insulin resistance [37]. However, the differential results of RYGB and other types of bariatric surgery seem to point that RYGB has (at least) an additive effect to starvation and calorie restriction

[37, 43, 44]. In a long-term follow-up study, Pournaras *et al* [45] have concluded that in spite of similar weight loss at 2 years, patients with RYGB were more likely to be in remission of diabetes than patients with GB, which suggests a direct metabolic role of the surgery not related to calorie restriction or weight loss. Similarly, Woelnerhanssen *et al* reported that the improvement in insulin resistance after RYGB "does not parallel" the weight loss and when compared with a very low calorie diet, RYGB has been shown to lead to a greater improvement in insulin resistance, especially in diabetic patients [35, 46].

However, other studies concluded that the improvement in insulin resistance is directly related to post-operative weight loss and calorie restriction [47 - 50]. The report that in the sub-acute setting (3 months) there is a slight increase in insulin resistance, supports that calorie restriction might play a role in the early improvements widely reported [33].

Several studies concluded that RYGB leads to an increase in glucagon-like protein 1 (GLP1) expression, and that this will regulate and improve β-cell function [35, 45, 51 - 57] and β-cell proliferation [58, 59]. In this regard, two major theories have arisen. According to the "foregut" theory [60], it is the exclusion of the duodenum that is responsible for this improvement; while according to the "hindgut" theory [61], it is the rapid arrival of undigested food to the ileum that drives the metabolic improvement. The results in human subjects have been conflicting [62], but whatever the prevailing theory proves to be, it appears that RYGB surgery "fundamentally alters the physiology of the foregut" [33].

It has been reported [33, 41, 63] that the improvement in insulin resistance after RYGB is not related to a modification of the production of insulin in response to a glucose challenge, but rather due to a decrease in the fasting production of insulin. Indeed, Reed *et al* [64] concluded that RYGB corrected the fasting hyperinsulinemia associated with obesity, without significant changes in glucose tolerance. Even more, weight stable patients after RYGBP had lower fasting insulin levels than weight-matched controls.

Similar results have been found in T2DM patients with BMI < 35 kg/m^2 such that euglycemia is achieved in a variable number of patients (but higher than any non-surgical method), without excessive weight loss [65 - 67].

IMPACT OF BARIATRIC SURGERY ON COMORBIDITIES

Weight loss is not the only measure of success after bariatric surgery. It has been reported that a modest 10% reduction in excess weight is associated with significant metabolic improvement and resolution of co-morbid diseases [68, 69].

These metabolic improvements ultimately lead to a significant reduction of up to 90% in all-cause mortality after bariatric surgery [20, 70].

A longitudinal observational study concluded that overall %EWL after bariatric surgery was 67% at 5 years and produced significant reductions in cardiovascular, endocrine, respiratory, infectious and psychiatric comorbidities [20]. The impact on comorbidities is dependent on the procedure and on the corresponding changes in digestive physiology, weight loss, alteration of eating habits and the relation of obesity on the comorbidities.

According to the IFSO Global Registry 3rd Annual Report [26], there is a significant improvement in all obesity-associated comorbidities Fig. (**1**).

The term Metabolic Syndrome (MetS) clusters the most dangerous cardiovascular disease (CVD) risk factors: dysglycemia, abdominal obesity, DLP and HBP [59]. It is an important societal burden with 20-25% of the world's adult population affected [71, 72]. These people are more likely to die, suffer a heart attack or stroke or develop T2DM [59, 72, 73].

Several studies have reported that MetS is a reversible condition after bariatric surgery, and that the ~80% remission rates after surgery are significantly higher than after medical management [4, 70, 74 - 83].

As with insulin resistance [33, 39, 40], MetS improvement is seen early after surgery, so that more than 50% of obese patients with a BMI < 50 kg/m^2 experience remission of MetS 1 month after surgery [84]. This suggests that the metabolic improvement is not entirely dependent on weight loss. The remission of MetS and improvement in CVD risk factors might offer an explanation to the reduction in overall mortality after bariatric surgery [20, 70].

We previously reported that the remission of MetS is dependent on the severity of the underlying metabolic disease and that a 10-point Metabolic Score comprising duration of obesity, HBP, low HDL-cholesterol and fasting blood glucose (FBG) levels could predict patients at risk of disease persistence [83].

Effect on type 2 diabetes *mellitus*

The first meta-analysis of the impact of bariatric surgery on diabetes [25] reported complete resolution and improvement of diabetes in 78.1% and 86.6% of the patients. Hemoglobin A1c (HbA1c), FBG and insulin levels were significantly reduced after surgery.

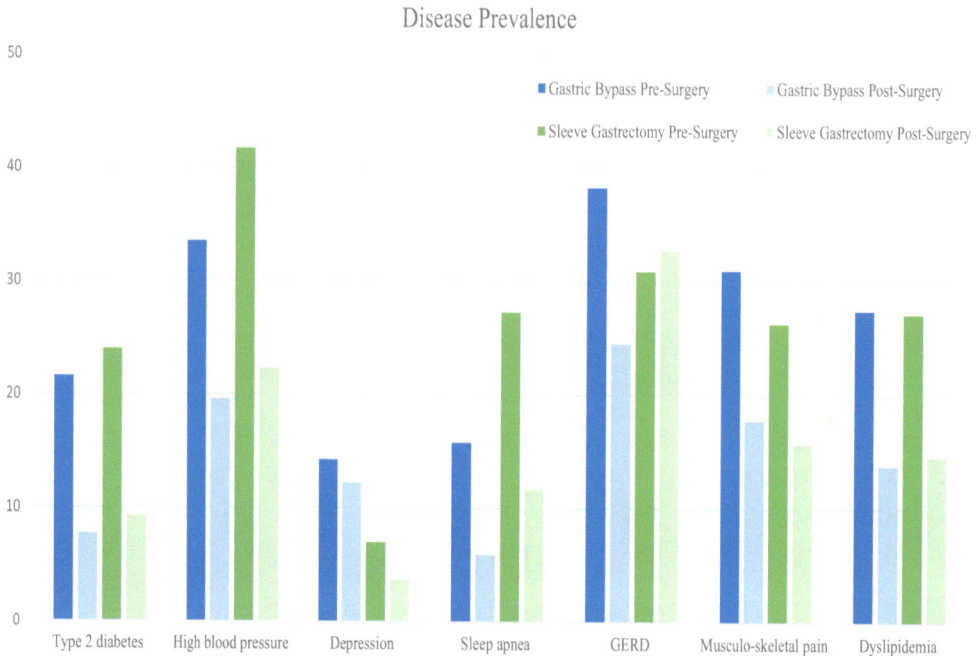

Fig. (1). Prevalence of Obesity-associated diseases before and 12 months after Bariatric Surgery. GERD: gastroesophageal reflux disease. Adapted from 3rd IFSO Global Registry [26].

One of the major problems regarding the evaluation of T2DM remission is the very own definition of remission mostly regarding HbA1c levels. Slight differences in the HbA1c threshold might impact significantly in the remission rates reported: for instance reducing the threshold for remission from 6.0% to 5.7% can cut remission rates in half [85, 86].

Interestingly, T2DM resolution has been reported early after surgery, even before significant weight loss occurred [87]. Although not completely understood, several mechanisms have been implicated in T2DM resolution, such as [88]:

- Calorie restriction,
- Appetite suppression,
- Weight loss,
- Decreased hepatic glucose production and increased uptake,
- Rapid gastric emptying,
- Decreased leptin levels and increased leptin sensitivity,
- Increased insulin levels and enhanced insulin sensitivity,
- Reduced ghrelin levels, and

• Change in gastric inhibitory peptide levels and increased levels of GLP1.

Bariatric surgery has proven superior to medical management in the treatment of T2DM, reducing the need for medication and even achieving complete disease remission [85, 86, 89 - 94]. Despite the long-term effects on the complications of T2DM not being completely understood [95], a recent meta-analysis concluded that RYGB significantly reduces micro- and macrovascular complications of T2DM [96].

Several randomized control trials (RCTs) have concluded that although the results are not as impressive as some earlier prospective cohort studies had suggested, T2DM improvement and remission are significantly better after surgery than with optimized medical management for patients with BMI > 30 kg/m^2 [91, 97 - 103]. Even in patients with moderate obesity (BMI 30-40 kg/m^2), the odds for full (OR=17) or partial (OR=20) T2DM remission were significantly higher after surgery than with best medical management for at least 5 years after surgery [104].

A 2014 meta-analysis found an improvement in T2DM control in more than 3/4 of patients after RYGB surgery as well as a remission rate of 50% among insulin users and of almost 90% in the group of patients with no preoperative use of insulin [90]. A 2016 meta-analysis of RCTs comparing RYGB with medical treatment concluded that there is a significant difference in disease control between groups (55% remission in the surgical group *vs.* 0% in the medical management) [3].

Severity and control of T2DM are related to the resolution rates after surgery. The remission rates are of up to 90% for patients with diet-controlled T2DM, 83% for those on oral hypoglycaemic agents and 53% for those on insulin. Also, C-peptide levels and duration of T2DM strongly affect remission rates, such that more severe ß-cell dysfunction impairs T2DM remission. Both good glycemic control and short-duration of T2DM significantly increase the rate of T2DM remission [34, 88, 90, 105 - 111].

Although there is no clear consensus regarding the choice of the surgical procedure for control of the metabolic disease, most studies report the best results for mal-absorptive procedures, such as BPD, followed by metabolic procedures, like RYGB, and finally restrictive procedures, such as SG (and to a lesser extent GB) [86, 89, 90]. The comparison of the results between the most popular surgeries (SG and RYGB) seems to indicate that both surgeries achieve good results regarding glycemic control. Although the results are slightly better after RYGB the difference is statistically different [112, 113]. Despite similar weight loss with SG, RYGB uniquely restores pancreatic β-cell function and reduces truncal fat, thus reversing the core defects in diabetes [102].

Overall, patients with higher BMIs seem to achieve greater remission of T2DM after surgery. The search for the cure for diabetes in lower weight patients has led to the selection of some of the most severe forms of T2DM and such, the results of the surgical treatment of mild obesity are not as impressive as those previously reported. Furthermore, RCTs have selected only the group of patients with more severe T2DM (uncontrolled despite optimal medical treatment). This bias leads to the conclusion that RYGB is "not that" effective in T2DM treatment, while a more correct interpretation would be that "even in the worst cases of T2DM, about half the patients might achieve long-term remission".

Preoperative BMI and weight loss are not directly related to the improvement in glycemic control and although remission rates may be different, HbA1c levels 12 months after surgery were not different between patients with BMI < 35 kg/m^2 or BMI ≥ 35 kg/m^2 [103, 114 - 116]. Interestingly, even patients with failed weight loss (%EWL<25%) achieved significant control of T2DM but also of HBP and DLP [117].

Older age has been reported to decrease the chances of remission and is included in most validated scores. However, if age plays an independent role or is only a surrogate marker of more severe T2DM is still under debate [90, 118 - 121].

Several scores to predict the chances of T2DM remission after surgery have been proposed and the most used are the ABCD and the DiaRem [120, 121]. The ABCD score has been validated for Asian populations and includes Age, BMI, C-peptide and Disease duration. The DiaRem score includes Age, HbA1c, Insulin Use and Metformin use. As can be seen, both try to capture the "severity" of the metabolic disease and most important than choosing a single score is to understand that the chances of remission are higher for less severe and shorter disease duration.

T2DM is a chronic disease of increasing resistance to insulin and decreasing pancreatic function. As such, even for patients with disease remission, progressing pancreatic failure might ultimately lead to relapse. Increasing follow-up after surgery to 5 years increases relapse rate to 1/3 of the patients with post-operative remission and can be even higher with increasing follow-up time [85, 122, 123].

As for remission, relapse rates are higher for longer duration of the disease, older patients and pre-operative poor metabolic control [95]. Patients with insufficient weight loss or with weight regain are also more prone to T2DM relapse [2, 92, 122]. However, even in patients with disease relapse, glycemic control is easier to achieve, there is less medication required and there are improvements in other surrogate markers of metabolic disease (HBP and DLP) [85, 86, 95].

Effect on High Blood Pressure

Between 40-70% of bariatric surgery patients have HBP [88, 124] and bariatric surgery improves HBP in 37%-53% of patients significantly reducing the need for medication [88]. The higher cardiovascular risk associated with obesity and HBP can be reduced by bariatric surgery, to rates lower than the age- and gender-adjusted rates for the general population [125]. The prevalence of hypertension decreases with time elapsed from surgery. In a study from Cremieux *et al* [126], the prevalence of HBP was 38.8% in the preoperative period, 21.1% up to 4 months after surgery and 12.3% at 3 years after surgery. Even for patients who did not achieve complete remission (systolic blood pressure < 140 mmHg and diastolic blood pressure < 90 mmHg, without medication use), there is a significant improvement in blood pressure and medication requirements [2, 90, 117, 122, 127].

Specifically for RYGB, resolution rates of HBP have been reported between 65% and 91% [124, 128]. Although improvement of HBP is not as fast as the improvement in resistance to insulin, it has been reported that patients have a significantly lower systolic and diastolic blood pressure 10 days after RYGB [129].

The best results were achieved in patients not on active treatment for HBP and in those with HBP for less than 4 years. As for T2DM, the best results were achieved in patients with less antihypertensive medication, younger age and shorter disease duration. HBP relapse affects up to 20% of patients and is related with increasing number of drugs pre-operatively and not only less weight loss but also weight regain. Bariatric surgery is also effective in achieving long-term remission of HBP in adolescents and in the prevention of HBP [88, 122, 130]. Conversely, normotensive patients did not show any significant reduction in blood pressure [131].

Regarding differences in remission rates between SG and RYGB, the results are conflicting. Several papers report higher remission rates for RYGB and 2 different meta-analysis concluded that remission is more likely after RYGB [113] or not significantly different between the procedures [132].

Effect on Dislipidemia

DLP refers to high levels of total and LDL-cholesterol, diminished HDL-cholesterol and increased serum triglycerides. It is present in up to 50% of morbidly obese patients and is one of the most important modifiable cardiovascular risk factors and a major risk factor for the development of atherosclerosis and coronary heart disease. The improvement after medically induced weight lost is modest, but it is significantly better after surgical treatment, especially for the HDL-cholesterol [4, 88, 133, 134].

RYGB causes a reduction in enterocolic circulation and reabsorption of cholesterol, resulting in an optimization of cholesterol and triglyceride profiles within 6 months after surgery and the effect lasts up to 6 years. Mal-absorptive procedures have higher rates of medication discontinuation, which overall ranges from 40% to 100% at 12 months. Total cholesterol reduction is around 20% 6-12 months after surgery, which contrasts to non-significant reductions after lifestyle changes and medical weight loss; the reduction seems to be correlated with weight loss and weight regain [10, 88, 134, 135].

There are reports of improvement in the lipid profile as early as 1 month after surgery, which supports the hypothesis that DLP improves through weight independent mechanisms. Several hypotheses ranging from reduced intake, reduced lipid absorption, modulation of bile acids production, changes in gut microbiota or reduced cholesterol synthesis have been proposed. Comparing RYGB with statins for the control of DLP renders that RYGB is more effective than statins especially in reducing triglycerides and increasing HDL-cholesterol [136].

A direct comparison of lipid changes after surgery between SG and RYGB showed that RYGB is the only surgery that decreases total cholesterol and LDL-cholesterol, after matching for age, sex, BMI and %EWL but triglycerides and HDL-cholesterol are similarly improved with both surgeries after adjusting for weight loss [137, 138]. However, as for other metabolic diseases, even patients with failed weight loss may see a significant improvement in DLP with almost 70% of patients achieving the goal of LDL-cholesterol levels < 100 mg/dL [117].

Effects on Other Comorbidities

Bariatric surgery results in improvement of several cardiovascular morbidities, such as congestive heart disease, coronary artery disease and atherosclerosis.

Increased adipose cells and lean mass in obese patients lead to a high cardiac output state and an increased circulating volume that ultimately impairs cardiac function. Weight loss promotes favorable hemodynamic changes and after bariatric surgery, a decrease in left-ventricle thickness and overall ventricular mass have been reported, even after weight loss has stopped. Patients with severe cardiomyopathy and low ejection fraction have also been reported to improve the cardiac function and some authors suggest that weight loss surgery might serve as a bridge to heart transplantation [139 - 141].

In patients with coronary artery disease, both coronary microvascular function and peripheral vasodilatation improve after bariatric surgery, independent of the improvement in other cardiovascular risk factors. The SOS study has concluded that bariatric surgery is a safe treatment and might be used as a strategy for secondary prevention in CVD, since it significantly reduces the risk of cardiovascular events, both fatal and non-fatal [14, 142, 143].

Improvement or reversal in plaque progression have been reported. Both carotid intima thickness and peripheral vascular flow were improved at 18 months after bariatric surgery. A significant improvement in inflammatory markers, such as C-reactive protein and in nitric oxide levels, is also observed after bariatric surgery [88, 144 - 146].

Respiratory problems are also improved after bariatric surgery. Obstructive sleep apnea is very common among obese individuals, with prevalence rates as high as 77%. The resolution rates have been reported between 52.9% to 100%, 1 to 3 years after surgery. Although not much studied, also asthma and chronic obstructive pulmonary disease are reported to be improved after weight control surgery [88, 147].

Renal impairment is also improved after bariatric surgery, with improvements in albuminuria and creatinine clearance up to 2 years after surgery, which has been recommended for prevention of progression or improvement of renal disease [88, 146]. Also, there have been some recent suggestions that RYGB might slow the progression of diabetic retinopathy [148].

Hepatic steatosis, non-alcoholic fatty liver disease (NAFLD) and non-alcoholic steatohepatitis (NASH) are strongly associated with obesity and significantly improve after surgery, with decreased incidence of liver cirrhosis [88, 149]. NAFLD might affect up to 50% of morbid obese patients undergoing surgery and RYGB and bariatric surgery can lead to histological improvement in steatosis, fibrosis and inflammation. NASH resolution is expected in 85% of the patients 1 year after surgery and is thought to be related both with disease severity and weight loss [150, 151].

Obese patients have an increased prevalence of gastroesophageal reflux disease (GERD) and more severe reflux episodes. GERD is expected to improve after RYGB but on the other hand SG might increase reflux. RYGB has shown excellent results in difficult-to-treat GERD in obese patients and has been used as salvage surgery for reflux symptoms after restrictive surgery [88, 152 - 154].

Bariatric surgery is also beneficial in weight-dependent morbidities such as joint pain. Weight loss surgery is recommended for obese patients, before joint replacement surgery [155].

Just in the USA, it is estimated that each year 85000 new cases of cancer are related to obesity and metabolic surgery has a proven effect on decreasing the incidence of new cancers. This effect is strongest for obesity-related cancers in women and the underlying causes include the improvement in insulin resistance, decreased oxidative stress and inflammation and a modulation of sex steroids, adipokines, immune system and gut hormones [88].

CONCLUDING REMARKS

Obesity is a proinflammatory condition increasing cardiovascular risk factors through several pathways. Obesity might cause disease by metabolic pathways, deregulation of hormonal balance, increasing intra-abdominal pressure or just exerting extra pressure on soft-tissues.

There is a lack of options to treat obesity and bariatric surgery has emerged as the most effective and lasting treatment for this disease. The major end-point of bariatric surgery has been weight loss; however, this might not be the most important clinical marker of disease. After bariatric surgery, even in the absence of successful weight loss or after weight regain, there is a significant improvement in obesity-associated comorbidities.

It is possible to achieve long-term remission of the metabolic disease (T2DM, HBP and DLP) but it seems that surgery is most effective in early-stage disease. Currently, we propose surgery to the most severe forms of obesity and metabolic disease but understanding the pathophysiology of the disease and the clinical implications of metabolic improvement might lead, in the near future, to indicate surgery earlier in the course of the disease, before irreversible metabolic damage has been settled. Understanding the mechanisms of improvement after bariatric surgery has led to new fields of research in the development of obesity in itself.

Overall, bariatric surgery is related to a significant improvement or resolution of the obesity-associated comorbidities and efforts should be made to offer this treatment to an increasing population of morbidly obese patients.

CONSENT FOR PUBLICATION

Not applicable.

CONFLICT OF INTEREST

The authors confirm that this chapter contents have no conflict of interest.

ACKNOWLEDGEMENTS

Declared none.

REFERENCES

[1]   Balakumar P, Maung-U K, Jagadeesh G. Prevalence and prevention of cardiovascular disease and diabetes mellitus. Pharmacol Res 2016; 113(Pt A): 600-9..
[http://dx.doi.org/10.1016/j.phrs.2016.09.040]

[2]   Corcelles R, Daigle CR, Schauer PR. MANAGEMENT OF ENDOCRINE DISEASE: Metabolic effects of bariatric surgery. Eur J Endocrinol 2016; 174(1): R19-28.
[http://dx.doi.org/10.1530/EJE-15-0533] [PMID: 26340972]

[3]   Yan Y, Sha Y, Yao G, *et al.* Roux-en-Y Gastric Bypass Versus Medical Treatment for Type 2 Diabetes Mellitus in Obese Patients: A Systematic Review and Meta-Analysis of Randomized Controlled Trials. Medicine (Baltimore) 2016; 95(17)e3462
[http://dx.doi.org/10.1097/MD.0000000000003462] [PMID: 27124041]

[4]   Sjöström L, Lindroos A-K, Peltonen M, *et al.* Swedish Obese Subjects Study Scientific Group. Lifestyle, diabetes, and cardiovascular risk factors 10 years after bariatric surgery. N Engl J Med 2004; 351(26): 2683-93.
[http://dx.doi.org/10.1056/NEJMoa035622] [PMID: 15616203]

[5]   Adams TD, Gress RE, Smith SC, *et al.* Long-term mortality after gastric bypass surgery. N Engl J Med 2007; 357(8): 753-61.
[http://dx.doi.org/10.1056/NEJMoa066603] [PMID: 17715409]

[6]   Eligar VS, Narayanaswamy AKP. Bariatric surgery and remission of type 2 diabetes mellitus. Curr Opin Lipidol 2016; 27(1): 97-8.
[http://dx.doi.org/10.1097/MOL.0000000000000265] [PMID: 26655295]

[7]   Campos J, Ramos A, Szego T, Zilberstein B, Feitosa H, Cohen R. The role of metabolic surgery for patients with obesity grade I and type 2 diabetes not controlled clinically. Arq Bras Cir Dig 2016; 29 (1): 102-6.
[http://dx.doi.org/10.1590/0102-6720201600s10025]

[8]   Eisenberg D, Duffy A-J, Bell R-L. Update on Obes Surg World J Gastroenterol 2006; 12(20): 3196-203.
[http://dx.doi.org/10.3748/wjg.v12.i20.3196]

[9]   Cummings DE, Overduin J, Foster-Schubert KE. Gastric bypass for obesity: mechanisms of weight loss and diabetes resolution. J Clin Endocrinol Metab 2004; 89(6): 2608-15.
[http://dx.doi.org/10.1210/jc.2004-0433] [PMID: 15181031]

[10]   Brolin RE. Bariatric surgery and long-term control of morbid obesity. JAMA 2002; 288(22): 2793-6.
[http://dx.doi.org/10.1001/jama.288.22.2793] [PMID: 12472304]

[11]   Mun EC, Blackburn GL, Matthews JB. Current status of medical and surgical therapy for obesity. Gastroenterology 2001; 120(3): 669-81.
[http://dx.doi.org/10.1053/gast.2001.22430] [PMID: 11179243]

[12]   Pontiroli AE, Morabito A. Long-term prevention of mortality in morbid obesity through bariatric surgery. a systematic review and meta-analysis of trials performed with gastric banding and gastric bypass. Ann Surg 2011; 253(3): 484-7.
[http://dx.doi.org/10.1097/SLA.0b013e31820d98cb] [PMID: 21245741]

[13] Johnson RJ, Johnson BL, Blackhurst DW, *et al.* Bariatric surgery is associated with a reduced risk of mortality in morbidly obese patients with a history of major cardiovascular events. Am Surg 2012; 78(6): 685-92.
[PMID: 22643265]

[14] Sjöström L, Peltonen M, Jacobson P, *et al.* Bariatric surgery and long-term cardiovascular events. JAMA 2012; 307(1): 56-65.
[http://dx.doi.org/10.1001/jama.2011.1914] [PMID: 22215166]

[15] Dumon KR, Murayama KM. Bariatric surgery outcomes. Surg Clin North Am 2011; 91(6): 1313-1338, x.
[http://dx.doi.org/10.1016/j.suc.2011.08.014] [PMID: 22054156]

[16] Buchwald H, Oien DM. Metabolic/bariatric surgery worldwide 2011. Obes Surg 2013; 23(4): 427-36.
[http://dx.doi.org/10.1007/s11695-012-0864-0] [PMID: 23338049]

[17] Sun S, Borisenko O, Spelman T, Ahmed AR. Patient Characteristics, Procedural and Safety Outcomes of Bariatric Surgery in England: a Retrospective Cohort Study-2006-2012. Obes Surg 2017; 24: 437-11.
[PMID: 29076010]

[18] Buchwald H, Estok R, Fahrbach K, Banel D, Sledge I. Trends in mortality in bariatric surgery: a systematic review and meta-analysis. Surgery 2007; 142(4): 621-32.
[http://dx.doi.org/10.1016/j.surg.2007.07.018] [PMID: 17950357]

[19] Smith MD, Patterson E, Wahed AS, *et al.* Relationship between surgeon volume and adverse outcomes after RYGB in Longitudinal Assessment of Bariatric Surgery (LABS) study. Surg Obes Relat Dis 2010; 6(2): 118-25.
[http://dx.doi.org/10.1016/j.soard.2009.09.009] [PMID: 19969507]

[20] Sjöström L, Narbro K, Sjöström CD, *et al.* Swedish Obese Subjects Study. Effects of bariatric surgery on mortality in Swedish obese subjects. N Engl J Med 2007; 357(8): 741-52.
[http://dx.doi.org/10.1056/NEJMoa066254] [PMID: 17715408]

[21] Picot J, Jones J, Colquitt JL, *et al.* The clinical effectiveness and cost-effectiveness of bariatric (weight loss) surgery for obesity: a systematic review and economic evaluation. Health Technol Assess 2009; 13(41): 1-190, 215-357, iii-iv.
[http://dx.doi.org/10.3310/hta13410] [PMID: 19726018]

[22] Buddeberg-Fischer B, Klaghofer R, Krug L, *et al.* Physical and psychosocial outcome in morbidly obese patients with and without bariatric surgery: a 4 1/2-year follow-up. Obes Surg 2006; 16(3): 321-30.
[http://dx.doi.org/10.1381/096089206776116471] [PMID: 16545164]

[23] O'Brien PE, Dixon JB, Laurie C, *et al.* Treatment of mild to moderate obesity with laparoscopic adjustable gastric banding or an intensive medical program: a randomized trial. Ann Intern Med 2006; 144(9): 625-33.
[http://dx.doi.org/10.7326/0003-4819-144-9-200605020-00005] [PMID: 16670131]

[24] Colquitt JL, Picot J, Loveman E, Clegg AJ. Surgery for obesity. Cochrane Database Syst Rev 2009; (2): CD003641
[PMID: 19370590]

[25] Buchwald H, Avidor Y, Braunwald E, *et al.* Bariatric surgery: a systematic review and meta-analysis. JAMA 2004; 292(14): 1724-37.
[http://dx.doi.org/10.1001/jama.292.14.1724] [PMID: 15479938]

[26] Higa K, Himpens J, Welbourn R, Dixon J, Kinsman R, Walton P, Eds. The IFSO Global Registry Third IFSO Global Registry Report. Oxfordshire: Dendrite Clinical Systems 2017.

[27] Christou NV, MacLean LD. Effect of bariatric surgery on long-term mortality. Adv Surg 2005; 39: 165-79.

[http://dx.doi.org/10.1016/j.yasu.2005.04.005] [PMID: 16250551]

[28]   Herpertz S, Kielmann R, Wolf AMA, Langkafel M, Senf W, Hebebrand J. Does obesity surgery improve psychosocial functioning? A systematic review. Int J Obes Relat Metab Disord 2003; 27(11): 1300-14.
[http://dx.doi.org/10.1038/sj.ijo.0802410] [PMID: 14574339]

[29]   Faria G, Nunes Santos JM, Simonson DC. Quality of life after gastric sleeve and gastric bypass for morbid obesity. Porto Biomedical Journal 2017; 2(2): 40-6.
[http://dx.doi.org/10.1016/j.pbj.2016.12.006]

[30]   Mohos E, Schmaldienst E, Prager M. Quality of life parameters, weight change and improvement of co-morbidities after laparoscopic Roux Y gastric bypass and laparoscopic gastric sleeve resection--comparative study. Obes Surg 2011; 21(3): 288-94.
[http://dx.doi.org/10.1007/s11695-010-0227-7] [PMID: 20628831]

[31]   Campos GM, Rabl C, Roll GR, *et al.* Better weight loss, resolution of diabetes, and quality of life for laparoscopic gastric bypass vs banding: results of a 2-cohort pair-matched study. Arch Surg 2011; 146(2): 149-55.
[http://dx.doi.org/10.1001/archsurg.2010.316] [PMID: 21339424]

[32]   Reaven GM. Insulin resistance: the link between obesity and cardiovascular disease. Med Clin North Am 2011; 95(5): 875-92.
[http://dx.doi.org/10.1016/j.mcna.2011.06.002] [PMID: 21855697]

[33]   Wickremesekera K, Miller G, Naotunne TD, Knowles G, Stubbs RS. Loss of insulin resistance after Roux-en-Y gastric bypass surgery: a time course study. Obes Surg 2005; 15(4): 474-81.
[http://dx.doi.org/10.1381/0960892053723402] [PMID: 15946424]

[34]   Nannipieri M, Mari A, Anselmino M, *et al.* The role of beta-cell function and insulin sensitivity in the remission of type 2 diabetes after gastric bypass surgery. J Clin Endocrinol Metab 2011; 96(9): E1372-9.
[http://dx.doi.org/10.1210/jc.2011-0446] [PMID: 21778221]

[35]   Woelnerhanssen B, Peterli R, Steinert RE, Peters T, Borbély Y, Beglinger C. Effects of postbariatric surgery weight loss on adipokines and metabolic parameters: comparison of laparoscopic Roux-en-Y gastric bypass and laparoscopic sleeve gastrectomy--a prospective randomized trial. Surg Obes Relat Dis 2011; 7(5): 561-8.
[http://dx.doi.org/10.1016/j.soard.2011.01.044] [PMID: 21429816]

[36]   Braun S, Bitton-Worms K, LeRoith D. The link between the metabolic syndrome and cancer. Int J Biol Sci 2011; 7(7): 1003-15.
[http://dx.doi.org/10.7150/ijbs.7.1003] [PMID: 21912508]

[37]   Foo J, Krebs J, Hayes MT, *et al.* Studies in insulin resistance following very low calorie diet and/or gastric bypass surgery. Obes Surg 2011; 21(12): 1914-20.
[http://dx.doi.org/10.1007/s11695-011-0527-6] [PMID: 22002509]

[38]   Wallace TM, Levy JC, Matthews DR. Use and abuse of HOMA modeling. Diabetes Care 2004; 27(6): 1487-95.
[http://dx.doi.org/10.2337/diacare.27.6.1487] [PMID: 15161807]

[39]   Faria G, Preto J, da Costa EL, Guimarães JT, Calhau C, Taveira-Gomes A. Acute improvement in insulin resistance after laparoscopic Roux-en-Y gastric bypass: is 3 days enough to correct insulin metabolism? Obes Surg 2013; 23(1): 103-10.
[http://dx.doi.org/10.1007/s11695-012-0803-0] [PMID: 23114971]

[40]   Rao RS, Yanagisawa R, Kini S. Insulin resistance and bariatric surgery. Obes Rev 2012; 13(4): 316-28.
[http://dx.doi.org/10.1111/j.1467-789X.2011.00955.x] [PMID: 22106981]

[41]   Lima MMO, Pareja JC, Alegre SM, *et al.* Acute effect of roux-en-y gastric bypass on whole-body

insulin sensitivity: a study with the euglycemic-hyperinsulinemic clamp. J Clin Endocrinol Metab 2010; 95(8): 3871-5.
[http://dx.doi.org/10.1210/jc.2010-0085] [PMID: 20484482]

[42]   Rubino F, Gagner M, Gentileschi P, *et al.* The early effect of the Roux-en-Y gastric bypass on hormones involved in body weight regulation and glucose metabolism. Ann Surg 2004; 240(2): 236-42.
[http://dx.doi.org/10.1097/01.sla.0000133117.12646.48] [PMID: 15273546]

[43]   Ashrafian H, Athanasiou T, Li JV, *et al.* Diabetes resolution and hyperinsulinaemia after metabolic Roux-en-Y gastric bypass. Obes Rev 2011; 12(5): e257-72.
[http://dx.doi.org/10.1111/j.1467-789X.2010.00802.x] [PMID: 20880129]

[44]   Mingrone G, Castagneto M. Bariatric surgery: unstressing or boosting the beta-cell? Diabetes Obes Metab 2009; 11 (Suppl. 4): 130-42.
[http://dx.doi.org/10.1111/j.1463-1326.2009.01120.x] [PMID: 19817795]

[45]   Pournaras DJ, Osborne A, Hawkins SC, *et al.* Remission of type 2 diabetes after gastric bypass and banding: mechanisms and 2 year outcomes. Ann Surg 2010; 252(6): 966-71.
[http://dx.doi.org/10.1097/SLA.0b013e3181efc49a] [PMID: 21107106]

[46]   Plum L, Ahmed L, Febres G, *et al.* Comparison of glucostatic parameters after hypocaloric diet or bariatric surgery and equivalent weight loss. Obesity (Silver Spring) 2011; 19(11): 2149-57.
[http://dx.doi.org/10.1038/oby.2011.134] [PMID: 21593800]

[47]   Ballantyne GH, Wasielewski A, Saunders JK. The surgical treatment of type II diabetes mellitus: changes in HOMA Insulin resistance in the first year following laparoscopic Roux-en-Y gastric bypass (LRYGB) and laparoscopic adjustable gastric banding (LAGB). Obes Surg 2009; 19(9): 1297-303.
[http://dx.doi.org/10.1007/s11695-009-9870-2] [PMID: 19629603]

[48]   Lee W-J, Lee Y-C, Ser K-H, Chen J-C, Chen SC. Improvement of insulin resistance after obesity surgery: a comparison of gastric banding and bypass procedures. Obes Surg 2008; 18(9): 1119-25.
[http://dx.doi.org/10.1007/s11695-008-9457-3] [PMID: 18317853]

[49]   Ballantyne GH, Farkas D, Laker S, Wasielewski A. Short-term changes in insulin resistance following weight loss surgery for morbid obesity: laparoscopic adjustable gastric banding versus laparoscopic Roux-en-Y gastric bypass. Obes Surg 2006; 16(9): 1189-97.
[http://dx.doi.org/10.1381/096089206778392158] [PMID: 16989703]

[50]   Gumbs AA, Modlin IM, Ballantyne GH. Changes in insulin resistance following bariatric surgery: role of caloric restriction and weight loss. Obes Surg 2005; 15(4): 462-73.
[http://dx.doi.org/10.1381/0960892053723367] [PMID: 15946423]

[51]   Kashyap SR, Daud S, Kelly KR, *et al.* Acute effects of gastric bypass versus gastric restrictive surgery on beta-cell function and insulinotropic hormones in severely obese patients with type 2 diabetes. Int J Obes 2010; 34(3): 462-71.
[http://dx.doi.org/10.1038/ijo.2009.254] [PMID: 20029383]

[52]   Liu Y, Zhou Y, Wang Y, Geng D, Liu J. Roux-en-Y gastric bypass-induced improvement of glucose tolerance and insulin resistance in type 2 diabetic rats are mediated by glucagon-like peptide-1. Obes Surg 2011; 21(9): 1424-31.
[http://dx.doi.org/10.1007/s11695-011-0388-z] [PMID: 21479766]

[53]   Perugini RA, Malkani S. Remission of type 2 diabetes mellitus following bariatric surgery: review of mechanisms and presentation of the concept of 'reversibility'. Curr Opin Endocrinol Diabetes Obes 2011; 18(2): 119-28.
[http://dx.doi.org/10.1097/MED.0b013e3283446c1f] [PMID: 21522001]

[54]   Laferrère B. Diabetes remission after bariatric surgery: is it just the incretins? Int J Obes 2011; 35 (Suppl. 3): S22-5.
[http://dx.doi.org/10.1038/ijo.2011.143] [PMID: 21912382]

[55]   Yin DP, Gao Q, Ma LL, *et al.* Assessment of different bariatric surgeries in the treatment of obesity and insulin resistance in mice. Ann Surg 2011; 254(1): 73-82.
[http://dx.doi.org/10.1097/SLA.0b013e3182197035] [PMID: 21522012]

[56]   Laferrère B. Effect of gastric bypass surgery on the incretins. Diabetes Metab 2009; 35(6 Pt 2): 513-7.
[http://dx.doi.org/10.1016/S1262-3636(09)73458-5] [PMID: 20152736]

[57]   Hofsø D, Jenssen T, Bollerslev J, *et al.* Beta cell function after weight loss: a clinical trial comparing gastric bypass surgery and intensive lifestyle intervention. Eur J Endocrinol 2011; 164(2): 231-8.
[http://dx.doi.org/10.1530/EJE-10-0804] [PMID: 21078684]

[58]   Scheen AJ, De Flines J, De Roover A, Paquot N. Bariatric surgery in patients with type 2 diabetes: benefits, risks, indications and perspectives. Diabetes Metab 2009; 35(6 Pt 2): 537-43.
[http://dx.doi.org/10.1016/S1262-3636(09)73463-9] [PMID: 20152741]

[59]   Alberti KGMM, Eckel RH, Grundy SM, *et al.* Harmonizing the metabolic syndrome: a joint interim statement of the International Diabetes Federation Task Force on Epidemiology and Prevention; National Heart, Lung, and Blood Institute; American Heart Association; World Heart Federation; International Atherosclerosis Society; and International Association for the Study of Obesity. Circulation 2009; 120(16): 1640-5.
[http://dx.doi.org/10.1161/CIRCULATIONAHA.109.192644] [PMID: 19805654]

[60]   Rubino F, Forgione A, Cummings DE, *et al.* The mechanism of diabetes control after gastrointestinal bypass surgery reveals a role of the proximal small intestine in the pathophysiology of type 2 diabetes. Ann Surg 2006; 244(5): 741-9.
[http://dx.doi.org/10.1097/01.sla.0000224726.61448.1b] [PMID: 17060767]

[61]   Morínigo R, Lacy AM, Casamitjana R, Delgado S, Gomis R, Vidal J. GLP-1 and changes in glucose tolerance following gastric bypass surgery in morbidly obese subjects. Obes Surg 2006; 16(12): 1594-601.
[http://dx.doi.org/10.1381/096089206779319338] [PMID: 17217635]

[62]   Laferrère B. Do we really know why diabetes remits after gastric bypass surgery? Endocrine 2011; 40(2): 162-7.
[http://dx.doi.org/10.1007/s12020-011-9514-x] [PMID: 21853297]

[63]   de Carvalho CP, Marin DM, de Souza AL, *et al.* GLP-1 and adiponectin: effect of weight loss after dietary restriction and gastric bypass in morbidly obese patients with normal and abnormal glucose metabolism. Obes Surg 2009; 19(3): 313-20.
[http://dx.doi.org/10.1007/s11695-008-9678-5] [PMID: 18815849]

[64]   Reed MA, Pories WJ, Chapman W, *et al.* Roux-en-Y gastric bypass corrects hyperinsulinemia implications for the remission of type 2 diabetes. J Clin Endocrinol Metab 2011; 96(8): 2525-31.
[http://dx.doi.org/10.1210/jc.2011-0165] [PMID: 21593117]

[65]   Maggard-Gibbons M, Maglione M, Livhits M, *et al.* Bariatric surgery for weight loss and glycemic control in nonmorbidly obese adults with diabetes: a systematic review. JAMA 2013; 309(21): 2250-61.
[http://dx.doi.org/10.1001/jama.2013.4851] [PMID: 23736734]

[66]   Ikramuddin S, Korner J, Lee W-J, *et al.* Roux-en-Y gastric bypass vs intensive medical management for the control of type 2 diabetes, hypertension, and hyperlipidemia: the Diabetes Surgery Study randomized clinical trial. JAMA 2013; 309(21): 2240-9.
[http://dx.doi.org/10.1001/jama.2013.5835] [PMID: 23736733]

[67]   Fried M, Ribaric G, Buchwald JN, Svacina S, Dolezalova K, Scopinaro N. Metabolic surgery for the treatment of type 2 diabetes in patients with BMI <35 kg/m2: an integrative review of early studies. Obes Surg 2010; 20(6): 776-90.
[http://dx.doi.org/10.1007/s11695-010-0113-3] [PMID: 20333558]

[68]   Bray GA, Ryan DH, Harsha DW. Diet, Weight Loss, and Cardiovascular Disease Prevention. Curr

Treat Options Cardiovasc Med 2003; 5(4): 259-69.
[http://dx.doi.org/10.1007/s11936-003-0025-9] [PMID: 12834563]

[69] Busetto L, Tregnaghi A, De Marchi F, *et al.* Liver volume and visceral obesity in women with hepatic steatosis undergoing gastric banding. Obes Res 2002; 10(5): 408-11.
[http://dx.doi.org/10.1038/oby.2002.56] [PMID: 12006641]

[70] Batsis JA, Romero-Corral A, Collazo-Clavell ML, Sarr MG, Somers VK, Lopez-Jimenez F. Effect of bariatric surgery on the metabolic syndrome: a population-based, long-term controlled study. Mayo Clin Proc 2008; 83(8): 897-907.
[http://dx.doi.org/10.1016/S0025-6196(11)60766-0] [PMID: 18674474]

[71] Alberti KGMM, Zimmet P, Shaw J. Metabolic syndrome--a new world-wide definition. A Consensus Statement from the International Diabetes Federation. Diabet Med 2006; 23(5): 469-80.
[http://dx.doi.org/10.1111/j.1464-5491.2006.01858.x] [PMID: 16681555]

[72] Williams S, Cunningham E, Pories WJ. Surgical treatment of metabolic syndrome. Med Princ Pract 2012; 21(4): 301-9.
[http://dx.doi.org/10.1159/000334480] [PMID: 22222561]

[73] Lee W-J, Huang M-T, Wang W, Lin C-M, Chen T-C, Lai I-R. Effects of obesity surgery on the metabolic syndrome. Arch Surg 2004; 139(10): 1088-92.
[http://dx.doi.org/10.1001/archsurg.139.10.1088] [PMID: 15492149]

[74] Hofsø D, Nordstrand N, Johnson LK, *et al.* Obesity-related cardiovascular risk factors after weight loss: a clinical trial comparing gastric bypass surgery and intensive lifestyle intervention. Eur J Endocrinol 2010; 163(5): 735-45.
[http://dx.doi.org/10.1530/EJE-10-0514] [PMID: 20798226]

[75] Madan AK, Orth W, Ternovits CA, Tichansky DS. Metabolic syndrome: yet another co-morbidity gastric bypass helps cure. Surg Obes Relat Dis 2006; 2(1): 48-51.
[http://dx.doi.org/10.1016/j.soard.2005.09.014] [PMID: 16925317]

[76] Mattar SG, Velcu LM, Rabinovitz M, *et al.* Surgically-induced weight loss significantly improves nonalcoholic fatty liver disease and the metabolic syndrome. Ann Surg 2005; 242(4): 610-7.
[PMID: 16192822]

[77] Gazzaruso C, Giordanetti S, La Manna A, *et al.* Weight loss after Swedish Adjustable Gastric Banding: relationships to insulin resistance and metabolic syndrome. Obes Surg 2002; 12(6): 841-5.
[http://dx.doi.org/10.1381/096089202320995673] [PMID: 12568192]

[78] Alexandrides TK, Skroubis G, Kalfarentzos F. Resolution of diabetes mellitus and metabolic syndrome following Roux-en-Y gastric bypass and a variant of biliopancreatic diversion in patients with morbid obesity. Obes Surg 2007; 17(2): 176-84.
[http://dx.doi.org/10.1007/s11695-007-9044-z] [PMID: 17476868]

[79] Inabnet WB III, Winegar DA, Sherif B, Sarr MG. Early outcomes of bariatric surgery in patients with metabolic syndrome: an analysis of the bariatric outcomes longitudinal database. J Am Coll Surg 2012; 214(4): 550-6.
[http://dx.doi.org/10.1016/j.jamcollsurg.2011.12.019] [PMID: 22321517]

[80] Ali MR, Fuller WD, Rasmussen J. Detailed description of early response of metabolic syndrome after laparoscopic Roux-en-Y gastric bypass. Surg Obes Relat Dis 2009; 5(3): 346-51.
[http://dx.doi.org/10.1016/j.soard.2008.10.014] [PMID: 19362060]

[81] Gracia-Solanas JA, Elia M, Aguilella V, *et al.* Metabolic syndrome after bariatric surgery. Results depending on the technique performed. Obes Surg 2011; 21(2): 179-85.
[http://dx.doi.org/10.1007/s11695-010-0309-6] [PMID: 21080097]

[82] de Carvalho PS, Moreira CL de CB, Barelli MDC, *et al.* [Can bariatric surgery cure metabolic syndrome?]. Arq Bras Endocrinol Metabol 2007; 51(1): 79-85.
[http://dx.doi.org/10.1590/S0004-27302007000100013] [PMID: 17435859]

[83] Faria G, Pestana D, Aral M, *et al*. Metabolic score: insights on the development and prediction of remission of metabolic syndrome after gastric bypass. Ann Surg 2014; 260(2): 279-86. [http://dx.doi.org/10.1097/SLA.0000000000000686] [PMID: 24743628]

[84] Saboya C, Arasaki CH, Matos D, Lopes-Filho GJ. Relationship between the preoperative body mass index and the resolution of metabolic syndrome following Roux-en-Y gastric bypass. Metab Syndr Relat Disord 2012; 10(4): 292-6. [http://dx.doi.org/10.1089/met.2012.0014] [PMID: 22545590]

[85] Brito JP, Montori VM, Davis AM. Metabolic Surgery in the Treatment Algorithm for Type 2 Diabetes: A Joint Statement by International Diabetes Organizations. JAMA 2017; 317(6): 635-6. [http://dx.doi.org/10.1001/jama.2016.20563] [PMID: 28196240]

[86] Amouyal C, Andreelli F. What is the evidence for metabolic surgery for type 2 diabetes? A critical perspective. Diabetes Metab 2017; 43(1): 9-17. [http://dx.doi.org/10.1016/j.diabet.2016.06.005] [PMID: 27400671]

[87] Pories WJ, Swanson MS, MacDonald KG, *et al*. Who would have thought it? An operation proves to be the most effective therapy for adult-onset diabetes mellitus. Ann Surg 1995; 222(3): 339-50. [http://dx.doi.org/10.1097/00000658-199509000-00011] [PMID: 7677463]

[88] Kaul A, Sharma J. Impact of bariatric surgery on comorbidities. Surg Clin North Am 2011; 91(6): 1295-1312, ix. [http://dx.doi.org/10.1016/j.suc.2011.08.003] [PMID: 22054155]

[89] Vidal J, Jiménez A, de Hollanda A, Flores L, Lacy A. Metabolic Surgery in Type 2 Diabetes: Roux-en-Y Gastric Bypass or Sleeve Gastrectomy as Procedure of Choice? Curr Atheroscler Rep 2015; 17(10): 58. [http://dx.doi.org/10.1007/s11883-015-0538-1] [PMID: 26303455]

[90] Chen Y, Zeng G, Tan J, Tang J, Ma J, Rao B. Impact of roux-en Y gastric bypass surgery on prognostic factors of type 2 diabetes mellitus: meta-analysis and systematic review. Diabetes Metab Res Rev 2015; 31(7): 653-62. [http://dx.doi.org/10.1002/dmrr.2622] [PMID: 25387821]

[91] Schauer PR, Bhatt DL, Kirwan JP, *et al*. Bariatric surgery versus intensive medical therapy for diabetes--3-year outcomes. N Engl J Med 2014; 370(21): 2002-13. [http://dx.doi.org/10.1056/NEJMoa1401329] [PMID: 24679060]

[92] Arterburn D, McCulloch D. Bariatric Surgery for Type 2 Diabetes: Getting Closer to the Long-term Goal. JAMA 2016; 315(12): 1276-7. [http://dx.doi.org/10.1001/jama.2016.1884] [PMID: 27002449]

[93] Panunzi S, Carlsson L, De Gaetano A, *et al*. Determinants of Diabetes Remission and Glycemic Control After Bariatric Surgery. Diabetes Care 2016; 39(1): 166-74. [http://dx.doi.org/10.2337/dc15-0575] [PMID: 26628418]

[94] Yska JP, van Roon EN, de Boer A, *et al*. Remission of Type 2 Diabetes Mellitus in Patients After Different Types of Bariatric Surgery: A Population-Based Cohort Study in the United Kingdom. JAMA Surg 2015; 150(12): 1126-33. [http://dx.doi.org/10.1001/jamasurg.2015.2398] [PMID: 26422580]

[95] Brethauer SA, Aminian A, Romero-Talamás H, *et al*. Can diabetes be surgically cured? Long-term metabolic effects of bariatric surgery in obese patients with type 2 diabetes mellitus. Ann Surg 2013; 258(4): 628-36. [http://dx.doi.org/10.1097/SLA.0b013e3182a5034b] [PMID: 24018646]

[96] Sheng B, Truong K, Spitler H, Zhang L, Tong X, Chen L. The Long-Term Effects of Bariatric Surgery on Type 2 Diabetes Remission, Microvascular and Macrovascular Complications, and Mortality: a Systematic Review and Meta-Analysis. Obes Surg 2017; 27(10): 2724-32. [http://dx.doi.org/10.1007/s11695-017-2866-4] [PMID: 28801703]

[97] Courcoulas AP, Belle SH, Neiberg RH, *et al.* Three-Year Outcomes of Bariatric Surgery vs Lifestyle Intervention for Type 2 Diabetes Mellitus Treatment: A Randomized Clinical Trial. JAMA Surg 2015; 150(10): 931-40.
[http://dx.doi.org/10.1001/jamasurg.2015.1534] [PMID: 26132586]

[98] Ikramuddin S, Billington CJ, Lee W-J, *et al.* Roux-en-Y gastric bypass for diabetes (the Diabetes Surgery Study): 2-year outcomes of a 5-year, randomised, controlled trial. Lancet Diabetes Endocrinol 2015; 3(6): 413-22.
[http://dx.doi.org/10.1016/S2213-8587(15)00089-3] [PMID: 25979364]

[99] Parikh M, Chung M, Sheth S, *et al.* Randomized pilot trial of bariatric surgery versus intensive medical weight management on diabetes remission in type 2 diabetic patients who do NOT meet NIH criteria for surgery and the role of soluble RAGE as a novel biomarker of success. Ann Surg 2014; 260(4): 617-22.
[http://dx.doi.org/10.1097/SLA.0000000000000919] [PMID: 25203878]

[100] Halperin F, Ding S-A, Simonson DC, *et al.* Roux-en-Y gastric bypass surgery or lifestyle with intensive medical management in patients with type 2 diabetes: feasibility and 1-year results of a randomized clinical trial. JAMA Surg 2014; 149(7): 716-26.
[http://dx.doi.org/10.1001/jamasurg.2014.514] [PMID: 24899464]

[101] Liang Z, Wu Q, Chen B, Yu P, Zhao H, Ouyang X. Effect of laparoscopic Roux-en-Y gastric bypass surgery on type 2 diabetes mellitus with hypertension: a randomized controlled trial. Diabetes Res Clin Pract 2013; 101(1): 50-6.
[http://dx.doi.org/10.1016/j.diabres.2013.04.005] [PMID: 23706413]

[102] Kashyap SR, Bhatt DL, Wolski K, *et al.* Metabolic effects of bariatric surgery in patients with moderate obesity and type 2 diabetes: analysis of a randomized control trial comparing surgery with intensive medical treatment. Diabetes Care 2013; 36(8): 2175-82.
[http://dx.doi.org/10.2337/dc12-1596] [PMID: 23439632]

[103] Mingrone G, Panunzi S, De Gaetano A, *et al.* Bariatric surgery versus conventional medical therapy for type 2 diabetes. N Engl J Med 2012; 366(17): 1577-85.
[http://dx.doi.org/10.1056/NEJMoa1200111] [PMID: 22449317]

[104] Cohen R, Le Roux CW, Junqueira S, Ribeiro RA, Luque A. Roux-En-Y Gastric Bypass in Type 2 Diabetes Patients with Mild Obesity: a Systematic Review and Meta-analysis. Obes Surg 2017; 27(10): 2733-9.
[http://dx.doi.org/10.1007/s11695-017-2869-1] [PMID: 28785975]

[105] Carbonell AM, Wolfe LG, Meador JG, Sugerman HJ, Kellum JM, Maher JW. Does diabetes affect weight loss after gastric bypass? Surg Obes Relat Dis 2008; 4(3): 441-4.
[http://dx.doi.org/10.1016/j.soard.2007.10.001] [PMID: 18065289]

[106] Lee W-J, Chong K, Ser K-H, *et al.* C-peptide predicts the remission of type 2 diabetes after bariatric surgery. Obes Surg 2012; 22(2): 293-8.
[http://dx.doi.org/10.1007/s11695-011-0565-0] [PMID: 22139820]

[107] Lee W-J, Hur KY, Lakadawala M, Kasama K, Wong SKH, Lee Y-C. Gastrointestinal metabolic surgery for the treatment of diabetic patients: a multi-institutional international study. J Gastrointest Surg 2012; 16(1): 45-51.
[http://dx.doi.org/10.1007/s11605-011-1740-2] [PMID: 22042564]

[108] Ramos-Levi A, Sanchez-Pernaute A, Matia P, *et al.* Diagnosis of diabetes remission after bariatric surgery may be jeopardized by remission criteria and previous hypoglycemic treatment. Obes Surg 2013; 23(10): 1520-6.
[http://dx.doi.org/10.1007/s11695-013-0995-y] [PMID: 23702908]

[109] Dixon JB, Chuang L-M, Chong K, *et al.* Predicting the glycemic response to gastric bypass surgery in patients with type 2 diabetes. Diabetes Care 2013; 36(1): 20-6.
[http://dx.doi.org/10.2337/dc12-0779] [PMID: 23033249]

[110] Lee W-J, Chong K, Chen J-C, *et al.* Predictors of diabetes remission after bariatric surgery in Asia. Asian J Surg 2012; 35(2): 67-73.
[http://dx.doi.org/10.1016/j.asjsur.2012.04.010] [PMID: 22720861]

[111] Robert M, Ferrand-Gaillard C, Disse E, *et al.* Predictive factors of type 2 diabetes remission 1 year after bariatric surgery: impact of surgical techniques. Obes Surg 2013; 23(6): 770-5.
[http://dx.doi.org/10.1007/s11695-013-0868-4] [PMID: 23355293]

[112] Cho J-M, Kim HJ, Lo Menzo E, Park S, Szomstein S, Rosenthal RJ. Effect of sleeve gastrectomy on type 2 diabetes as an alternative treatment modality to Roux-en-Y gastric bypass: systemic review and meta-analysis. Surg Obes Relat Dis 2015; 11(6): 1273-80.
[http://dx.doi.org/10.1016/j.soard.2015.03.001] [PMID: 26071847]

[113] Li J, Lai D, Wu D. Laparoscopic Roux-en-Y Gastric Bypass Versus Laparoscopic Sleeve Gastrectomy to Treat Morbid Obesity-Related Comorbidities: a Systematic Review and Meta-analysis. Obes Surg 2016; 26(2): 429-42.
[http://dx.doi.org/10.1007/s11695-015-1996-9] [PMID: 26661105]

[114] Schauer PR, Bhatt DL, Kirwan JP, *et al.* Bariatric Surgery versus Intensive Medical Therapy for Diabetes - 5-Year Outcomes. N Engl J Med 2017; 376(7): 641-51.
[http://dx.doi.org/10.1056/NEJMoa1600869] [PMID: 28199805]

[115] Sjöström L. Review of the key results from the Swedish Obese Subjects (SOS) trial - a prospective controlled intervention study of bariatric surgery. J Intern Med 2013; 273(3): 219-34.
[http://dx.doi.org/10.1111/joim.12012] [PMID: 23163728]

[116] Panunzi S, De Gaetano A, Carnicelli A, Mingrone G. Predictors of remission of diabetes mellitus in severely obese individuals undergoing bariatric surgery: do BMI or procedure choice matter? A meta-analysis. Ann Surg 2015; 261(3): 459-67.
[http://dx.doi.org/10.1097/SLA.0000000000000863] [PMID: 25361217]

[117] Aminian A, Jamal M, Augustin T, *et al.* Failed Surgical Weight Loss Does Not Necessarily Mean Failed Metabolic Effects. Diabetes Technol Ther 2015; 17(10): 682-4.
[http://dx.doi.org/10.1089/dia.2015.0064] [PMID: 26177379]

[118] Palmisano S, Silvestri M, Giuricin M, *et al.* Preoperative Predictive Factors of Successful Weight Loss and Glycaemic Control 1 Year After Gastric Bypass for Morbid Obesity. Obes Surg 2015; 25(11): 2040-6.
[http://dx.doi.org/10.1007/s11695-015-1662-2] [PMID: 25845353]

[119] Park JY, Kim YJ. Prediction of Diabetes Remission in Morbidly Obese Patients After Roux-en-Y Gastric Bypass. Obes Surg 2016; 26(4): 749-56.
[http://dx.doi.org/10.1007/s11695-015-1823-3] [PMID: 26205218]

[120] Lee W-J, Hur KY, Lakadawala M, *et al.* Predicting success of metabolic surgery: age, body mass index, C-peptide, and duration score. Surg Obes Relat Dis 2013; 9(3): 379-84.
[http://dx.doi.org/10.1016/j.soard.2012.07.015] [PMID: 22963817]

[121] Still CD, Wood GC, Benotti P, *et al.* Preoperative prediction of type 2 diabetes remission after Roux-en-Y gastric bypass surgery: a retrospective cohort study. Lancet Diabetes Endocrinol 2014; 2(1): 38-45.
[http://dx.doi.org/10.1016/S2213-8587(13)70070-6] [PMID: 24579062]

[122] Benaiges D, Sagué M, Flores-Le Roux JA, *et al.* Predictors of Hypertension Remission and Recurrence After Bariatric Surgery. Am J Hypertens 2016; 29(5): 653-9.
[http://dx.doi.org/10.1093/ajh/hpv153] [PMID: 26350297]

[123] Abbasi J. Unveiling the "Magic" of Diabetes Remission After Weight-Loss Surgery. JAMA 2017; 317(6): 571-4.
[http://dx.doi.org/10.1001/jama.2017.0020] [PMID: 28196253]

[124] Hinojosa MW, Varela JE, Smith BR, Che F, Nguyen NT. Resolution of systemic hypertension after

laparoscopic gastric bypass. J Gastrointest Surg 2009; 13(4): 793-7.
[http://dx.doi.org/10.1007/s11605-008-0759-5] [PMID: 19050981]

[125] Vogel JA, Franklin BA, Zalesin KC, *et al.* Reduction in predicted coronary heart disease risk after substantial weight reduction after bariatric surgery. Am J Cardiol 2007; 99(2): 222-6.
[http://dx.doi.org/10.1016/j.amjcard.2006.08.017] [PMID: 17223422]

[126] Crémieux P-Y, Ledoux S, Clérici C, Cremieux F, Buessing M. The impact of bariatric surgery on comorbidities and medication use among obese patients. Obes Surg 2010; 20(7): 861-70.
[http://dx.doi.org/10.1007/s11695-010-0163-6] [PMID: 20440579]

[127] Fouse T, Brethauer S. Resolution of Comorbidities and Impact on Longevity Following Bariatric and Metabolic Surgery. Surg Clin North Am 2016; 96(4): 717-32.
[http://dx.doi.org/10.1016/j.suc.2016.03.007] [PMID: 27473797]

[128] Benaiges D, Goday A, Ramon JM, Hernandez E, Pera M, Cano JF. Laparoscopic sleeve gastrectomy and laparoscopic gastric bypass are equally effective for reduction of cardiovascular risk in severely obese patients at one year of follow-up. Surg Obes Relat Dis 2011; 7(5): 575-80.
[http://dx.doi.org/10.1016/j.soard.2011.03.002] [PMID: 21546321]

[129] Pedersen JS, Borup C, Damgaard M, *et al.* Early 24-hour blood pressure response to Roux-en-Y gastric bypass in obese patients. Scand J Clin Lab Invest 2017; 77(1): 53-9.
[http://dx.doi.org/10.1080/00365513.2016.1258725] [PMID: 27905219]

[130] Vilallonga R, Himpens J, van de Vrande S. Long-Term (7 Years) Follow-Up of Roux-en-Y Gastric Bypass on Obese Adolescent Patients (<18 Years). Obes Facts 2016; 9(2): 91-100.
[http://dx.doi.org/10.1159/000442758] [PMID: 27035348]

[131] Fernstrom JD, Courcoulas AP, Houck PR, Fernstrom MH. Long-term changes in blood pressure in extremely obese patients who have undergone bariatric surgery. Arch Surg 2006; 141(3): 276-83.
[http://dx.doi.org/10.1001/archsurg.141.3.276] [PMID: 16549693]

[132] Shoar S, Saber AA. Long-term and midterm outcomes of laparoscopic sleeve gastrectomy versus Roux-en-Y gastric bypass: a systematic review and meta-analysis of comparative studies. Surg Obes Relat Dis 2017; 13(2): 170-80.
[http://dx.doi.org/10.1016/j.soard.2016.08.011] [PMID: 27720197]

[133] Schauer PR, Burguera B, Ikramuddin S, *et al.* Effect of laparoscopic Roux-en Y gastric bypass on type 2 diabetes mellitus. Ann Surg 2003; 238(4): 467-84.
[PMID: 14530719]

[134] Jamal M, Wegner R, Heitshusen D, Liao J, Samuel I. Resolution of hyperlipidemia follows surgical weight loss in patients undergoing Roux-en-Y gastric bypass surgery: a 6-year analysis of data. Surg Obes Relat Dis 2011; 7(4): 473-9.
[http://dx.doi.org/10.1016/j.soard.2010.08.009] [PMID: 21036105]

[135] Nguyen NT, Varela E, Sabio A, Tran C-L, Stamos M, Wilson SE. Resolution of hyperlipidemia after laparoscopic Roux-en-Y gastric bypass. J Am Coll Surg 2006; 203(1): 24-9.
[http://dx.doi.org/10.1016/j.jamcollsurg.2006.03.019] [PMID: 16798484]

[136] Carswell KA, Belgaumkar AP, Amiel SA, Patel AG. A Systematic Review and Meta-analysis of the Effect of Gastric Bypass Surgery on Plasma Lipid Levels. Obes Surg 2016; 26(4): 843-55.
[http://dx.doi.org/10.1007/s11695-015-1829-x] [PMID: 26210195]

[137] Cunha FM, Oliveira J, Preto J, *et al.* The Effect of Bariatric Surgery Type on Lipid Profile: An Age, Sex, Body Mass Index and Excess Weight Loss Matched Study. Obes Surg 2016; 26(5): 1041-7.
[http://dx.doi.org/10.1007/s11695-015-1825-1] [PMID: 26220239]

[138] Nosso G, Griffo E, Cotugno M, *et al.* Comparative Effects of Roux-en-Y Gastric Bypass and Sleeve Gastrectomy on Glucose Homeostasis and Incretin Hormones in Obese Type 2 Diabetic Patients: A One-Year Prospective Study. Horm Metab Res 2016; 48(5): 312-7.
[http://dx.doi.org/10.1055/s-0041-111505] [PMID: 26788926]

[139] Jhaveri RR, Pond KK, Hauser TH, *et al.* Cardiac remodeling after substantial weight loss: a prospective cardiac magnetic resonance study after bariatric surgery. Surg Obes Relat Dis 2009; 5(6): 648-52.
[http://dx.doi.org/10.1016/j.soard.2009.01.011] [PMID: 19833561]

[140] Algahim MF, Lux TR, Leichman JG, *et al.* Progressive regression of left ventricular hypertrophy two years after bariatric surgery. Am J Med 2010; 123(6): 549-55.
[http://dx.doi.org/10.1016/j.amjmed.2009.11.020] [PMID: 20569762]

[141] McCloskey CA, Ramani GV, Mathier MA, *et al.* Bariatric surgery improves cardiac function in morbidly obese patients with severe cardiomyopathy. Surg Obes Relat Dis 2007; 3(5): 503-7.
[http://dx.doi.org/10.1016/j.soard.2007.05.006] [PMID: 17903770]

[142] Nerla R, Tarzia P, Sestito A, *et al.* Effect of bariatric surgery on peripheral flow-mediated dilation and coronary microvascular function. Nutr Metab Cardiovasc Dis 2012; 22(8): 626-34.
[http://dx.doi.org/10.1016/j.numecd.2010.10.004] [PMID: 21186109]

[143] Delling L, Karason K, Olbers T, *et al.* Feasibility of bariatric surgery as a strategy for secondary prevention in cardiovascular disease: a report from the Swedish obese subjects trial J Obes 2010; 2010

[144] Wang Y, Zhang C. Bariatric Surgery to Correct Morbid Obesity Also Ameliorates Atherosclerosis in Patients with Type 2 Diabetes Mellitus. Am J Biomed Sci 2009; 1(1): 56-69.
[http://dx.doi.org/10.5099/aj090100056] [PMID: 19915685]

[145] Sturm W, Tschoner A, Engl J, *et al.* Effect of bariatric surgery on both functional and structural measures of premature atherosclerosis. Eur Heart J 2009; 30(16): 2038-43.
[http://dx.doi.org/10.1093/eurheartj/ehp211] [PMID: 19502233]

[146] Agrawal V, Krause KR, Chengelis DL, Zalesin KC, Rocher LL, McCullough PA. Relation between degree of weight loss after bariatric surgery and reduction in albuminuria and C-reactive protein. Surg Obes Relat Dis 2009; 5(1): 20-6.
[http://dx.doi.org/10.1016/j.soard.2008.07.011] [PMID: 18951068]

[147] Sareli AE, Cantor CR, Williams NN, *et al.* Obstructive sleep apnea in patients undergoing bariatric surgery--a tertiary center experience. Obes Surg 2011; 21(3): 316-27.
[http://dx.doi.org/10.1007/s11695-009-9928-1] [PMID: 19669842]

[148] Banks J, Adams ST, Laughlan K, *et al.* Roux-en-Y gastric bypass could slow progression of retinopathy in type 2 diabetes: a pilot study. Obes Surg 2015; 25(5): 777-81.
[http://dx.doi.org/10.1007/s11695-014-1476-7] [PMID: 25416083]

[149] McCarty TR, Echouffo-Tcheugui JB, Lange A, Haque L, Njei B. Impact of bariatric surgery on outcomes of patients with nonalcoholic fatty liver disease: a nationwide inpatient sample analysis, 2004-2012. Surg Obes Relat Dis 2018; 14(1): 74-80.
[http://dx.doi.org/10.1016/j.soard.2017.09.511] [PMID: 29055669]

[150] Kalinowski P, Paluszkiewicz R, Ziarkiewicz-Wróblewska B, *et al.* Liver Function in Patients With Nonalcoholic Fatty Liver Disease Randomized to Roux-en-Y Gastric Bypass Versus Sleeve Gastrectomy: A Secondary Analysis of a Randomized Clinical Trial. Ann Surg 2017; 266(5): 738-45.
[http://dx.doi.org/10.1097/SLA.0000000000002397] [PMID: 28767558]

[151] Shouhed D, Steggerda J, Burch M, Noureddin M. The role of bariatric surgery in nonalcoholic fatty liver disease and nonalcoholic steatohepatitis. Expert Rev Gastroenterol Hepatol 2017; 11(9): 797-811.
[http://dx.doi.org/10.1080/17474124.2017.1355731] [PMID: 28712339]

[152] El-Serag HB, Ergun GA, Pandolfino J, Fitzgerald S, Tran T, Kramer JR. Obesity increases oesophageal acid exposure. Gut 2007; 56(6): 749-55.
[http://dx.doi.org/10.1136/gut.2006.100263] [PMID: 17127706]

[153] Himpens J, Dapri G, Cadière GB. A prospective randomized study between laparoscopic gastric banding and laparoscopic isolated sleeve gastrectomy: results after 1 and 3 years. Obes Surg 2006; 16(11): 1450-6.

[http://dx.doi.org/10.1381/096089206778869933] [PMID: 17132410]

[154]   Foster A, Laws HL, Gonzalez QH, Clements RH. Gastrointestinal symptomatic outcome after laparoscopic Roux-en-Y gastric bypass. J Gastrointest Surg 2003; 7(6): 750-3.
[http://dx.doi.org/10.1016/S1091-255X(03)00092-1] [PMID: 13129551]

[155]   Parvizi J, Trousdale RT, Sarr MG. Total joint arthroplasty in patients surgically treated for morbid obesity. J Arthroplasty 2000; 15(8): 1003-8.
[http://dx.doi.org/10.1054/arth.2000.9054] [PMID: 11112195]

CHAPTER 10

The Role of Macronutrients in Diets for Weight Control

Cátia Braga-Pontes[1,2], **Vânia S. Ribeiro**[1,2] and **Cidália D. Pereira**[1,2,*]

[1] *School of Health Sciences, Polytechnic of Leiria, Leiria, Portugal*

[2] *Center for Innovative Care and Health Technology (ciTechCare), Polytechnic of Leiria, Leiria, Portugal*

Abstract: Obesity has reached epidemic proportions in the last decades and as so successful weight loss diets have been pursuit. Different dietary approaches, with distinct macronutrients distribution, have been studied. Low-fat, low-carbohydrate and/or high-protein diets are among the most used diets for obesity research and in clinical practice. However, their effects on obesity management, including in metabolic complications often associated, are not completely clarified. Moreover, additional questions arose inside each macronutrient group, being the following ones just a few: are all sugars equal for weight control? How does saturated *vs.* unsaturated fatty acids ingestion affect weight loss? What are the differences between animal or vegetable protein intake, regarding weight management? Taking all evidence together, it seems impossible to define an ideal macronutrients' distribution for weight loss and maintenance that fits everyone. Energy-restricted diets continue to be the most successful weight loss strategy, independently of macronutrient distribution. However, severe restriction of fat or carbohydrates do not seem to have an additional benefit for weight control as compared to a more balanced macronutrient distribution, as occurs in Mediterranean diet. Importantly, diets must be individualized and based on the personal and cultural preferences in order to promote a successful weight loss and maintenance in the long-term.

Keywords: Animal protein, Conjugated linoleic acid, Energy-restricted diet, Fibre, Fructose, Glycemic index, High-fructose corn syrup, High-protein diets, Ketogenic diets, Low-carbohydrate diets, Low-fat diets, n-3 fatty acids, n-6 fatty acids, Saturated fatty acid, Sugar addiction, Trans fatty acid, Unsaturated fatty acid, Vegetable protein, Weight loss, Weight maintenance.

INTRODUCTION

Weight control is a subject of increasing investigation since the 1970's [1] and it

* **Corresponding author Cidália D. Pereira:** School of Health Sciences, Polytechnic of Leiria, Leiria, Portugal; Tel/Fax: +351 244845300; E-mail: cidalia.pereira@ipleiria.pt

Rosário Monteiro and Maria João Martins (Eds.)

continues to grow as currently more than 2 billion people worldwide are overweight or obese [2].

Weight loss and weight maintenance are difficult, as they imply, among others, a good diet compliance, which may be very difficult especially if strict energy-restricted diets are recommended. Numerous dietary approaches have, therefore, been designed: low-carbohydrate, low-fat diets and/or high-protein diets continue to be tested and their efficiency for weight management is still being discussed. Moreover, the particularities of each macronutrient group for weight control beyond their energy value, *i.e.*, their specific subtypes or components (different protein sources, specific sugars, amino acids or fatty acids), are still under debate [3].

As overweight and obesity are often associated to metabolic disturbances (as insulin resistance, hypertension, dyslipidemia or central adiposity), the effects of each dietary intervention in these features are also important to understand. Additionally, it is most relevant to recognize the best approach for lean mass preservation, an important issue regarding weight loss intervention [3].

In this chapter, we review evidence regarding the contribution of each macronutrient, and their specific subtypes or components, in weight management in an attempt to understand their impact on weight loss and weight maintenance and the rationale beyond many dietary approaches applied in clinical practice.

FATS

Fats and fatty acids are identified as essential nutrients in both human and animal diets. Nutritionally, they are the highest source of energy (9 kcal/g or 37 kJ/g) [4]. Humans can use fatty acids as a source of energy or to produce other biologically important metabolites for normal body functioning [4].

Fats can be characterized by the specific content, saturation or chain length characteristics of their fatty acids; origin (animal *vs.* vegetable) and food sources of fats are also most relevant [5]. Fatty acids are classified as saturated (SFA) or unsaturated, the latter being further subdivided into monounsaturated (MUFA) or polyunsaturated fatty acids (PUFA) [4].

The complex nature of fatty acid food composition may be exemplified by lard, which consists of 40% SFA, 45% MUFA and 15% PUFA. This may be compared with olive oil which is 14% SFA, 74% MUFA, and 12% PUFA. Lard, like other examples of animal fat that are solid at room temperature, is often considered highly saturated, when in fact MUFA is more prevalent [5, 6].

The role of different types of dietary fat and its relation with metabolic regulation and weight is far from being unanimous in the scientific literature [5].

Saturated and Unsaturated Fatty Acids and Weight Control

Increasing evidence has established a link between chronic inflammation and many chronic diseases and metabolic disorders, including obesity-induced insulin resistance [7, 8]. *In vivo* and *in vitro* studies have demonstrated the proinflammatory effects of saturated fats [9, 10]. Indeed, the intake of a meal enriched with SFA induces a postprandial proinflammatory response through upregulation of several inflammatory genes in subcutaneous adipose tissue [11]. Many studies indicate the relationship between SFA and Toll-like receptor 4 (TLR4) as being associated with the subclinical inflammation often seen in obese individuals [8].

In addition, SFA decreases lipolytic activity in adipocytes because of its impact on membrane fluidity, thus hindering the ability to use the stored fats [5, 12, 13].

The oxidation rates of fats are differentiated, depending on the saturation characteristics of the fatty acids, as well as their polarity. According to Hunsberger *et al*, there seems to be a positive association between unsaturated fatty acids and fat oxidation [5]. Unsaturated fatty acids are more easily oxidized than SFA with similar chain length, while chain length tends to be inversely associated to the oxidation rate [6]. In fact, PUFA, unlike SFA, increase the fatty acid oxidative capacity of tissues through their ability to induce several transcription factors, such as peroxisome proliferator activated receptor α (PPARα), involved in fatty acid oxidation. On the other hand, PUFA suppress lipid synthesis by inhibiting transcription factors, such as sterol regulatory element-binding protein 1 (SREBP1), that mediate the insulin and carbohydrate control of lipogenic and glycolytic genes [14].

Despite those positive effects of PUFA, experimental studies have demonstrated that omega-3 (ω-3 or n-3) and omega-6 (ω-6 or n-6) fatty acids may elicit divergent effects on body fat mass, through mechanisms of adipogenesis, browning of adipose tissue, modulation of lipid homeostasis, modulation of brain-gut-adipose tissue axis and, mainly, systemic inflammation [15]. A recent review summarizing studies upon the association between n-6 fatty acids intake and obesity indicates that n-6 fatty acids might have proadipogenic properties as well as a potential role in fetal programming of obesity [16]. On the opposite, the n-3 fatty acids have been suggested to reduce the risk of a number of non-communicable metabolic diseases, including obesity. Eicosapentaenoic acid (EPA; 20: 5n-3) and docosahexaenoic acid (DHA; 22: 6n-3) have been suggested to play a role in adipose tissue/adipocyte metabolism, inducing anti-obesity and anti-inflammatory effects [17, 18]. It has been demonstrated (in animal models) that long-chain n-3 fatty acids, particularly EPA and DHA, may reduce lipogenesis, increase lipolysis and decrease inflammation by mechanisms that should include changes in the expression of genes involved in fat oxidation and energy expenditure [17, 19]. Interestingly, fish oil diets (1% or 3%, w/w) significantly reduce the levels of araquidonic acid-derived endocannabinoids and, at the same time, increase the levels of docosahexaenoyl ethanolamide and eicosapentaenoyl ethanolamide in plasma and adipose tissue as compared with mice receiving equivalent amounts of high oleic sunflower oil in diets. Animals that consume fish oil also produce fewer n-6 eicosanoids and larger volumes of n-3 eicosanoids [20]. Genetically obese Zucker rats fed with fish oil or krill oil diets have lower levels of triglycerides in the liver, and the collected peritoneal macrophages dictionaries have less inflammatory response to lipopolysaccharides (LPS) in culture, compared to animals that received a control diet without (n-3) long-chain PUFA [21].

Of concern, in the last decades, the n-6 fatty acids intake has been increasing and, in the opposite direction, the n-3 fatty acids intake has been decreasing, resulting in a large enhancement in the n-6/n-3 ratio from 1:1 to 20:1 [15]. Prospective studies clearly demonstrate an increased risk of obesity as the n-6 fatty acids level and the n-6/n-3 ratio increase in red blood cell (RBC) membrane phospholipids, while high levels of omega-3 in RBC membrane phospholipids levels lower the risk of obesity [15]. Current studies in humans demonstrate that, in addition to absolute amounts of n-6 and n-3 fatty acids intake, the n-6/n-3 ratio plays a relevant role in the development of obesity through arachidonic acid (AA) eicosanoid metabolites and hyperactivity of the cannabinoid system, which can be reversed with increased intake of EPA and DHA [15]. Therefore, a balanced n-6/n-3 ratio is important for health and in the prevention and management of overweight and obesity [15]. The current recommendation for n-3 fatty acid intake (in humans) is between 0.5% and 2% of total energy intake [19]. However, the duration and dose required for the favourable effects of EPA and DHA in overweight and/or obese individuals have not yet been clarified [17].

Regarding MUFA, there are many studies showing their positive effects not only on body weight control but also in the amelioration of the metabolic profile under obesity (both in rodents and in humans) [22 - 24]. In a similar way as PUFA, MUFA seem also capable to control gene expression. In a rodent obesity model, a high-MUFA diet decrease white adipose tissue accumulation by a) decreasing adipose peroxisome proliferator-activated receptor γ (PPARγ) and lipoprotein lipase mRNA expression, b) mediating phosphorylation of hormone-sensitive lipase, and c) improving hepatic lipolytic enzyme activities and mRNA expression involved in β-oxidation [23]. In addition, high-MUFA diets may also reverse

SFA-induced inflammation [22]. Interestingly, olive oil, an excellent source of MUFA, may be particularly beneficial to obese individuals. In post-menopausal and abdominally obese women, olive oil promotes postprandial fat oxidation and stimulates dietary thermogenesis [25].

Trans Fatty Acids

The unsaturated *trans* fatty acids (TFA), contain at least one double bond in the *trans* configuration. TFAs can be generated with the use of microbial fermentation or through the industrial process of hydrogenation of oil (vegetable oils). Thermal processes such as frying and edible oil refining promote the formation of TFA [26]. Animal studies have shown conflicting data regarding TFA ingestion and obesity [27]. However, a randomized controlled study in green monkeys for 6 years concluded that animals with a high-TFA diet (reaching 8% of total energy intake) have a higher weight gain and higher visceral fat deposition than animals with a high-*cis*-MUFA diet [28]. Epidemiological studies provide limited, though consistent, evidence to support that high-TFA ingestion may induce a slight increase of body weight [29]. Interestingly, diets with TFA during gestation and lactation activate hypothalamic inflammation in rodents, contributing to weight gain in adult life [30].

Conjugated Linoleic Acids

The conjugated linoleic acids (CLA) refer to a group of conjugated octadecadienoic acid isomers derived from linoleic acid, a fatty acid that contains 18 carbons and two double bonds, in the *cis* configuration, at the 9th and 12th carbons [31]. Most of the CLAs' physiologic effects are supported by both the *cis*-9, *trans*-11 isomer (the main dietary form of CLA), and *trans*-10, *cis*-12 isomer, which have been linked to CLA's weight control effects. The *trans*-10, *cis*-12 isomer seems to mediate CLA effects on body composition [31]. CLA intake from dietary sources is generally < 600 mg/day and it occurs naturally in beef and dairy products [32].

There are several studies on CLA supplementation, both in animals and humans, demonstrating the positive effects of CLA, particularly on body composition [33 - 36]. Studies on CLA supplementation and weight control in human subjects, have shown that daily intake of 3.4 g of CLA (equal parts of both isomers) reduce total body fat [37]. Despite data from animal studies are consistent, supporting the beneficial effect of CLA supplementation, results from humans studies are still quite discordant and some side effects (such as constipation, diarrhoea and soft stools) were pointed [38]. According to Lehnen *et al* [39], selected foods naturally enriched with CLA (and not from supplementation) would be an alternative to reduce adiposity, without the unwanted side effects [40].

There are no clinical evidences or consistent effects on health to conclude that CLA can be considered a functional or medical food. Further research is needed to evaluate the benefits of CLA dietary supplementation and also the potential long-term health risks.

Are Low-fat Diets Effective for Weight Loss?

Dietary guidelines recommend a reduction in total fat content to less than 30% of the energy intake for obesity prevention [41].

High-fat diets (generally ≥ 30% of energy from fat) have been linked to increased body weight, which has led to the adoption of low-fat diets, with the inclusion of low-fat products. High-fat diets have been for long identified as the cause of the obesity epidemic because fat is the most energy dense macronutrient [5]. In addition, high-fat diets (within the range of 30-78% of total energy intake) have been used to induce obesity (and some of its metabolic complications) in animals [42].

There are many physiological mechanisms that seem to be involved in high-fat diet-induced obesity such as food overconsumption due to low satiating effects and high palatability of fat [5, 41, 43] as well as the high efficiency of dietary fat in being stored in the body and the alterations in the hormones involved in energy balance. In this regard, high-fat diets induce hyperleptinemia and hyperinsulinemia with consequent leptin and insulin resistance; additionally, a decrease of the suppression of ghrelin secretion following high-fat diets has been observed [42 - 44]. Moreover, high-fat diet-induced dysbiosis and systemic inflammation may also contribute to obesity [45].

Thus, fat intake has been blamed for the adiposity increase and has led to a worldwide effort to decrease the amount of fat in the diet. However, the efficacy of this approach is questionable. Short-term dietary intervention studies reveal that low-fat diets (within ≤ 10-30% of energy from fat) lead to weight loss in both healthy and overweight individuals. However, in the long-term, it is less clear if a decrease in fat intake is more effective than other dietary restrictions [5, 41].

Some studies have shown that there are no significant differences on weight loss between low-fat and other diets [46, 47]. A review conducted in 2008 by Summerbell *et al* [48] allowed to evaluate the effects of low-fat diets on overweight or clinically obese participants (12 randomized controlled clinical trials) and suggested that fat-restricted diets are no better than other calorie-restricted diets.

The results of a more recent systematic review showed that low- and high-fat interventions (under energy restriction) have a similar effect on weight loss. The same review also showed that low-fat interventions only led to greater weight loss when compared with the usual diet. Evidence from randomised controlled trials (RCTs) does not support the efficiency of low-fat diets over other dietary interventions on long-term weight loss [49]. The long-term compliance with low-fat diets seems to be difficult, particularly with very-low-fat diets, which may partially explain these results [50].

CARBOHYDRATES

Carbohydrates are present in the major food sources in the human diet, providing 17 kJ/g (4.0 kcal/g) [51]. Among them, "free sugars" have been considered the culprits of the obesity epidemic for decades, in the same way as high-fat diets. Although many other factors have been recognized to be involved in obesity aetiology, efforts have also been made regarding sugar restriction in the diet [52]. Accordingly, many guidelines emerged from different international organizations. World Health Organization (WHO) strongly recommends reducing the intake of free sugars to less than 10% of total energy intake (in both adults and children). WHO suggests that a further reduction of free sugar intake to below 5% of total energy intake (conditional recommendation) would provide additional health benefits [53]. Free sugars include monosaccharaides and disaccharides added to foods and beverages by the manufacturer, cook or consumer as well as sugars naturally present in honey, syrups, fruit juices and fruit juice concentrates [53]. The UK Scientific Advisory Committee on Nutrition (SACN) report on Dietary Carbohydrates and Health [54] also recommends that free sugar intake should not exceed 5% of total energy, maintaining total carbohydrate intake at 50% of total dietary energy. These guidelines are based on the well-established relationship between the frequent consumption of sugar containing foods and dental caries, particularly, in children rather than evidence regarding obesity prevention. In fact, discussion remains about the relationship between sugar intake and obesity, particularly if consumed under isoenergetic controlled conditions [52].

Are all Sugars Equal for Weight Control?

Regarding sugar consumption, fructose ingestion, particularly through high-fructose corn syrup (HFCS) as present in sugar-sweetened beverages (SSB), has emerged as an etiological factor not only for obesity, but also for the frequent obesity-associated metabolic abnormalities [55, 56]. So, the question arose: are fructose, HFCS, sucrose or glucose differently implicated in obesity development?

Fructose and glucose are differently metabolized in the human body and these well-known differences may account for the controversy. Over 90% of fructose ingested is absorbed through the small intestine and metabolized in the liver on first pass. In contrast, glucose is metabolized by a variety of organs. It is important to note, however, that the pathways are interactive. In fact, numerous studies have shown that roughly 50% of fructose is converted to glucose within the liver, 15%-20% is converted to glycogen, 20%-25% to lactate, and a few percent to carbon dioxide. Multiple studies have shown that only 1%-5% of consumed fructose may follow the pathway of *de novo* lipogenesis and be converted into fatty acids which are then packaged as triglycerides and either stored in the liver or released in the bloodstream. The amount of fat produced through this process is in the order of one gram per day compared to the 100-125 g typically consumed each day in the human diet. In certain animals, *de novo* lipogenesis can be a major pathway, however in humans, it is minimal. These facts have not always been considered, leading for claims of fructose as an inducer of non-alcoholic fatty liver disease (NAFLD) and insulin resistance in humans. Moreover, some of the studies that found differences regarding fructose and glucose metabolism compared the ingestion of pure fructose *vs.* pure glucose, which does not properly represent human nutrition, as either pure fructose or pure glucose are rarely consumed in the human diet [56 - 59].

Regarding HFCS ingestion, the controversy came from an opinion paper published in 2004, in the American Journal of Clinical Nutrition, by Bray *et al*, where it was mentioned that "the increase in consumption of HFCS has a temporal relation to the epidemic of obesity, and the overconsumption of HFCS in calorically sweetened beverages may play a role in the epidemic of obesity" [60]. Although the authors have recognized only a temporal association, the idea of a causal relationship emerged. However, subsequent research has shown that HFCS and sucrose have indistinguishable metabolic effects and health consequences in human beings. These results are not completely surprising as sucrose and HFCS are very similar in their composition. Sucrose contains 50% fructose and 50% glucose and HFCS generally appears through HFCS-55 (containing 55% fructose, 42% glucose and 3% other carbohydrates which are readily hydrolysable polymers of glucose) or HFCS-42 (containing 42% fructose and 53% glucose as well as 5% polymers which are hydrolysable to glucose). HFCS-55 is the form of HFCS commonly used in soft drinks and other sugar sweetened beverages in the United States; HFCS-42 is the common form of fructose used in solid foods and other applications [57 - 59]. To dissipate any concern, the American Medical Association [61] and the Academy of Nutrition and Dietetics [62] produced statements indicating that there are no differences between HFCS and sucrose in their likelihood of causing obesity or its related metabolic complications.

WHO commissioned a systematic literature review to clarify some doubts about the effect of sugar intake on body weight and adiposity. Results from RCTs indicate that in adults under *ad libitum* diets, a decrease in dietary sugar intake is associated with a significant reduction on body weight [−0.80kg (95% confidence interval −1.21 to −0.39), p < 0.001] by comparison with no reduction or an increase in sugar intake (intervention period ranging from 10 weeks to 8 months). Conversely, an increase of sugar intake, mostly through SSB, is associated with a significant rise on body weight [0.75kg (95% confidence interval 0.30 to 1.19), p = 0.001] by comparison with no increase in sugar intake. Importantly, when isoenergetic exchanges of dietary sugar with other carbohydrates (sucrose or fructose-sweeten food or liquids) or other macronutrient sources were analysed, no evidence of differences on body weight changes were found. This finding strongly suggests that energy imbalance is a major determinant for the increase on body weight often associated to sugar intake [63].

Regarding metabolic dysfunction often associated to obesity, large prospective cohort studies have shown no association between sugar intake with diabetes, hypertension and coronary heart disease (CHD). One exception is gout, which was associated with fructose consumption in a systematic review and meta-analysis of prospective cohort studies [64].

Sugars from SSB might, however, be a special case. In fact, regular consumption of SSB indicates that it can lead to weight gain both in children and adults [65, 66]. Significant relationship of SSB also exists with type 2 diabetes [67], metabolic syndrome [68], hypertension [69], coronary heart disease [70, 71], stroke [72] and gout [73]. However, it is important to mention that this association might be related to energy as the observed associations between SSB and cardiometabolic diseases only remain significant at the highest quintiles of exposures, the exception being gout. On the other hand, it is possible that liquid calories from SSB are poorly compensated for by a decrease in total energy intake compared to solid calories, leading to weight gain and downstream cardiometabolic diseases. Additionally, SSB ingestion might be associated to an unhealthy lifestyle, particularly to a worse dietary pattern and to a sedentary behavior [64].

Therefore, despite the continuing concern regarding fructose's unique metabolic effects, which stems from low-quality ecological studies, animal models and a few human studies, the highest level of evidence from systematic review and meta-analysis does not support a direct causal relationship with cardiometabolic disease. Considering the highest quality evidence from controlled feeding trials, fructose-containing sugars can lead to weight gain and increase in cardiometabolic risk factors only under a positive energy balance. Under isocaloric conditions, fructose-containing sugars do not appear to cause weight gain compared to other forms of macronutrients including complex carbohydrates, fats and protein, and in low doses fructose might even show benefit. Prospective cohort studies have shown an association between fructose-containing sugars and cardiometabolic risk including weight gain, cardiovascular disease outcomes and diabetes only when restricted to SSB and not for sugars from other sources [57 - 59, 64, 74].

Glycemic Index: Does it Really Matters for Weight Loss?

There is increasing interest in the possibility that the glycemic characteristics of carbohydrates may also be of importance regarding weight control. However, the efficiency of glycemic index (GI) *per se* for obesity treatment remains controversial [75 - 78]. Sloth and Astrup, reviewing the literature, stated that there is no convincing evidence to suggest that a low-GI diet is superior for cardiovascular health and weight loss in healthy subjects, when compared to professional dietary advice. However, data on cardiovascular risk factors tend to be somewhat more extensive in insulin-resistant subjects and in this particular population the results are more coincident, favouring low-GI diets [79].

In a systematic review by Thomas *et al* [80], that included 6 RCTs (n=202), low-GI or low-glycemic load diets, compared to control diets (diets with a higher GI or glycemic load; or even other diets), induced a greater decrease on body mass, total fat mass and body mass index (BMI) as well as in total cholesterol and LDL-cholesterol. Additionally, in studies comparing *ad libitum* low-GI or glycemic load diets to conventional restricted energy low-fat diets, participants in the former group have similar or better results. The authors concluded that lowering the glycemic load of the diet appears to be an effective method of promoting weight loss and improving lipid profile, but further research with longer-term follow-up will determine whether improvement continues. It is important to mention, however, that many of these studies did not adjust for potential confounders, such as protein or total fibre intake.

The GLYNDIET study [81] was a 6-month RCT designed to assess the effect of dietary GI on weight loss, satiety, glucose and insulin metabolism, lipid profile, inflammation, and other emergent metabolic risk markers. This clinical trial included men and women aged between 30 and 60 years with BMI between 27 and 35 kg/m^2, without obesity-related diseases. The participants were randomly assigned to one of the three isocaloric energy-restricted diets: low-GI (LGI, n=41), high-GI (HGI, n=40) and low-fat diet (LF, n=40, 18% protein, 52% carbohydrates and 30% fat). The LGI and HGI diets had a comparable macronutrient distribution (18% protein, 42% carbohydrates and 40% fat) but included foods with different GI (34 *vs.* 62). Results from this RCT showed that the LGI diet reduced weight more effectively than did a traditional LF diet.

Moreover, the LGI diet led to a significantly greater improvement in insulin sensitivity than did the LF diet. LGI and HGI diets, however, did not have different effects on body weight and insulin metabolism. Postprandial satiety and hunger rates, lipid profile, inflammation and related peripheral metabolic risk markers were similarly affected by the 3 dietary interventions.

In agreement, a more recent systematic review and meta-analysis demonstrated that low-GI/glycemic load diets do not lead to significantly more weight loss than higher GI/glycemic load diets over the moderate-term, as compared to an isocaloric control diet, in overweight or obese people [82].

Nonetheless, the International Scientific Consensus Summit from the International Carbohydrate Quality Consortium, regarding GI, glycemic load and glycemic response recommended that "the quality of carbohydrate-rich foods as defined by GI/glycemic load is particularly important for individuals who are sedentary, overweight and at increased risk of type 2 diabetes" and "probable evidence exists for low-GI/glycemic load diets in reducing total body fat mass and in weight management" [83].

Fibre and Weight Management

The established adequate intake of dietary fibre (14 g of total fibre/1000 kcal or 35 g/day for adult men and 25 g/day for adult women) is increasingly being recommended as evidence from epidemiological studies found an inverse association between dietary fibre consumption and the risk of some chronic diseases, such as cardiovascular disease, obesity, type 2 diabetes or some cancers. However, the results of intervention studies in humans regarding the effect of fibre intake on body weight or satiety were less consensual [84 - 86].

In a systematic review by Clark and Slavin [87], studies measuring appetite, food and/or energy intake with a treatment period of ≤ 24 hours, a low- or no-fibre control and healthy human participants, as well as reporting fibre type and amount, were included. In this review, the percentage of treatments that significantly reduced subjective appetite rating and food or energy intake was 39% and 22%, respectively, as compared with the control. The satiety-enhancing effects of β-glucans, lupin kernel fibre, rye bran, whole grain rye, or a mixed high-fibre diet were supported in more than one publication. Most isolated fibres, however, do not reduce appetite or energy intake in acute study designs.

In a systematic review of RCTs, Wanders *et al* [88] found clear differences for appetite, acute energy intake, long-term energy intake and body weight, depending on chemical structure of fibre. In fact, fibres characterized as being more viscous (*e.g.* pectins, β-glucans and guar gum) reduce appetite more often than those less viscous (59% *vs.* 14%), which also applies to acute energy intake (69% *vs.* 30%). Overall, effects on energy intake and body weight are relatively small, but may be of clinical significance.

More recently, a RCT compared the effectiveness of two approaches for dietary change in adults with metabolic syndrome (n=240): a fibre-focused diet ($\geq$ 30 g/day), and the American Heart Association diet (AHA). The intervention consisted of two individual sessions and 12 group sessions where participants received instructions on how to increase their fibre intake (fibre-focused diet) or to follow the AHA diet, which also includes a high-fibre intake (AHA diet). At 3 months, mean change in weight in the high-fibre group was −3.5 pounds as compared to −4.4 in the AHA group [95% confidence interval (CI)]. Weight loss was maintained in both groups at 6 and 12 months. At 12 months, weight loss for the high-fibre group was −4.6 pounds (−6.4, −2.9, 95% CI) and for the AHA group was −6.0 (−7.7, −4.3, 95% CI). Additionally, participants in both treatment groups decreased their total calorie intake over the 1-year study duration [−200.0 (−313.2, −86.9) kcal/day for high-fibre group *vs.* −464.6 (−578.0, −351.2) kcal/day for the AHA group]. Both diastolic and systolic blood pressure decreased during the trial with no difference between the two groups. Changes in glucose metabolism, lipid profile and inflammatory markers were also not different between the two groups. Accordingly, the authors concluded that a single component dietary intervention, specifically a recommendation to increase fibre intake, can achieve clinically meaningful weight loss as compared to a more complex approach as the AHA diet [89].

Although many mechanisms may explain the potential association between high-fibre consumption and a decrease on body weight, satiety is one of the most cited [86, 90, 91].

Additionally, some fibres are well recognized to modulate gut microbiota which has been also implicated in obesity development and treatment. These particular fibres known as prebiotics may exert beneficial effects in gut microbiota and consequently may led to positive changes not only on body weight and composition but also in satiety and in metabolic parameters often deregulated in overweight and obese individuals [92]. However, this subject is beyond the scope of the present chapter and will be discussed in another chapter of this book.

Dietary fibre is not an uniform entity, but rather a diverse group of polysaccharides including resistant starch, other glucose polymers with alpha or beta linkages, polymers based on specific sugars such as pectins, fructans and xylans; fibre of marine origin such as alginate and chitosan; and complex fibres rich in pectin, arabinoxylan or β-glucan [85, 90]. As a result, the particular benefits in weight management of this heterogeneous group viewed as a whole may be difficult to prove. In agreement, the CARMEN study [93], a multicentre RCT that evaluated the effect of simple *vs.* complex carbohydrates in association with a low-fat diet, found no significant differences on weight loss nor fat mass between the 2 groups, after 6 months.

Hence, long-term studies with particular types of fibre will be useful in the understanding the association between fibre intake and weight management. Meanwhile, it seems reasonable that diets for weight loss should also include fibre-rich foods, as their composition in micronutrients and other bioactive components may be beneficial as a whole health approach [85, 94].

Sugar Addiction: Myth or Reality?

The concept of "food addiction" was first defined by Randolph, almost 60 years ago, as "[…] a specific adaptation to one or more regularly consumed foods to which a person is highly sensitive, produces a common pattern of symptoms descriptively similar to those of other addictive processes" [95]. With the increase in the worldwide prevalence of obesity over the past decades, the concept of "food addiction" has regained popularity both among the public and professionals, probably by the greater importance that has been given to environmental obesogenic factors, such as calorie-dense sweet and/or fatty foods. In this context, the hedonic rewarding characteristic of sugar has been recently suggested for abuse potential similar to classical drugs of abuse by stimulating shared brain reward pathways involved in drug addiction [96, 97]. However, by now, this sugar-addiction hypothesis comes mainly from rodent experiments [98 - 100] and its translational value for human eating behavior is highly controversial in the current scientific community [96, 97]. In fact, evidence from systematic reviews and meta-analysis of controlled human dietary trials do not support that a specific macronutrient as sugar causes binge eating more than other food sources [96, 101].

In a recent cross-sectional study by Markus *et al,* 1495 university students were assessed for Diagnostic and Statistical Manual of Mental Disorders (DSM)-related signs of food addiction for particular food categories (Yale Food Addiction Scale – YFAS). Results revealed that 95% of participants experienced at least one symptom of food dependence and 12.6% met the YFAS diagnosis for food addiction. These problems were mostly reported for the combined high-fat savoury (30%) and high-fat sweet foods (25%), whereas only a minority experienced such problems for low-fat and savoury (2%) and mainly sugar-containing foods (5%). Furthermore, "withdrawal" and/or "adaptation" signs were more frequently reported for high-fat savoury and high-fat sweet foods than for sugar-specific foods. This study also revealed a high positive correlation between depression symptomatology and YFAS symptom scores. Importantly, depression symptoms predicted increases in YFAS scores markedly in participants who reported addiction symptoms for the high-fat savoury and high-fat sweet foods. The authors concluded that consuming palatable energy-dense foods and drinks can become an emotionally rewarding experience that promotes additional energy intake, particularly under individual adverse circumstances. Although this emotional rewarding value of food will be reflected by altered brain reward pathways, including the endogenous opioid and/or dopamine systems, this does not validate the hypothesis of "sugar addiction", as the brain does not appear to respond to food and/or sugar in the same way as to drugs of abuse [96].

Pursey *et al*, reviewing the current evidence on this subject, concluded that highly processed, hyper-palatable foods with combinations of fat and sugar may potentiate an addictive-like response. Total fat content and GI also appear to be important factors in the addictive potential of foods. However, few studies have reported an association between sugar and addictive-like eating. Consequently, due to the paucity of studies, it is difficult to conclusively identify a specific food or ingredient as capable of triggering an addictive-like response in humans [102]. Meanwhile, a concept of "eating addiction/dependence" instead of "food addiction" has been suggested as superior for educational purposes. "Eating addiction" stresses the behavioral component, whereas "food addiction" seems a passive process which simply befalls an individual [96, 103].

Low-carbohydrate Diets *vs.* High-fat Diets

Low-carbohydrate diets gained increased popularity in the last decades for obesity prevention and treatment. This dietetic approach involves carbohydrate replacement by a greater intake of fat and/or protein. Low-carbohydrate, high-fat diets become a concern regarding potential detrimental effects on cardiovascular risk factors due to a more liberal fat intake [104]. Low-carbohydrate, high-protein diets seemed quite promising [105, 106], but again questions arose for the potential health threats of a high-protein intake [107]. This subject will be discussed later in this chapter, on the proteins topic.

Bazzano *et al* [108] conducted a RCT to assess the effects of a low-carbohydrate diet compared with a low-fat diet on body weight and cardiovascular risk factors. Participants (n=148) were randomly assigned to a low-fat group [less than 30% of daily energy intake from total fat (with < 7% from saturated fat) and 55% from carbohydrates] or to a low-carbohydrate group [intake of digestible carbohydrates (total carbohydrates minus total fibre) of less than 40 g/d]. Neither diet included a specific calorie or energy goal. However, during the follow-up period (12 months), total energy intake was similar between groups. The reduction on body weight and the proportional reductions in fat mass were significantly greater while the proportional increases in lean mass were significantly greater in the low-carbohydrate group as compared with the low-fat group. Participants in both groups significantly reduced waist circumference. Although changes in waist circumference were more favourable in the low-carbohydrate group at 3 and 6 months, they did not differ significantly from those in the low-fat group at 12 months. Concerning the lipid profile, at 12 months, serum levels of total and LDL-cholesterol had not significantly changed among participants in either group. However, HDL-cholesterol levels increased significantly more in the low-carbohydrate group than in the low-fat group. Serum levels of triglycerides also decreased significantly in both groups, with greater decreases among participants in the low-carbohydrate group. Although systolic and diastolic blood pressures did not significantly decrease among participants in either group, participants in the low-carbohydrate group had significant reductions in the estimated 10-year risk for CHD (10-Year Framingham CHD Risk Score) at 6 and 12 months, as compared to the low-fat group.

A recent meta-analysis of RCTs [104] compared also the effects of low-carbohydrate diets (defined as an intake of only 20–40 g/d of carbohydrates in the first phase or carbohydrate intake of < 20% of total energy intake) with low-fat diets (< 30% of total energy as fat) on weight loss and cardiovascular risk factors, only with intervention periods of at least of 6 months up to 2 years. Individuals in the low-carbohydrate group had significantly greater weight loss, greater triglyceride reduction and greater HDL-cholesterol increase, as compared to the low-fat group. However, LDL-cholesterol significantly increased in the low-carbohydrate group (*vs.* the low-fat group). In fact, the LDL-cholesterol increase induced by low-carbohydrate diets was corroborated by different studies [109, 110] and was also mentioned in the current guidelines for the management of overweight and obesity in adults [111], raising the question if cardiovascular risk reduction previously found may outweigh the potential increase in LDL-cholesterol.

PROTEINS

Proteins are essential elements of a healthy diet and provide 17 kJ/g (4.0 kcal/g) [51]. Proteins have been widely studied in the management of weight and body composition in overweight subjects [112]. Although a growing body of evidence highlights their positive effects on weight loss (and weight loss maintenance), potential adverse effects of high-protein diets also arise [105 - 107].

Protein Role on Weight Loss Diets

Scientific evidence suggests that adequate protein intake plays an important role in regulating body weight through the following metabolic mechanisms: a) promoting satiety [113 - 115], b) increasing energy expenditure [115 - 118], and c) sparing fat-free mass [113, 115, 119]. Studies in animals and humans suggest that macronutrients have a hierarchical effect on short-term food intake and satiety, with proteins promoting more satiety and lower intakes of food than carbohydrates or fats [114]. A longitudinal study [120] that followed the same subjects for 23 years found a decrease in energy intake of 125 kJ and 152 kJ in men and women, respectively, for each 1% increase in the percentage of daily protein intake. In addition, the negative association between protein intake and energy intake is three times stronger than the positive association between fat intake and energy intake [121]. In 1956, Mellinkoff *et al* [122] suggested that one of the mechanisms that contributes to protein satiating capacity is the resultant high concentration of amino acids in plasma or blood which, not being used for protein synthesis, act as a sign of satiety and as a depressor mechanism of food intake. It is now known that protein intake and amino acid profile contribute significantly to the decrease in food intake due to the release of bioactive anorexigenic peptides that are involved in the satiety cascade, namely the glucagon-like peptide 1 (GLP1), cholecystokinin (CCK) and peptide YY [114, 123]. The satiating capacity of proteins is independent of diet energy [124] and contributes both to a greater adherence to diet and to a positive "attitude-towar--eating" [113].

Regarding protein intake and energy expenditure, the effect of this macronutrient involves both basal metabolic rate and the thermogenic effect of food [113, 124]. The thermogenic effect of food is different for each macronutrient (0 to 3% for fat, 5 to 10% for carbohydrates and 20 to 30% for protein), representing for total energy intake about 10% of daily energy expenditure [113, 124]. The effects of protein intake on basal metabolic rate have been well studied, especially for high-protein diets, and, in this context, it has been concluded that the increase in basal metabolic rate is related to increased gluconeogenesis [113, 117, 125]. The gluconeogenesis which occurs in low-carbohydrate and high-protein diets, requires ATP for the initial processes of protein metabolism and oxidation, including urea synthesis, which partially explains the increase in energy expenditure with this type of diet. In addition, there is still an increase of long-term basal metabolic rate due to increased protein synthesis and protein turnover [113, 116]. Regarding the relationship between protein consumption and energy expenditure, different studies showed that protein intake causes an acute increase in diet-induced energy expenditure and when this increased protein intake is longer than three days, it also results in an increase in the sleeping metabolic rate

[113, 117]. Additionally, the effects of protein consumption on energy expenditure are stronger with consumption of complete proteins, as shown by casein, and high-biological value proteins producing a higher thermogenic effect than low-biological value proteins, which may explain the lower protein synthesis that occurs during the ingestion of plant proteins [113].

Sparing fat-free mass is another mechanism that positively contributes for the role of protein on weight loss and weight maintenance. Studies designed to evaluate the relationship between protein intake and weight management demonstrate an improvement on body composition through an increase of fat-free mass and a healthier metabolic profile. These beneficial changes occur in diets with a negative energy balance, where protein contributes with 20 to 30% of total energy intake, as long as an adequate protein intake is ensured [113, 124]. Scientific evidence shows that during weight loss, as well as weight maintenance, a relatively high-protein diet (within recommended intake values) maintains or increases muscle mass and reduces fat mass, contributing to the improvement of the metabolic profile [113, 115]. Several studies have shown that increasing protein intake (30% of total energy intake) and decreasing carbohydrate intake (40% of total energy intake) may favour the reduction of fat mass, especially abdominal fat mass [126, 127]. Under energy restriction, the amount of protein required to maintain muscle mass is greater, and it is sometimes advisable to follow diets with 30 to 35% of protein, despite this advice is not suitable for individuals with renal disease [126, 128].

The evaluation of the metabolic profile during the follow-up of high-protein diets demonstrated an improvement of plasma lipids and lipoproteins, particularly when associated with a low-carbohydrate diet. Such diets have not only been associated with a reduction in risk factors for heart disease (by reducing blood pressure as well as serum triglycerides and by increasing both HDL-cholesterol and the size of LDL particles) but also revealed their particular suitability for individuals with atherogenic dyslipidemia [126]. Protein intake also plays an important role in insulin mediation and glucagon secretion, as protein consumption has an insulinotropic effect, promoting clearance of blood glucose into peripheral tissues. Although in healthy individuals, a protein intake higher than the recommendations (above 0.83 g/kg/day) could lead to hyperinsulinemia and, in the long-term, causes insulin resistance, in obese individuals the consumption of high-protein non-energy restricted diets, containing more than 20% of energy derived from proteins, may favourably reduce body weight, increasing insulin sensitivity [105, 129]. Further, diets with a suitable amount of protein improve calcium balance resulting in the preservation of the mineral content of bones [115]. These results are extremely important, especially during weight loss after bariatric surgery, due to the higher risk of protein malnutrition in this situation [115].

Considering the beneficial effects previously reported, it is possible to conclude that protein is a determinant nutrient on weight loss diets. Furthermore, high-protein diets associate to complacency of individuals on weight loss process. In studies carried out over 12 months, individuals on high-protein diets are more compliant with diet and have lower drop-out rate, with greater capacity to maintain weight loss, less adverse effects and lower cardiovascular risk [113, 130 - 134].

How much Protein for Weight Loss?

The recommended level of protein intake is usually determined by the daily minimum required to maintain nitrogen balance, that is, the quantity and quality of protein sufficient to prevent the catabolism of protein reserves. However, this recommendation may not be adequate to ensure good health, and there is increasing evidence that high-protein diets can prevent and treat diseases such as obesity, metabolic syndrome, type 2 diabetes and atherosclerotic cardiovascular disease [135]. The determination of protein requirements through recent methods, such as stable isotope-based methods, suggest that current protein recommendations are underestimated, highlighting the need to re-evaluate the existing guidelines [112].

The protein content of normal or high-protein diets needs to be evaluated both in relative terms of the daily energy balance and in absolute terms of the amount of daily protein intake. On weight loss diets, total energy intake is decreased and, although the protein contribution may be relatively high (20 to 30% of total energy intake), in absolute terms the amount of protein intake remains sufficient to assure the nitrogen balance. In these diets, the absolute amount of protein is similar to that provided in normal-protein diets under neutral energy balance, where protein contributes with 10 to 15% of total daily energy. Diets providing approximately 60 g of daily protein maintain the satiety effect, preserve muscle mass and increase energy expenditure as in high-protein diets. However, when the diet does not ensure a sufficient amount of protein, a rapid recovery of the weight lost occurs [136 - 140]. An absolute amount of protein equivalent to 0.8 g/kg/day is sufficient for both weight and fat mass loss, and consequent weight maintenance. However, to increase muscle mass and basal metabolic rate an absolute amount of protein equivalent to 1.2 g/kg/day is required [112, 136, 138 - 140]. In addition, moderate consumption (25-35 g) of high-biological value protein at each meal stimulates muscle protein synthesis and preserves fat-free mass [112] as well as improves appetite control, satiety and body weight management [141]. The beneficial effects of increased protein intake are even higher when combined with exercise [112, 119].

High-protein Diets

Considering the potential benefits of increasing protein intake for weight loss, high-protein diets have emerged. Traditionally characterized by the replacement of carbohydrates by proteins, high-protein diets have led to a huge scientific interest regarding their effects and efficacy. One of the crucial factors to be clarified is the definition of "high-protein diet" wherein the protein composition of the diet may be addressed in several ways: absolute daily amount of protein (in grams), the percentage of protein to total daily energy intake or protein intake per kg of body weight per day [142]. High-protein weight loss diets considered in literature reviews include mostly 30% of the energy intake from protein. However, the absolute amount of protein intake only increases about 20%, as there is a decrease in daily energy intake [142].

High-protein-low-carbohydrate diets can be categorized into: a) very-lo-
-carbohydrate, high-protein diets, simultaneously with a high proportion of saturated fat, also called ketogenic diets, being an example the "Atkins Diet" and the "Protein Power", and b) reduced carbohydrate, high-protein diets, which are also characterized by fat restriction, for example "The Zone Diet" and "Sugar Busters". The ketogenic diets includes only about 20 g of carbohydrates per day, in order to generate the production of ketone bodies – β-hydroxybutyrate and acetoacetate – which are produced by the liver as an alternative fuel for the brain. Under these conditions, the liver transforms fat into fatty acids and ketone bodies. Ketone bodies are an alternative source of energy to the body, especially to the brain, in situations where carbohydrate intake is insufficient to account for glucose needs [113, 142]. Additionally, this type of diet causes an increase in gluconeogenesis, resulting in a higher energy expenditure, as previously mentioned [113]. Some studies have shown that following a ketogenic diet for four weeks induces a decrease on body weight, insulin levels and glycemia. However, some adverse effects of low-carbohydrate-high-protein diets (most probably also high in saturated fat), like constipation, halitosis, headache and dehydration may be related to increased production of ketone bodies [107]. Although this dietetic approach can be effective for weight loss and subsequent maintenance [105, 106], it is important to note that the loss of water and muscle mass, rather than fat mass, mostly account for the initial weight loss. Furthermore, these diets restrict too much food groups with great nutritional richness, which makes it hard to comply with the recommendations of some macro- and micronutrients. Some high-protein diets, like "Atkins Diet" and "Protein Power", promote the consumption of excess amounts of saturated fat (greater than 10% of total energy intake) and are strongly associated with an increase of cardiovascular

risk factors (dyslipidemia and endothelial dysfunction) [143, 144].

The possible adverse effects related to excessive protein consumption are related to renal damage caused by the excretion of nitrogenous products generated during protein metabolism, increasing glomerular pressure and hyperfiltration mainly when excessive protein intake is maintained for a long period of time. In healthy individuals, increased protein intake causes adaptive changes in renal size and function, without adverse effects; renal parameters are maintained at normal reference values and weight loss results in a decrease in diastolic and systolic blood pressure. However, individuals with subclinical kidney disease, such as individuals with metabolic syndrome or type 2 diabetes, or elderly individuals are more susceptible to an increase in blood pressure caused by acidifying amino acids [113, 136]. Other possible adverse effects of high-protein diets are changes in liver function. However, scientific evidence shows that in obesity-induced fatty liver, weight loss has beneficial effects on liver function biomarkers [142]. Although some of the adverse effects that are often associated with high-protein diets only occur in particular cases, such as in renal patients, the consumption of a high-protein diet for long-term has been associated with an increased risk of developing type 2 diabetes [105]. Another concern of high-protein diets is bone health. High-protein intake induces hypercalciuria at constant levels of calcium intake, although the effect may depend on the nature of the dietary protein. On the other hand, individuals on high-protein diets have lower urinary pH. Thereby, hypercalciuria and low urinary pH induced by high-protein diets were suspected of unfavourably affecting bone health. However, it is also known that high-protein diets may increase intestinal calcium absorption; so the hypercalciuria may result from this increased absorption instead of impaired calcium balance. Furthermore, there are no clinical data supporting detrimental effects of high-protein diets on bone health, except under inadequate calcium supply [115, 145, 146]. In the same direction, a recent meta-analysis and systematic review [147] found that although the majority of studies have demonstrated a significant decrease in bone quantity following active weight loss (62%), high-protein weight loss diet neither exacerbate nor attenuate bone loss.

High-protein diets have been shown to be more effective at long-term in *ad libitum* energy intake compared to energy-restricted diets. In studies in which energy intake occurs *ad libitum*, high-protein diets show more favourable results on body weight and fat mass loss, as well as on weight loss maintenance [114]. The effects of high-protein diets with restricted calorie intake are inconsistent due to the high drop-out rate in the studies performed [114].

Animal or Vegetable Protein?

The effect of protein on satiety and food intake seems to depend on the amino acid profile, the origin (animal or vegetable) and energy intake, as well as the characteristics of digestion and absorption of the protein. Nonetheless, the existing data on this subject are still inconclusive. Proteins that are rapidly digested and absorbed, such as whey and soy, decrease short-term food intake (up to 1h) more than slowly absorbed proteins, such as casein and egg albumin. However, this effect disappears when food intake occurs *ad libitum*. After all, the hydrolysed form of the protein, which is more easily digested, further decreases food intake as compared with the protein in its intact form [114]. Some studies have demonstrated a greater satiating effect of whey protein and fish proteins compared to other protein sources. In fact, scientific evidence suggests that animal protein, particularly whey protein, promotes muscle mass gain and improves satiety and appetite control more than vegetable protein [141, 148 - 150]. However, the effects of different protein sources on body weight are inconclusive and sometimes incomplete (the effect of proteins from legumes and nuts on body weight have not been extensively studied, yet), and it cannot be stated that a particular protein source has a greater effect on weight loss or subsequent maintenance [112, 142, 151].

MACRONUTRIENTS: IS THERE AN OPTIMAL PROPORTION FOR WEIGHT LOSS?

The Food and Nutrition Board of the Institute of Medicine established in 2005 the "Acceptable Macronutrient Distribution Ranges" and regarding adults, fat should represent 20 to 35% of total energy intake, protein 10 to 35% and carbohydrates 45 to 65%. These macronutrient distribution ranges were defined in the context of a healthy diet that prevents chronic disease [152]. Regarding obesity management, many dietary approaches, with different macronutrients distribution have been proposed and investigated, as earlier described, but consensus about the best proportion for weight loss is still lacking [153].

In 2009, Sacks *et al* [154] conducted a clinical trial trying to answer this question. They randomly assigned 811 overweight adults to one of four diets with the following targeted percentages of energy derived from fat, protein and carbohydrates, respectively: 20, 15 and 65% (low-fat, average-protein); 20, 25 and 55% (low-fat, high-protein); 40, 15 and 45% (high-fat, average-protein); and 40, 25 and 35% (high-fat, high-protein). The diets consisted of similar foods and met guidelines for cardiovascular health (≤ 8% of saturated fat, at least 20 g of dietary fibre per day, and ≤ 150 mg of cholesterol per 1000 kcal) and carbohydrate-rich foods with a low-GI were recommended. Each participant's caloric prescription represented a deficit of 750 kcal per day from baseline values. Participants were followed for 2 years and during this period they had individual and group sessions regarding diet compliance. After 2 years of intervention, weight loss was similar for all diets. The change in waist circumference did not differ significantly among the diet groups. Interestingly, most of the weight loss occurred in the first 6 months, and after 12 months, all groups, on average, slowly regained body weight. Regarding cardiovascular disease, all diets reduced risk factors both at 6 months and 2 years. The two low-fat diets and the highest-carbohydrate diet decreased LDL-cholesterol levels more than did the high-fat diets or the lowest-carbohydrate diet, after 2 years. The lowest-carbohydrate diet increased HDL-cholesterol levels more than the highest-carbohydrate diet. All the diets decreased triglyceride levels in a similar way. Moreover, craving, fullness, and hunger and diet-satisfaction scores were similar at 6 months and at 2 years among all diets. Thus, it was concluded that energy-restricted diets result in clinically meaningful weight loss and maintenance regardless of macronutrient distribution.

Corroborating those findings, a systematic review and meta-analysis [155] (including 19 RCTs with 3209 participants) comparing low-carbohydrate diets with isoenergetic balanced diets (fat 25 to 35%, protein 10 to 20% and carbohydrates 45 to 65%) found that there is probably little or no difference in changes in weight as well as cardiovascular and diabetes risk factors when considering the low-carbohydrate diet *vs.* balanced diet. This was in both overweight and obese adults, with and without diabetes, with follow-up for up to two years.

By now, it seems very reasonable that the best dietary approach to treat obesity will be the one with energy restriction and with a macronutrient distribution that takes into account the individual's preferences, in order to increase diet adherence in the long-term. In this regard, extreme macronutrient restrictions either in the form of fat or carbohydrates may compromise diet adherence and are not supported by high quality scientific evidence as having any advantages when compared to a more balanced diet [153]. In line with this, adherence to the Mediterranean diet [which has a more balanced macronutrient distribution (approximately 35-40% of energy from fat and particularly rich in MUFA and PUFA; about 20% of protein; and 40-45% of carbohydrates [5])] compares favourably to adherence to low-fat diets and similarly to adherence to low-carbohydrate diets [156]. Regarding protein, an energy-restricted diet with moderate-protein content seems also a reasonable option for weight loss and maintenance, as long-term safety of very-high-protein diets is still questionable and the beneficial effects of protein ingestion do not seem to be potentiated with this dietary approach [111, 154].

Table 1. Suggested macronutrient distribution range for obesity treatment. *Percentages of macronutrients are presented regarding total energy intake and are based in different cited studies along the chapter, particularly Sacks *et al* [154].

	Energy-restricted diets		
Must consider	Individuals' clinical and sociocultural conditions		
Suggested macronutrient recomendations	Proteins (15-25%)*	Fats (25-35%)*	Carbohydrates (45-55%)*
Some considerations	• Energy-restricted diets may not meet protein requirements • 0.8 g protein/kg of body weight is sufficient for body weight loss and maintenance, but to increase muscle mass 1.2 g protein/kg is required • 25-30 g of high biological value proteins per meal seem beneficial • High-protein diets seem safe for healthy individuals, but may be a threat for individuals with (or at great risk of) renal disease	• Severe restriction of total fat may decrease the ingestion of essential fatty acids • Diets should decrease SFA ingestion and increase MUFA and PUFA ingestion • Among PUFA, n-3 and n-6 fatty acid may have divergent effects on body fat mass: n-3 should be preferred • *Trans* fatty acid intake should be limited • There are no clinical evidences or consistent effects on health to recommend CLA supplementation in obese individuals	• The ingestion of "free-sugars" should be limited, but there is no high quality evidence that glucose, fructose, HFCS and sucrose have distinct effects on body weight (under isocaloric conditions) • SSB should be limited in weight loss diets • Low GI diets do not seem superior to high GI diets (under isocaloric conditions) for weight loss, exception maybe for insulin-resistant obese individuals • Diets should include high-fibre food • "Sugar addiction" is not supported by high quality scientific evidence • Severe carbohydrate restriction may increase LDL-cholesterol
Potential mechanisms	Increase satiety and diet adherence Decrease fat mass and increase fat-free mass Increase energy expenditure Improve metabolic profile (lipids, glycaemic control) Decrease inflammatory markers Induce favourable alterations of gut microbiota		
May contribute to	Sucessful weight loss and maintenance		

Abbreviations: conjugated linoleic acids (CLA), high fructose corn syrup (HFCS), low-density lipoprotein (LDL), monounsaturated fatty acid (MUFA), polyunsaturated fatty acid (PUFA), saturated fatty acid (SFA), sugar sweetened beverage (SSB).

CONCLUDING REMARKS

It is impossible to define an ideal macronutrient distribution for weight loss and maintenance that fits everyone. Calorie restriction continues to be the most successful weight loss strategy, whether by reducing fat, carbohydrates, or increasing protein content of the diet. Apparently, the best diet will be the one that is kept long enough for weight loss and maintenance [153]. For this purpose, diets that are individualized and based on the personal and cultural preferences are the best ones to promote and maintain weight loss. Such diets, whatever the macronutrient composition, have beneficial effects on risk factors for cardiovascular disease and promote psychological health [142, 157]. Moreover, severe restrictions of either fat or carbohydrates besides have no scientific support in the literature (as compared to a more balanced macronutrient distribution, like in the Mediterranean diet) may certainly compromise individual's diet adherence and, consequently, weight loss success. Table **1** presents an integrated overview of the main contents of this chapter.

CONSENT FOR PUBLICATION

Not applicable.

CONFLICT OF INTEREST

The authors confirm that this chapter contents have no conflict of interest.

ACKNOWLEDGEMENTS

Declared none.

REFERENCES

[1]   Bray GA, Siri-Tarino PW. The Role of Macronutrient Content in the Diet for Weight Management. Endocrinol Metab Clin North Am 2016; 45(3): 581-604.
[http://dx.doi.org/10.1016/j.ecl.2016.04.009] [PMID: 27519132]

[2]   González-Muniesa P, Mártinez-González MA, Hu FB, *et al.* Obesity. Nat Rev Dis Primers 2017; 3: 17034.
[http://dx.doi.org/10.1038/nrdp.2017.34] [PMID: 28617414]

[3]   Martinez JA, Navas-Carretero S, Saris WH, Astrup A. Personalized weight loss strategies-the role of macronutrient distribution. Nat Rev Endocrinol 2014; 10(12): 749-60.
[http://dx.doi.org/10.1038/nrendo.2014.175] [PMID: 25311395]

[4]   Moghadasian MH, Shahidi F. Fatty Acids.International Encyclopedia of Public Health. 2nd ed. Oxford: Academic Press 2017; pp. 114-22.
[http://dx.doi.org/10.1016/B978-0-12-803678-5.00157-0]

[5]   Hunsberger M, Tognon G, Lissner L. Low-fat diets in obesity management and weight control.Managing and Preventing Obesity. Woodhead Publishing 2015; pp. 91-107.
[http://dx.doi.org/10.1533/9781782420996.2.91]

[6]   DeLany JP, Windhauser MM, Champagne CM, Bray GA. Differential oxidation of individual dietary fatty acids in humans. Am J Clin Nutr 2000; 72(4): 905-11.
[http://dx.doi.org/10.1093/ajcn/72.4.905] [PMID: 11010930]

[7]   Hermsdorff HH, Puchau B, Zulet MA, Martínez JA. Association of body fat distribution with proinflammatory gene expression in peripheral blood mononuclear cells from young adult subjects. OMICS 2010; 14(3): 297-307.
[http://dx.doi.org/10.1089/omi.2009.0125] [PMID: 20450441]

[8]   Rocha DM, Caldas AP, Oliveira LL, Bressan J, Hermsdorff HH. Saturated fatty acids trigger TLR4-

mediated inflammatory response. Atherosclerosis 2016; 244: 211-5.
[http://dx.doi.org/10.1016/j.atherosclerosis.2015.11.015] [PMID: 26687466]

[9] Nicholas DA, Zhang K, Hung C, *et al*. Palmitic acid is a toll-like receptor 4 ligand that induces human dendritic cell secretion of IL-1β. PLoS One 2017; 12(5)e0176793
[http://dx.doi.org/10.1371/journal.pone.0176793] [PMID: 28463985]

[10] Wang Z, Liu D, Wang F, *et al*. Saturated fatty acids activate microglia via Toll-like receptor 4/NF-κB signalling. Br J Nutr 2012; 107(2): 229-41.
[http://dx.doi.org/10.1017/S0007114511002868] [PMID: 21733316]

[11] Rocha DM, Bressan J, Hermsdorff HH. The role of dietary fatty acid intake in inflammatory gene expression: a critical review. Sao Paulo Med J 2017; 135(2): 157-68.
[http://dx.doi.org/10.1590/1516-3180.2016.008607072016] [PMID: 28076613]

[12] Matsuo T, Sumida H, Suzuki M. Beef tallow diet decreases β-adrenergic receptor binding and lipolytic activities in different adipose tissues of rat. Metabolism 1995; 44(10): 1271-7.
[http://dx.doi.org/10.1016/0026-0495(95)90028-4] [PMID: 7476283]

[13] Awad AB, Chattopadhyay JP. Effect of dietary saturated fatty acids on hormone-sensitive lipolysis in rat adipocytes. J Nutr 1986; 116(6): 1088-94.
[http://dx.doi.org/10.1093/jn/116.6.1088] [PMID: 3014093]

[14] Clarke SD. Polyunsaturated fatty acid regulation of gene transcription: a molecular mechanism to improve the metabolic syndrome. J Nutr 2001; 131(4): 1129-32.
[http://dx.doi.org/10.1093/jn/131.4.1129] [PMID: 11285313]

[15] Simopoulos AP. An Increase in the Omega-6/Omega-3 Fatty Acid Ratio Increases the Risk for Obesity. Nutrients 2016; 8(3): 128.
[http://dx.doi.org/10.3390/nu8030128] [PMID: 26950145]

[16] Muhlhausler BS, Ailhaud GP. Omega-6 polyunsaturated fatty acids and the early origins of obesity. Curr Opin Endocrinol Diabetes Obes 2013; 20(1): 56-61.
[http://dx.doi.org/10.1097/MED.0b013e32835c1ba7] [PMID: 23249760]

[17] Todorčević M, Hodson L. The Effect of Marine Derived n-3 Fatty Acids on Adipose Tissue Metabolism and Function. J Clin Med 2015; 5(1): 3.
[http://dx.doi.org/10.3390/jcm5010003] [PMID: 26729182]

[18] Buckley JD, Howe PRC. Long-chain omega-3 polyunsaturated fatty acids may be beneficial for reducing obesity-a review. Nutrients 2010; 2(12): 1212-30.
[http://dx.doi.org/10.3390/nu2121212] [PMID: 22254005]

[19] Aranceta J, Pérez-Rodrigo C. Recommended dietary reference intakes, nutritional goals and dietary guidelines for fat and fatty acids: a systematic review. Br J Nutr 2012; 107 (Suppl. 2): S8-S22.
[http://dx.doi.org/10.1017/S0007114512001444] [PMID: 22591906]

[20] Balvers MG, Verhoeckx KC, Bijlsma S, *et al*. Fish oil and inflammatory status alter the n-3 to n-6 balance of the endocannabinoid and oxylipin metabolomes in mouse plasma and tissues. Metabolomics 2012; 8(6): 1130-47.
[http://dx.doi.org/10.1007/s11306-012-0421-9] [PMID: 23136559]

[21] Batetta B, Griinari M, Carta G, *et al*. Endocannabinoids may mediate the ability of (n-3) fatty acids to reduce ectopic fat and inflammatory mediators in obese Zucker rats. J Nutr 2009; 139(8): 1495-501.
[http://dx.doi.org/10.3945/jn.109.104844] [PMID: 19549757]

[22] Finucane OM, Lyons CL, Murphy AM, *et al*. Monounsaturated fatty acid-enriched high-fat diets impede adipose NLRP3 inflammasome-mediated IL-1β secretion and insulin resistance despite obesity. Diabetes 2015; 64(6): 2116-28.
[http://dx.doi.org/10.2337/db14-1098] [PMID: 25626736]

[23] Liao FH, Liou TH, Chiu WC, Shieh MJ, Chien YW. Differential effects of high MUFA with high or low P/S ratio (polyunsaturated to saturated fatty acids) on improving hepatic lipolytic enzymes and

mediating PPARγ related with lipoprotein lipase and hormone-sensitive lipase of white adipose tissue in diet-induced obese hamster. Int J Obes 2010; 34(11): 1608-17.
[http://dx.doi.org/10.1038/ijo.2010.88] [PMID: 20458324]

[24]　Bos MB, de Vries JH, Feskens EJ, *et al.* Effect of a high monounsaturated fatty acids diet and a Mediterranean diet on serum lipids and insulin sensitivity in adults with mild abdominal obesity. Nutr Metab Cardiovasc Dis 2010; 20(8): 591-8.
[http://dx.doi.org/10.1016/j.numecd.2009.05.008] [PMID: 19692213]

[25]　Soares MJ, Cummings SJ, Mamo JC, Kenrick M, Piers LS. The acute effects of olive oil v. cream on postprandial thermogenesis and substrate oxidation in postmenopausal women. Br J Nutr 2004; 91(2): 245-52.
[http://dx.doi.org/10.1079/BJN20031047] [PMID: 14756910]

[26]　Bhardwaj S, Passi SJ, Misra A. Overview of trans fatty acids: biochemistry and health effects. Diabetes Metab Syndr 2011; 5(3): 161-4.
[http://dx.doi.org/10.1016/j.dsx.2012.03.002] [PMID: 22813572]

[27]　Ochiai M, Fujii K, Takeuchi H, Matsuo T. Effects of dietary trans fatty acids on fat accumulation and metabolic rate in rat. J Oleo Sci 2013; 62(2): 57-64.
[http://dx.doi.org/10.5650/jos.62.57] [PMID: 23391528]

[28]　Kavanagh K, Jones KL, Sawyer J, *et al.* Trans fat diet induces abdominal obesity and changes in insulin sensitivity in monkeys. Obesity (Silver Spring) 2007; 15(7): 1675-84.
[http://dx.doi.org/10.1038/oby.2007.200] [PMID: 17636085]

[29]　Thompson AK, Minihane AM, Williams CM. Trans fatty acids and weight gain. Int J Obes 2011; 35(3): 315-24.
[http://dx.doi.org/10.1038/ijo.2010.141] [PMID: 20644558]

[30]　Vogt MC, Paeger L, Hess S, *et al.* Neonatal insulin action impairs hypothalamic neurocircuit formation in response to maternal high-fat feeding. Cell 2014; 156(3): 495-509.
[http://dx.doi.org/10.1016/j.cell.2014.01.008] [PMID: 24462248]

[31]　Pariza MW, Park Y, Cook ME. The biologically active isomers of conjugated linoleic acid. Prog Lipid Res 2001; 40(4): 283-98.
[http://dx.doi.org/10.1016/S0163-7827(01)00008-X] [PMID: 11412893]

[32]　Kovacs EM, Mela DJ. Metabolically active functional food ingredients for weight control. Obes Rev 2006; 7(1): 59-78.
[http://dx.doi.org/10.1111/j.1467-789X.2006.00203.x] [PMID: 16436103]

[33]　Cho K, Kwon D, Park J, Song Y. Serum levels of appetite-regulating hormones and pro-inflammatory cytokines are ameliorated by a CLA diet and endurance exercise in rats fed a high-fat diet. J Exerc Nutrition Biochem 2015; 19(4): 303-9.
[http://dx.doi.org/10.5717/jenb.2015.15120905] [PMID: 27274463]

[34]　Nall JL, Wu G, Kim KH, Choi CW, Smith SB. Dietary supplementation of L-arginine and conjugated linoleic acid reduces retroperitoneal fat mass and increases lean body mass in rats. J Nutr 2009; 139(7): 1279-85.
[http://dx.doi.org/10.3945/jn.108.102301] [PMID: 19439462]

[35]　Segovia SA, Vickers MH, Zhang XD, Gray C, Reynolds CM. Maternal supplementation with conjugated linoleic acid in the setting of diet-induced obesity normalises the inflammatory phenotype in mothers and reverses metabolic dysfunction and impaired insulin sensitivity in offspring. J Nutr Biochem 2015; 26(12): 1448-57.
[http://dx.doi.org/10.1016/j.jnutbio.2015.07.013] [PMID: 26318151]

[36]　López-Plaza B, Bermejo LM, Koester Weber T, *et al.* Effects of milk supplementation with conjugated linoleic acid on weight control and body composition in healthy overweight people. Nutr Hosp 2013; 28(6): 2090-8.
[PMID: 24506387]

[37]　Blankson H, Stakkestad JA, Fagertun H, Thom E, Wadstein J, Gudmundsen O. Conjugated linoleic acid reduces body fat mass in overweight and obese humans. J Nutr 2000; 130(12): 2943-8.
[http://dx.doi.org/10.1093/jn/130.12.2943] [PMID: 11110851]

[38]　Onakpoya IJ, Posadzki PP, Watson LK, Davies LA, Ernst E. The efficacy of long-term conjugated linoleic acid (CLA) supplementation on body composition in overweight and obese individuals: a systematic review and meta-analysis of randomized clinical trials. Eur J Nutr 2012; 51(2): 127-34.
[http://dx.doi.org/10.1007/s00394-011-0253-9] [PMID: 21990002]

[39]　Lehnen TE, da Silva MR, Camacho A, Marcadenti A, Lehnen AM. A review on effects of conjugated linoleic fatty acid (CLA) upon body composition and energetic metabolism. J Int Soc Sports Nutr 2015; 12: 36.
[http://dx.doi.org/10.1186/s12970-015-0097-4] [PMID: 26388708]

[40]　Benjamin S, Prakasan P, Sreedharan S, Wright A-DG, Spener F. Pros and cons of CLA consumption: an insight from clinical evidences. Nutr Metab (Lond) 2015; 12: 4.
[http://dx.doi.org/10.1186/1743-7075-12-4] [PMID: 25972911]

[41]　Astrup A, Grunwald GK, Melanson EL, Saris WH, Hill JO. The role of low-fat diets in body weight control: a meta-analysis of ad libitum dietary intervention studies. Int J Obes Relat Metab Disord 2000; 24(12): 1545-52.
[http://dx.doi.org/10.1038/sj.ijo.0801453] [PMID: 11126204]

[42]　Hariri N, Thibault L. High-fat diet-induced obesity in animal models. Nutr Res Rev 2010; 23(2): 270-99.
[http://dx.doi.org/10.1017/S0954422410000168] [PMID: 20977819]

[43]　Blundell JE, MacDiarmid JI. Fat as a risk factor for overconsumption: satiation, satiety, and patterns of eating. J Am Diet Assoc 1997; 97(7) (Suppl.): S63-9.
[http://dx.doi.org/10.1016/S0002-8223(97)00733-5] [PMID: 9216571]

[44]　Bray GA, Popkin BM. Dietary fat intake does affect obesity! Am J Clin Nutr 1998; 68(6): 1157-73.
[http://dx.doi.org/10.1093/ajcn/68.6.1157] [PMID: 9846842]

[45]　Araújo JR, Tomas J, Brenner C, Sansonetti PJ. Impact of high-fat diet on the intestinal microbiota and small intestinal physiology before and after the onset of obesity. Biochimie 2017; 141: 97-106.
[http://dx.doi.org/10.1016/j.biochi.2017.05.019] [PMID: 28571979]

[46]　Hu T, Mills KT, Yao L, et al. Effects of low-carbohydrate diets versus low-fat diets on metabolic risk factors: a meta-analysis of randomized controlled clinical trials. Am J Epidemiol 2012; 176 (Suppl. 7): S44-54.
[http://dx.doi.org/10.1093/aje/kws264] [PMID: 23035144]

[47]　Pirozzo S, Summerbell C, Cameron C, Glasziou P. Should we recommend low-fat diets for obesity? Obes Rev 2003; 4(2): 83-90.
[http://dx.doi.org/10.1046/j.1467-789X.2003.00099.x] [PMID: 12760443]

[48]　Summerbell CD, Cameron C, Glasziou PP. WITHDRAWN: Advice on low-fat diets for obesity. Cochrane Database Syst Rev 2008; (3): CD003640
[PMID: 18646093]

[49]　Tobias DK, Chen M, Manson JE, Ludwig DS, Willett W, Hu FB. Effect of low-fat diet interventions versus other diet interventions on long-term weight change in adults: a systematic review and meta-analysis. Lancet Diabetes Endocrinol 2015; 3(12): 968-79.
[http://dx.doi.org/10.1016/S2213-8587(15)00367-8] [PMID: 26527511]

[50]　McClain AD, Otten JJ, Hekler EB, Gardner CD. Adherence to a low-fat vs. low-carbohydrate diet differs by insulin resistance status. Diabetes Obes Metab 2013; 15(1): 87-90.
[http://dx.doi.org/10.1111/j.1463-1326.2012.01668.x] [PMID: 22831182]

[51]　Food and Agriculture Organization of the United Nations. Food energy - methods of analysis and conversion factors; Food and Agriculture Organization of the United Nations paper 77. Rome: Food

and Agriculture Organization of the United Nations 2003.

[52]   Sanders TA. How important is the relative balance of fat and carbohydrate as sources of energy in relation to health? Proc Nutr Soc 2016; 75(2): 147-53.
[http://dx.doi.org/10.1017/S0029665115004188] [PMID: 26564394]

[53]   World Health Organization. Guideline: Sugar Intakes for Adults and Children. Geneva: World Health Organization 2015.

[54]   Scientific Advisory Committee on Nutrition. Carbohydrates and Health. London: TSO 2015.

[55]   Stanhope KL. Sugar consumption, metabolic disease and obesity: The state of the controversy. Crit Rev Clin Lab Sci 2016; 53(1): 52-67.
[http://dx.doi.org/10.3109/10408363.2015.1084990] [PMID: 26376619]

[56]   van Buul VJ, Tappy L, Brouns FJ. Misconceptions about fructose-containing sugars and their role in the obesity epidemic. Nutr Res Rev 2014; 27(1): 119-30.
[http://dx.doi.org/10.1017/S0954422414000067] [PMID: 24666553]

[57]   Rippe JM, Angelopoulos TJ. Relationship between Added Sugars Consumption and Chronic Disease Risk Factors: Current Understanding. Nutrients 2016; 8(11)E697
[http://dx.doi.org/10.3390/nu8110697] [PMID: 27827899]

[58]   Rippe JM, Angelopoulos TJ. Sugars, obesity, and cardiovascular disease: results from recent randomized control trials. Eur J Nutr 2016; 55 (Suppl. 2): 45-53.
[http://dx.doi.org/10.1007/s00394-016-1257-2] [PMID: 27418186]

[59]   Rippe JM, Saltzman E. Sweetened beverages and health: current state of scientific understandings. Adv Nutr 2013; 4(5): 527-9.
[http://dx.doi.org/10.3945/an.113.004143] [PMID: 24038246]

[60]   Bray GA, Nielsen SJ, Popkin BM. Consumption of high-fructose corn syrup in beverages may play a role in the epidemic of obesity. Am J Clin Nutr 2004; 79(4): 537-43.
[http://dx.doi.org/10.1093/ajcn/79.4.537] [PMID: 15051594]

[61]   Association Medical Association. The Health Effects of High Fructose Corn Syrup. Chicago: American Medical Association 2008.

[62]   Fitch C, Keim KS. Position of the Academy of Nutrition and Dietetics: use of nutritive and nonnutritive sweeteners. J Acad Nutr Diet 2012; 112(5): 739-58.
[http://dx.doi.org/10.1016/j.jand.2012.03.009] [PMID: 22709780]

[63]   Te Morenga L, Mallard S, Mann J. Dietary sugars and body weight: systematic review and meta-analyses of randomised controlled trials and cohort studies. BMJ 2012; 346e7492
[http://dx.doi.org/10.1136/bmj.e7492] [PMID: 23321486]

[64]   Khan TA, Sievenpiper JL. Controversies about sugars: results from systematic reviews and meta-analyses on obesity, cardiometabolic disease and diabetes. Eur J Nutr 2016; 55 (Suppl. 2): 25-43.
[http://dx.doi.org/10.1007/s00394-016-1345-3] [PMID: 27900447]

[65]   Hu FB. Resolved: there is sufficient scientific evidence that decreasing sugar-sweetened beverage consumption will reduce the prevalence of obesity and obesity-related diseases. Obes Rev 2013; 14(8): 606-19.
[http://dx.doi.org/10.1111/obr.12040] [PMID: 23763695]

[66]   Malik VS, Pan A, Willett WC, Hu FB. Sugar-sweetened beverages and weight gain in children and adults: a systematic review and meta-analysis. Am J Clin Nutr 2013; 98(4): 1084-102.
[http://dx.doi.org/10.3945/ajcn.113.058362] [PMID: 23966427]

[67]   Imamura F, O'Connor L, Ye Z, *et al.* Consumption of sugar sweetened beverages, artificially sweetened beverages, and fruit juice and incidence of type 2 diabetes: systematic review, meta-analysis, and estimation of population attributable fraction. BMJ 2015; 351: h3576.
[http://dx.doi.org/10.1136/bmj.h3576] [PMID: 26199070]

[68] Malik VS, Popkin BM, Bray GA, Després JP, Willett WC, Hu FB. Sugar-sweetened beverages and risk of metabolic syndrome and type 2 diabetes: a meta-analysis. Diabetes Care 2010; 33(11): 2477-83.
[http://dx.doi.org/10.2337/dc10-1079] [PMID: 20693348]

[69] Jayalath VH, de Souza RJ, Ha V, *et al.* Sugar-sweetened beverage consumption and incident hypertension: a systematic review and meta-analysis of prospective cohorts. Am J Clin Nutr 2015; 102(4): 914-21.
[http://dx.doi.org/10.3945/ajcn.115.107243] [PMID: 26269365]

[70] de Koning L, Malik VS, Kellogg MD, *et al.* Sweetened beverage consumption, incident coronary heart disease, and biomarkers of risk in men. Circulation 2012; 125(14): 1735-41, s1.
[http://dx.doi.org/10.1161/CIRCULATIONAHA.111.067017]

[71] Huang C, Huang J, Tian Y, Yang X, Gu D. Sugar sweetened beverages consumption and risk of coronary heart disease: a meta-analysis of prospective studies. Atherosclerosis 2014; 234(1): 11-6.
[http://dx.doi.org/10.1016/j.atherosclerosis.2014.01.037] [PMID: 24583500]

[72] Bernstein AM, de Koning L, Flint AJ, Rexrode KM, Willett WC. Soda consumption and the risk of stroke in men and women. Am J Clin Nutr 2012; 95(5): 1190-9.
[http://dx.doi.org/10.3945/ajcn.111.030205] [PMID: 22492378]

[73] Batt C, Phipps-Green AJ, Black MA, *et al.* Sugar-sweetened beverage consumption: a risk factor for prevalent gout with SLC2A9 genotype-specific effects on serum urate and risk of gout. Ann Rheum Dis 2014; 73(12): 2101-6.
[http://dx.doi.org/10.1136/annrheumdis-2013-203600] [PMID: 24026676]

[74] Macdonald IA. A review of recent evidence relating to sugars, insulin resistance and diabetes. Eur J Nutr 2016; 55 (Suppl. 2): 17-23.
[http://dx.doi.org/10.1007/s00394-016-1340-8] [PMID: 27882410]

[75] Juanola-Falgarona M, Salas-Salvadó J, Buil-Cosiales P, *et al.* Dietary Glycemic Index and Glycemic Load Are Positively Associated with Risk of Developing Metabolic Syndrome in Middle-Aged and Elderly Adults. J Am Geriatr Soc 2015; 63(10): 1991-2000.
[http://dx.doi.org/10.1111/jgs.13668] [PMID: 26480969]

[76] Karl JP, Roberts SB, Schaefer EJ, *et al.* Effects of carbohydrate quantity and glycemic index on resting metabolic rate and body composition during weight loss. Obesity (Silver Spring) 2015; 23(11): 2190-8.
[http://dx.doi.org/10.1002/oby.21268] [PMID: 26530933]

[77] Pereira EV, Costa JdeA, Alfenas RdeC. Effect of glycemic index on obesity control. Arch Endocrinol Metab 2015; 59(3): 245-51.
[http://dx.doi.org/10.1590/2359-3997000000045] [PMID: 26154093]

[78] Schwingshackl L, Hobl LP, Hoffmann G. Effects of low glycaemic index/low glycaemic load *vs.* high glycaemic index/ high glycaemic load diets on overweight/obesity and associated risk factors in children and adolescents: a systematic review and meta-analysis. Nutr J 2015; 14: 87.
[http://dx.doi.org/10.1186/s12937-015-0077-1] [PMID: 26489667]

[79] Sloth B, Astrup A. Low glycemic index diets and body weight. Int J Obes 2006; 30: S47-51.
[http://dx.doi.org/10.1038/sj.ijo.0803492]

[80] Thomas DE, Elliott EJ, Baur L. Low glycaemic index or low glycaemic load diets for overweight and obesity. Cochrane Database Syst Ver 2007; (3): Cd005105
[http://dx.doi.org/10.1002/14651858.CD005105.pub2]

[81] Juanola-Falgarona M, Salas-Salvadó J, Ibarrola-Jurado N, *et al.* Effect of the glycemic index of the diet on weight loss, modulation of satiety, inflammation, and other metabolic risk factors: a randomized controlled trial. Am J Clin Nutr 2014; 100(1): 27-35.
[http://dx.doi.org/10.3945/ajcn.113.081216] [PMID: 24787494]

[82]   Braunstein CR, Mejia SB, Stoiko E, *et al.* Effect of Low-Glycemic Index/Load Diets on Body Weight: A Systematic Review and Meta-Analysis. FASEB J 2016; 30 (1) 906.9.

[83]   Augustin LS, Kendall CW, Jenkins DJ, *et al.* Glycemic index, glycemic load and glycemic response: An International Scientific Consensus Summit from the International Carbohydrate Quality Consortium (ICQC). Nutr Metab Cardiovasc Dis 2015; 25(9): 795-815.
[http://dx.doi.org/10.1016/j.numecd.2015.05.005] [PMID: 26160327]

[84]   Fogelholm M, Anderssen S, Gunnarsdottir I, Lahti-Koski M. Dietary macronutrients and food consumption as determinants of long-term weight change in adult populations: a systematic literature review. Food Nutr Res 2012; 56: 56.
[http://dx.doi.org/10.3402/fnr.v56i0.19103] [PMID: 22893781]

[85]   Dahl WJ, Stewart ML. Position of the Academy of Nutrition and Dietetics: Health Implications of Dietary Fiber. J Acad Nutr Diet 2015; 115(11): 1861-70.
[http://dx.doi.org/10.1016/j.jand.2015.09.003] [PMID: 26514720]

[86]   Brownawell AM, Caers W, Gibson GR, *et al.* Prebiotics and the health benefits of fiber: current regulatory status, future research, and goals. J Nutr 2012; 142(5): 962-74.
[http://dx.doi.org/10.3945/jn.112.158147] [PMID: 22457389]

[87]   Clark MJ, Slavin JL. The effect of fiber on satiety and food intake: a systematic review. J Am Coll Nutr 2013; 32(3): 200-11.
[http://dx.doi.org/10.1080/07315724.2013.791194] [PMID: 23885994]

[88]   Wanders AJ, van den Borne JJ, de Graaf C, *et al.* Effects of dietary fibre on subjective appetite, energy intake and body weight: a systematic review of randomized controlled trials. Obes Rev 2011; 12(9): 724-39.
[http://dx.doi.org/10.1111/j.1467-789X.2011.00895.x] [PMID: 21676152]

[89]   Ma Y, Olendzki BC, Wang J, *et al.* Single-component *versus* multicomponent dietary goals for the metabolic syndrome: a randomized trial. Ann Intern Med 2015; 162(4): 248-57.
[http://dx.doi.org/10.7326/M14-0611] [PMID: 25686165]

[90]   Du H, van der A DL, Boshuizen HC, *et al.* Dietary fiber and subsequent changes in body weight and waist circumference in European men and women. Am J Clin Nutr 2010; 91(2): 329-36.
[http://dx.doi.org/10.3945/ajcn.2009.28191] [PMID: 20016015]

[91]   Slavin J. Fiber and prebiotics: mechanisms and health benefits. Nutrients 2013; 5(4): 1417-35.
[http://dx.doi.org/10.3390/nu5041417] [PMID: 23609775]

[92]   Kellow NJ, Coughlan MT, Reid CM. Metabolic benefits of dietary prebiotics in human subjects: a systematic review of randomised controlled trials. Br J Nutr 2014; 111(7): 1147-61.
[http://dx.doi.org/10.1017/S0007114513003607] [PMID: 24230488]

[93]   Saris WH, Astrup A, Prentice AM, *et al.* Randomized controlled trial of changes in dietary carbohydrate/fat ratio and simple vs complex carbohydrates on body weight and blood lipids: the CARMEN study. The Carbohydrate Ratio Management in European National diets. Int J Obes Relat Metab Disord 2000; 24(10): 1310-8.
[http://dx.doi.org/10.1038/sj.ijo.0801451] [PMID: 11093293]

[94]   Liu RH. Dietary bioactive compounds and their health implications. J Food Sci 2013; 78 (Suppl. 1): A18-25.
[http://dx.doi.org/10.1111/1750-3841.12101] [PMID: 23789932]

[95]   Randolph TG. The descriptive features of food addiction; addictive eating and drinking. Q J Stud Alcohol 1956; 17(2): 198-224.
[PMID: 13336254]

[96]   Markus CR, Rogers PJ, Brouns F, Schepers R. Eating dependence and weight gain; no human evidence for a 'sugar-addiction' model of overweight. Appetite 2017; 114: 64-72.
[http://dx.doi.org/10.1016/j.appet.2017.03.024] [PMID: 28330706]

[97] Westwater ML, Fletcher PC, Ziauddeen H. Sugar addiction: the state of the science. Eur J Nutr 2016; 55 (Suppl. 2): 55-69.
[http://dx.doi.org/10.1007/s00394-016-1229-6] [PMID: 27372453]

[98] Bocarsly ME, Berner LA, Hoebel BG, Avena NM. Rats that binge eat fat-rich food do not show somatic signs or anxiety associated with opiate-like withdrawal: implications for nutrient-specific food addiction behaviors. Physiol Behav 2011; 104(5): 865-72.
[http://dx.doi.org/10.1016/j.physbeh.2011.05.018] [PMID: 21635910]

[99] Johnson PM, Kenny PJ. Dopamine D2 receptors in addiction-like reward dysfunction and compulsive eating in obese rats. Nat Neurosci 2010; 13(5): 635-41.
[http://dx.doi.org/10.1038/nn.2519] [PMID: 20348917]

[100] Papacostas-Quintanilla H, Ortiz-Ortega VM, López-Rubalcava C. Wistar-Kyoto Female Rats Are More Susceptible to Develop Sugar Binging: A Comparison with Wistar Rats. Front Nutr 2017; 4: 15.
[http://dx.doi.org/10.3389/fnut.2017.00015] [PMID: 28536692]

[101] Benton D, Young HA. A meta-analysis of the relationship between brain dopamine receptors and obesity: a matter of changes in behavior rather than food addiction? Int J Obes 2016; 40 (Suppl. 1): S12-21.
[http://dx.doi.org/10.1038/ijo.2016.9] [PMID: 27001642]

[102] Pursey KM, Davis C, Burrows TL. Nutritional Aspects of Food Addiction. Curr Addict Rep 2017; 4(2): 142-50.
[http://dx.doi.org/10.1007/s40429-017-0139-x]

[103] Hebebrand J, Albayrak Ö, Adan R, *et al.* "Eating addiction", rather than "food addiction", better captures addictive-like eating behavior. Neurosci Biobehav Rev 2014; 47: 295-306.
[http://dx.doi.org/10.1016/j.neubiorev.2014.08.016] [PMID: 25205078]

[104] Mansoor N, Vinknes KJ, Veierød MB, Retterstøl K. Effects of low-carbohydrate diets v. low-fat diets on body weight and cardiovascular risk factors: a meta-analysis of randomised controlled trials. Br J Nutr 2016; 115(3): 466-79.
[http://dx.doi.org/10.1017/S0007114515004699] [PMID: 26768850]

[105] Rietman A, Schwarz J, Tomé D, Kok FJ, Mensink M. High dietary protein intake, reducing or eliciting insulin resistance? Eur J Clin Nutr 2014; 68(9): 973-9.
[http://dx.doi.org/10.1038/ejcn.2014.123] [PMID: 24986822]

[106] Johnston BC, Kanters S, Bandayrel K, *et al.* Comparison of weight loss among named diet programs in overweight and obese adults: a meta-analysis. JAMA 2014; 312(9): 923-33.
[http://dx.doi.org/10.1001/jama.2014.10397] [PMID: 25182101]

[107] Kappagoda CT, Hyson DA, Amsterdam EA. Low-carbohydrate-high-protein diets: is there a place for them in clinical cardiology? J Am Coll Cardiol 2004; 43(5): 725-30.
[http://dx.doi.org/10.1016/j.jacc.2003.06.022] [PMID: 14998607]

[108] Bazzano LA, Hu T, Reynolds K, *et al.* Effects of low-carbohydrate and low-fat diets: a randomized trial. Ann Intern Med 2014; 161(5): 309-18.
[http://dx.doi.org/10.7326/M14-0180] [PMID: 25178568]

[109] Wood TR, Hansen R, Sigurðsson AF, Jóhannsson GF. The cardiovascular risk reduction benefits of a low-carbohydrate diet outweigh the potential increase in LDL-cholesterol. Br J Nutr 2016; 115(6): 1126-8.
[http://dx.doi.org/10.1017/S0007114515005450] [PMID: 26858234]

[110] Mansoor N, Vinknes KJ, Veierød MB, Retterstøl K. Low-carbohydrate diets increase LDL-cholesterol, and thereby indicate increased risk of CVD. Br J Nutr 2016; 115(12): 2264-6.
[http://dx.doi.org/10.1017/S0007114516001343] [PMID: 27376624]

[111] Jensen MD, Ryan DH, Apovian CM, *et al.* 2013 AHA/ACC/TOS guideline for the management of overweight and obesity in adults: a report of the American College of Cardiology/American Heart

Association Task Force on Practice Guidelines and The Obesity Society. J Am Coll Cardiol 2014; 63 (25 Pt B): 2985-3023.
[http://dx.doi.org/10.1016/j.jacc.2013.11.004] [PMID: 24239920]

[112]   Arentson-Lantz E, Clairmont S, Paddon-Jones D, Tremblay A, Elango R. Protein: A nutrient in focus. Appl Physiol Nutr Metab 2015; 40(8): 755-61.
[http://dx.doi.org/10.1139/apnm-2014-0530] [PMID: 26197807]

[113]   Westerterp-Plantenga MS, Lemmens SG, Westerterp KR. Dietary protein - its role in satiety, energetics, weight loss and health. Br J Nutr 2012; 108 (Suppl. 2): S105-12.
[http://dx.doi.org/10.1017/S0007114512002589] [PMID: 23107521]

[114]   Bellissimo N, Akhavan T. Effect of macronutrient composition on short-term food intake and weight loss. Adv Nutr 2015; 6(3): 302S-8S.
[http://dx.doi.org/10.3945/an.114.006957] [PMID: 25979503]

[115]   Keller U. Dietary proteins in obesity and in diabetes. Int J Vitam Nutr Res 2011; 81(2-3): 125-33.
[http://dx.doi.org/10.1024/0300-9831/a000059] [PMID: 22139563]

[116]   Mikkelsen PB, Toubro S, Astrup A. Effect of fat-reduced diets on 24-h energy expenditure: comparisons between animal protein, vegetable protein, and carbohydrate. Am J Clin Nutr 2000; 72(5): 1135-41.
[http://dx.doi.org/10.1093/ajcn/72.5.1135] [PMID: 11063440]

[117]   Veldhorst MA, Westerterp-Plantenga MS, Westerterp KR. Gluconeogenesis and energy expenditure after a high-protein, carbohydrate-free diet. Am J Clin Nutr 2009; 90(3): 519-26.
[http://dx.doi.org/10.3945/ajcn.2009.27834] [PMID: 19640952]

[118]   Bray GA, Redman LM, de Jonge L, *et al.* Effect of protein overfeeding on energy expenditure measured in a metabolic chamber. Am J Clin Nutr 2015; 101(3): 496-505.
[http://dx.doi.org/10.3945/ajcn.114.091769] [PMID: 25733634]

[119]   Cava E, Yeat NC, Mittendorfer B. Preserving Healthy Muscle during Weight Loss. Adv Nutr 2017; 8(3): 511-9.
[http://dx.doi.org/10.3945/an.116.014506] [PMID: 28507015]

[120]   Koppes LL, Boon N, Nooyens AC, van Mechelen W, Saris WH. Macronutrient distribution over a period of 23 years in relation to energy intake and body fatness. Br J Nutr 2009; 101(1): 108-15.
[http://dx.doi.org/10.1017/S0007114508986864] [PMID: 18466652]

[121]   Pedersen AN, Kondrup J, Børsheim E. Health effects of protein intake in healthy adults: a systematic literature review. Food Nutr Res 2013; 57: 57.
[http://dx.doi.org/10.3402/fnr.v57i0.21245] [PMID: 23908602]

[122]   Mellinkoff SM, Frankland M, Boyle D, Greipel M. Relationship between serum amino acid concentration and fluctuations in appetite. J Appl Physiol 1956; 8(5): 535-8.
[http://dx.doi.org/10.1152/jappl.1956.8.5.535] [PMID: 13295170]

[123]   Moran TH. Gut peptides in the control of food intake. Int J Obes 2009; 33 (Suppl. 1): S7-S10.
[http://dx.doi.org/10.1038/ijo.2009.9] [PMID: 19363513]

[124]   Westerterp-Plantenga MS, Nieuwenhuizen A, Tomé D, Soenen S, Westerterp KR. Dietary protein, weight loss, and weight maintenance. Annu Rev Nutr 2009; 29: 21-41.
[http://dx.doi.org/10.1146/annurev-nutr-080508-141056] [PMID: 19400750]

[125]   Veldhorst MA, Westerterp KR, van Vught AJ, Westerterp-Plantenga MS. Presence or absence of carbohydrates and the proportion of fat in a high-protein diet affect appetite suppression but not energy expenditure in normal-weight human subjects fed in energy balance. Br J Nutr 2010; 104(9): 1395-405.
[http://dx.doi.org/10.1017/S0007114510002060] [PMID: 20565999]

[126]   Abete I, Astrup A, Martínez JA, Thorsdottir I, Zulet MA. Obesity and the metabolic syndrome: role of different dietary macronutrient distribution patterns and specific nutritional components on weight loss

and maintenance. Nutr Rev 2010; 68(4): 214-31.
[http://dx.doi.org/10.1111/j.1753-4887.2010.00280.x] [PMID: 20416018]

[127] Lee K, Lee J, Bae WK, Choi JK, Kim HJ, Cho B. Efficacy of low-calorie, partial meal replacement diet plans on weight and abdominal fat in obese subjects with metabolic syndrome: a double-blind, randomised controlled trial of two diet plans - one high in protein and one nutritionally balanced. Int J Clin Pract 2009; 63(2): 195-201.
[http://dx.doi.org/10.1111/j.1742-1241.2008.01965.x] [PMID: 19196357]

[128] Layman DK. Protein quantity and quality at levels above the RDA improves adult weight loss. J Am Coll Nutr 2004; 23(6) (Suppl.): 631S-6S.
[http://dx.doi.org/10.1080/07315724.2004.10719435] [PMID: 15640518]

[129] Ricci G, Canducci E, Pasini V, *et al.* Nutrient intake in Italian obese patients: relationships with insulin resistance and markers of non-alcoholic fatty liver disease. Nutrition 2011; 27(6): 672-6.
[http://dx.doi.org/10.1016/j.nut.2010.07.014] [PMID: 20961734]

[130] Paddon-Jones D, Westman E, Mattes RD, Wolfe RR, Astrup A, Westerterp-Plantenga M. Protein, weight management, and satiety. Am J Clin Nutr 2008; 87(5): 1558S-61S.
[http://dx.doi.org/10.1093/ajcn/87.5.1558S] [PMID: 18469287]

[131] Due A, Toubro S, Skov AR, Astrup A. Effect of normal-fat diets, either medium or high in protein, on body weight in overweight subjects: a randomised 1-year trial. Int J Obes Relat Metab Disord 2004; 28(10): 1283-90.
[http://dx.doi.org/10.1038/sj.ijo.0802767] [PMID: 15303109]

[132] Clifton P. The science behind weight loss diets--a brief review. Aust Fam Physician 2006; 35(8): 580-2.
[PMID: 16894429]

[133] Clifton P. Value of high-protein diet is clearer than drawbacks. Nature 2006; 439(7074): 266.
[http://dx.doi.org/10.1038/439266b] [PMID: 16421545]

[134] Campos-Nonato I, Hernandez L, Barquera S. Effect of a High-Protein Diet *versus* Standard-Protein Diet on Weight Loss and Biomarkers of Metabolic Syndrome: A Randomized Clinical Trial. Obes Facts 2017; 10(3): 238-51.
[http://dx.doi.org/10.1159/000471485] [PMID: 28601864]

[135] Astrup A, Raben A, Geiker N. The role of higher protein diets in weight control and obesity-related comorbidities. Int J Obes 2015; 39(5): 721-6.
[http://dx.doi.org/10.1038/ijo.2014.216] [PMID: 25540980]

[136] Soenen S, Martens EA, Hochstenbach-Waelen A, Lemmens SG, Westerterp-Plantenga MS. Normal protein intake is required for body weight loss and weight maintenance, and elevated protein intake for additional preservation of resting energy expenditure and fat free mass. J Nutr 2013; 143(5): 591-6.
[http://dx.doi.org/10.3945/jn.112.167593] [PMID: 23446962]

[137] Noakes M, Keogh JB, Foster PR, Clifton PM. Effect of an energy-restricted, high-protein, low-fat diet relative to a conventional high-carbohydrate, low-fat diet on weight loss, body composition, nutritional status, and markers of cardiovascular health in obese women. Am J Clin Nutr 2005; 81(6): 1298-306.
[http://dx.doi.org/10.1093/ajcn/81.6.1298] [PMID: 15941879]

[138] Martin WF, Armstrong LE, Rodriguez NR. Dietary protein intake and renal function. Nutr Metab (Lond) 2005; 2: 25.
[http://dx.doi.org/10.1186/1743-7075-2-25] [PMID: 16174292]

[139] Westerterp-Plantenga M, Luscombe-Marsh N, Lejeune MPGM, *et al.* Dietary protein, metabolism, and body-weight regulation: dose-response effects. Int J Obes 2006; 30(S16-23): 16-23.
[http://dx.doi.org/10.1038/sj.ijo.0803487]

[140] Weigle DS, Breen PA, Matthys CC, *et al.* A high-protein diet induces sustained reductions in appetite, ad libitum caloric intake, and body weight despite compensatory changes in diurnal plasma leptin and

ghrelin concentrations. Am J Clin Nutr 2005; 82(1): 41-8.
[http://dx.doi.org/10.1093/ajcn/82.1.41] [PMID: 16002798]

[141] Phillips SM, Chevalier S, Leidy HJ. Protein "requirements" beyond the RDA: implications for optimizing health. Appl Physiol Nutr Metab 2016; 41(5): 565-72.
[http://dx.doi.org/10.1139/apnm-2015-0550] [PMID: 26960445]

[142] Johnstone AM. Safety and efficacy of high-protein diets for weight loss. Proc Nutr Soc 2012; 71(2): 339-49.
[http://dx.doi.org/10.1017/S0029665112000122] [PMID: 22397883]

[143] Clifton P. High protein diets and weight control. Nutr Metab Cardiovasc Dis 2009; 19(6): 379-82.
[http://dx.doi.org/10.1016/j.numecd.2009.02.011] [PMID: 19369046]

[144] Luscombe-Marsh ND. High protein diets in obesity management and weight control.Managing and Preventing Obesity - Behavioural Factors and Dietary Interventions. Cambridge: Elsevier 2015; pp. 79-90.
[http://dx.doi.org/10.1533/9781782420996.2.79]

[145] Calvez J, Poupin N, Chesneau C, Lassale C, Tomé D. Protein intake, calcium balance and health consequences. Eur J Clin Nutr 2012; 66(3): 281-95.
[http://dx.doi.org/10.1038/ejcn.2011.196] [PMID: 22127335]

[146] Tang M, O'Connor LE, Campbell WW. Diet-induced weight loss: the effect of dietary protein on bone. J Acad Nutr Diet 2014; 114(1): 72-85.
[http://dx.doi.org/10.1016/j.jand.2013.08.021] [PMID: 24183993]

[147] Wright CS, Li J, Campbell WW. The Effect of Dietary Protein on Bone during Weight Loss: A Meta-Analysis and Systematic Review. FASEB J 2016; 30(Suppl): 415.4..

[148] Hector AJ, Marcotte GR, Churchward-Venne TA, *et al.* Whey protein supplementation preserves postprandial myofibrillar protein synthesis during short-term energy restriction in overweight and obese adults. J Nutr 2015; 145(2): 246-52.
[http://dx.doi.org/10.3945/jn.114.200832] [PMID: 25644344]

[149] Veldhorst MA, Nieuwenhuizen AG, Hochstenbach-Waelen A, *et al.* Dose-dependent satiating effect of whey relative to casein or soy. Physiol Behav 2009; 96(4-5): 675-82.
[http://dx.doi.org/10.1016/j.physbeh.2009.01.004] [PMID: 19385022]

[150] Volek JS, Volk BM, Gómez AL, *et al.* Whey protein supplementation during resistance training augments lean body mass. J Am Coll Nutr 2013; 32(2): 122-35.
[http://dx.doi.org/10.1080/07315724.2013.793580] [PMID: 24015719]

[151] Beavers KM, Gordon MM, Easter L, *et al.* Effect of protein source during weight loss on body composition, cardiometabolic risk and physical performance in abdominally obese, older adults: a pilot feeding study. J Nutr Health Aging 2015; 19(1): 87-95.
[http://dx.doi.org/10.1007/s12603-015-0438-7] [PMID: 25560821]

[152] Institute of Medicine. Dietary Reference Intakes for Energy, Carbohydrate, Fiber, Fat, Fatty Acids, Cholesterol, Protein, and Amino Acids. Washington, DC: National Academy Press 2006.

[153] Thom G, Lean M. Is There an Optimal Diet for Weight Management and Metabolic Health? Gastroenterology 2017; 152(7): 1739-51.
[http://dx.doi.org/10.1053/j.gastro.2017.01.056] [PMID: 28214525]

[154] Sacks FM, Bray GA, Carey VJ, *et al.* Comparison of weight-loss diets with different compositions of fat, protein, and carbohydrates. N Engl J Med 2009; 360(9): 859-73.
[http://dx.doi.org/10.1056/NEJMoa0804748] [PMID: 19246357]

[155] Naude CE, Schoonees A, Senekal M, Young T, Garner P, Volmink J. Low carbohydrate *versus* isoenergetic balanced diets for reducing weight and cardiovascular risk: a systematic review and meta-analysis. PLoS One 2014; 9(7)e100652
[http://dx.doi.org/10.1371/journal.pone.0100652] [PMID: 25007189]

[156] Shai I, Schwarzfuchs D, Henkin Y, *et al.* Weight loss with a low-carbohydrate, Mediterranean, or low-fat diet. N Engl J Med 2008; 359(3): 229-41.
[http://dx.doi.org/10.1056/NEJMoa0708681] [PMID: 18635428]

[157] Stelmach-Mardas M, Walkowiak J. Dietary Interventions and Changes in Cardio-Metabolic Parameters in Metabolically Healthy Obese Subjects: A Systematic Review with Meta-Analysis. Nutrients 2016; 8(8): 455.
[http://dx.doi.org/10.3390/nu8080455] [PMID: 27483307]

Recent Advances in Obesity Research, 2020, Vol. 1, 271-307

CHAPTER 11

The Relevance of Polyphenols in Obesity Therapy

Ana Faria[1,2,3], **Cristina Pereira-Wilson**[4,5,6] and **Rita Negrão**[7,8,*]

[1] *Nutrição e Metabolismo, NOVA Medical School, Faculdade de Ciências Médicas, Universidade Nova de Lisboa, Lisboa, Portugal*

[2] *CINTESIS - Center for Health Technology and Services Research, ProNutri - Clinical Nutrition & Disease Programming, Univeristy of Porto, Porto, Portugal*

[3] *REQUIMTE/LAQV, Faculty of Sciences, University of Porto, Porto, Portugal*

[4] *Department of Biology, University of Minho, Braga, Portugal*

[5] *CITAB-UM - Center for the Research and Technology of Agro-Environmental and Biological Sciences, University of Minho, Braga, Portugal*

[6] *Center for Biological Engineering, University of Minho, Braga, Portugal*

[7] *Department of Biomedicine, Biochemistry Unit, Faculty of Medicine, University of Porto, Porto, Portugal*

[8] *i3S - Instituto de Investigação e Inovação em Saúde, University of Porto, Porto, Portugal*

Abstract: Polyphenols are secondary metabolites from plant metabolism, widely distributed in nature. The major dietary sources of polyphenols are fruits, vegetables, chocolate and plant-derived beverages like tea, coffee and wine. Polyphenols are mostly absorbed in the small intestine, extensively and quickly metabolized in the liver and appear in the circulation or are excreted into bile and urine as both intact and metabolized forms. Much attention has been given to polyphenols in the last decades, mainly due to the positive association between the consumption of polyphenol-rich foods and the low risk of chronic diseases like cardiovascular diseases, type 2 diabetes and obesity. In fact, obesity has increased enormously worldwide and is becoming a threat to public health. Several studies suggest that polyphenols and polyphenol-rich foods have very interesting properties regarding the management of obesity and weight loss. Polyphenols promote a healthy profile of intestinal microbiota, decreasing *Firmicutes* and increasing *Bacteroidetes*. Polyphenols may modulate carbohydrate digestion, glucose absorption and gluconeogenesis, thereby helping contain postprandial hyperglycemic excursions. They improve lipid metabolism by decreasing adipogenesis and inhibiting lipogenesis, and stimulating lipolysis and beta-oxidation. Polyphenol ingestion was also associated with decreased food-intake and thermogenesis stimulation. Nevertheless, the effects described are still subject to debate because human studies are scarce and some results are inconsistent. Further research is needed before recommending the use of polyphenols as regulators of weight and/or modulators of obesity.

* **Corresponding author Rita Negrão:** Department of Biomedicine, Biochemistry Unit, Faculty of Medicine, University of Porto, 4200-319 Porto, Portugal; Tel/Fax: +351 225513624; E-mail: ritabsn@med.up.pt

Rosário Monteiro and Maria João Martins (Eds.)

Keywords: Absorption, Adipogenesis, Adipose tissue browning, Flavonoids, Food, Food-intake, Lipogenesis, Lipolysis, Metabolism, Microbiota, Polyphenols, Peroxisome proliferator-activated receptor alpha, Peroxisome proliferator-activated receptor gamma, Sterol regulatory element-binding protein, Obesity, Thermogenesis, Uncoupling protein 1, Weight loss.

INTRODUCTION

Polyphenols are secondary metabolites from plant metabolism. These compounds are widely distributed in nature and ubiquitous in food from vegetal origin [1].

Much attention has been given to polyphenols in the last two decades, mainly due to the positive association between the consumption of fruits and vegetables (good sources of polyphenols) with low risk for chronic diseases [2 - 4].

Due to the antioxidant theory in the 1980s and the potential for polyphenols to act as direct antioxidants derived from their chemical features, there was over a decade in which the antioxidant capacity of polyphenols was explored in a wide range of concentrations, using simple and complex mixtures of compounds in various models [5 - 7]. Nevertheless, this antioxidant activity has failed to be the main justification for the epidemiologic association observed. It has become clear that the concentration in which these compounds are ingested (mM range) are very different from the ones absorbed (in the nM range) and the concentrations tested in *in vitro* models (in the μM range) are unattainable *in vivo*, what compromises the conclusions drawn from this type of studies. So, it was proposed that the antioxidant activity of polyphenols and their actual beneficial effect could occur in the gastrointestinal tract before absorption [8, 9].

Nowadays, the paradigm that the health beneficial properties of polyphenols are due to their antioxidant activity has changed and the role of these compounds and its metabolites in a variety of cellular pathways responsible for positively modulating biological processes and hence promoting health is increasingly accepted [10, 11]. This has become emphasised knowing that they can accumulate in several cells and tissues, reaching concentrations much higher than it was expected taking into account the low plasma concentration [12, 13].

The beneficial effects of polyphenols on metabolic diseases and obesity have been reported numerous times and the mechanisms of action are emerging and include effects on macronutrient digestion and absorption, through modulation of digestive enzymes and membrane transporters, modulation of gut microbiota, alterations of carbohydrate and lipid metabolism, appetite regulation and stimulation of thermogenesis, among others. These mechanisms of action will be discussed in the present chapter, highlighting the potential benefits of polyphenols in the management of obesity.

POLYPHENOL STRUCTURE

Chemically, polyphenols are defined by the presence of polyhydroxylphenyl units and vary from simple monomeric units to complex polymeric structures. There are thousands of identified polyphenols that are classified according to their chemical structure into two subgroups: flavonoids and non-flavonoids (Fig. 1). Flavonoids are characterized by the flavan nucleus, which consists of a C6-C3-C6 structure constituted by two aromatic rings linked by a heterocyclic ring, labelled A, B and C (Fig. (2).

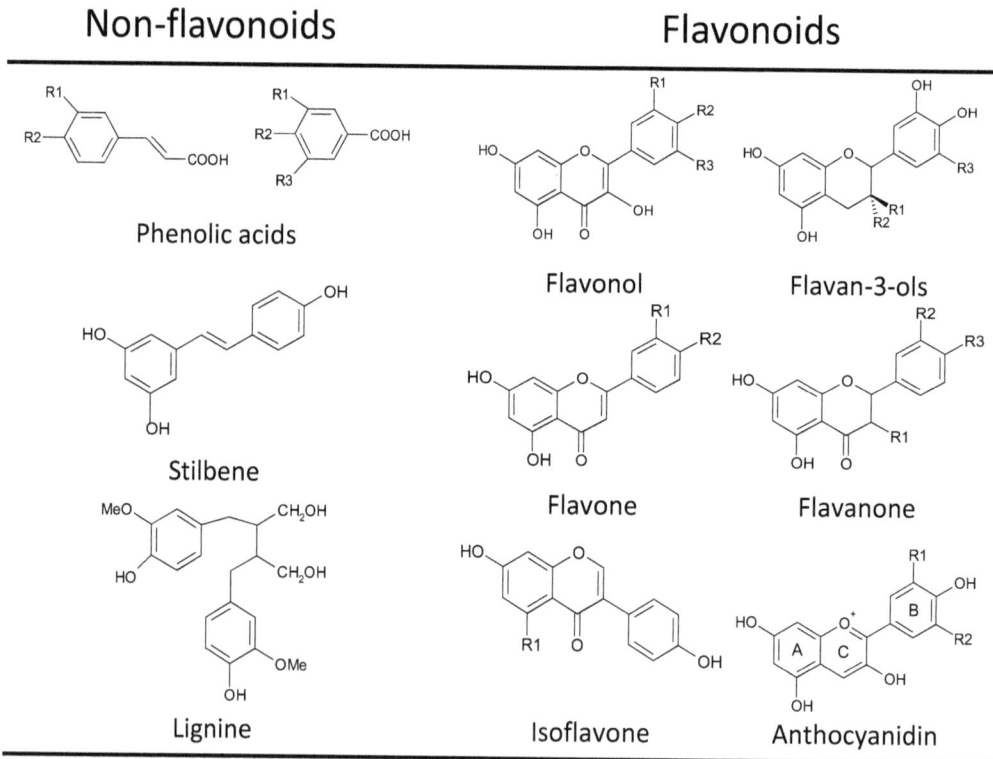

Fig. (1). Schematic representation of the most common polyphenols in food (R1, R2, R3 = H or OH or OCH$_3$).

The different classes of flavonoids differ in the level of oxidation and pattern of substitution in the C ring (Fig. (1)). Individual compounds within a class differ in the arrangements of hydroxyl, methoxyl and glycosidic groups. Flavonols, flavanones and anthocyanidins exist in nature as glycosides, and the predominant sugar moiety is glucose and rhamnose.

The most abundant classes of compounds present in food are represented in (Fig. (1); because of its predominance they are the most studied ones and with more consolidated information.

POLYPHENOLS SOURCES AND OCCURRENCE

The major dietary sources of polyphenols are fruits, vegetables, chocolate and plant-derived beverages like tea, coffee and wine as described in Table 1.

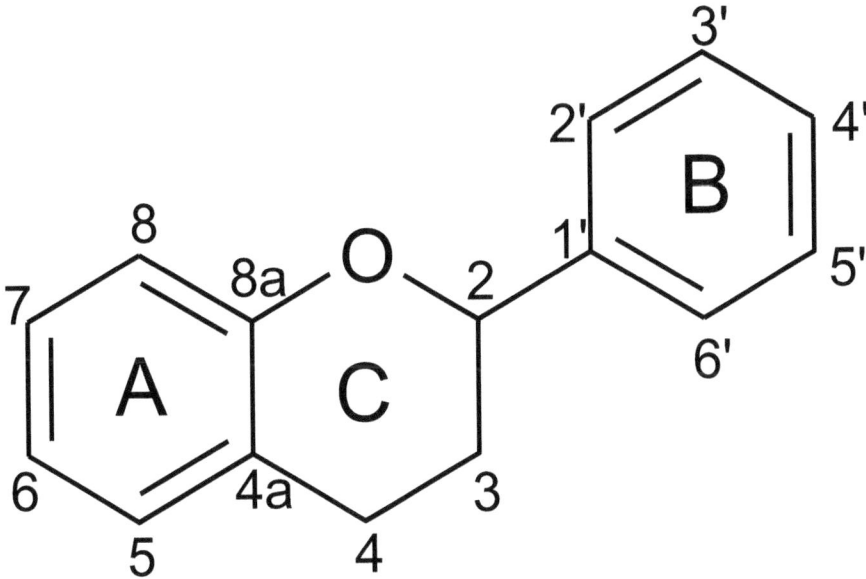

Fig. (2). Representation of the flavan nucleus.

Flavonoids are the most abundant and studied polyphenols. Some are ubiquitous in plants like quercetin, while others are specific of a plant like the flavanones in citrus fruits and isoflavones in soy. Flavanols appear in nature as monomers (catechins) and as dimers, oligomers and polymers of catechins (proanthocyanidins), also known as condensed tannins. They provide astringency and bitterness to red wine, fruits and chocolate. Anthocyanins are glycosides of anthocyanidins. They are pigments of flowers and fruits, responsible for pink, red, blue and purple colors and are abundant in all types of berries, red fruits (as grapes) and red wine [14, 15].

The composition and concentration of polyphenols depends not only on the plant, the local where it is grown, the climate and sun exposure, but also on the processing and storage conditions of food, among other factors [16].

Also, major dietary sources depend on the type of the diet and although fruits, specially berries, have higher content of polyphenols, beverages like tea, coffee and wine may be nowadays important sources due to their higher consumption.

It has been estimated that the average daily intake of polyphenols is about 1 gram per day [15]. Data obtained from the European Prospective Investigation into Cancer and Nutrition (EPIC) study, involving 35628 subjects recruited between 1992 and 2000, has not found differences in total flavonoid intake between European Mediterranean and non-Mediterranean countries. Subjects consumed about 370 mg flavonoids/day, flavanols being the most ingested flavonoids. In Mediterranean countries, the major contributors were proanthocyanidins (59%) and catechin monomers (13%) while in non-Mediterranean countries proanthocyanidins contributed to 48% and catechin monomers to 25% of total flavonoid intake. In non-Mediterranean countries, fruits (33%) and tea (26%) were the main flavonoid sources while in Mediterranean countries the major contributors were fruits (55%) and wine (17%) [17]. Another very recent study, using National Health and Nutrition Examination Survey (NHANES) food consumption data of 18634 subjects between 1999-2002 and 2007-2010 in the USA, revealed that total flavonoid intake was about 200 mg/day and did not change between these two periods. However, the intake of anthocyanidins increased in the USA due to higher ingestion patterns of berries and wine in the last years [18]. These studies demonstrated that, in general, flavonoid intake seems to be higher in Europe and also that flavonoid sources and classes vary between different regions and countries.

Polyphenols are a group of compounds chemically very different and the most ingested polyphenols, present in higher levels in foods and beverages, are not always the most absorbed and bioactive compounds.

Table 1. Main human food sources of most abundant polyphenols.

Polyphenols	Main food sources
Non-flavonoids	
Phenolic acids	
Hydroxybenzoic acids	Blackberry
Gallic acid	Raspberry
p-Hydroxybenzoic acid	Black currant
	Strawberry
	Tea
Hydroxycinnamic acids	Blueberry
Caffeic acid	Coffee
Ferulic acid	Kiwi
Chlorogenic acid	Cherry
Coumaric acid	Aubergine
	Plum
	Apple
	Pear
	Chicory
	Wheat
Stilbene	Black grape
Resveratrol	Red wine
Lignine	Linseed
Enterodiol	Lentils
	Cereals
Flavonoids	
Flavonols	Yellow onion
Quercetin	Curly kale
Kaempferol	Tomato
Myricetin	Broccoli
	Blueberry
	Black currant
	Apricot
	Apple
	Beans
	Black grape
	Black tea
	Green tea
	Red wine
Flavan-3-ols	Chocolate
Catechin	Green tea
Epicatechin	Beans
Epigallocatechin	Apricot
Epigallocatechin gallate	Black tea
	Red wine
	Blackberry
	Cherry
	Grape
	Apple
	Peach
Flavones	Sweet red pepper
Apigenin	Celery
Luteolin	Parsley
Flavanones	Orange
Hesperetin	Grapefruit
Naringenin	Lemon
Isoflavones	Soybeans
Daidzein	Miso
Genistein	Tofu
	Soy milk
Anthocyanidins	Blackberry
Cyanidin	Black currant
Delphinidin	Strawberry
Pelargonidin	cherry
Malvidin	Chocolate
	Red grape
	Apple
	Red wine

ABSORPTION AND METABOLISM OF POLYPHENOLS

Despite the extensive literature available regarding fruits and vegetable consumption, and consequently polyphenol rich-food, one crucial point has not yet been fully understood: polyphenol absorption.

Due to its enormous chemical diversity, several hypotheses regarding the site and the mechanism for polyphenol absorption have been raised. It has become clear that the hydroxylation and methoxylation pattern along with the glucoside substitution have great influence in the absorption pattern as well as in biotransformation in the gastrointestinal (GI) tract [8, 19].

Polyphenols' concentration in the blood stream and their availability in target tissues are, as expected, highly dependent on their absorption. The forms of the compounds that reach the tissues will be a consequence of the modifications suffered by the compounds in the GI tract and in other tissues, such as the liver [20, 21].

The oral cavity is the first site where absorption process of polyphenols may occur. It is worth noticing that polyphenols, unless taken as supplements, are part of food, being inserted in a complex matrix of substances that will certainly exert influence on their absorption [22].

In this site, polyphenols that were able to be released from the food matrix may interact with salivary proteins (proline-rich proteins) [23, 24]. These interactions may occur through hydrogen bonds or hydrophobic interactions, thus forming polyphenol-protein aggregates that are able to bind together creating bigger protein complexes capable to precipitate in solution. Also, these interactions with proteins will have an impact on protein activity as a result of protein structure modifications [23].

It has been reported that (+)-catechin has a higher affinity toward the salivary proteins than (-)-epicatechin, whereas proanthocyanidin dimers coupled by a C-4−C-8 bond exhibit a higher affinity towards those proteins than dimers having a C-4−C-6 bond [25]. Also, a significant interaction between salivary proteins and both condensed tannins and ellagitannins has been reported [23] as well as with anthocyanins [26] and pyranoanthocyanins [27].

In addition to protein interaction, polyphenols can also suffer enzyme activity in the oral cavity. In a work with healthy volunteers, black raspberry anthocyanins have been detected in their hydrolyzed aglycon form in the oral cavity, resulting from the activity of beta-glucosidase derived both from oral bacteria and epithelial cells [28]. Also, the parent anthocyanins and the cyanidin-3-glucoside microbiota metabolite, protocatechuic acid, have been detected in the saliva. Furthermore, saliva samples contain glucuronidated anthocyanin conjugates, consistent with intracellular uptake and phase II conversion of anthocyanins [28].

Nevertheless, the relevance of these oral transformations for local effects, given the relatively short residence time of most foods in the oral cavity, is still to be determined.

The stomach is not, by definition, a local for absorption but several studies have shown that important transformations with impact on polyphenol availability occur at this site [20, 25]. The strong acidic pH of the stomach might affect polyphenol stability. Nevertheless, studies with resveratrol, quercetin and catechin have shown that the compounds were stable at low pH [29 - 31]. It has been proposed that proanthocyanins could be degraded to monomers in acidic conditions [32]. However, further studies have shown that these compounds were stable in these conditions [33, 34].

The ability of anthocyanins to cross the gastric mucosa has been suggested in early 2000 due to its rapid appearance in the blood stream [35] and it was demonstrated that anthocyanin glycosides are quickly and efficiently absorbed in the stomach (approximately 25%) [36]. However, their absorption varies greatly according to the anthocyanin structure and they are rapidly excreted into the bile either intact or metabolized [36]. Also, anthocyanins are unstable and degraded easily under certain conditions. Two hours after ingestion of pelargonidin only the presence of p-hydroxybenzoic acid was detected in stomach [37].

Several other studies report anthocyanin absorption in the stomach with lack of anthocyanin metabolites [38, 39]. To notice that, unlike other flavonoids, anthocyanins are absorbed in its glycosidic form, without hydrolysis of the sugar moiety. Nevertheless, the mechanism of anthocyanin gastric absorption remains unknown. Several hypotheses have been raised, for example, transport through bilitranslocase, which is expressed in stomach [40, 41], and has its *in vitro* transport activity competitively inhibited by quinoidal forms of dietary anthocyanins, despite the experimental conditions used (pH 8) did not simulate the stomach environment. Other possibilities include the glucose transporters (GLUT) 1 and 3, monocarboxylate transporter 1 (MCT1), the organic anion uptake transporter 2 (OAT2) and the sodium-coupled monocarboxylate transporters (SMCT) 1 and 2, since the expression of these transporters has already been detected in the stomach tissue [42 - 45].

Quercetin, but not quercetin 3-O-glucoside nor quercetin 3-O-rutinoside, was found to be absorbed in the stomach of the rat [46]. Similarly, the isoflavones genistein and daidzein, but not their glucosides, were also found to be absorbed in the rat stomach [47]. Finally, some phenolic acids were also found to be absorbed at the rat gastric epithelium [48 - 51].

Also, stomach is rarely seen as a metabolizing organ and the importance of the metabolic transformations that may occur at this site are often neglected. Nevertheless, stomach possesses conjugative enzyme activities [UDP-glucuronosyltransferase (UGT), sulphotransferase (SULT) and catechol-O-methyl transferase (COMT)] [20, 52 - 55] and some *in vitro* studies have shown that flavonoids could be metabolized into glucuronidated, sulphated and methylated metabolites in the gastric wall [20, 47, 56].

Even after possible interference of the stomach, the majority of the polyphenols ingested reach the small intestine intact. At this site, they can suffer a variety of reactions that will depend on the chemistry and the structure of the polyphenol. Aglycones are transported easily into the cells, possible by passive diffusion due to their lipophilicity. In glycosylated flavonoids, the sugar moiety could be removed at the brush border of intestinal cells, by lactase-phlorizin hydrolase (LPH), or inside the cells, by cytosolic beta-glucosidase (CBG), to originate the aglycone (which has higher lipophilicity that the glycoside) that may cross cell membranes by passive transport [22].

Hesperidin (hesperetin-7-O-rhamnoglucoside) is the rutinoside of hesperetin [57]. Intact hesperidin is not absorbed across the small intestine epithelium [58] but if the terminal rhamnose moiety is hydrolyzed before consumption, the product, hesperetin-7-O-glucoside, becomes a substrate for LPH and the resulting hesperetin is efficiently absorbed [58]. Intact hesperidin is not absorbed passively, but hesperetin, after removal of the two sugars, is readily absorbed [59].

The same mechanism occurs with quercetin. This flavonol is found in nature attached to sugar moieties, such as the 3-O-glucoside and 3,4'-O-diglucoside forms found in onions [60], the 3-O-rutinoside found in tea [61, 62] and various glycosides in apples [63]. The glucoside is absorbed rapidly and efficiently in the small intestine, but the rutinoside is absorbed only after hydrolysis of the sugars [64, 65].

Furthermore, glucose transporters also participate in the transport of polyphenols. Quercetin 3-glucoside transport has been associated with GLUT2 [66] while GLUT4 has been involved in the transport of genistein, myricetin, and quercetin [67]; in the transport of quercetin, GLUT1 is also involved [68].

Anthocyanin glycosides are rapidly and efficiently absorbed in the small intestine and appear intact in the blood stream [69 - 71]. The potential mechanisms of anthocyanin glycoside absorption in the small intestine may involve glucose transporters, such as the sodium-dependent glucose cotransporter 1 (SGLT1), as previously suggested for other flavonoids [64] or GLUT2 [72]. Accordingly, the transport rate of cyanidin-3-glucose was found to be significantly decreased after SGLT1 or GLUT2 siRNA transfection in Caco-2 cells [73].

Epicatechin, as most of the flavanol monomers, is found in most foods in the free form [74] and is absorbed in the small intestine without any prior transformation [75]. Also, simple phenolic acids are absorbed through the small intestinal epithelium [76], although some hydrolysis may occur in esterified compounds, through the action of esterases, before absorption occurs [77].

Polyphenols are rapidly and extensively metabolized after ingestion. Sometimes this metabolism starts in the oral cavity and may have a participation of the stomach as described before. The small intestine, besides being a site of absorption, is also a place where active metabolism occurs, with particular importance for UGT, COMT and SULT. Anthocyanins, for example, are quickly metabolized and appear in the circulation or are excreted into bile and urine as both intact and metabolized forms (glucuronidated, sulfated or methylated derivatives) [36, 69, 70, 78 - 81]. Also, phenolic acids are rapidly sulfated, to form sulfate derivatives, or simultaneously sulfated and methylated, sometimes resulting in other phenolic acid [82].

Glucuronides and sulfates of polyphenolic compounds are too hydrophilic to enter the cell by simple diffusion. Some studies have proposed the ATP-binding cassette (ABC) transporters to participate in this process [83, 84].

ABC transporters are a family that includes multidrug resistance proteins (MRPs), breast cancer resistance protein (BCRP) and P-glycoprotein [20, 83], all with low specificity to substrates. Nevertheless, they have a critical role in limiting substances into the cell [84], being involved either in the flux of compounds from the intestinal cells to the basolateral (blood) side as to the intestinal lumen.

Trans-resveratrol glucuronide was shown to be transported to the blood stream by MRP3 [85]. Also, MRP2 in the apical membrane of Caco-2 cells is involved in the transport of polyphenols conjugated with glucuronide and/or sulfate [86]. P-glycoprotein as well as MRP2 have been shown to be involved in naringenin and quercetin transport [20, 87, 88].

POLYPHENOLS AND INTESTINAL MICROBIOTA

Of all the polyphenols that are ingested, a part is absorbed intact and another part is metabolized and absorbed in the GI tract, but a great amount of these polyphenols reach the colon intact. The colon is no longer seen as a simple excretion route and is being considered an active site for metabolism, receiving much attention from the scientific community [89]. Although the colon is colonized by microorganisms that have not been fully described, it is clear that the human gut is home for an ecosystem of around 10^{13}-10^{14} bacterial cells [90]. Evidence has been accumulating regarding the composition of human intestinal microbiota and the influence on health and the incidence of disease [91].

In human subjects, high-fat diet (HFD) feeding triggers the development of obesity, inflammation, insulin resistance, type 2 diabetes *mellitus* (T2DM) and atherosclerosis, associates with the development of metabolic endotoxemia and induces low-grade inflammation, a mechanism associated with the development of atherogenic markers [92, 93].

The evidence that the gut microbiota composition can be different between healthy and obese or T2DM patients [94, 95] has led to the study of this factor as a key link between the pathophysiology of metabolic diseases and the gut bacteria composition, as it has been explored in another chapter of this book. Among other variables, obesity has been associated with changes in gut microbiota composition [96]. Although some studies diverge, given the use of different methodologies, it seems that, in obesity, the abundance of *Firmicutes* increase at the expense of *Bacteroidetes* [97]. The change in the *Firmicutes/Bacteroidetes* ratio can be related to the expression of genes encoding key enzymes involved in the digestion of polysaccharides [98].

There are several reviews in the literature concerning the beneficial effects of polyphenols in obesity progression [99, 100], but the interaction between polyphenols and microbiota has not yet been completely described. If in one hand, polyphenols are subjected to metabolism by microbiota, on the other hand, they and/or their metabolites may modulate growth of specific bacteria from microbiota.

Different polyphenols have been suggested to affect the relative viability of colonic bacterial groups [101, 102], implying that dietary modulation with polyphenols may play a role in reshaping the gut microbial community and enhance host microbial interactions to provide beneficial effects such as weight loss [103]. Thus, polyphenols should be considered to have a prebiotic action.

Malvidin-3-glucoside, and anthocyanin, incubated *in vitro* with fecal slurry increased the growth of total bacteria and *Bifidobaterium spp.* and *Lactobacillus spp* [104]; when together with other anthocyanins showed a synergistic effect on benefic bacteria growth [104]. Anthocyanin-enriched apple-supplemented mice showed a greater number of bacteria than in control animals as well as a significant increase in *Bifidobaterium spp* [105]. Accordingly, a six-week consumption of a blueberry drink by human volunteers significantly increased *Bifidobaterium spp* [106].

The distribution ratio of different genera within *Bacteroidetes* and *Firmicutes* phyla was different between baseline and intake periods [107], *Firmicutes* concentration increasing after red wine consumption in volunteers.

A study with pigs fed a diet supplemented with cocoa husks for 3 weeks showed a decrease in *Firmicutes* and an increase in *Bacteroidetes*, without any changes in food intake and weight gain. Cocoa-husk intake reduced *Lactobacillus-Enterococcus* group and *Clostridium histolyticum* and increased the *Bacteroides-Prevotella* group and *Faecalibacterium prausnitzii* [108]. In the same animal model, but this time supplemented with a flavonoid-enriched cocoa powder for 27 days, the *Lactobacillus* species abundance was greater in feces and *Bifidobacterium* was greater in proximal colon content from supplemented animals, highlighting the effect of this supplementation on microbiota modulation [109]. The results of these two studies are quite different but, despite the common use of cocoa-derived products, the product composition is not similar and the type and quantity of compounds in the supplement can make the difference.

In vivo and clinical studies have shown that urolithin-A, the main metabolite of ellagitannins, significantly increased the growth of *Bifidobacterium* and *Lactobacillus spp*. in a rat model of colitis [110]. Also, this compound relates with the reduction of *Firmicutes* levels and the induction of growth of *Enterobacter, Lactobacillus, E. coli*, and *Verrucomicrobia (A. muciphila)* in volunteers able to metabolize ellagitannins to urolithin-A [111].

Firmicutes/Bacteroidetes ratio was reduced after administration of both quercetin and resveratrol (in rats) [112], or resveratrol alone (in mice) [113]. Also, polymeric apple procyanidins showed the same effect on mice fed high-fat/hig--sugar diet [114].

Nevertheless, the biologic activity of polyphenols in obesity may not be exclusively due to modulation of microbiota, but also to conversion of polyphenols in the colon into active metabolites by microbiota, which are different from parent compounds and may influence other biological pathways [106, 115].

EFFECTS OF POLYPHENOLS ON MACRONUTRIENT ABSORPTION AND GLYCEMIC CONTROL

There is growing evidence that dietary polyphenols help in the regulation of glucose homeostasis and insulin sensitivity thereby having a role in the prevention and management of metabolic diseases, including T2DM [116].

Dietary polyphenols may function as digestive enzyme inhibitors (alpha-amylase and alpha-glucosidade) as well as modulators of intestinal glucose absorption through effects both on SGLT1 and/or GLUT2. Polyphenols may additionally reduce endogenous glucose production by gluconeogenesis, increase peripheral glucose uptake or protect insulin-producing pancreatic beta cells against glucotoxicity [116].

Starch, the main carbohydrate in the human diet, contains amylose and amylopectin (polymers of glucose linked by alpha-1,4 glycosidic bonds, with additional alpha-1,6 branch points in amylopectin). The disaccharides sucrose and lactose are also important components of human diet as well as the monosaccharide fructose, today widely used as sweetener by the food industry.

Alpha-amylase (EC 3.2.1.1) is responsible for the digestion of starch but hydrolyses only the alpha-1,4 glycosidic bonds. The products of alpha-amylase digestion of starch include fragments with two or more alpha-1,4-linked glucose molecules (maltose) as well as dextrins which contain the alpha-1,6 linked glucose branch points [117].

Sucrase (sucrose alpha-glucosidase, included in the sucrase-isomaltase protein) and maltase (alpha-glucosidase, included in the maltase-glucoamylase protein) hydrolyse the disaccharides sucrose and maltose, respectively. Proteins containing sucrase and maltase are bound to the brush-border membrane (BBM) of enterocytes, where the enzymes act on the substrates present in the gut lumen. Lactose, a milk disaccharide composed of glucose and galactose, is hydrolysed by the brush-border enzyme lactase (included in the LPH protein) [117].

Although less is known about the inhibitory effects of polyphenols on lipid digestive enzymes, green tea (GT) catechins have been shown to inhibit pancreatic and gastric lipases and lipid emulsification [118, 119].

After digestion, the monosaccharides glucose, fructose and galactose are taken up into the enterocytes from which they are delivered to the circulation. Enterocytes are equipped with BBM SGLT1 for glucose and galactose transport and GLUT5 for fructose transport. GLUT2 is present in enterocyte basolateral membrane [120]. In diabetic patients there is a paradoxical increase of carbohydrate digestion and intestinal uptake efficiency as a result of increased alpha-amylase activity and SGLT1 and GLUT2 expression in BBM [120 - 122]. Adaptive responses to dietary carbohydrates also exist that adjust glucose intestinal uptake to digestible carbohydrate intake with the diet [120]. Increased digestive efficiency and nutrient uptake play a major role in the positive energy balance of metabolic syndrome patients and contribute to increased fat deposition.

The effects of polyphenols on carbohydrate digestion and absorption have been reviewed by Williamson [117]. Theaflavins and gallate esters present in black tea, but not (-)-epicatechin or (-)-epigallocatechin, inhibit alpha-amylase from human saliva [123]. Chlorogenic acid (5-caffeoylquinic acid) inhibits pancreatic pig alpha-amylase and is 4-5 times more potent than caffeic acid [124].

Polyphenol-rich extracts from berries, such as raspberry and strawberry, are more efficient than blackcurrant and blueberry as inhibitors of pancreatic alpha-amylase [125, 126]. Berry anthocyanins also inhibit alpha-glucosidases. Acarbose and viglibose are therapeutic alpha-glucosidase inhibitors used in the management of T2DM due to their glucose lowering effects which suggests that plant polyphenols may play an important role in dietary strategies for the prevention of metabolic diseases [117, 125].

In GLUT2 expressing *Xenopus* oocytes, myricetin, fisetin and quercetin have been shown to inhibit the transport of glucose [66]. In pig intestinal BBM vesicles, quercetin glucosides inhibit glucose uptake [127]. In Caco-2 cells GT polyphenols decrease radiolabeled glucose uptake by inhibiting both SGLT1 and GLUT2 [117]. Phlorizin inhibits SGLT1-dependent glucose uptake whereas quercetin and myricetin inhibit GLUT2-dependent transport [128].

Effects on BBM expression levels of SGLT1 have shown that this transporter is modulated by rosmarinic acid with impact on diabetes progression and on increased glucose uptake capacity induced by manipulation of dietary carbohydrates [120].

Blood glucose levels are prevented from declining below acceptable basal values by hepatic gluconeogenesis. In insulin resistant or T2DM patients there is a defective inhibition of gluconeogenesis whereby endogenous production of glucose in the liver aggravates hyperglycemia. In these cases, metformin is used as a prescription drug to inhibit hepatic gluconeogenesis [129].

Individual polyphenols or polyphenol mixtures contribute to blood glucose regulation by inhibiting gluconeogenesis. Epigallocatechin-3-gallate (EGCG), a GT polyphenol, suppresses liver gluconeogenesis and decreases phosphoenolpyruvate carboxykinase (PEPCK) mRNA in mice. Naringin and areca nut procyanidins also decrease PEPCK and hepatic *de novo* glucose production in mice, thereby contributing to plasma glucose regulation [116].

Consumption of common sage herbal tea had a metformin-like effect in rat hepatic glucose production [130].

In summary, plant polyphenols may modulate carbohydrate digestion and glucose absorption and gluconeogenesis thereby helping contain postprandial hyperglycemic excursions which are known to negatively contribute to metabolic diseases and obesity.

POLYPHENOLS ON LIPID METABOLISM

Adipose tissue stores excess dietary energy as triacylglycerols and releases fatty acids and glycerol into the blood stream whenever needed, thereby working as an important player in energy metabolism and homeostasis. Obesity is associated with unhealthy increases in fat deposits and altered energy homeostasis which increase the risk of insulin resistance, T2DM and cardiovascular diseases (CVD).

Adipogenesis, the process by which precursor cells differentiate into adipocytes increasing cell mass in adipose tissue, is regulated by nuclear hormone receptor transcription factors. The most important one is the peroxisome proliferator-activated receptor (PPAR) gamma that is particularly expressed in adipose tissue and belongs to a family of transcription factors to which PPARalpha and PPARbeta/delta also belong. PPARs function as heterodimers with the retinoid X receptor and bind to specific DNA sequences to regulate the transcription of target genes. PPAR activity is regulated by ligand binding and dissociation or recruitment of corepressor or coactivator molecules [131]. The promoter regions of genes involved in lipid deposition and the differentiation of adipocytes, such as GLUT4, lipoprotein lipase (LPL), stearyl-Coa-desaturase (SCD) and fatty acid synthase (FAS), have PPARgamma binding sites [132]. Ligands may function as agonists or antagonists. In the case of PPARgamma, thiazolidinediones (also known as glitazones), such as rosiglitazone, are pharmacologically-developed agonists used in the treatment of T2DM due to their effects on glucose homeostasis and insulin sensitivity, that result from stimulation of lipid removal from circulation due to increased uptake into the adipose tissue. These drugs, however, are not suitable in the case of obese patients since they increase fat deposition and weight gain [133].

On the other hand, negatively regulating PPARgamma, both by decreasing its expression and/or inhibiting its transcriptional activity, results in decreased adipogenesis and constitute an attractive strategy in the fight against obesity [131].

The histone deacetylase sirtuin 1 (SIRT1) has been suggested as a corepressor of PPARgamma [134]. SIRT1, which plays a wide variety of important roles, including the response to calorie restriction, has been shown to play a role as inhibitor of adipogenesis in 3T3-L1 adipocytes, where overexpression of SIRT1 also led to lipolysis, an effect mediated by PPARgamma repression [132, 134]. In addition, SIRT1 is also known to affect mitochondrial biogenesis and fatty acid oxidation, through effects on PPARgamma coactivator 1-alpha (PGC1alpha) [134].

Activation of AMP-activated protein kinase (AMPK), a serine/threonine kinase, promotes energy production and inhibits energy consuming pathways [135]. AMPK inhibits the energy consuming process of adipogenesis, through phosphorylation-mediated inhibition of PPARgamma [136, 137].

Other negative regulators of PPARgamma and adipogenesis include the kruppel-like factor 2 (KLF2), the GATA2 and the GATA3 zinc finger proteins, preadipocyte factor-1 (Pref-1) and the transcriptional-coactivator with PDZ-binding motif (TAZ) [132].

The effects of botanicals in the regulation of PPARgamma and inhibition of adipogenesis have recently been reviewed [134]. Screening for natural compounds that function as direct antagonists of PPARgamma has revealed that piperine, an alkaloide in black pepper, significantly decreased both PPARgamma mRNA as well as its rosiglitazone-induced transcriptional activity. Indole-3-carbinol, a breakdown product of glucobrassicin, a glucosinolate abundant in broccoli and cabbage, is a SIRT1 activator that decreases adipogenesis in 3T3-L1 cells. Curcumin decreases adipogenesis through AMPK activation and downregulation of PPARgamma transcriptional activity. Also, the isoflavone genistein and the triterpene saponin from *Panax ginseng*, ginsenoside Rh2, as well as the triterpenoid ursolic acid, increase activation of AMPK thereby inhibiting adipogenesis [134]. Resveratrol (3,4',5-trihydroxystilbene) has been shown to activate SIRT1 and inhibit adipogenic differentiation [138].

Signaling pathways affecting adipogenesis such as Wnt/beta catenin and mitogen-activated protein kinase (MAPK) may also be targeted for decreased adipogenesis [136]. MAPK activity seems to inhibit adipocyte differentiation through phosphorylation-mediated decreased PPARgamma transcriptional activity [136]. EGCG seems to regulate adipogenesis through decreased MAPK activity [139]. Genistein appears to regulate both expression and transcriptional activity of PPARgamma in addition to the effects on AMPK and Wnt/beta-catenin signaling, thereby decreasing adipogenesis [134].

While adipogenesis refers to adipocyte differentiation, the actual lipid synthesis is called lipogenesis and lipid degradation for ATP generation is known as lipolysis. Fat deposits in adipose tissue are the result of the balance between lipid deposition and lipid mobilization. Lipogenesis involves the upregulation of the expression of genes dependent on the transcription factor sterol regulatory element-binding protein 1c (SREBP1c), such as FAS, and is activated by insulin. Although less is known about the involvement of SREBP1c activation and lipogenesis in adipose tissue, it is believed to be similar to what happens in the liver [131, 140]. Coffee polyphenols have been reported to decrease visceral and liver fat accumulation in HFD fed mice, through a SREBP1c-dependent mechanism with decreased expression of lipogenic enzymes such as FAS [141].

Also, resveratrol has been reported to decrease lipogenesis in hepatocytes (HepG2 cells) through a decrease in the expression of SREBP1 [142]. Grape seed proanthocyanidins reduce SREBP mRNA expression in the liver of high-fructose fed rats [143] and anthocyanidins also modulate liver lipid metabolism by decreasing the expression of SREBP1 in male C57BL/6J mice [144].

When ATP generation is required, triacylglycerols stored in the adipose tissue are hydrolyzed by lipases, as lipid catabolism is initiated. In peroxisomes, long-chain fatty acids are converted into acyl-CoA. The fatty acid beta-oxidation takes place in mitochondria and the first requirement for this to occur is the transport of acyl-CoA into the mitochondria, the rate limiting step of beta-oxidation, that is facilitated, among others, by carnitine palmitoyltransferase-1 (CPT1) (short-chain fatty acids are activated inside the mitochondria) [145].

However, lipogenesis and lipolysis should not be activated simultaneously and malonyl-CoA, produced by acetyl-CoA carboxylase (ACC), while being a substrate for fatty acid biosynthesis, is an inhibitor of CPT1 (and, consequently, of beta-oxidation of longer fatty acids). The metabolic regulator AMPK can change the phosphorylation and activation state of ACC, thereby inhibiting the production of malonyl-CoA and fatty acid synthesis as it induces fatty acid beta-oxidation [145].

PPARalpha is highly expressed in muscles, liver, heart and kidney where it regulates the expression of genes encoding proteins involved in fat mobilization and fatty acid beta-oxidation. Lipid accumulation in the liver of subjects with fatty liver disease strongly impacts blood lipoproteins and cholesterol, severely increasing the risk of CVD [146, 147]. Drugs known as fibrates are pharmacological agonists of PPARalpha used to treat dyslipidemia. PPARalpha activation stimulates LPL activity and reduces triacylglycerol levels in circulation while increasing high-density lipoprotein (HDL) cholesterol [148]. In addition to ligand activation, PPARalpha may also be stimulated by phosphorylation through MAPK, protein-kinase C (PKC) and AMPK [149].

Natural products as activators of PPARalpha have recently been reviewed [150]. The stilbene resveratrol decreases adipogenesis and lipogenesis and increases lipolysis in mature adipocytes while preventing weight gain in mice fed a HFD [138, 151].

The citrus flavonoid naringenin activates PPARalpha and produces an increase in hepatic fatty acid oxidation *in vivo* [152, 153]. Green tea EGCG also increases PPARalpha expression [154]. With regard to isoflavones, daidzein and genistein protect against hepatic steatosis through a mechanism involving increased PPARalpha expression (with 3'-hydroxygenistein being more efficient than genistein itself) [155, 156]. In spite of structural similarities, formononetin is more potent than daidzein in its effects [157]. Sesamin, a lignan from sesame seeds, improves hepatic steatosis, through induction of PPARalpha [158]. On the other hand, the positive effects of bilobetin, a compound isolated from *Gingko biloba*, on hyperlipidemia and lipotoxicity could not be attributed to PPARalpha-related mechanisms [159].

The dietary flavone luteolin-7-glucoside (L7G), abundant in many aromatic herbs and other Mediterranean diet foods, has recently been shown to induce the hepatic expression of PPARalpha and of its target gene CPT1 in rats [146]. L7G also has a positive effect on plasma lipoproteins in rats [160].

Although limited, human studies report that dietary polyphenols hold great promise as aids in weight reducing strategies [145].

POLYPHENOLS AND APPETITE REGULATION

The hypothalamus is a key regulator of energy metabolism, as it contains nuclei that coordinate food intake and energy expenditure (EE), by changing the expression of neuromodulators in response to peripheral hormones. The arcuate nucleus contains the ventromedial nuclei, an orexigenic center, with neurons expressing neuropeptide Y (NPY) and Agouti-related protein (AgRP). The production of these neuropeptides is inhibited by insulin, leptin and peptide YY3-36 (PYY) and stimulated by ghrelin. The arcuate nucleus also contains the ventrolateral nuclei, with anorexigenic neurons, expressing proopiomelanocortin (POMC)/alpha-melanocyte stimulating hormone (alphaMSH) and cocaine- and amphetamine regulated transcript (CART) that are stimulated by insulin and leptin and inhibited by the orexigenic hormone ghrelin [161]. Although with an important and established role in energy metabolism, in the hypothalamus, AMPK is regulated by these hormones, regulating feeding, what is stimulated by its phosphorylation [162].

Polyphenols have been reported to cross the blood-brain barrier [163], but the concentration they can reach in the brain is still controversial and seems to depend on the polyphenol, the period of treatment and the species used in the study. The results obtained for long periods of exposition, as occurs in human life, may be different from those regarding an acute exposure to these compounds. In fact,

Ferruzzi *et al* demonstrated that the brain concentration of several polyphenols increased with chronic exposure to these compounds [164].

Several research groups presented evidence that polyphenols may interfere with appetite regulation, although there are still many controversial studies regarding this issue. Intra-peritoneal injection of GT EGCG in obese Zucker and in Sprague-Dawley rats decreased food intake by 50%, in a process independent of leptin-signaling [165], but this effect was reduced or absent when EGCG was administered orally. On the contrary, *Xu et al* observed a weight reduction in mice treated simultaneously with HFD and tea polyphenols, with a concomitant reversion of serum leptin levels in these animals compared to HFD-treated animals [166]. In another study conducted with healthy volunteers, a reduction in food intake of about 8% was observed in the group treated for 12 weeks with a GT extract supplement [167]. Decreased hunger feelings and energy intake were also described in a study involving overweight volunteers consuming beverages containing GT catechins or beverages containing GT catechins, caffeine and fibers [168].

In a very interesting study, Kim *et al* demonstrated that in mice treated with resveratrol, the expression of the orexigenic genes NPY and AgRP was inhibited and that a single injection of resveratrol decreased food intake until 17% for 48 hours [169]. Resveratrol also reversed the increase in body weight as well as leptin resistance resulting from early weaning, suggesting that the regulation of leptin levels by resveratrol may be an interesting target in obesity and weight maintenance treatments [170]. Zhang *et al* demonstrated that treatment with isoflavones for 4 weeks was able to reduce body weight and food intake through the decrease in ghrelin and NPY levels of female ovariectomized rats [171]. In another study with female rats, daidzein, an isoflavone, decreased food intake by avoiding the usually post-prandial increase in NPY expression [172]. Nevertheless, in a clinical trial, the supplementation of 34 healthy postmenopausal women with soy isoflavone during 8 weeks did not reduce food intake or body weight, although it increased the satiety peptide PYY in the plasma [173]. However, many human studies regarding appetite regulation or food ingestion use a self-reported diet which may not be sensitive enough to detect changes in food intake that may occur in long-term interventions, despite favorable outcomes regarding weight loss [174]. In another study, Badshah *et al* demonstrated that anthocyanins from black soybeans diminished food intake and body weight, and decreased NPY expression in the hypothalamus, when administered for 40 days to rats [175]. Myoung *et al* reported, in an interesting study, that apigenin, a flavone, stimulated POMC and CART activity in neuronal cells, and that one single intraperitoneal injection of apigenin in mice decreased food ingestion by 28% during 48 hours. These authors also observed a decrease in food intake and body weight after treating mice with a HFD and oral apigenin administration; nevertheless, this effect was much less pronounced [175].

Although studies regarding polyphenols and appetite regulation are still scarce, polyphenols seem to have potential in the modulation of neuropeptides relevant for food intake and satiety regulation. Due to the obvious difficulty in the access to human brain tissues, cellular and animal experimental studies are of huge importance to elucidate the possibility of using polyphenols as nutrition supplements with satiety properties. Also, clinical trials should clarify the pertinence of this possibility.

THERMOGENESIS MODULATION AND BROWNING OF ADIPOSE TISSUE BY POLYPHENOLS

While white adipose tissue (WAT) functions as energy storage, brown adipose tissue (BAT) dissipates it through heat production. In fact, brown adipocytes oxidize glucose and fatty acids to produce heat as a response to stimulus like cold exposure or food ingestion, in a process called non-shivering thermogenesis. Brown adipocytes are characterized by the presence of multi-locular lipid vacuoles and high mitochondria content, rich in uncoupling protein (UCP) 1 or thermogenin [176]. When activated, UCP1 catalyses the uncoupling of oxidative respiration from ATP synthesis, by allowing the passage of protons into the mitochondria matrix, according to the proton gradient, with concomitant production of heat [177]. The discovery that adult individuals also have BAT depots [178] and that thermogenic stimulation can also induce the development "beige" adipocytes (WAT adipocytes expressing UCP1), in a process designated by WAT "browning" [179], has caught the attention of pharmaceutical and nutraceutical industries due to the possibility of counteracting the development of obesity by thermogenesis stimulation through increasing basal EE. In fact, beige adipocytes seem to have an adaptive phenotype, according to environmental stimulus, functioning as energy depots or as heat producers [180].

Thermogenesis is mainly regulated by the sympathetic nervous system. The release of adrenaline or noradrenaline (NA) and their binding to beta 3-adrenergic receptors in adipocyte membrane stimulates cyclic-AMP production that activates protein kinase A (PKA), increasing lipolysis and UCP1 expression and activity in mitochondria [181]. Fatty acids released during lipolysis are important not only as substrate for oxidation but also regulators of UCP1 proton permeability [182]. Several hormones can also function as stimulators of BAT thermogenesis or WAT browning, such as thyroid hormones, natriuretic peptides, leptin, adiponectin, as well as several cytokines. PGC1alpha is a transcription coactivator that interacts with several transcription factors, including PPARgamma, and regulates many biological processes, including thermogenesis through the promotion of UCP1 expression [183]. AMPK, another important metabolic modulator, increases the expression of PGC1alpha, SIRT1 and UCP1.

After water, tea has been considered the most consumed drink worldwide and it has been attributed several health promoting properties, specially GT. GT is a rich source of polyphenols, specially flavanols, namely catechin and EGCG, but also flavonols. The initial interest regarding polyphenols and GT on thermogenesis regulation was triggered by the discovery that thermogenesis stimulation after GT ingestion by human individuals was superior than expected (24-hour EE increased 4%), taking into account the correspondent caffeine content of GT [184]. Many other studies have been done since then, in order to obtain better results or to understand the molecular processes involved. *In vitro* studies confirm that EGCG inhibits COMT, decreasing NA metabolism and, thus, improves the sympathetic nervous system stimulation and thermogenesis [185]. Choo *et al* observed that the simultaneous ingestion of a HFD and GT by rats decrease fat accumulation, probably by stimulating thermogenesis [186]. Chen *et al* suggested that EGCG may be involved in the aforementioned regulation increasing UCP2 and PPARgamma expression in AT [187]. Theaflavins from black tea are also involved in tea-induced thermogenesis as they were able to increase PGC1alpha and UCP1 genes expression in BAT of mice [188], improving EE. Although human studies regarding the modulation of obesity by GT are not abundant, thermogenesis has been the mechanism of action most studied [189]. The thermogenic potential of products so far experimented in humans vary between 2-5% for most studies [184, 190, 191], suggesting that catechins and caffeine may be important molecules involved in increased EE and that they activate BAT thermogenesis, probably by COMT inhibition [184, 192]. Nevertheless, in a meta-analysis, Hursel *et al* suggested that the thermogenic effects of tea catechins may be more pronounced in the Asian population due to a genetic polymorphism [193], justifying the lack of results sometimes observed in Western populations.

During these years, other polyphenols have also been studied regarding thermogenesis. Resveratrol-treated mice survived longer time in cold conditions and even when fed with HFD had decreased fat deposition and increased thermogenesis, with larger mitochondria and increased expression of SIRT1, PGC1alpha and UCP1 [194]. The AMPK pathway may be also involved in this process and mitochondrial number was elevated after resveratrol treatment [195, 196]. In fact, other authors suggest that the association of resveratrol and quercetin may be more potent in the browning of WAT, increasing the number of multi-locular lipid vacuoles and the expression of UCP1 in rat adipocytes [197]. Myricetin, another polyphenol, improved mouse EE and mitochondrial function by modulation of PGC1alpha, in a process dependent on SIRT1. This effect seems to be tissue-specific and occurs only in BAT and skeletal muscle [198]. Naringenin, a citrus polyphenol, was also capable to increase PPARalpha, PPARgamma and PGC1alpha activity and, thus, UCP1 when administered to mice [199]. The ingestion of soy protein diets, rich in isoflavones, has also been studied as these polyphenols seem promising in the regulation of weight gain. In fact, they increase UCP1 mRNA levels in BAT of rats [200], suggesting that isoflavones may also regulate thermogenesis. Daidzein presents similar effects in rats [201]. Interestingly enough, another isoflavone, genistein, seems to programme 3T3-L1 adipocyte differentiation into beige adipocytes [202], in a process mediated by UCP1 and SIRT1 proteins. Chrysin also induced browning of 3T3-L1 adipocytes, improving PGC1alpha and UCP1 protein levels, in a process dependent on AMPK activation [203]. Proanthocyanidins from grape seed extract were also able to modulate mitochondrial function of BAT in rats, improving thermogenesis, reversing the effects of cafeteria diet in experimental animals, increasing SIRT1 and PGC1alpha gene expression and increasing UCP1 activity [204]. Matsumura *et al* verified that mRNA levels of PGC1alpha and UCP1 increased after ingestion of flavanols from cocoa extract, but not after administration of epicatechin alone in mice [205], suggesting that procyanidins may be the molecules involved in the process. However, other authors demonstrat that flavanols from cocoa are indeed able to increase UCP1 expression in rat BAT, improving thermogenesis and reversing the effects of a HFD [206].

The majority of the results here presented were obtained with experimental animals, and it should be noted that polyphenol metabolism and mechanisms of action differ between human and animals. Also, some authors defend that the *in vivo* concentrations of catechins are not high enough to inhibit COMT activity and observed no impaired enzyme activity after human exposure to high EGCG doses [207]. So, although promising, the results described for animals should be confirmed in clinical trials and the molecular targets involved should be elucidated.

CONCLUDING REMARKS

Data published until now indicate that polyphenols and polyphenol-rich foods, have very interesting properties regarding the management of obesity and weight loss. Several mechanisms involved in these effects have been described:
i) impaired carbohydrate digestion, ii) decreased intestinal glucose absorption,
iii) inhibition of gluconeogenesis, iv) decreased adipogenesis,
v) inhibition of lipogenesis, vi) stimulation of lipolysis,
vii) stimulation of beta-oxidation, viii) modulation of intestinal microflora,
ix) decreased appetite and x) stimulation of thermogenesis.

Nevertheless, the effects described are still subject to debate because human studies are scarce and some results are inconsistent. Further research is needed before recommending the use of polyphenols as regulators of weight and modulators of obesity.

CONSENT FOR PUBLICATION

Not applicable.

CONFLICT OF INTEREST

The authors confirm that this chapter contents have no conflict of interest.

ACKNOWLEDGEMENTS

Declared none.

REFERENCES

[1]   Cooper-Driver GA, Bhattacharya M. Role of phenolics in plant evolution. Phytochemistry 1998; 49(5): 1165-74.

[2]   Hollman PC, Katan MB. Dietary flavonoids: intake, health effects and bioavailability. Food Chem Toxicol 1999; 37(9-10): 937-42.
[http://dx.doi.org/10.1016/S0278-6915(99)00079-4] [PMID: 10541448]

[3]   Kaur C, Kapoor HC. Antioxidants in fruits and vegetables - the millennium's health. Int J Food Sci Technol 2001; 36(7): 703-25.
[http://dx.doi.org/10.1046/j.1365-2621.2001.00513.x]

[4]   Van Duyn MA, Pivonka E. Overview of the health benefits of fruit and vegetable consumption for the dietetics professional: selected literature. J Am Diet Assoc 2000; 100(12): 1511-21.
[http://dx.doi.org/10.1016/S0002-8223(00)00420-X] [PMID: 11138444]

[5]   Rice-Evans C. Flavonoid antioxidants. Curr Med Chem 2001; 8(7): 797-807.
[http://dx.doi.org/10.2174/0929867013373011] [PMID: 11375750]

[6]   Hu JP, Calomme M, Lasure A, *et al*. Structure-activity relationship of flavonoids with superoxide scavenging activity. Biol Trace Elem Res 1995; 47(1-3): 327-31.
[http://dx.doi.org/10.1007/BF02790134] [PMID: 7779566]

[7]   Rice-Evans CA, Miller NJ, Paganga G. Structure-antioxidant activity relationships of flavonoids and phenolic acids. Free Radic Biol Med 1996; 20(7): 933-56.
[http://dx.doi.org/10.1016/0891-5849(95)02227-9] [PMID: 8743980]

[8]   Williamson G, Clifford MN. Role of the small intestine, colon and microbiota in determining the metabolic fate of polyphenols. Biochem Pharmacol 2017; 139: 24-39.
[http://dx.doi.org/10.1016/j.bcp.2017.03.012] [PMID: 28322745]

[9]   Del Rio D, Rodriguez-Mateos A, Spencer JP, Tognolini M, Borges G, Crozier A. Dietary (poly)phenolics in human health: structures, bioavailability, and evidence of protective effects against chronic diseases. Antioxid Redox Signal 2013; 18(14): 1818-92.
[http://dx.doi.org/10.1089/ars.2012.4581] [PMID: 22794138]

[10]   Fraga CG, Galleano M, Verstraeten SV, Oteiza PI. Basic biochemical mechanisms behind the health benefits of polyphenols. Mol Aspects Med 2010; 31(6): 435-45.
[http://dx.doi.org/10.1016/j.mam.2010.09.006] [PMID: 20854840]

[11]   Hollman PC. Unravelling of the health effects of polyphenols is a complex puzzle complicated by metabolism. Arch Biochem Biophys 2014; 559: 100-5.
[http://dx.doi.org/10.1016/j.abb.2014.04.013] [PMID: 24796225]

[12]   Kawai Y, Nishikawa T, Shiba Y, *et al.* Macrophage as a target of quercetin glucuronides in human atherosclerotic arteries: implication in the anti-atherosclerotic mechanism of dietary flavonoids. J Biol Chem 2008; 283(14): 9424-34.
[http://dx.doi.org/10.1074/jbc.M706571200] [PMID: 18199750]

[13]   Wolff H, Motyl M, Hellerbrand C, Heilmann J, Kraus B. Xanthohumol uptake and intracellular kinetics in hepatocytes, hepatic stellate cells, and intestinal cells. J Agric Food Chem 2011; 59(24): 12893-901.
[http://dx.doi.org/10.1021/jf203689z] [PMID: 22088086]

[14]   Manach C, Scalbert A, Morand C, Rémésy C, Jiménez L. Polyphenols: food sources and bioavailability. Am J Clin Nutr 2004; 79(5): 727-47.
[http://dx.doi.org/10.1093/ajcn/79.5.727] [PMID: 15113710]

[15]   Scalbert A, Williamson G. Dietary intake and bioavailability of polyphenols Nutr 2000; (8S Suppl)2073S-85S.

[16]   Bravo L. Polyphenols: chemistry, dietary sources, metabolism, and nutritional significance. Nutr Rev 1998; 56(11): 317-33.
[http://dx.doi.org/10.1111/j.1753-4887.1998.tb01670.x] [PMID: 9838798]

[17]   Zamora-Ros R, Knaze V, Luján-Barroso L, *et al.* Differences in dietary intakes, food sources and determinants of total flavonoids between Mediterranean and non-Mediterranean countries participating in the European Prospective Investigation into Cancer and Nutrition (EPIC) study. Br J Nutr 2013; 109(8): 1498-507.
[http://dx.doi.org/10.1017/S0007114512003273] [PMID: 22980437]

[18]   Kim K, Vance TM, Chun OK. Estimated intake and major food sources of flavonoids among US adults: changes between 1999-2002 and 2007-2010 in NHANES. Eur J Nutr 2016; 55(2): 833-43.
[http://dx.doi.org/10.1007/s00394-015-0942-x] [PMID: 26026481]

[19]   Fernandes I, Faria A, Calhau C, de Freitas V, Mateus N. Bioavailability of anthocyanins and derivatives. J Funct Foods 2014; 7 (Suppl. C): 54-66.
[http://dx.doi.org/10.1016/j.jff.2013.05.010]

[20]   Fernandes I, Faria A, de Freitas V, Calhau C, Mateus N. Multiple-approach studies to assess anthocyanin bioavailability. Phytochem Rev 2015; 14(6): 899-919.
[http://dx.doi.org/10.1007/s11101-015-9415-3]

[21]   Rubió L, Macià A, Motilva MJ. Impact of various factors on pharmacokinetics of bioactive polyphenols: an overview. Curr Drug Metab 2014; 15(1): 62-76.
[http://dx.doi.org/10.2174/1389200214666131210144115] [PMID: 24328690]

[22]   Faria A, Fernandes I, Mateus N, Calhau C. Bioavailability of Anthocyanins.Natural Products: Phytochemistry, Botany and Metabolism of Alkaloids, Phenolics and Terpenes. Berlin, Heidelberg: Springer Berlin Heidelberg 2013; pp. 2465-87.
[http://dx.doi.org/10.1007/978-3-642-22144-6_75]

[23]   Silva MS, García-Estévez I, Brandão E, Mateus N, de Freitas V, Soares S. Molecular Interaction Between Salivary Proteins and Food Tannins. J Agric Food Chem 2017; 65(31): 6415-24.
[http://dx.doi.org/10.1021/acs.jafc.7b01722] [PMID: 28589723]

[24]   Soares S, Vitorino R, Osório H, *et al.* Reactivity of human salivary proteins families toward food polyphenols. J Agric Food Chem 2011; 59(10): 5535-47.
[http://dx.doi.org/10.1021/jf104975d] [PMID: 21417408]

[25]   Spencer JP. Metabolism of tea flavonoids in the gastrointestinal tract. J Nutr 2003; 133(10): 3255S-61S.

[http://dx.doi.org/10.1093/jn/133.10.3255S] [PMID: 14519823]

[26]   Ferrer-Gallego R, Soares S, Mateus N, Rivas-Gonzalo J, Escribano-Bailón MT, de Freitas V. New Anthocyanin-Human Salivary Protein Complexes. Langmuir 2015; 31(30): 8392-401.
[http://dx.doi.org/10.1021/acs.langmuir.5b01122] [PMID: 26162056]

[27]   García-Estévez I, Cruz L, Oliveira J, Mateus N, de Freitas V, Soares S. First evidences of interaction between pyranoanthocyanins and salivary proline-rich proteins. Food Chem 2017; 228: 574-81.
[http://dx.doi.org/10.1016/j.foodchem.2017.02.030] [PMID: 28317766]

[28]   Mallery SR, Budendorf DE, Larsen MP, *et al.* Effects of human oral mucosal tissue, saliva, and oral microflora on intraoral metabolism and bioactivation of black raspberry anthocyanins. Cancer Prev Res (Phila) 2011; 4(8): 1209-21.
[http://dx.doi.org/10.1158/1940-6207.CAPR-11-0040] [PMID: 21558412]

[29]   Boyer J, Brown D, Liu RH. In vitro digestion and lactase treatment influence uptake of quercetin and quercetin glucoside by the Caco-2 cell monolayer. Nutr J 2005; 4: 1.
[http://dx.doi.org/10.1186/1475-2891-4-1] [PMID: 15644141]

[30]   Tagliazucchi D, Verzelloni E, Bertolini D, Conte A. In vitro bio-accessibility and antioxidant activity of grape polyphenols. Food Chem 2010; 120(2): 7.
[http://dx.doi.org/10.1016/j.foodchem.2009.10.030]

[31]   Record IR, Lane JM. Simulated intestinal digestion of green and black teas. Food Chem 2001; 73(4): 481-6.
[http://dx.doi.org/10.1016/S0308-8146(01)00131-5]

[32]   Spencer JP, Chaudry F, Pannala AS, Srai SK, Debnam E, Rice-Evans C. Decomposition of cocoa procyanidins in the gastric milieu. Biochem Biophys Res Commun 2000; 272(1): 236-41.
[http://dx.doi.org/10.1006/bbrc.2000.2749] [PMID: 10872833]

[33]   Rios LY, Bennett RN, Lazarus SA, Rémésy C, Scalbert A, Williamson G. Cocoa procyanidins are stable during gastric transit in humans. Am J Clin Nutr 2002; 76(5): 1106-10.
[http://dx.doi.org/10.1093/ajcn/76.5.1106] [PMID: 12399286]

[34]   Stoupi S, Williamson G, Viton F, *et al.* In vivo bioavailability, absorption, excretion, and pharmacokinetics of [14C]procyanidin B2 in male rats. Drug Metab Dispos 2010; 38(2): 287-91.
[http://dx.doi.org/10.1124/dmd.109.030304] [PMID: 19910517]

[35]   Passamonti S, Vrhovsek U, Vanzo A, Mattivi F. The stomach as a site for anthocyanins absorption from food. FEBS Lett 2003; 544(1-3): 210-3.
[http://dx.doi.org/10.1016/S0014-5793(03)00504-0] [PMID: 12782318]

[36]   Talavéra S, Felgines C, Texier O, Besson C, Lamaison JL, Rémésy C. Anthocyanins are efficiently absorbed from the stomach in anesthetized rats. J Nutr 2003; 133(12): 4178-82.
[http://dx.doi.org/10.1093/jn/133.12.4178] [PMID: 14652368]

[37]   El Mohsen MA, Marks J, Kuhnle G, *et al.* Absorption, tissue distribution and excretion of pelargonidin and its metabolites following oral administration to rats. Br J Nutr 2006; 95(1): 51-8.
[http://dx.doi.org/10.1079/BJN20051596] [PMID: 16441916]

[38]   Felgines C, Talavéra S, Texier O, *et al.* Absorption and metabolism of red orange juice anthocyanins in rats. Br J Nutr 2006; 95(5): 898-904.
[http://dx.doi.org/10.1079/BJN20061728] [PMID: 16611379]

[39]   Talavéra S, Felgines C, Texier O, *et al.* Anthocyanin metabolism in rats and their distribution to digestive area, kidney, and brain. J Agric Food Chem 2005; 53(10): 3902-8.
[http://dx.doi.org/10.1021/jf050145v] [PMID: 15884815]

[40]   Battiston L, Macagno A, Passamonti S, Micali F, Sottocasa GL. Specific sequence-directed anti-bilitranslocase antibodies as a tool to detect potentially bilirubin-binding proteins in different tissues of the rat. FEBS Lett 1999; 453(3): 351-5.
[http://dx.doi.org/10.1016/S0014-5793(99)00736-X] [PMID: 10405174]

[41] Nicolin V, Grill V, Micali F, Narducci P, Passamonti S. Immunolocalisation of bilitranslocase in mucosecretory and parietal cells of the rat gastric mucosa. J Mol Histol 2005; 36(1-2): 45-50.
[http://dx.doi.org/10.1007/s10735-004-2920-0] [PMID: 15703998]

[42] Yoshikawa T, Inoue R, Matsumoto M, Yajima T, Ushida K, Iwanaga T. Comparative expression of hexose transporters (SGLT1, GLUT1, GLUT2 and GLUT5) throughout the mouse gastrointestinal tract. Histochem Cell Biol 2011; 135(2): 183-94.
[http://dx.doi.org/10.1007/s00418-011-0779-1] [PMID: 21274556]

[43] Eraly SA, Bush KT, Sampogna RV, Bhatnagar V, Nigam SK. The molecular pharmacology of organic anion transporters: from DNA to FDA? Mol Pharmacol 2004; 65(3): 479-87.
[http://dx.doi.org/10.1124/mol.65.3.479] [PMID: 14978224]

[44] Garcia CK, Brown MS, Pathak RK, Goldstein JL. cDNA cloning of MCT2, a second monocarboxylate transporter expressed in different cells than MCT1. J Biol Chem 1995; 270(4): 1843-9.
[http://dx.doi.org/10.1074/jbc.270.4.1843] [PMID: 7829520]

[45] Oliveira H, Fernandes I, Brás NF, *et al.* Experimental and Theoretical Data on the Mechanism by Which Red Wine Anthocyanins Are Transported through a Human MKN-28 Gastric Cell Model. J Agric Food Chem 2015; 63(35): 7685-92.
[http://dx.doi.org/10.1021/acs.jafc.5b00412] [PMID: 25858301]

[46] Crespy V, Morand C, Besson C, Manach C, Demigne C, Remesy C. Quercetin, but not its glycosides, is absorbed from the rat stomach. J Agric Food Chem 2002; 50(3): 618-21.
[http://dx.doi.org/10.1021/jf010919h] [PMID: 11804539]

[47] Piskula MK, Yamakoshi J, Iwai Y. Daidzein and genistein but not their glucosides are absorbed from the rat stomach. FEBS Lett 1999; 447(2-3): 287-91.
[http://dx.doi.org/10.1016/S0014-5793(99)00307-5] [PMID: 10214963]

[48] Konishi Y, Zhao Z, Shimizu M. Phenolic acids are absorbed from the rat stomach with different absorption rates. J Agric Food Chem 2006; 54(20): 7539-43.
[http://dx.doi.org/10.1021/jf061554+] [PMID: 17002419]

[49] Lafay S, Gil-Izquierdo A, Manach C, Morand C, Besson C, Scalbert A. Chlorogenic acid is absorbed in its intact form in the stomach of rats. J Nutr 2006; 136(5): 1192-7.
[http://dx.doi.org/10.1093/jn/136.5.1192] [PMID: 16614403]

[50] Vanzo A, Cecotti R, Vrhovsek U, Torres AM, Mattivi F, Passamonti S. The fate of trans-caftaric acid administered into the rat stomach. J Agric Food Chem 2007; 55(4): 1604-11.
[http://dx.doi.org/10.1021/jf0626819] [PMID: 17300159]

[51] Zhao Z, Egashira Y, Sanada H. Ferulic acid is quickly absorbed from rat stomach as the free form and then conjugated mainly in liver. J Nutr 2004; 134(11): 3083-8.
[http://dx.doi.org/10.1093/jn/134.11.3083] [PMID: 15514279]

[52] Harris RM, Picton R, Singh S, Waring RH. Activity of phenolsulfotransferases in the human gastrointestinal tract. Life Sci 2000; 67(17): 2051-7.
[http://dx.doi.org/10.1016/S0024-3205(00)00791-8] [PMID: 11057755]

[53] Strassburg CP, Nguyen N, Manns MP, Tukey RH. Polymorphic expression of the UDP-glucuronosyltransferase UGT1A gene locus in human gastric epithelium. Mol Pharmacol 1998; 54(4): 647-54.
[PMID: 9765507]

[54] Strassburg CP, Oldhafer K, Manns MP, Tukey RH. Differential expression of the UGT1A locus in human liver, biliary, and gastric tissue: identification of UGT1A7 and UGT1A10 transcripts in extrahepatic tissue. Mol Pharmacol 1997; 52(2): 212-20.
[http://dx.doi.org/10.1124/mol.52.2.212] [PMID: 9271343]

[55] Karhunen T, Tilgmann C, Ulmanen I, Julkunen I, Panula P. Distribution of catechol--methyltransferase enzyme in rat tissues. J Histochem Cytochem 1994; 42(8): 1079-90.

[http://dx.doi.org/10.1177/42.8.8027527] [PMID: 8027527]

[56]   Déchelotte P, Varrentrapp M, Meyer HJ, Schwenk M. Conjugation of 1-naphthol in human gastric epithelial cells. Gut 1993; 34(2): 177-80.
[http://dx.doi.org/10.1136/gut.34.2.177] [PMID: 8432468]

[57]   Vallejo F, Larrosa M, Escudero E, *et al.* Concentration and solubility of flavanones in orange beverages affect their bioavailability in humans. J Agric Food Chem 2010; 58(10): 6516-24.
[http://dx.doi.org/10.1021/jf100752j] [PMID: 20441150]

[58]   Actis-Goretta L, Dew TP, Lévèques A, *et al.* Gastrointestinal absorption and metabolism of hesperetin-7-O-rutinoside and hesperetin-7-O-glucoside in healthy humans. Mol Nutr Food Res 2015; 59(9): 1651-62.
[http://dx.doi.org/10.1002/mnfr.201500202] [PMID: 26018925]

[59]   Takumi H, Mukai R, Ishiduka S, Kometani T, Terao J. Tissue distribution of hesperetin in rats after a dietary intake. Biosci Biotechnol Biochem 2011; 75(8): 1608-10.
[http://dx.doi.org/10.1271/bbb.110157] [PMID: 21821945]

[60]   Rhodes MJC, Price KR. Analytical problems in the study of flavonoid compounds in onions. Food Chem 1996; 57(1): 113-7.
[http://dx.doi.org/10.1016/0308-8146(96)00147-1]

[61]   Price KR, Prosser T, Richetin AMF, Rhodes MJC. A comparison of the flavonol content and composition in dessert, cooking and cider-making apples; distribution within the fruit and effect of juicing. Food Chem 1999; 66(4): 489-94.
[http://dx.doi.org/10.1016/S0308-8146(99)00099-0]

[62]   Price KR, Rhodes MJC, Barnes KA. Flavonol Glycoside Content and Composition of Tea Infusions Made from Commercially Available Teas and Tea Products. J Agric Food Chem 1998; 46(7): 2517-22.
[http://dx.doi.org/10.1021/jf9800211]

[63]   Lommen A, Godejohann M, Venema DP, Hollman PC, Spraul M. Application of directly coupled HPLC-NMR-MS to the identification and confirmation of quercetin glycosides and phloretin glycosides in apple peel. Anal Chem 2000; 72(8): 1793-7.
[http://dx.doi.org/10.1021/ac9912303] [PMID: 10784143]

[64]   Hollman PC, Bijsman MN, van Gameren Y, Cnossen EP, de Vries JH, Katan MB. The sugar moiety is a major determinant of the absorption of dietary flavonoid glycosides in man. Free Radic Res 1999; 31(6): 569-73.
[http://dx.doi.org/10.1080/10715769900301141] [PMID: 10630681]

[65]   Hollman PC, van Trijp JM, Buysman MN, *et al.* Relative bioavailability of the antioxidant flavonoid quercetin from various foods in man. FEBS Lett 1997; 418(1-2): 152-6.
[http://dx.doi.org/10.1016/S0014-5793(97)01367-7] [PMID: 9414116]

[66]   Kwon O, Eck P, Chen S, *et al.* Inhibition of the intestinal glucose transporter GLUT2 by flavonoids. FASEB J 2007; 21(2): 366-77.
[http://dx.doi.org/10.1096/fj.06-6620com] [PMID: 17172639]

[67]   Strobel P, Allard C, Perez-Acle T, Calderon R, Aldunate R, Leighton F. Myricetin, quercetin and catechin-gallate inhibit glucose uptake in isolated rat adipocytes. Biochem J 2005; 386(Pt 3): 471-8.
[http://dx.doi.org/10.1042/BJ20040703] [PMID: 15469417]

[68]   Cunningham P, Afzal-Ahmed I, Naftalin RJ. Docking studies show that D-glucose and quercetin slide through the transporter GLUT1. J Biol Chem 2006; 281(9): 5797-803.
[http://dx.doi.org/10.1074/jbc.M509422200] [PMID: 16407180]

[69]   Talavéra S, Felgines C, Texier O, *et al.* Anthocyanins are efficiently absorbed from the small intestine in rats. J Nutr 2004; 134(9): 2275-9.
[http://dx.doi.org/10.1093/jn/134.9.2275] [PMID: 15333716]

[70]   Miyazawa T, Nakagawa K, Kudo M, Muraishi K, Someya K. Direct intestinal absorption of red fruit anthocyanins, cyanidin-3-glucoside and cyanidin-3,5-diglucoside, into rats and humans. J Agric Food Chem 1999; 47(3): 1083-91.
[http://dx.doi.org/10.1021/jf9809582] [PMID: 10552420]

[71]   Tsuda T, Horio F, Osawa T. Absorption and metabolism of cyanidin 3-O-β-D-glucoside in rats. FEBS Lett 1999; 449(2-3): 179-82.
[http://dx.doi.org/10.1016/S0014-5793(99)00407-X] [PMID: 10338127]

[72]   Faria A, Pestana D, Azevedo J, *et al.* Absorption of anthocyanins through intestinal epithelial cells - Putative involvement of GLUT2. Mol Nutr Food Res 2009; 53(11): 1430-7.
[http://dx.doi.org/10.1002/mnfr.200900007] [PMID: 19785001]

[73]   Zou TB, Feng D, Song G, Li HW, Tang HW, Ling WH. The role of sodium-dependent glucose transporter 1 and glucose transporter 2 in the absorption of cyanidin-3-o-β-glucoside in Caco-2 cells. Nutrients 2014; 6(10): 4165-77.
[http://dx.doi.org/10.3390/nu6104165] [PMID: 25314643]

[74]   de Pascual-Teresa S, Santos-Buelga C, Rivas-Gonzalo JC. Quantitative analysis of flavan-3-ols in Spanish foodstuffs and beverages. J Agric Food Chem 2000; 48(11): 5331-7.
[http://dx.doi.org/10.1021/jf000549h] [PMID: 11087482]

[75]   Kuhnle G, Spencer JP, Schroeter H, *et al.* Epicatechin and catechin are O-methylated and glucuronidated in the small intestine. Biochem Biophys Res Commun 2000; 277(2): 507-12.
[http://dx.doi.org/10.1006/bbrc.2000.3701] [PMID: 11032751]

[76]   Olthof MR, Hollman PC, Katan MB. Chlorogenic acid and caffeic acid are absorbed in humans. J Nutr 2001; 131(1): 66-71.
[http://dx.doi.org/10.1093/jn/131.1.66] [PMID: 11208940]

[77]   da Encarnação JA, Farrell TL, Ryder A, Kraut NU, Williamson G. In vitro enzymic hydrolysis of chlorogenic acids in coffee. Mol Nutr Food Res 2015; 59(2): 231-9.
[http://dx.doi.org/10.1002/mnfr.201400498] [PMID: 25380542]

[78]   Ichiyanagi T, Rahman MM, Kashiwada Y, *et al.* Absorption and metabolism of delphinidin 3-O--D-glucopyranoside in rats. Free Radic Biol Med 2004; 36(7): 930-7.
[http://dx.doi.org/10.1016/j.freeradbiomed.2004.01.005] [PMID: 15019977]

[79]   Ichiyanagi T, Shida Y, Rahman MM, Hatano Y, Konishi T. Extended glucuronidation is another major path of cyanidin 3-O-β-D-glucopyranoside metabolism in rats. J Agric Food Chem 2005; 53(18): 7312-9.
[http://dx.doi.org/10.1021/jf051002b] [PMID: 16131148]

[80]   Ichiyanagi T, Shida Y, Rahman MM, *et al.* Metabolic pathway of cyanidin 3-O-β-D-glucopyranoside in rats. J Agric Food Chem 2005; 53(1): 145-50.
[http://dx.doi.org/10.1021/jf0485943] [PMID: 15631521]

[81]   McGhie TK, Ainge GD, Barnett LE, Cooney JM, Jensen DJ. Anthocyanin glycosides from berry fruit are absorbed and excreted unmetabolized by both humans and rats. J Agric Food Chem 2003; 51(16): 4539-48.
[http://dx.doi.org/10.1021/jf026206w] [PMID: 14705874]

[82]   Stalmach A, Mullen W, Barron D, *et al.* Metabolite profiling of hydroxycinnamate derivatives in plasma and urine after the ingestion of coffee by humans: identification of biomarkers of coffee consumption. Drug Metab Dispos 2009; 37(8): 1749-58.
[http://dx.doi.org/10.1124/dmd.109.028019] [PMID: 19460943]

[83]   Alvarez AI, Real R, Pérez M, Mendoza G, Prieto JG, Merino G. Modulation of the activity of ABC transporters (P-glycoprotein, MRP2, BCRP) by flavonoids and drug response. J Pharm Sci 2010; 99(2): 598-617.
[http://dx.doi.org/10.1002/jps.21851] [PMID: 19544374]

[84]   Brand W, Schutte ME, Williamson G, *et al*. Flavonoid-mediated inhibition of intestinal ABC transporters may affect the oral bioavailability of drugs, food-borne toxic compounds and bioactive ingredients. Biomed Pharmacother 2006; 60(9): 508-19.
[http://dx.doi.org/10.1016/j.biopha.2006.07.081] [PMID: 16978825]

[85]   van de Wetering K, Burkon A, Feddema W, *et al*. Intestinal breast cancer resistance protein (BCRP)/Bcrp1 and multidrug resistance protein 3 (MRP3)/Mrp3 are involved in the pharmacokinetics of resveratrol. Mol Pharmacol 2009; 75(4): 876-85.
[http://dx.doi.org/10.1124/mol.108.052019] [PMID: 19114588]

[86]   Kaldas MI, Walle UK, Walle T. Resveratrol transport and metabolism by human intestinal Caco-2 cells. J Pharm Pharmacol 2003; 55(3): 307-12.
[http://dx.doi.org/10.1211/002235702612] [PMID: 12724035]

[87]   Nait Chabane M, Al Ahmad A, Peluso J, Muller CD, Ubeaud G. Quercetin and naringenin transport across human intestinal Caco-2 cells. J Pharm Pharmacol 2009; 61(11): 1473-83.
[http://dx.doi.org/10.1211/jpp.61.11.0006] [PMID: 19903372]

[88]   Williamson G, Aeberli I, Miguet L, *et al*. Interaction of positional isomers of quercetin glucuronides with the transporter ABCC2 (cMOAT, MRP2). Drug Metab Dispos 2007; 35(8): 1262-8.
[http://dx.doi.org/10.1124/dmd.106.014241] [PMID: 17478601]

[89]   Aura A-M. Microbial metabolism of dietary phenolic compounds in the colon. Phytochem Rev 2008; 7(3): 407-29.
[http://dx.doi.org/10.1007/s11101-008-9095-3]

[90]   Cani PD, Delzenne NM. The role of the gut microbiota in energy metabolism and metabolic disease. Curr Pharm Des 2009; 15(13): 1546-58.
[http://dx.doi.org/10.2174/138161209788168164] [PMID: 19442172]

[91]   Sekirov I, Russell SL, Antunes LC, Finlay BB. Gut microbiota in health and disease. Physiol Rev 2010; 90(3): 859-904.
[http://dx.doi.org/10.1152/physrev.00045.2009] [PMID: 20664075]

[92]   Moreira AP, Texeira TF, Ferreira AB, Peluzio MdoC, Alfenas RdeC. Influence of a high-fat diet on gut microbiota, intestinal permeability and metabolic endotoxaemia. Br J Nutr 2012; 108(5): 801-9.
[http://dx.doi.org/10.1017/S0007114512001213] [PMID: 22717075]

[93]   Cani PD, Amar J, Iglesias MA, *et al*. Metabolic endotoxemia initiates obesity and insulin resistance. Diabetes 2007; 56(7): 1761-72.
[http://dx.doi.org/10.2337/db06-1491] [PMID: 17456850]

[94]   Armougom F, Henry M, Vialettes B, Raccah D, Raoult D. Monitoring bacterial community of human gut microbiota reveals an increase in Lactobacillus in obese patients and Methanogens in anorexic patients. PLoS One 2009; 4(9)e7125
[http://dx.doi.org/10.1371/journal.pone.0007125] [PMID: 19774074]

[95]   Ley RE, Turnbaugh PJ, Klein S, Gordon JI. Microbial ecology: human gut microbes associated with obesity. Nature 2006; 444(7122): 1022-3.
[http://dx.doi.org/10.1038/4441022a] [PMID: 17183309]

[96]   Ley RE, Bäckhed F, Turnbaugh P, Lozupone CA, Knight RD, Gordon JI. Obesity alters gut microbial ecology. Proc Natl Acad Sci USA 2005; 102(31): 11070-5.
[http://dx.doi.org/10.1073/pnas.0504978102] [PMID: 16033867]

[97]   Mathur R, Barlow GM. Obesity and the microbiome. Expert Rev Gastroenterol Hepatol 2015; 9(8): 1087-99.
[http://dx.doi.org/10.1586/17474124.2015.1051029] [PMID: 26082274]

[98]   Turnbaugh PJ, Ley RE, Mahowald MA, Magrini V, Mardis ER, Gordon JI. An obesity-associated gut microbiome with increased capacity for energy harvest. Nature 2006; 444(7122): 1027-31.
[http://dx.doi.org/10.1038/nature05414] [PMID: 17183312]

[99] González-Castejón M, Rodriguez-Casado A. Dietary phytochemicals and their potential effects on obesity: a review. Pharmacol Res 2011; 64(5): 438-55.
[http://dx.doi.org/10.1016/j.phrs.2011.07.004] [PMID: 21798349]

[100] Meydani M, Hasan ST. Dietary polyphenols and obesity. Nutrients 2010; 2(7): 737-51.
[http://dx.doi.org/10.3390/nu2070737] [PMID: 22254051]

[101] Selma MV, Espín JC, Tomás-Barberán FA. Interaction between phenolics and gut microbiota: role in human health. J Agric Food Chem 2009; 57(15): 6485-501.
[http://dx.doi.org/10.1021/jf902107d] [PMID: 19580283]

[102] Parkar SG, Trower TM, Stevenson DE. Fecal microbial metabolism of polyphenols and its effects on human gut microbiota. Anaerobe 2013; 23: 12-9.
[http://dx.doi.org/10.1016/j.anaerobe.2013.07.009] [PMID: 23916722]

[103] Rastmanesh R. High polyphenol, low probiotic diet for weight loss because of intestinal microbiota interaction. Chem Biol Interact 2011; 189(1-2): 1-8.
[http://dx.doi.org/10.1016/j.cbi.2010.10.002] [PMID: 20955691]

[104] Hidalgo M, Oruna-Concha MJ, Kolida S, *et al.* Metabolism of anthocyanins by human gut microflora and their influence on gut bacterial growth. J Agric Food Chem 2012; 60(15): 3882-90.
[http://dx.doi.org/10.1021/jf3002153] [PMID: 22439618]

[105] Espley RV, Butts CA, Laing WA, *et al.* Dietary flavonoids from modified apple reduce inflammation markers and modulate gut microbiota in mice. J Nutr 2014; 144(2): 146-54.
[http://dx.doi.org/10.3945/jn.113.182659] [PMID: 24353343]

[106] Vendrame S, Guglielmetti S, Riso P, Arioli S, Klimis-Zacas D, Porrini M. Six-week consumption of a wild blueberry powder drink increases bifidobacteria in the human gut. J Agric Food Chem 2011; 59(24): 12815-20.
[http://dx.doi.org/10.1021/jf2028686] [PMID: 22060186]

[107] Queipo-Ortuño MI, Boto-Ordóñez M, Murri M, *et al.* Influence of red wine polyphenols and ethanol on the gut microbiota ecology and biochemical biomarkers. Am J Clin Nutr 2012; 95(6): 1323-34.
[http://dx.doi.org/10.3945/ajcn.111.027847] [PMID: 22552027]

[108] Magistrelli D, Zanchi R, Malagutti L, Galassi G, Canzi E, Rosi F. Effects of Cocoa Husk Feeding on the Composition of Swine Intestinal Microbiota. J Agric Food Chem 2016; 64(10): 2046-52.
[http://dx.doi.org/10.1021/acs.jafc.5b05732] [PMID: 26877143]

[109] Jang S, Sun J, Chen P, *et al.* Flavanol-Enriched Cocoa Powder Alters the Intestinal Microbiota, Tissue and Fluid Metabolite Profiles, and Intestinal Gene Expression in Pigs. J Nutr 2016; 146(4): 673-80.
[http://dx.doi.org/10.3945/jn.115.222968] [PMID: 26936136]

[110] Larrosa M, González-Sarrías A, Yáñez-Gascón MJ, *et al.* Anti-inflammatory properties of a pomegranate extract and its metabolite urolithin-A in a colitis rat model and the effect of colon inflammation on phenolic metabolism. J Nutr Biochem 2010; 21(8): 717-25.
[http://dx.doi.org/10.1016/j.jnutbio.2009.04.012] [PMID: 19616930]

[111] Zhang Y, Zhang H. Microbiota associated with type 2 diabetes and its related complications. Food Sci Hum Wellness 2013; 2(3): 167-72.
[http://dx.doi.org/10.1016/j.fshw.2013.09.002]

[112] Etxeberria U, Arias N, Boqué N, *et al.* Metabolic faecal fingerprinting of trans-resveratrol and quercetin following a high-fat sucrose dietary model using liquid chromatography coupled to high-resolution mass spectrometry. Food Funct 2015; 6(8): 2758-67.
[http://dx.doi.org/10.1039/C5FO00473J] [PMID: 26156396]

[113] Qiao Y, Sun J, Xia S, Tang X, Shi Y, Le G. Effects of resveratrol on gut microbiota and fat storage in a mouse model with high-fat-induced obesity. Food Funct 2014; 5(6): 1241-9.
[http://dx.doi.org/10.1039/c3fo60630a] [PMID: 24722352]

[114] Masumoto S, Terao A, Yamamoto Y, Mukai T, Miura T, Shoji T. Non-absorbable apple procyanidins prevent obesity associated with gut microbial and metabolomic changes. Sci Rep 2016; 6: 31208.
[http://dx.doi.org/10.1038/srep31208] [PMID: 27506289]

[115] Landete JM. Updated knowledge about polyphenols: functions, bioavailability, metabolism, and health. Crit Rev Food Sci Nutr 2012; 52(10): 936-48.
[http://dx.doi.org/10.1080/10408398.2010.513779] [PMID: 22747081]

[116] Kim Y, Keogh JB, Clifton PM. Polyphenols and Glycemic Control. Nutrients 2016; 8(1)E17
[http://dx.doi.org/10.3390/nu8010017] [PMID: 26742071]

[117] Williamson G. Possible effects of dietary polyphenols on sugar absorption and digestion. Mol Nutr Food Res 2013; 57(1): 48-57.
[http://dx.doi.org/10.1002/mnfr.201200511] [PMID: 23180627]

[118] Janssens PL, Hursel R, Westerterp-Plantenga MS. Nutraceuticals for body-weight management: The role of green tea catechins. Physiol Behav 2016; 162: 83-7.
[http://dx.doi.org/10.1016/j.physbeh.2016.01.044] [PMID: 26836279]

[119] Wang S, Moustaid-Moussa N, Chen L, *et al.* Novel insights of dietary polyphenols and obesity. J Nutr Biochem 2014; 25(1): 1-18.
[http://dx.doi.org/10.1016/j.jnutbio.2013.09.001] [PMID: 24314860]

[120] Azevedo MF, Lima CF, Fernandes-Ferreira M, Almeida MJ, Wilson JM, Pereira-Wilson C. Rosmarinic acid, major phenolic constituent of Greek sage herbal tea, modulates rat intestinal SGLT1 levels with effects on blood glucose. Mol Nutr Food Res 2011; 55 (Suppl. 1): S15-25.
[http://dx.doi.org/10.1002/mnfr.201000472] [PMID: 21433280]

[121] Dyer J, Wood IS, Palejwala A, Ellis A, Shirazi-Beechey SP. Expression of monosaccharide transporters in intestine of diabetic humans. Am J Physiol Gastrointest Liver Physiol 2002; 282(2): G241-8.
[http://dx.doi.org/10.1152/ajpgi.00310.2001] [PMID: 11804845]

[122] Aydin S. A comparison of ghrelin, glucose, alpha-amylase and protein levels in saliva from diabetics. J Biochem Mol Biol 2007; 40(1): 29-35.
[PMID: 17244479]

[123] Hara Y, Honda M. The Inhibition of α-Amylase by Tea Polyphenols. Agric Biol Chem 1990; 54(8): 1939-45.
[http://dx.doi.org/10.1080/00021369.1990.10870239]

[124] Narita Y, Inouye K. Kinetic analysis and mechanism on the inhibition of chlorogenic acid and its components against porcine pancreas alpha-amylase isozymes I and II. J Agric Food Chem 2009; 57(19): 9218-25.
[http://dx.doi.org/10.1021/jf9017383] [PMID: 19807164]

[125] McDougall GJ, Stewart D. The inhibitory effects of berry polyphenols on digestive enzymes. Biofactors 2005; 23(4): 189-95.
[http://dx.doi.org/10.1002/biof.5520230403] [PMID: 16498205]

[126] Gee JM, DuPont MS, Rhodes MJ, Johnson IT. Quercetin glucosides interact with the intestinal glucose transport pathway. Free Radic Biol Med 1998; 25(1): 19-25.
[http://dx.doi.org/10.1016/S0891-5849(98)00020-3] [PMID: 9655517]

[127] Cermak R, Landgraf S, Wolffram S. Quercetin glucosides inhibit glucose uptake into brush-borde--membrane vesicles of porcine jejunum. Br J Nutr 2004; 91(6): 849-55.
[http://dx.doi.org/10.1079/BJN20041128] [PMID: 15182388]

[128] Johnston K, Sharp P, Clifford M, Morgan L. Dietary polyphenols decrease glucose uptake by human intestinal Caco-2 cells. FEBS Lett 2005; 579(7): 1653-7.
[http://dx.doi.org/10.1016/j.febslet.2004.12.099] [PMID: 15757656]

[129]   Madiraju AK, Erion DM, Rahimi Y, *et al.* Metformin suppresses gluconeogenesis by inhibiting mitochondrial glycerophosphate dehydrogenase. Nature 2014; 510(7506): 542-6.
[http://dx.doi.org/10.1038/nature13270] [PMID: 24847880]

[130]   Lima CF, Azevedo MF, Araujo R, Fernandes-Ferreira M, Pereira-Wilson C. Metformin-like effect of Salvia officinalis (common sage): is it useful in diabetes prevention? Br J Nutr 2006; 96(2): 326-33.
[http://dx.doi.org/10.1079/BJN20061832] [PMID: 16923227]

[131]   Desvergne B, Michalik L, Wahli W. Transcriptional regulation of metabolism. Physiol Rev 2006; 86(2): 465-514.
[http://dx.doi.org/10.1152/physrev.00025.2005] [PMID: 16601267]

[132]   Moseti D, Regassa A, Kim WK. Molecular Regulation of Adipogenesis and Potential Anti-Adipogenic Bioactive Molecules. Int J Mol Sci 2016; 17(1)E124
[http://dx.doi.org/10.3390/ijms17010124] [PMID: 26797605]

[133]   Ji Q. Treatment Strategy for Type 2 Diabetes with Obesity: Focus on Glucagon-like Peptide-1 Receptor Agonists. Clin Ther 2017; 39(6): 1244-64.
[http://dx.doi.org/10.1016/j.clinthera.2017.03.013] [PMID: 28526416]

[134]   Feng S, Reuss L, Wang Y. Potential of Natural Products in the Inhibition of Adipogenesis through Regulation of PPARγ Expression and/or Its Transcriptional Activity. Molecules 2016; 21(10)E1278
[http://dx.doi.org/10.3390/molecules21101278] [PMID: 27669202]

[135]   Carling D. AMPK signalling in health and disease. Curr Opin Cell Biol 2017; 45: 31-7.
[http://dx.doi.org/10.1016/j.ceb.2017.01.005] [PMID: 28232179]

[136]   Hu E, Kim JB, Sarraf P, Spiegelman BM. Inhibition of adipogenesis through MAP kinase-mediated phosphorylation of PPARgamma. Science 1996; 274(5295): 2100-3.
[http://dx.doi.org/10.1126/science.274.5295.2100] [PMID: 8953045]

[137]   Diradourian C, Girard J, Pégorier JP. Phosphorylation of PPARs: from molecular characterization to physiological relevance. Biochimie 2005; 87(1): 33-8.
[http://dx.doi.org/10.1016/j.biochi.2004.11.010] [PMID: 15733734]

[138]   Baile CA, Yang JY, Rayalam S, *et al.* Effect of resveratrol on fat mobilization. Ann N Y Acad Sci 2011; 1215: 40-7.
[http://dx.doi.org/10.1111/j.1749-6632.2010.05845.x] [PMID: 21261640]

[139]   Hung PF, Wu BT, Chen HC, *et al.* Antimitogenic effect of green tea (-)-epigallocatechin gallate on 3T3-L1 preadipocytes depends on the ERK and Cdk2 pathways. Am J Physiol Cell Physiol 2005; 288(5): C1094-108.
[http://dx.doi.org/10.1152/ajpcell.00569.2004] [PMID: 15647388]

[140]   Czech MP, Tencerova M, Pedersen DJ, Aouadi M. Insulin signalling mechanisms for triacylglycerol storage. Diabetologia 2013; 56(5): 949-64.
[http://dx.doi.org/10.1007/s00125-013-2869-1] [PMID: 23443243]

[141]   Murase T, Misawa K, Minegishi Y, *et al.* Coffee polyphenols suppress diet-induced body fat accumulation by downregulating SREBP-1c and related molecules in C57BL/6J mice. Am J Physiol Endocrinol Metab 2011; 300(1): E122-33.
[http://dx.doi.org/10.1152/ajpendo.00441.2010] [PMID: 20943752]

[142]   Wang GL, Fu YC, Xu WC, Feng YQ, Fang SR, Zhou XH. Resveratrol inhibits the expression of SREBP1 in cell model of steatosis via Sirt1-FOXO1 signaling pathway. Biochem Biophys Res Commun 2009; 380(3): 644-9.
[http://dx.doi.org/10.1016/j.bbrc.2009.01.163] [PMID: 19285015]

[143]   Yogalakshmi B, Sreeja S, Geetha R, Radika MK, Anuradha CV. Grape seed proanthocyanidin rescues rats from steatosis: a comparative and combination study with metformin. J Lipids 2013; 2013153897
[http://dx.doi.org/10.1155/2013/153897] [PMID: 24307947]

[144] Tsuda T, Horio F, Uchida K, Aoki H, Osawa T. Dietary cyanidin 3-O-beta-D-glucoside-rich purple corn color prevents obesity and ameliorates hyperglycemia in mice. J Nutr 2003; 133(7): 2125-30.
[http://dx.doi.org/10.1093/jn/133.7.2125] [PMID: 12840166]

[145] Rupasinghe HP, Sekhon-Loodu S, Mantso T, Panayiotidis MI. Phytochemicals in regulating fatty acid β-oxidation: Potential underlying mechanisms and their involvement in obesity and weight loss. Pharmacol Ther 2016; 165: 153-63.
[http://dx.doi.org/10.1016/j.pharmthera.2016.06.005] [PMID: 27288729]

[146] Sá C, Oliveira AR, Machado C, Azevedo M, Pereira-Wilson C. Effects on Liver Lipid Metabolism of the Naturally Occurring Dietary Flavone Luteolin-7-glucoside. Evid Based Complement Alternat Med 2015; 2015647832
[http://dx.doi.org/10.1155/2015/647832] [PMID: 26113868]

[147] Liu H, Lu HY. Nonalcoholic fatty liver disease and cardiovascular disease. World J Gastroenterol 2014; 20(26): 8407-15.
[http://dx.doi.org/10.3748/wjg.v20.i26.8407] [PMID: 25024598]

[148] Staels B, Fruchart JC. Therapeutic roles of peroxisome proliferator-activated receptor agonists. Diabetes 2005; 54(8): 2460-70.
[http://dx.doi.org/10.2337/diabetes.54.8.2460] [PMID: 16046315]

[149] Burns KA, Vanden Heuvel JP. Modulation of PPAR activity via phosphorylation. Biochim Biophys Acta 2007; 1771(8): 952-60.
[http://dx.doi.org/10.1016/j.bbalip.2007.04.018] [PMID: 17560826]

[150] Rigano D, Sirignano C, Taglialatela-Scafati O. The potential of natural products for targeting PPARα. Acta Pharm Sin B 2017; 7(4): 427-38.
[http://dx.doi.org/10.1016/j.apsb.2017.05.005] [PMID: 28752027]

[151] Aguirre L, Fernández-Quintela A, Arias N, Portillo MP. Resveratrol: anti-obesity mechanisms of action. Molecules 2014; 19(11): 18632-55.
[http://dx.doi.org/10.3390/molecules191118632] [PMID: 25405284]

[152] Liu L, Shan S, Zhang K, Ning ZQ, Lu XP, Cheng YY. Naringenin and hesperetin, two flavonoids derived from Citrus aurantium up-regulate transcription of adiponectin. Phytother Res 2008; 22(10): 1400-3.
[http://dx.doi.org/10.1002/ptr.2504] [PMID: 18690615]

[153] Cho KW, Kim YO, Andrade JE, Burgess JR, Kim YC. Dietary naringenin increases hepatic peroxisome proliferators-activated receptor α protein expression and decreases plasma triglyceride and adiposity in rats. Eur J Nutr 2011; 50(2): 81-8.
[http://dx.doi.org/10.1007/s00394-010-0117-8] [PMID: 20567977]

[154] Zhang S, Yang X, Luo J, *et al.* PPARα activation sensitizes cancer cells to epigallocatechin-3-gallate (EGCG) treatment via suppressing heme oxygenase-1. Nutr Cancer 2014; 66(2): 315-24.
[http://dx.doi.org/10.1080/01635581.2014.868909] [PMID: 24447094]

[155] Hou S, Wu D, Jiang Z. Effect of genistein on the changes of PPARalpha expression and glycolipid level in the oleic acid induced steatosis in HepG2 cells. Acta Nutr Sin 2014; 36: 49-52.

[156] Mueller M, Hobiger S, Jungbauer A. Red clover extract: a source for substances that activate peroxisome proliferator-activated receptor alpha and ameliorate the cytokine secretion profile of lipopolysaccharide-stimulated macrophages. Menopause 2010; 17(2): 379-87.
[http://dx.doi.org/10.1097/gme.0b013e3181c94617] [PMID: 20142789]

[157] Shen P, Liu MH, Ng TY, Chan YH, Yong EL. Differential effects of isoflavones, from Astragalus membranaceus and Pueraria thomsonii, on the activation of PPARalpha, PPARgamma, and adipocyte differentiation in vitro. J Nutr 2006; 136(4): 899-905.
[http://dx.doi.org/10.1093/jn/136.4.899] [PMID: 16549448]

[158] Zhang R, Yu Y, Hu S, *et al.* Sesamin ameliorates hepatic steatosis and inflammation in rats on a high-

fat diet via LXRα and PPARα. Nutr Res 2016; 36(9): 1022-30.
[http://dx.doi.org/10.1016/j.nutres.2016.06.015] [PMID: 27632923]

[159] Kou XH, Zhu MF, Chen D, *et al.* Bilobetin ameliorates insulin resistance by PKA-mediated phosphorylation of PPARα in rats fed a high-fat diet. Br J Pharmacol 2012; 165(8): 2692-706.
[http://dx.doi.org/10.1111/j.1476-5381.2011.01727.x] [PMID: 22091731]

[160] Azevedo MF, Camsari C, Sá CM, Lima CF, Fernandes-Ferreira M, Pereira-Wilson C. Ursolic acid and luteolin-7-glucoside improve lipid profiles and increase liver glycogen content through glycogen synthase kinase-3. Phytother Res 2010; 24 (Suppl. 2): S220-4.
[http://dx.doi.org/10.1002/ptr.3118] [PMID: 20127879]

[161] Schwartz MW, Woods SC, Porte D Jr, Seeley RJ, Baskin DG. Central nervous system control of food intake. Nature 2000; 404(6778): 661-71.
[http://dx.doi.org/10.1038/35007534] [PMID: 10766253]

[162] Andersson U, Filipsson K, Abbott CR, *et al.* AMP-activated protein kinase plays a role in the control of food intake. J Biol Chem 2004; 279(13): 12005-8.
[http://dx.doi.org/10.1074/jbc.C300557200] [PMID: 14742438]

[163] Faria A, Pestana D, Teixeira D, *et al.* Flavonoid transport across RBE4 cells: A blood-brain barrier model. Cell Mol Biol Lett 2010; 15(2): 234-41.
[http://dx.doi.org/10.2478/s11658-010-0006-4] [PMID: 20140760]

[164] Ferruzzi MG, Lobo JK, Janle EM, *et al.* Bioavailability of gallic acid and catechins from grape seed polyphenol extract is improved by repeated dosing in rats: implications for treatment in Alzheimer's disease. J Alzheimers Dis 2009; 18(1): 113-24.
[http://dx.doi.org/10.3233/JAD-2009-1135] [PMID: 19625746]

[165] Kao YH, Hiipakka RA, Liao S. Modulation of endocrine systems and food intake by green tea epigallocatechin gallate. Endocrinology 2000; 141(3): 980-7.
[http://dx.doi.org/10.1210/endo.141.3.7368] [PMID: 10698173]

[166] Xu Y, Zhang M, Wu T, Dai S, Xu J, Zhou Z. The anti-obesity effect of green tea polysaccharides, polyphenols and caffeine in rats fed with a high-fat diet. Food Funct 2015; 6(1): 297-304.
[http://dx.doi.org/10.1039/C4FO00970C] [PMID: 25431018]

[167] Belza A, Frandsen E, Kondrup J. Body fat loss achieved by stimulation of thermogenesis by a combination of bioactive food ingredients: a placebo-controlled, double-blind 8-week intervention in obese subjects. Int J Obes 2007; 31(1): 121-30.
[http://dx.doi.org/10.1038/sj.ijo.0803351] [PMID: 16652130]

[168] Carter BE, Drewnowski A. Beverages containing soluble fiber, caffeine, and green tea catechins suppress hunger and lead to less energy consumption at the next meal. Appetite 2012; 59(3): 755-61.
[http://dx.doi.org/10.1016/j.appet.2012.08.015] [PMID: 22922604]

[169] Kim SJ, Lee YH, Han MD, Mar W, Kim WK, Nam KW. Resveratrol, purified from the stem of Vitis coignetiae Pulliat, inhibits food intake in C57BL/6J Mice. Arch Pharm Res 2010; 33(5): 775-80.
[http://dx.doi.org/10.1007/s12272-010-0518-5] [PMID: 20512477]

[170] Franco JG, Lisboa PC, da Silva Lima N, *et al.* Resveratrol prevents hyperleptinemia and central leptin resistance in adult rats programmed by early weaning. Horm Metab Res 2014; 46(10): 728-35.
[http://dx.doi.org/10.1055/s-0034-1375688] [PMID: 24956416]

[171] Zhang Y, Na X, Zhang Y, Li L, Zhao X, Cui H. Isoflavone reduces body weight by decreasing food intake in ovariectomized rats. Ann Nutr Metab 2009; 54(3): 163-70.
[http://dx.doi.org/10.1159/000217812] [PMID: 19420908]

[172] Fujitani M, Mizushige T, Bhattarai K, *et al.* Dynamics of appetite-mediated gene expression in daidzein-fed female rats in the meal-feeding method. Biosci Biotechnol Biochem 2015; 79(8): 1342-9.
[http://dx.doi.org/10.1080/09168451.2015.1025034] [PMID: 25952775]

[173] Weickert MO, Reimann M, Otto B, *et al.* Soy isoflavones increase preprandial peptide YY (PYY), but

have no effect on ghrelin and body weight in healthy postmenopausal women. J Negat Results Biomed 2006; 5: 11.
[http://dx.doi.org/10.1186/1477-5751-5-11] [PMID: 16907966]

[174] Rains TM, Agarwal S, Maki KC. Antiobesity effects of green tea catechins: a mechanistic review. J Nutr Biochem 2011; 22(1): 1-7.
[http://dx.doi.org/10.1016/j.jnutbio.2010.06.006] [PMID: 21115335]

[175] Myoung HJ, Kim G, Nam KW. Apigenin isolated from the seeds of Perilla frutescens britton var crispa (Benth.) inhibits food intake in C57BL/6J mice. Arch Pharm Res 2010; 33(11): 1741-6.
[http://dx.doi.org/10.1007/s12272-010-1105-5] [PMID: 21116776]

[176] Ricquier D, Kader JC. Mitochondrial protein alteration in active brown fat: a sodium dodecyl sulfate-polyacrylamide gel electrophoretic study. Biochem Biophys Res Commun 1976; 73(3): 577-83.
[http://dx.doi.org/10.1016/0006-291X(76)90849-4] [PMID: 1008874]

[177] Cannon B, Nedergaard J. Brown adipose tissue: function and physiological significance. Physiol Rev 2004; 84(1): 277-359.
[http://dx.doi.org/10.1152/physrev.00015.2003] [PMID: 14715917]

[178] Cypess AM, Lehman S, Williams G, *et al.* Identification and importance of brown adipose tissue in adult humans. N Engl J Med 2009; 360(15): 1509-17.
[http://dx.doi.org/10.1056/NEJMoa0810780] [PMID: 19357406]

[179] Nedergaard J, Cannon B. The browning of white adipose tissue: some burning issues. Cell Metab 2014; 20(3): 396-407.
[http://dx.doi.org/10.1016/j.cmet.2014.07.005] [PMID: 25127354]

[180] Sidossis L, Kajimura S. Brown and beige fat in humans: thermogenic adipocytes that control energy and glucose homeostasis. J Clin Invest 2015; 125(2): 478-86.
[http://dx.doi.org/10.1172/JCI78362] [PMID: 25642708]

[181] Lowell BB, Spiegelman BM. Towards a molecular understanding of adaptive thermogenesis. Nature 2000; 404(6778): 652-60.
[http://dx.doi.org/10.1038/35007527] [PMID: 10766252]

[182] De Meis L, Ketzer LA, Camacho-Pereira J, Galina A. Brown adipose tissue mitochondria: modulation by GDP and fatty acids depends on the respiratory substrates. Biosci Rep 2012; 32(1): 53-9.
[http://dx.doi.org/10.1042/BSR20100144] [PMID: 21561434]

[183] Liang H, Ward WF. PGC-1alpha: a key regulator of energy metabolism. Adv Physiol Educ 2006; 30(4): 145-51.
[http://dx.doi.org/10.1152/advan.00052.2006] [PMID: 17108241]

[184] Dulloo AG, Duret C, Rohrer D, *et al.* Efficacy of a green tea extract rich in catechin polyphenols and caffeine in increasing 24-h energy expenditure and fat oxidation in humans. Am J Clin Nutr 1999; 70(6): 1040-5.
[http://dx.doi.org/10.1093/ajcn/70.6.1040] [PMID: 10584049]

[185] Lu H, Meng X, Yang CS. Enzymology of methylation of tea catechins and inhibition of catechol--methyltransferase by (-)-epigallocatechin gallate. Drug Metab Dispos 2003; 31(5): 572-9.
[http://dx.doi.org/10.1124/dmd.31.5.572] [PMID: 12695345]

[186] Choo JJ. Green tea reduces body fat accretion caused by high-fat diet in rats through beta-adrenoceptor activation of thermogenesis in brown adipose tissue. J Nutr Biochem 2003; 14(11): 671-6.
[http://dx.doi.org/10.1016/j.jnutbio.2003.08.005] [PMID: 14629899]

[187] Chen N, Bezzina R, Hinch E, *et al.* Green tea, black tea, and epigallocatechin modify body composition, improve glucose tolerance, and differentially alter metabolic gene expression in rats fed a high-fat diet. Nutr Res 2009; 29(11): 784-93.
[http://dx.doi.org/10.1016/j.nutres.2009.10.003] [PMID: 19932867]

[188] Kudo N, Arai Y, Suhara Y, Ishii T, Nakayama T, Osakabe N. A Single Oral Administration of

Theaflavins Increases Energy Expenditure and the Expression of Metabolic Genes. PLoS One 2015; 10(9)e0137809
[http://dx.doi.org/10.1371/journal.pone.0137809] [PMID: 26375960]

[189] Komatsu T, Nakamori M, Komatsu K, *et al.* Oolong tea increases energy metabolism in Japanese females. J Med Invest 2003; 50(3-4): 170-5.
[PMID: 13678386]

[190] Rudelle S, Ferruzzi MG, Cristiani I, *et al.* Effect of a thermogenic beverage on 24-hour energy metabolism in humans. Obesity (Silver Spring) 2007; 15(2): 349-55.
[http://dx.doi.org/10.1038/oby.2007.529] [PMID: 17299107]

[191] Yoneshiro T, Matsushita M, Hibi M, *et al.* Tea catechin and caffeine activate brown adipose tissue and increase cold-induced thermogenic capacity in humans. Am J Clin Nutr 2017; 105(4): 873-81.
[http://dx.doi.org/10.3945/ajcn.116.144972] [PMID: 28275131]

[192] Thavanesan N. The putative effects of green tea on body fat: an evaluation of the evidence and a review of the potential mechanisms. Br J Nutr 2011; 106(9): 1297-309.
[http://dx.doi.org/10.1017/S0007114511003849] [PMID: 21810286]

[193] Hursel R, Viechtbauer W, Westerterp-Plantenga MS. The effects of green tea on weight loss and weight maintenance: a meta-analysis. Int J Obes 2009; 33(9): 956-61.
[http://dx.doi.org/10.1038/ijo.2009.135] [PMID: 19597519]

[194] Lagouge M, Argmann C, Gerhart-Hines Z, *et al.* Resveratrol improves mitochondrial function and protects against metabolic disease by activating SIRT1 and PGC-1alpha. Cell 2006; 127(6): 1109-22.
[http://dx.doi.org/10.1016/j.cell.2006.11.013] [PMID: 17112576]

[195] Baur JA, Pearson KJ, Price NL, *et al.* Resveratrol improves health and survival of mice on a high-calorie diet. Nature 2006; 444(7117): 337-42.
[http://dx.doi.org/10.1038/nature05354] [PMID: 17086191]

[196] Wang S, Liang X, Yang Q, *et al.* Resveratrol induces brown-like adipocyte formation in white fat through activation of AMP-activated protein kinase (AMPK) α1. Int J Obes 2015; 39(6): 967-76.
[http://dx.doi.org/10.1038/ijo.2015.23] [PMID: 25761413]

[197] Arias N, Picó C, Teresa Macarulla M, *et al.* A combination of resveratrol and quercetin induces browning in white adipose tissue of rats fed an obesogenic diet. Obesity (Silver Spring) 2017; 25(1): 111-21.
[http://dx.doi.org/10.1002/oby.21706] [PMID: 27874268]

[198] Jung HY, Lee D, Ryu HG, *et al.* Myricetin improves endurance capacity and mitochondrial density by activating SIRT1 and PGC-1α. Sci Rep 2017; 7(1): 6237.
[http://dx.doi.org/10.1038/s41598-017-05303-2] [PMID: 28740165]

[199] Goldwasser J, Cohen PY, Yang E, Balaguer P, Yarmush ML, Nahmias Y. Transcriptional regulation of human and rat hepatic lipid metabolism by the grapefruit flavonoid naringenin: role of PPARalpha, PPARgamma and LXRalpha. PLoS One 2010; 5(8)e12399
[http://dx.doi.org/10.1371/journal.pone.0012399] [PMID: 20811644]

[200] Takahashi Y, Ide T. Effects of soy protein and isoflavone on hepatic fatty acid synthesis and oxidation and mRNA expression of uncoupling proteins and peroxisome proliferator-activated receptor gamma in adipose tissues of rats. J Nutr Biochem 2008; 19(10): 682-93.
[http://dx.doi.org/10.1016/j.jnutbio.2007.09.003] [PMID: 18328687]

[201] Crespillo A, Alonso M, Vida M, *et al.* Reduction of body weight, liver steatosis and expression of stearoyl-CoA desaturase 1 by the isoflavone daidzein in diet-induced obesity. Br J Pharmacol 2011; 164(7): 1899-915.
[http://dx.doi.org/10.1111/j.1476-5381.2011.01477.x] [PMID: 21557739]

[202] Aziz SA, Wakeling LA, Miwa S, Alberdi G, Hesketh JE, Ford D. Metabolic programming of a beige adipocyte phenotype by genistein. Mol Nutr Food Res 2017; 61(2)

[http://dx.doi.org/10.1002/mnfr.201600574] [PMID: 27670404]

[203] Choi JH, Yun JW. Chrysin induces brown fat-like phenotype and enhances lipid metabolism in 3T3-L1 adipocytes. Nutrition 2016; 32(9): 1002-10.
[http://dx.doi.org/10.1016/j.nut.2016.02.007] [PMID: 27133810]

[204] Pajuelo D, Quesada H, Díaz S, *et al.* Chronic dietary supplementation of proanthocyanidins corrects the mitochondrial dysfunction of brown adipose tissue caused by diet-induced obesity in Wistar rats. Br J Nutr 2012; 107(2): 170-8.
[http://dx.doi.org/10.1017/S0007114511002728] [PMID: 21733324]

[205] Matsumura Y, Nakagawa Y, Mikome K, Yamamoto H, Osakabe N. Enhancement of energy expenditure following a single oral dose of flavan-3-ols associated with an increase in catecholamine secretion. PLoS One 2014; 9(11)e112180
[http://dx.doi.org/10.1371/journal.pone.0112180] [PMID: 25375880]

[206] Osakabe N, Hoshi J, Kudo N, Shibata M. The flavan-3-ol fraction of cocoa powder suppressed changes associated with early-stage metabolic syndrome in high-fat diet-fed rats. Life Sci 2014; 114(1): 51-6.
[http://dx.doi.org/10.1016/j.lfs.2014.07.041] [PMID: 25132363]

[207] Lorenz M, Paul F, Moobed M, *et al.* The activity of catechol-O-methyltransferase (COMT) is not impaired by high doses of epigallocatechin-3-gallate (EGCG) in vivo. Eur J Pharmacol 2014; 740: 645-51.
[http://dx.doi.org/10.1016/j.ejphar.2014.06.014] [PMID: 24972245]

CHAPTER 12

Maternal Nutrition and Developmental Programming of Obesity

Fátima Martel[1,2] and **Elisa Keating[1,3,*]**

[1] *Department of Biomedicine, Biochemistry Unit, Faculty of Medicine, University of Porto, Porto, Portugal*

[2] *i3S - Instituto de Investigação e Inovação em Saúde, University of Porto, Porto, Portugal*

[3] *CINTESIS - Center for Research in Health Technologies and Information Systems, University of Porto, Porto, Portugal*

Abstract: The rapid increase in the incidence and prevalence of obesity and metabolic syndrome over the last decades cannot be explained solely by genetic and adult lifestyle factors. There is now considerable evidence that the fetal environment also strongly influences the risk of developing such diseases in later life. One of the principal environmental factors influencing the developing child is nutrient availability, which is dependent on maternal nourishment status and placental functionality. The influence of a nutritional insult to the fetus will not only depend on the type of maternal nutritional insult but will also depend on the maternal metabolic condition, the timing of maternal nutritional insult, and will occur when there is a mismatch between pregnancy and postnatal environments. Both human and animal studies have shown that maternal under- (caloric restriction, protein restriction or micronutrient restriction) or overnutrition (high-fat, high-carbohydrate or high-vitamin diets) can induce persistent changes in gene expression and metabolism in the offspring, resulting in an increased risk for obesity and metabolic disease. Because these changes are mediated by altered epigenetic regulation of specific genes, and given that epigenetic marks are reversible, nutritional or pharmaceutical interventions may be used to modify long-term obesity and cardio-metabolic disease risk.

Keywords: Caloric restriction, Developmental programming, DNA methylation, Epigenetics, Famine, Folic acid, High-fat diet, High-sugar diet, Histone modifications, Maternal nutrition, Metabolic syndrome, Non-coding RNA, Obesity, Pregnancy, Protein-restriction.

INTRODUCTION

The prevalence of obesity has been steadily increasing worldwide over the past 50

* **Corresponding author Elisa Keating:** Department of Biomedicine, Biochemistry Unit, Faculty of Medicine, University of Porto, 4200-319 Porto, Portugal; Tel/Fax: +351225513624; E-mail: keating@med.up.pt

Rosário Monteiro and Maria João Martins (Eds.)

years, with an estimated 18 million people dying from cardiovascular diseases (CVD) per year [1]. While this is partially due to changes in lifestyle and behavioral factors, such as consumption of caloric-dense, nutrient-low foods and sedentary behaviors [2, 3], an emerging body of evidence suggests that the interindividual variability in sensitivity to genetic and lifestyle factors may be triggered early in development.

During intrauterine development, the fetus is exposed to various external (maternal) factors. Maternal mental and physical status, the environment to which she is exposed and maternal physical activity and dietary habits can permanently affect health of the growing child. One of the principal environmental factors influencing the developing child is nutrient availability, which is dependent on maternal nourishment status and placental functionality [4, 5]. The mechanism(s) by which intrauterine nutrient availability is(are) transmitted to the fetus and the process(es) by which distinct and stable phenotypes are induced is(are) beginning to be understood.

The aim of this review is to analyze the influence of maternal nutrition during pregnancy on the long-term risk of obesity and metabolic syndrome for the offspring, and the involvement of epigenetic mechanisms in this process.

THE DEVELOPMENTAL PROGRAMMING OF DISEASE

The first description of a putative connection between environmental influence in early life and the disease risk in adulthood was done by Barker *et al*, who observed a strong geographical relationship between infant mortality and the incidence of coronary disease in adult life in the UK [6].

Large amounts of epidemiological data later showed a strong association between impaired intrauterine growth and an increased risk for hypertension, coronary heart disease, dyslipidemia, obesity, type 2 diabetes and insulin resistance (*e.g* [7 - 9].). So, a poor intrauterine environment, as induced by maternal diet deficiency, placental insufficiency or endocrine factors, such as stress, appear to induce changes in the embryo and fetus, increasing its future risk for metabolic diseases. Moreover, these findings have been replicated in animal models where restricted nutrition during pregnancy induces dyslipidemia, obesity, hypertension, hyperinsulinemia and hyperleptinemia in the offspring [10, 11].

According to the developmental origins of health and disease hypothesis, originally presented by Barker *et al*, the ability to respond to metabolic challenges during postnatal life is linked to environmental influences during fetal development – a concept also known as fetal programming of adult diseases [5, 12, 13].

Barker and Hales also provided the initial answer to the question of how birth weight and adult chronic diseases are connected, by formulating the "thrifty phenotype hypothesis". According to this theory, fetuses adapt to a poor intrauterine environment by changing their physiology and metabolism, causing an abnormal tissue structure and function in adult life. This adaptive response can be beneficial if postnatal environment remains poor. However, when a discrepancy exists between the prenatal and postnatal environments, namely if the postnatal ambient is a rich one, a metabolic mismatch occurs and a higher risk of developing metabolic diseases is then observed [14, 15] Fig. (**1**).

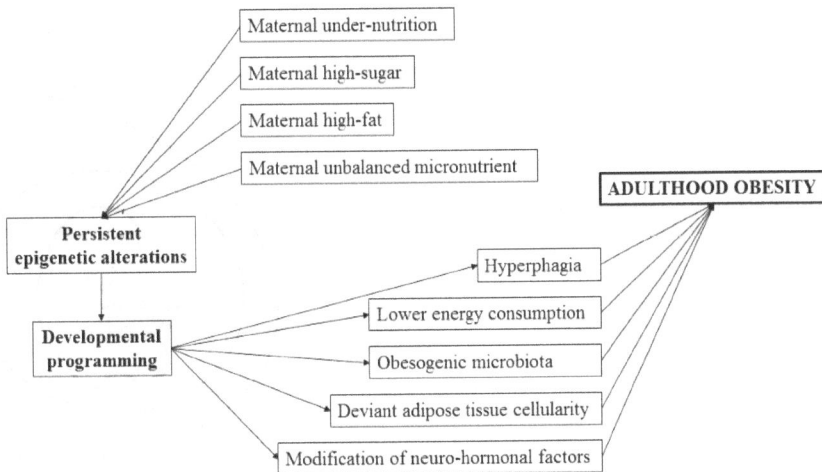

Fig. (1). Programming effects of an inadequate *in utero* nutrition on adulthood development of obesity and metabolic syndrome.

This concept of a relationship between birth weight and adult metabolic disease initially described in small-for-gestational age babies was further extended to large-for-gestational age babies, and the term of inappropriate gestational weight is now accepted as better illustrating changes in prenatal environment that contribute to the risk of obesity and metabolic syndrome in adulthood [16]. It is now clear that this association between birth weight and metabolic disease in later life is observed even within the normal birth weight; so, birth weight appears to have a continuous U- or J-shaped relationship with metabolic disease risk [7, 17].

EPIGENETICS AND DEVELOPMENTAL PROGRAMMING OF DISEASE

The above-mentioned developmental programming hypothesis proposes that environmental stimuli acting during critical periods of intrauterine development may cause a permanent alteration in the structure and functioning of the organism. This hypothesis thus suggests a close interaction between fetal and maternal environments and modulation of gene expression that starts very early in life and can even be passed across generations [18]. The precise mechanism through which developmental programming occurs is not fully understood, but epigenetics is considered to play a key and, eventually, a primary role.

Epigenetics refers to changes in gene expression that occur without a change in DNA sequence [19]. Multicellular organisms possess genotypically identical but phenotypically different cell types, as a result of differential gene expression patterns in different cell types. Tissue-specific gene expression is partially related to epigenetic control of expression. In contrast to the genetic code, epigenetic information maintains a certain level of plasticity and is inherently reversible [20].

Epigenetic modifications include DNA methylation, histone modifications (chromatin organization) and non-coding RNAs [19].

Methylation of mammalian DNA occurs on position 5 of the pyrimidine ring of a cytosine base followed by a guanine (known as CpG islands). Methylation of CpG islands represses gene transcription and controls gene expression. In human cells, most of CpG islands located outside promoters are hypermethylated, which results in transcriptional repression, whereas CpG islands located in the promoter regions of active genes are demethylated [21].

Nucleosomes, consisting of DNA wrapped around eight histone proteins, constitute the basic unit of chromatin. Covalent histone modifications affect the structural dynamics of the nucleosome and dictate gene expression patterns by changing the accessibility of the transcription machinery to genes. Covalent reversible histone modifications include methylation of lysine and arginine residues, phosphorylation of serine and threonine residues, acetylation, ubiquitinylation and ADP-ribosylation [22].

Micro-RNAs (miRNAs; small RNA molecules of about 22 nucleotides) constitute one class of small non-coding RNAs that plays an important role in the epigenetic control of gene expression. miRNAs bind to their target mRNAs and lead to target mRNAs degradation or translational suppression of the target genes. Additionally, miRNAs, as well as other classes on non-coding RNAs, namely small interfering RNAs (siRNAs) and Piwi-associated RNAs (piRNAs), have been shown to be involved in DNA methylation and histone modifications [21, 23].

Recent work has shown that epigenetic changes play critical roles in many biological processes related to intrauterine development, such as gene expression, chromatin accessibility, DNA replication, imprinting and human disease patterns [24]. Since the establishment of the epigenome during embryogenesis is a process that is dependent on environmental conditions, the epigenetic regulation of gene expression may function as a link between prenatal nutrition, gene expression, and health. Epigenetics thus emerged as the most suitable molecular explanation of developmental programming [18].

We will next review evidence that maternal nutrition during pregnancy influences the future onset of obesity and poor metabolic outcomes.

MATERNAL NUTRITIONAL INSULTS AND DEVELOPMENTAL PROGRAMMING OF OBESITY

An immense diversity of complex factors is known to condition and play a role in developmental programming and thus have to be considered when studying the effects of maternal nutrition upon developmental programming of obesity. These factors are deeply interrelated, influencing each other, and include but are not limited to:

- Maternal metabolic condition,
- Mismatch between pregnancy and postnatal environments,
- Timing of maternal nutritional insult, and
- Type of maternal nutritional insult.

The choice of the model for the study of developmental programming of disease is also critical. Although human studies are deeply valuable, they imply a long time period between the insult and the outcome observation as well as being subjected to a great amount of confounding factors, such as lifestyle, socioeconomic and cultural factors. On the other hand, the use of animal models enables access to tissue-specific research and shortage of observation periods, while avoiding confounding factors, being thus very useful and informative. Nevertheless, they also have limitations which rely essentially on disparities in the process of embryo and fetal development between species.

Maternal Metabolic Condition

A bad maternal metabolic condition (*e.g.,* pre-pregnancy obesity, gestational weight gain and diabetes) has for a long time been associated with increased risk of metabolic disease in the offspring. As recently reviewed by von Her and von

Versen-Hoynck [25], exposure to maternal diabetes during fetal life is known to increase the risk of several dysmetabolic outcomes in the offspring, such as obesity, type 2 diabetes and metabolic syndrome. In addition, pre-pregnancy maternal obesity is associated with higher body mass index (BMI) in school-aged offspring [25].

Mismatch Between Pregnancy and Postnatal Environments

As already referred in the above section "Epigenetics and developmental programming of disease", a mismatch between pre- and postnatal environments is known to be detrimental for metabolic function of the offspring.

Fetal development is a plastic period when environmental (maternal) cues drive persistent changes in phenotype that predict the future environment [26]. Whenever the postnatal environment differs from pregnancy environment, mismatch occurs and the developed phenotype has some degree of maladaptation which turns out to be detrimental to the individual throughout life [26, 27].

Mismatch occurs typically as a result of a combination of poor maternal diet during pregnancy, or maternal disease, with nutritional abundance (especially energy dense foods) after birth [26].

Timing of Nutritional Insult

Differential plasticity during *in utero* development creates temporal windows of increased susceptibility to environmental insults.

It has been claimed that nutritional insults occurring in early pregnancy will affect placental and fetal growth more severely while nutritional insults occurring in later periods of pregnancy will more likely impact fetal fat accretion and thus weight gain [28, 29]. It is thus plausible that nutritional insults occurring at different critical windows will also have different impacts in developmental programming of adulthood obesity and associated morbidities [28].

Data from the Dutch famine cohort reviewed by Symonds *et al* [28] stress some interesting differences in developmental programming induced by maternal undernutrition according to the period of exposure.

Exposure to famine in early gestation does not appear to induce changes in birth weight or body length at birth but is associated with higher BMI, weight and waist circumference in women at the age of 50 [30]. Increased atherogenic lipid profile (*e.g.,* an increase in the LDL-HDL cholesterol ratio), increased prevalence of CVD, and, more curiously, increased preference for fatty foods were other long-term consequences found to be related to early gestation famine exposure [31 -

33] (Table **1**).

On the other hand, exposure to famine in mid-to-late gestation was found to be related to decreased birth weight and other anthropometric measures at birth but was less frequently associated with poor metabolic outcomes, although a decrease in glucose tolerance was found [34 - 36].

As defended by Roseboom *et al* [37], the impact of famine during pregnancy seems to depend on the specific period of gestation and early gestation seems to be a critical window of greater susceptibility for developmental programming of poor metabolic outcomes.

Table 1. Developmental effects of maternal exposure to Dutch famine according to the period of exposure.

Period of exposure to famine	Neonatal period outcomes	Adulthood outcomes	Sex and age for outcome measures in adulthood	Reference
Early gestation	↔ BW ↔ BL	↑ BMI ↑ Waist circumference ↑ Weight	♀, 50 years old	[30]
	↔ BW ↔ BL	↑ Atherogenic lipid profile	♀ and ♂, 50-years-old	[31]
	↔ BW ↔ BL	↑ Prevalence of CVD	♀ and ♂, 50-years-old	[32]
	↔ BW ↔ BL	↑ Preference for fatty foods	♀ and ♂, 58-years-old	[33]
Mid gestation	↓ BW ↓ BL	↑ Prevalence of obstructive airway diseases	♀ and ♂, 50-years-old	[34]
	↓ BW ↓ BL	↑ Prevalence of obstructive airway diseases and microalbuminuria	♀ and ♂, 50-years-old	[35]
	↓ BW ↓ BL	↓ Glucose tolerance	♀ and ♂, 50-years-old	[36]
Late gestation	↓ BW ↓ Head circumference	↓ Glucose tolerance	♀ and ♂, 50-years-old	[36]

BW, birthweight; BL, body length at birth; BMI, body mass index; CVD, cardiovascular disease.

Type of Maternal Nutritional Insult

As defined by the World Health Organization, "nutrition is the intake of food, considered in relation to the body's dietary needs" [38]. So, studies on the effects of maternal nutrition on health outcomes of the offspring must have into consideration that different nutrients on a background of different food context or nutritional status may have different impacts.

In this context, maternal over- as well as undernutrition are often studied, with specific focus on low-protein, high-fat and high-sugar as well as low- or high-vitamin and mineral consumption.

Maternal Undernutrition

The above-referred studies of the Dutch famine (Table **1**) provide the most valuable evidence for the effects of undernutrition and severe caloric restriction, particularly during early pregnancy, in developmental programming of poor metabolic outcomes, most of them components of the metabolic syndrome.

Curiously, another study analyzing the effect of prenatal famine on the prevalence of metabolic syndrome (defined as a clustering of $\geq$ 3 of the following characteristics: waist circumference $\geq$ 102 cm in men and $\geq$ 88 cm in women, triacylglycerol $\geq$ 1.7 mmol/L, blood pressure $\geq$ 130/85 mm Hg or the use of antihypertensive medication, HDL cholesterol < 1.03 mmol/L in men and < 1.3 mmol/L in women and fasting glucose $\geq$ 6.1 mmol/L or the use of antidiabetic medication) at the age of 50, failed to show an association [39].

As referred in the section "Epigenetics and developmental programming of disease", epigenetic regulation of gene expression, particularly DNA methylation, is claimed to underlie developmental programming effects, and several works have demonstrated this relationship. By analyzing Table **2**, it is apparent that maternal undernutrition during pregnancy is indeed associated with changes in DNA methylation that seem to be *loci*-specific. Interestingly, early pregnancy exposure appears again as a particularly sensitive period, most likely because this period of development is characterized by a genome-wide demethylation and re-methylation cycle that may be more susceptible to epigenetic insults.

Table 2. *In utero* exposure to Dutch famine and DNA methylation patterns in different genome regions as assessed in whole blood samples at 58 years-old offspring.

Exposed (n)	Unexposed sibling control (n)	Unexposed time control (n)	Genome region	Alterations in DNA methylation?	Specific critical window in pregnancy	Ref.
350	307	290	LINE-1 and Sat2	No	Na	[44]
122	122	Na	IGF2 gene	Yes ($\downarrow$)	Early gestation	[45]
319	Na	440	GR; LPL PI3K PPARγ	No	Na	[46]

(Table 2) cont.....

Exposed (n)	Unexposed sibling control (n)	Unexposed time control (n)	Genome region	Alterations in DNA methylation?	Specific critical window in pregnancy	Ref.
60	60	Na	P-DMRs	Yes (↓ and ↑ dependent on the region)	Early gestation	[47]
60	60	Na	IGF2 DMRs	Yes (↓ and ↑ dependent on the region)	Early gestation	[48]
60	60	Na	H19 DMR	No	Na	[48]
422	303	160	FAM150B; SLC38A2; PPAP2C	Yes (↑)	Early gestation	[49]
422	303	160	OSBPL5/MRGPRG	Yes (↓)	Early gestation	[49]

Na, not applicable; Ref, reference.

Animal models of undernutrition are very well represented by maternal protein restriction in rodents. Studies with this model largely corroborate the conclusion that maternal undernutrition during pregnancy programs the offspring for bad metabolic outcomes, as recently extensively reviewed by Kereliuk *et al* [40].

Also, moderate to severe caloric restriction exposure during gestation has been shown to associate with dysmetabolism in the offspring. For example, pups exposed to moderate (50%) caloric restriction during gestation and nursed by non-restricted dams exhibited a rapid catch-up growth, resulting in higher weight gain, body fat percentage and leptin levels [41]. Curiously, restricted pups nursed by restricted dams failed to show these alterations, corroborating the importance of mismatch for developmental programing of dysmetabolism.

Similarly, Vickers *et al* have shown that rat pups exposed to severe (70%) caloric restriction during gestation developed hyperphagia, hyperinsulinemia, hyperleptinemia, hypertension and obesity in adulthood [42]. Importantly, these manifestations were aggravated by mismatch conferred by post-weaning hypercaloric diet.

As reviewed by Fernandez-Twinn *et al* [43], protein-restricted diet during pregnancy causing poor metabolic outcomes in the offspring has been demonstrated to cause epigenetic alterations of gene expression, either DNA methylation or expression of miRNAs, at several tissue levels.

Importantly, micronutrient shortage is also known to affect developmental programming of metabolic dysfunction, as demonstrated by the effect of low vitamin B_{12} or zinc restriction on the programming of glucose intolerance and insulin resistance [50 - 52].

Maternal Overnutrition

The study of the influence of overnutrition upon developmental programming of obesity may rely on human studies of maternal obesity. However, the study of the effect of excess of specific nutrients has mostly relied on animal models of high-fat, high-carbohydrate and high-vitamin diets. Informative reviews have been recently published and should be consulted for further details [5, 40, 43].

Overall, excess carbohydrate (either complex - dextrose, maltodextrin - or simple - sucrose and fructose) intake during pregnancy has been shown to program for increased body weight and obesity, worse lipid profile and adipose tissue cellularity, hyperphagia, hyperglycemia and hyperinsulinemia in the offspring [40, 53]. Also, maternal high-fat diet or a combined high-fat and high-sugar diet have been demonstrated to induce bad metabolic outcomes on the offspring [40].

Data regarding epigenetic mechanism involvement in those programming effects are still scarce comparing with data resulting from famine or protein restriction studies. However, some evidence has been found showing that maternal high-fat feeding induces hepatic steatosis in the offspring with reduction in hepatic histone methylation [54]. Additionally, maternal obesity has been found to program for offspring glucose intolerance and obesity, with overexpression of the miRNA miR-126-3p in adipose tissue [55].

In what concerns excessive micronutrient intake, interesting studies have been set up. Folic acid as a methyl-nutrient is believed to directly interfere with DNA methylation and thus to play an important role as an epigenetic regulator. As recently reviewed by Silva *et al* [56] folate intake has been associated with alterations in insulin-like growth factor 2 (IGF2) DNA methylation [57, 58]. This vitamin takes particular relevance during pregnancy given the important role of folic acid intake during this period in the prevention of the occurrence and recurrence of neural tube defects.

Importantly, a set of studies have demonstrated, both in humans and in rodents, that excessive folate intake during pregnancy may induce developmental programming of poor metabolic outcomes. Yajnik *et al* showed, in humans, that high maternal folate levels associates with insulin resistance in the offspring [52]. Accordingly, our group has shown that excessive folic acid exposure during the perigestational period, in the rat, induces developmental programming of an insulin-resistant state [59]. Finally, Huang *et al* have gathered evidence that excess folic acid intake by pregnant mice worsens adult offspring response to a metabolic challenge such as a high-fat diet [60].

CONCLUDING REMARKS

It is unquestionable that maternal nutritional imbalance during pregnancy can drive persistent alterations in the fetal genome that will program the new individual to develop obesity and other related metabolic outcomes later in life. It is also unquestionable that epigenetic mechanisms play an important role in developmental programming of obesity. Epigenetics represents a kind of molecular memory which relies in the persistence throughout life of epigenetic marks induced by environmental stressors [61]. These epigenetic marks may eventually result in an altered phenotype, when a second challenge is imposed to the organism, and this is one of the possible explanations for the appearance of disease in later stages of life, caused by *in utero* insults.

We cannot disregard, however, that developmental programming of obesity may also depend on specific physiological/molecular obesogenic processes such as hyperphagia, deviant adipose tissue cellularity, lower energy consumption and modification of neuro-hormonal factors, which in conjunction or by themselves increase the propensity for increased weight gain in the offspring later in life [62].

Importantly, microbiome modulation, another player in obesity development, is arising as a factor subjected to developmental programming [63, 64].

At the end, all these programmable factors may be under epigenetic regulation.

Further studies on the involvement of epigenetic mechanisms on the programming effect of specific nutritional stressors are warranted. Continuous research and knowledge on this area of research will be critical for the prevention and breaking of the still rising obesity and metabolic disease pandemic.

CONSENT FOR PUBLICATION

Not applicable.

CONFLICT OF INTEREST

The authors confirm that this chapter contents have no conflict of interest.

ACKNOWLEDGEMENTS

The authors thank Mr Ruy Lopez for his contribution to image conception of Fig. (**1**). This article was supported by National Funds through FCT - Fundação para a Ciência e a Tecnologia within i3S (UID/BIM/04293/2013)) and CINTESIS, R&D Unit (UID/IC/4255/2019).

REFERENCES

[1] WHO. Global Health Estimates. 2015. Geneva2015 [18th July 2017]. Available from: http://www.who.int/healthinfo/global_burden_disease/estimates/en/

[2] Johnson L, Mander AP, Jones LR, Emmett PM, Jebb SA. Energy-dense, low-fiber, high-fat dietary pattern is associated with increased fatness in childhood. Am J Clin Nutr 2008; 87(4): 846-54. [http://dx.doi.org/10.1093/ajcn/87.4.846] [PMID: 18400706]

[3] McAllister EJ, Dhurandhar NV, Keith SW, *et al.* Ten putative contributors to the obesity epidemic. Crit Rev Food Sci Nutr 2009; 49(10): 868-913. [http://dx.doi.org/10.1080/10408390903372599] [PMID: 19960394]

[4] Fleming TP, Kwong WY, Porter R, *et al.* The embryo and its future. Biol Reprod 2004; 71(4): 1046-54. [http://dx.doi.org/10.1095/biolreprod.104.030957] [PMID: 15215194]

[5] Marciniak A, Patro-Małysza J, Kimber-Trojnar Ż, Marciniak B, Oleszczuk J, Leszczyńska-Gorzelak B. Fetal programming of the metabolic syndrome. Taiwan J Obstet Gynecol 2017; 56(2): 133-8. [http://dx.doi.org/10.1016/j.tjog.2017.01.001] [PMID: 28420495]

[6] Barker DJ, Osmond C. Infant mortality, childhood nutrition, and ischaemic heart disease in England and Wales. Lancet 1986; 1(8489): 1077-81. [http://dx.doi.org/10.1016/S0140-6736(86)91340-1] [PMID: 2871345]

[7] Curhan GC, Willett WC, Rimm EB, Spiegelman D, Ascherio AL, Stampfer MJ. Birth weight and adult hypertension, diabetes mellitus, and obesity in US men. Circulation 1996; 94(12): 3246-50. [http://dx.doi.org/10.1161/01.CIR.94.12.3246] [PMID: 8989136]

[8] Harder T, Rodekamp E, Schellong K, Dudenhausen JW, Plagemann A. Birth weight and subsequent risk of type 2 diabetes: a meta-analysis. Am J Epidemiol 2007; 165(8): 849-57. [http://dx.doi.org/10.1093/aje/kwk071] [PMID: 17215379]

[9] McMillen IC, Robinson JS. Developmental origins of the metabolic syndrome: prediction, plasticity, and programming. Physiol Rev 2005; 85(2): 571-633. [http://dx.doi.org/10.1152/physrev.00053.2003] [PMID: 15788706]

[10] Armitage JA, Khan IY, Taylor PD, Nathanielsz PW, Poston L. Developmental programming of the metabolic syndrome by maternal nutritional imbalance: how strong is the evidence from experimental models in mammals? J Physiol 2004; 561(Pt 2): 355-77. [http://dx.doi.org/10.1113/jphysiol.2004.072009] [PMID: 15459241]

[11] Bertram CE, Hanson MA. Animal models and programming of the metabolic syndrome. Br Med Bull 2001; 60: 103-21. [http://dx.doi.org/10.1093/bmb/60.1.103]

[12] Barker DJ. The Wellcome Foundation Lecture, 1994. The fetal origins of adult disease. Proc Biol Sci 1995; 262(1363): 37-43. [http://dx.doi.org/10.1098/rspb.1995.0173] [PMID: 7479990]

[13] Gluckman PD, Hanson MA. Living with the past: evolution, development, and patterns of disease. Science 2004; 305(5691): 1733-6. [http://dx.doi.org/10.1126/science.1095292] [PMID: 15375258]

[14] Barker DJ. A new model for the origins of chronic disease. Med Health Care Philos 2001; 4(1): 31-5. [http://dx.doi.org/10.1023/A:1009934412988] [PMID: 11315417]

[15] Hales CN, Barker DJP. The thrifty phenotype hypothesis. Br Med Bull 2001; 60(1): 5-20. [http://dx.doi.org/10.1093/bmb/60.1.5] [PMID: 11809615]

[16] Poston L. Gestational weight gain: influences on the long-term health of the child. Curr Opin Clin Nutr Metab Care 2012; 15(3): 252-7. [http://dx.doi.org/10.1097/MCO.0b013e3283527cf2] [PMID: 22406744]

[17]   McCance DR, Pettitt DJ, Hanson RL, Jacobsson LT, Knowler WC, Bennett PH. Birth weight and non-insulin dependent diabetes: thrifty genotype, thrifty phenotype, or surviving small baby genotype? BMJ 1994; 308(6934): 942-5.
[http://dx.doi.org/10.1136/bmj.308.6934.942] [PMID: 8173400]

[18]   Sookoian S, Gianotti TF, Burgueño AL, Pirola CJ. Fetal metabolic programming and epigenetic modifications: a systems biology approach. Pediatr Res 2013; 73(4 Pt 2): 531-42.
[http://dx.doi.org/10.1038/pr.2013.2] [PMID: 23314294]

[19]   Kirchner H, Osler ME, Krook A, Zierath JR. Epigenetic flexibility in metabolic regulation: disease cause and prevention? Trends Cell Biol 2013; 23(5): 203-9.
[http://dx.doi.org/10.1016/j.tcb.2012.11.008] [PMID: 23277089]

[20]   Probst AV, Dunleavy E, Almouzni G. Epigenetic inheritance during the cell cycle. Nat Rev Mol Cell Biol 2009; 10(3): 192-206.
[http://dx.doi.org/10.1038/nrm2640] [PMID: 19234478]

[21]   Chmurzynska A. Fetal programming: link between early nutrition, DNA methylation, and complex diseases. Nutr Rev 2010; 68(2): 87-98.
[http://dx.doi.org/10.1111/j.1753-4887.2009.00265.x] [PMID: 20137054]

[22]   Munshi A, Shafi G, Aliya N, Jyothy A. Histone modifications dictate specific biological readouts. J Genet Genomics 2009; 36(2): 75-88.
[http://dx.doi.org/10.1016/S1673-8527(08)60094-6] [PMID: 19232306]

[23]   Guil S, Esteller M. DNA methylomes, histone codes and miRNAs: tying it all together. Int J Biochem Cell Biol 2009; 41(1): 87-95.
[http://dx.doi.org/10.1016/j.biocel.2008.09.005] [PMID: 18834952]

[24]   Heerwagen MJR, Miller MR, Barbour LA, Friedman JE. Maternal obesity and fetal metabolic programming: a fertile epigenetic soil. Am J Physiol Regul Integr Comp Physiol 2010; 299(3): R711-22.
[http://dx.doi.org/10.1152/ajpregu.00310.2010] [PMID: 20631295]

[25]   von Ehr J, von Versen-Höynck F. Implications of maternal conditions and pregnancy course on offspring's medical problems in adult life. Arch Gynecol Obstet 2016; 294(4): 673-9.
[http://dx.doi.org/10.1007/s00404-016-4178-7] [PMID: 27522600]

[26]   Godfrey KM, Inskip HM, Hanson MA. The long-term effects of prenatal development on growth and metabolism. Semin Reprod Med 2011; 29(3): 257-65.
[http://dx.doi.org/10.1055/s-0031-1275518] [PMID: 21769765]

[27]   Lakshmy R. Metabolic syndrome: Role of maternal undernutrition and fetal programming. Rev Endocr Metab Disord 2013; 14(3): 229-40.
[http://dx.doi.org/10.1007/s11154-013-9266-4] [PMID: 24005943]

[28]   Symonds ME, Sebert SP, Hyatt MA, Budge H. Nutritional programming of the metabolic syndrome. Nat Rev Endocrinol 2009; 5(11): 604-10.
[http://dx.doi.org/10.1038/nrendo.2009.195] [PMID: 19786987]

[29]   Villar J, Belizan JM. The timing factor in the pathophysiology of the intrauterine growth retardation syndrome. Obstet Gynecol Surv 1982; 37(8): 499-506.
[http://dx.doi.org/10.1097/00006254-198208000-00001] [PMID: 7050797]

[30]   Ravelli AC, van Der Meulen JH, Osmond C, Barker DJ, Bleker OP. Obesity at the age of 50 y in men and women exposed to famine prenatally. Am J Clin Nutr 1999; 70(5): 811-6.
[http://dx.doi.org/10.1093/ajcn/70.5.811] [PMID: 10539740]

[31]   Roseboom TJ, van der Meulen JH, Osmond C, Barker DJ, Ravelli AC, Bleker OP. Plasma lipid profiles in adults after prenatal exposure to the Dutch famine. Am J Clin Nutr 2000; 72(5): 1101-6.
[http://dx.doi.org/10.1093/ajcn/72.5.1101] [PMID: 11063435]

[32]   Roseboom TJ, van der Meulen JH, Osmond C, *et al.* Coronary heart disease after prenatal exposure to the Dutch famine, 1944-45. Heart 2000; 84(6): 595-8.
[http://dx.doi.org/10.1136/heart.84.6.595] [PMID: 11083734]

[33]   Lussana F, Painter RC, Ocke MC, Buller HR, Bossuyt PM, Roseboom TJ. Prenatal exposure to the Dutch famine is associated with a preference for fatty foods and a more atherogenic lipid profile. Am J Clin Nutr 2008; 88(6): 1648-52.
[http://dx.doi.org/10.3945/ajcn.2008.26140] [PMID: 19064527]

[34]   Lopuhaä CE, Roseboom TJ, Osmond C, *et al.* Atopy, lung function, and obstructive airways disease after prenatal exposure to famine. Thorax 2000; 55(7): 555-61.
[http://dx.doi.org/10.1136/thorax.55.7.555] [PMID: 10856314]

[35]   Painter RC, Roseboom TJ, Bleker OP. Prenatal exposure to the Dutch famine and disease in later life: an overview. Reprod Toxicol 2005; 20(3): 345-52.
[http://dx.doi.org/10.1016/j.reprotox.2005.04.005] [PMID: 15893910]

[36]   Ravelli AC, van der Meulen JH, Michels RP, *et al.* Glucose tolerance in adults after prenatal exposure to famine. Lancet 1998; 351(9097): 173-7.
[http://dx.doi.org/10.1016/S0140-6736(97)07244-9] [PMID: 9449872]

[37]   Roseboom TJ, Painter RC, van Abeelen AF, Veenendaal MV, de Rooij SR. Hungry in the womb: what are the consequences? Lessons from the Dutch famine. Maturitas 2011; 70(2): 141-5.
[http://dx.doi.org/10.1016/j.maturitas.2011.06.017] [PMID: 21802226]

[38]   WHO. Health Topics. Nutrition 2017. [cited 2017 27/07/2017].

[39]   de Rooij SR, Painter RC, Holleman F, Bossuyt PM, Roseboom TJ. The metabolic syndrome in adults prenatally exposed to the Dutch famine. Am J Clin Nutr 2007; 86(4): 1219-24.
[http://dx.doi.org/10.1093/ajcn/86.4.1219] [PMID: 17921405]

[40]   Kereliuk SM, Brawerman GM, Dolinsky VW. Maternal Macronutrient Consumption and the Developmental Origins of Metabolic Disease in the Offspring. Int J Mol Sci 2017; 18(7)E1451
[http://dx.doi.org/10.3390/ijms18071451] [PMID: 28684678]

[41]   Desai M, Gayle D, Babu J, Ross MG. Programmed obesity in intrauterine growth-restricted newborns: modulation by newborn nutrition. Am J Physiol Regul Integr Comp Physiol 2005; 288(1): R91-6.
[http://dx.doi.org/10.1152/ajpregu.00340.2004] [PMID: 15297266]

[42]   Vickers MH, Reddy S, Ikenasio BA, Breier BH. Dysregulation of the adipoinsular axis -- a mechanism for the pathogenesis of hyperleptinemia and adipogenic diabetes induced by fetal programming. J Endocrinol 2001; 170(2): 323-32.
[http://dx.doi.org/10.1677/joe.0.1700323] [PMID: 11479129]

[43]   Fernandez-Twinn DS, Constancia M, Ozanne SE. Intergenerational epigenetic inheritance in models of developmental programming of adult disease. Semin Cell Dev Biol 2015; 43: 85-95.
[http://dx.doi.org/10.1016/j.semcdb.2015.06.006]

[44]   Lumey LH, Terry MB, Delgado-Cruzata L, *et al.* Adult global DNA methylation in relation to pre-natal nutrition. Int J Epidemiol 2012; 41(1): 116-23.
[http://dx.doi.org/10.1093/ije/dyr137] [PMID: 22422450]

[45]   Heijmans BT, Tobi EW, Stein AD, *et al.* Persistent epigenetic differences associated with prenatal exposure to famine in humans. Proc Natl Acad Sci USA 2008; 105(44): 17046-9.
[http://dx.doi.org/10.1073/pnas.0806560105] [PMID: 18955703]

[46]   Veenendaal MV, Costello PM, Lillycrop KA, *et al.* Prenatal famine exposure, health in later life and promoter methylation of four candidate genes. J Dev Orig Health Dis 2012; 3(6): 450-7.
[http://dx.doi.org/10.1017/S2040174412000396] [PMID: 25084298]

[47]   Tobi EW, Goeman JJ, Monajemi R, *et al.* DNA methylation signatures link prenatal famine exposure to growth and metabolism. Nat Commun 2014; 5: 5592.

[http://dx.doi.org/10.1038/ncomms6592]

[48]   Tobi EW, Slagboom PE, van Dongen J, *et al.* Prenatal famine and genetic variation are independently and additively associated with DNA methylation at regulatory loci within IGF2/H19. PLoS One 2012; 7(5)e37933
[http://dx.doi.org/10.1371/journal.pone.0037933] [PMID: 22666415]

[49]   Tobi EW, Slieker RC, Stein AD, *et al.* Early gestation as the critical time-window for changes in the prenatal environment to affect the adult human blood methylome. Int J Epidemiol 2015; 44(4): 1211-23.
[http://dx.doi.org/10.1093/ije/dyv043] [PMID: 25944819]

[50]   Jou MY, Lönnerdal B, Philipps AF. Maternal zinc restriction affects postnatal growth and glucose homeostasis in rat offspring differently depending upon adequacy of their nutrient intake. Pediatr Res 2012; 71(3): 228-34.
[http://dx.doi.org/10.1038/pr.2011.44] [PMID: 22278188]

[51]   Muthayya S, Kurpad AV, Duggan CP, *et al.* Low maternal vitamin B12 status is associated with intrauterine growth retardation in urban South Indians. Eur J Clin Nutr 2006; 60(6): 791-801.
[http://dx.doi.org/10.1038/sj.ejcn.1602383] [PMID: 16404414]

[52]   Yajnik CS, Deshpande SS, Jackson AA, *et al.* Vitamin B12 and folate concentrations during pregnancy and insulin resistance in the offspring: the Pune Maternal Nutrition Study. Diabetologia 2008; 51(1): 29-38.
[http://dx.doi.org/10.1007/s00125-007-0793-y] [PMID: 17851649]

[53]   Cervantes-Rodríguez M, Martínez-Gómez M, Cuevas E, *et al.* Sugared water consumption by adult offspring of mothers fed a protein-restricted diet during pregnancy results in increased offspring adiposity: the second hit effect. Br J Nutr 2014; 111(4): 616-24.
[http://dx.doi.org/10.1017/S0007114513003000] [PMID: 24124655]

[54]   Li J, Huang J, Li J-S, Chen H, Huang K, Zheng L. Accumulation of endoplasmic reticulum stress and lipogenesis in the liver through generational effects of high fat diets. J Hepatol 2012; 56(4): 900-7.
[http://dx.doi.org/10.1016/j.jhep.2011.10.018] [PMID: 22173165]

[55]   Fernandez-Twinn DS, Alfaradhi MZ, Martin-Gronert MS, *et al.* Downregulation of IRS-1 in adipose tissue of offspring of obese mice is programmed cell-autonomously through post-transcriptional mechanisms. Mol Metab 2014; 3(3): 325-33.
[http://dx.doi.org/10.1016/j.molmet.2014.01.007] [PMID: 24749062]

[56]   Silva C, Keating E, Pinto E. The impact of folic acid supplementation on gestational and long term health: Critical temporal windows, benefits and risks. PBJ in press
[http://dx.doi.org/10.1016/j.pbj.2017.05.006]

[57]   Haggarty P, Hoad G, Campbell DM, Horgan GW, Piyathilake C, McNeill G. Folate in pregnancy and imprinted gene and repeat element methylation in the offspring. Am J Clin Nutr 2013; 97(1): 94-9.
[http://dx.doi.org/10.3945/ajcn.112.042572] [PMID: 23151531]

[58]   Hoyo C, Murtha AP, Schildkraut JM, *et al.* Methylation variation at IGF2 differentially methylated regions and maternal folic acid use before and during pregnancy. Epigenetics 2011; 6(7): 928-36.
[http://dx.doi.org/10.4161/epi.6.7.16263] [PMID: 21636975]

[59]   Azevedo C, Correia-Branco A, Araújo JR, Guimarães JT, Keating E, Martel F. The chemopreventive effect of the dietary compound kaempferol on the MCF-7 human breast cancer cell line is dependent on inhibition of glucose cellular uptake. Nutr Cancer 2015; 67(3): 504-13.
[http://dx.doi.org/10.1080/01635581.2015.1002625] [PMID: 25719685]

[60]   Huang Y, He Y, Sun X, He Y, Li Y, Sun C. Maternal high folic acid supplement promotes glucose intolerance and insulin resistance in male mouse offspring fed a high-fat diet. Int J Mol Sci 2014; 15(4): 6298-313.
[http://dx.doi.org/10.3390/ijms15046298] [PMID: 24736781]

[61]   Vineis P, Chatziioannou A, Cunliffe VT, *et al.* Epigenetic memory in response to environmental stressors. FASEB J 2017; 31(6): 2241-51.
[http://dx.doi.org/10.1096/fj.201601059RR] [PMID: 28280003]

[62]   Remacle C, Bieswal F, Bol V, Reusens B. Developmental programming of adult obesity and cardiovascular disease in rodents by maternal nutrition imbalance. Am J Clin Nutr 2011; 94(6) (Suppl.): 1846S-52S.
[http://dx.doi.org/10.3945/ajcn.110.001651] [PMID: 21543546]

[63]   Chu DM, Antony KM, Ma J, *et al.* The early infant gut microbiome varies in association with a maternal high-fat diet. Genome Med 2016; 8(1): 77.
[http://dx.doi.org/10.1186/s13073-016-0330-z] [PMID: 27503374]

[64]   Wang M, Monaco MH, Donovan SM. Impact of early gut microbiota on immune and metabolic development and function. Semin Fetal Neonatal Med 2016; 21(6): 380-7.
[http://dx.doi.org/10.1016/j.siny.2016.04.004] [PMID: 27132110]

CHAPTER 13

Targeting Gut Microbiota in Obesity Control

Cláudia Marques[1,2] and **Conceição Calhau**[1,2,*]

[1] *Nutrição e Metabolismo, NOVA Medical School, Faculdade de Ciências Médicas, Universidade Nova de Lisboa, Lisboa, Portugal*

[2] *CINTESIS - Center for Health Technology and Services Research, ProNutri - Clinical Nutrition & Disease Programming, University of Porto, Porto, Portugal*

Abstract: Despite the multifactorial etiology of obesity, the attention of the scientific community is now focused on the collection of microorganisms that inhabit the human gut (the gut microbiota) and on their effects upon energy harvest and metabolic signaling. The gut microbiota is involved in the pathophysiology of obesity and several mechanisms are behind this association, *e.g.* increased capacity to extract energy from undigested components of the diet, regulation of fat storage and fatty acid oxidation, bile acids transformation, endocannabinoid system modulation and metabolic endotoxemia. In this chapter, different therapeutic approaches (prebiotics, probiotics and fecal microbiota transplants) designed to modulate the gut microbiota composition towards better results and success rates in obesity management are reviewed and summarized. In conclusion, the gut microbiota might represent a useful marker for determining susceptibility to metabolic disease, as obesity, and be useful in disease diagnosis and monitoring of disease progression.

Keywords: Dysbiosis, Fecal microbiota transplant, Gut, Metabolic syndrome, Microbiome, Microbiota, Obesity, Prebiotics, Probiotics, Synbiotics.

INTRODUCTION

The human body harbors a collection of trillions of microorganisms. Bacteria, archaea, virus, fungi and other eukaryotes live inside different organs establishing a synbiotic relationship with the host [1 - 3]. The microbes that collectively inhabit the gut - the gut microbiota - constitute the largest and most diverse community in the body [4]. More than 90% of the bacterial species in our gut microbiota belong to only three phyla: *Firmicutes*, *Bacteroidetes* and *Actinobacteria*. The metabolic relationships that exist between host cells and microbiota are dynamic processes that have their origins in co-evolution and remain active throughout life [5].

---

[*] **Corresponding author Conceição Calhau:** Nutrição e Metabolismo, NOVA Medical School, Faculdade de Ciências Médicas, Universidade Nova de Lisboa, Lisboa, Portugal; Tel/Fax: +351 218803033; E-mail: ccalhau@nms.unl.pt

Rosário Monteiro and Maria João Martins (Eds.)

The gut microbiota is primarily responsible for the maintenance of the intestinal wall integrity and the protection against pathogens. The bacterial fermentation of non-digestible carbohydrates leads to the formation of short chain fatty acids (SCFA) which reduces luminal pH and inhibits the growth of pathogens. On the other hand, butyrate, one of the most abundant SCFA in the gut, regulates epithelial cell growth and differentiation, especially through epigenetic mechanisms (as histone deacetylase inhibition), thus contributing to the intestinal barrier reinforcement. Besides, the gut microbiota can synthesize certain vitamins, such as vitamin K and B group vitamins (including biotin, cobalamin, folates, nicotinic acid, pantothenic acid, pyridoxine, riboflavin and thiamine) [6]. Furthermore, the gut microbiota is involved in the bile acid transformation as some bacteria have the ability to hydrolyze the amide bond between the steroid nucleus and the conjugated amino acid (taurine or glycine). In addition to bile acid deconjugation, some bacteria can also convert primary bile acids into secondary bile acids through 7α-dehydroxylation, thus increasing the diversity of the bile acid pool.

These structural, protective and metabolic functions have long been attributed to the gut microbiota but the interest of the scientific and medical community upon this collection of microorganisms began to emerge when the first studies demonstrating its envelopment in obesity were published Fig. (**1**) [7, 8].

THE CAUSAL RELATIONSHIP BETWEEN GUT MICROBIOTA AND OBESITY

Obesity is defined by the World Health Organization (WHO) as an abnormal or excessive fat accumulation that presents a risk to health. The etiology of obesity is multifactorial, but in ultimate analysis it results from an energy imbalance in favor of body energy input. Dietary and genetic factors have only partial roles in the development of obesity, which is why the attention is now focused on the gut microbiota.

Until 2004, little attention was being paid to the gut microbiota when it appeared to be an environmental factor affecting predisposition towards obesity [7]. Using germ-free mice (mice raised without any exposure to microorganisms), Backhed *et al* found that mice lacking microbiota had about 40% less total body fat than conventionally raised mice [7]. In addition, the authors found that after colonizing germ-free animals with gut microbiota from conventionally raised mice, the body fat mass of 'germ-free animals' increased 60% in only two weeks [7]. These pioneering findings have linked the gut microbiota to the pathophysiology of obesity and encouraged subsequent research. Since then, a series of experiments have been conducted Fig. (**1**) showing that colonization of germ-free animals with gut microbiota either from *ob/ob* mice, high-fat diet induced obesity (DIO) animals or obese individuals, always result in increased fat mass and adiposity in comparison to colonization with gut microbiota from +/+ mice, chow animals or lean individuals [9 - 11]. Together, these data have shown that the 'obese microbiota' (which has specific characteristics and functions) participates *per se* in the accumulation of fat and body weight gain and have established a causal relationship between gut microbiota and obesity.

Gut microbiota and obesity: the underlying mechanisms

Several studies, using germ-free and conventionally raised mice have explored the mechanisms underlying the association between gut microbiota and adipogenesis [7, 12]. Backhed *et al* have shown that the gut microbiota promotes the absorption of monosaccharides from the gut lumen and increases the expression of key transcriptional factors [sterol regulatory element-binding transcription factor 1 (SREBP1) and carbohydrate-responsive element-binding protein (ChREBP)] in the liver that enhance *de novo* lipogenesis [7].

Furthermore, the gut microbiota suppresses the fasting-induced adipose factor production (Fiaf). Fiaf is released in response to fasting; it inhibits the activity of lipoprotein lipase (LPL) and prevents the storage of triacylglycerols in adipose tissue, functioning as a regulatory mechanism for energy supply [13]. The suppression of Fiaf production by the gut microbiota leads to opposite effects since LPL activity increases, enhancing adipogenesis [7].

In addition, the gut microbiota suppresses adenosine monophosphate-activated protein kinase (AMPK) activity, which has downstream effects on fatty acid oxidation [12].

These mechanisms have clarified why germ-free animals are resistant to DIO [12]. But, which mechanisms explain the increase in total body fat of germ-free mice, after transplanting the 'obese microbiota' (typical found in *ob/ob* and DIO mice) into these recipients? What are the characteristics of this disrupted microbiota?

Turnbaugh *et al* found that the 'obese' microbiome had an increased capacity to extract energy from food [9]. The intestinal fermentation of non-digested food components may lead to the formation of SCFA that, after absorption, can be utilized by the liver in *de novo* lipogenesis [9]. In addition, the authors proposed that the overexpression of microbial genes encoding key enzymes for polysaccharide digestion was related to alterations in the *Firmicutes* to *Bacteroidetes* ratio.

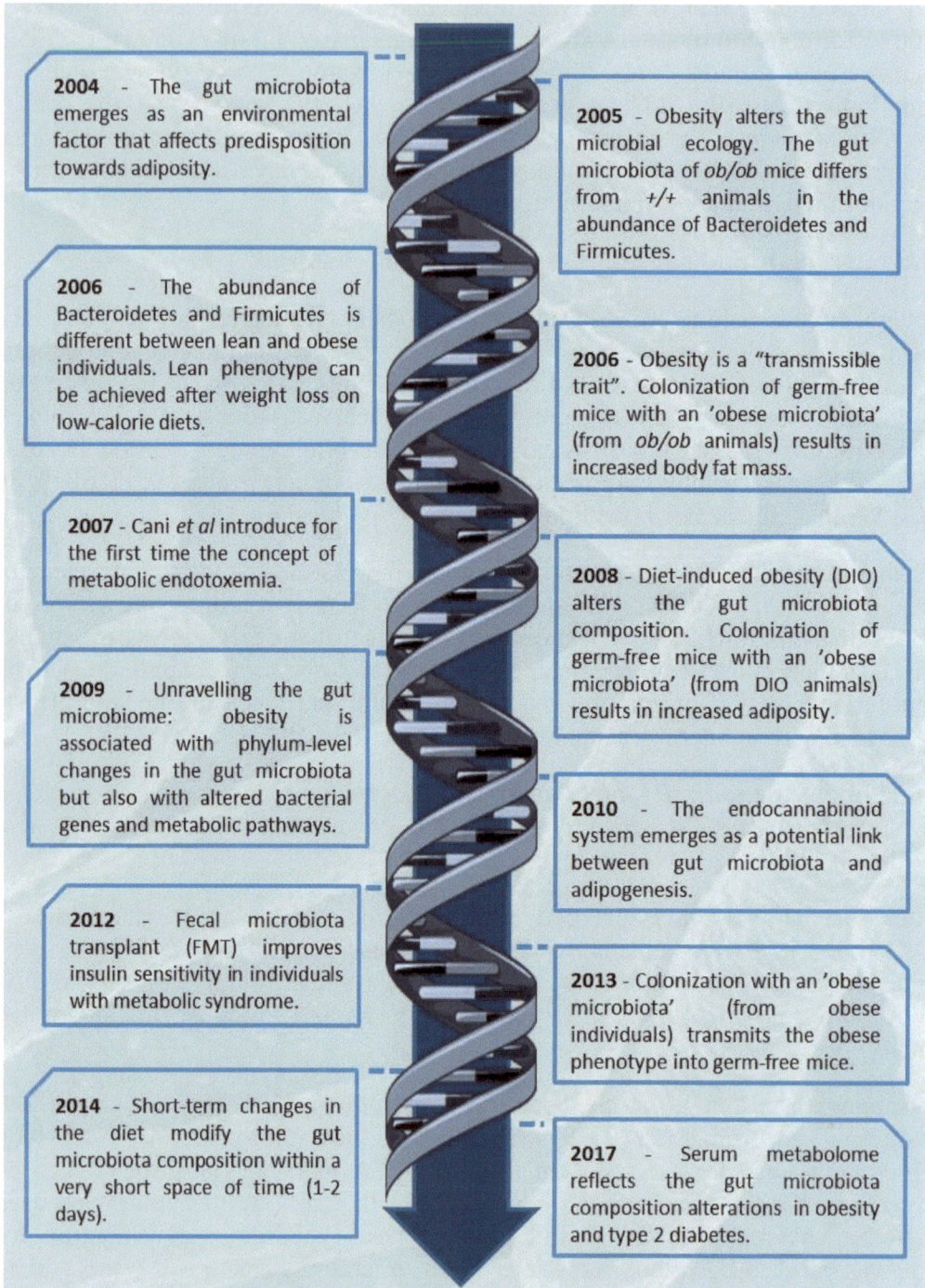

Fig. (1). Timeline of the research about gut microbiota and obesity.

In 2007, Cani *et al* presented lipopolysaccharide (LPS) as a triggering factor of obesity and metabolic diseases. LPS is a component of gram-negative bacteria that can activate an extensive inflammatory cell signaling pathway when it binds to Toll-like receptor 4 (TLR4), linking this endotoxin to insulin resistance [14]. Crossing the intestinal barrier via a paracellular or a transcellular route [15], LPS may reach the systemic circulation at concentrations five times lower than those observed in sepsis, inducing a state denominated as 'metabolic endotoxemia' [16]. In their work, the authors were successful in demonstrating that LPS infusions in chow-fed mice induce a metabolic response similar to high-fat (HF) diet feeding (increased body weight gain and adiposity). In the same line, both *ob/ob* and DIO mice have higher circulating levels of LPS than respective control mice, which is consistent with the increased gut permeability observed in these animals [16, 17]. Thus, it can be speculated that the 'obese microbiota' might induce alterations in the gut permeability of germ-free mice facilitating LPS transition into circulation what might, therefore, trigger the onset of obesity in these animals [18].

Endocannabinoids are produced in organs that contribute to the regulation of energy homeostasis, namely liver, brain and adipose tissue. The endocannabinoid system has a key role on adipose tissue metabolism by activating adipogenesis, adipose tissue expansion and, consequently, a proinflammatory effect. Thus, an overexpression of endocannabinoid system has been described in obesity. Among the putative mechanisms linking the gut microbiota and obesity, a role for the endocannabinoid system has been proposed: probably involving LPS permeability and its influence on cannabinoid receptor signaling [19].

Regarding the composition of the 'obese microbiota', it remains unclear which microbial taxa are actually altered in obesity. Looking at it as having a greater proportion of *Firmicutes* over *Bacteroidetes* is too reductive. The variation in the taxonomic composition of the gut microbiota between individuals is so large that it will be unlikely to find a 'core set' of microorganisms in all obese people. Therefore, characterizing the microbiota as 'healthy' or 'disease-specific' based on a set of specific microbes is no longer a practical definition [20, 21].

Nevertheless, an alternative hypothesis is that of a healthy 'functional core': a collection of beneficial metabolic functions and pathways that are assured by the gut microbiome (the gut microbiota genome) but are not necessarily provided by the same microorganisms in different people [20].

The resistance to ecological stress and the ability to recover from a stress-related perturbation (resilience) are characteristics of a healthy microbiome that empowers its maintenance throughout life [20]. When the microbial ecosystem is perturbed to an extent that exceeds its resistance and resilience capabilities, alterations in its composition and function may occur (dysbiosis) [22]. The expansion of pathobionts (commensal microorganisms that can cause pathology under uncontrolled proliferation), the loss of beneficial bacteria and the loss of diversity (microbial richness) are common characteristics of a dysbiotic state [22]. These features have detrimental consequences for the host (may initiate obesity and metabolic diseases) and can be caused by environmental factors such as dietary factors.

MODULATION OF GUT MICROBIOTA BY DIETARY APPROACHES

Diet is one of the most important factors that can modulate the gut microbiome and rapidly induce alterations in its composition [23].

HF and high-sucrose diets cause profound alterations in the gut microbial ecology, reducing bacterial diversity [24, 25]. One of the mechanisms that may explain these alterations is the increased production of bile acids stimulated by the HF content of the diet [26]. Since they have strong antimicrobial activity (bile acids damage bacterial cell membranes by interacting with membrane phospholipids), bile acids can reduce bacterial diversity. In addition, they can also contribute to gut barrier dysfunction, increasing gut permeability [27]. On the other hand, considering that bile acids are ligands for host cell receptors [namely farnesoid X receptor (FXR), G-protein-coupled bile acid receptor, Gpbar1 (TGR5) and Vitamin D Receptor] alterations in microbial enzymes, as a result of dysbiosis, will end up in changes in the bile acid signature. This will influence the signaling properties of the bile acid pool which may have expressive consequences for the host health.

In addition to HF diets, some environmental pollutants [28, 29] and food additives such as dietary emulsifiers [30 - 32] and non-caloric artificial sweeteners [33] have been shown to disrupt the gut microbiota (causing dysbiosis) in a similar way to what is observed in DIO. Dietary patterns that limit the exposure to these contaminants and food additives may be beneficial to prevent the development of obesity.

On the other hand, modulation of the gut microbiota composition by prebiotics may also be a strategy to reduce weight gain or encourage weight loss in obesity management.

The most commonly used prebiotics are fructooligosaccharides (FOS), galactooligosaccharides (GOS), lactulose and non-digestible carbohydrates: inulin, cellulose, resistant starches, hemicelluloses, gums and pectins [34]. In obesity control, inulin-type dietary fructans are particularly relevant since it has been demonstrated that they modulate gut peptides involved in appetite regulation, induce satiety and prompt the growth of *Bifidobacteria* and *Lactobacilli* [35 - 37].

The most studied prebiotics are non-digestible carbohydrates to fulfill the criteria of previous prebiotic definition [38]. However, the definition of prebiotics has been modified to 'a substrate that is selectively utilized by host microorganisms conferring a health benefit' [39]. Other substances, beyond carbohydrates, might fit the updated definition if convincing evidence demonstrates their health benefits. Compounds such as polyphenols, namely anthocyanins, whey peptide extracts and wheat germen may be considered prebiotics, according to this new definition [40 - 42].

MODULATION OF GUT MICROBIOTA BY PROBIOTICS

According to The Food and Agriculture Organization of the United Nations (FAO) and the World Health Organization (WHO), probiotics are 'live microorganisms that, when administered in adequate amounts, confer a health benefit on the host' [43]. Traditional fermented foods with undefined microbial content and for which there is no evidence of a health benefit are excluded from this definition, as well as fecal microbiota transplants [43].

Probiotic strains are usually isolated from the gut but can also be isolated from different body sites, as well as from fermented foods [44]. They should be resistant to gastrointestinal conditions (low pH and bile acids) and must be safe for their intended use [44]. After careful identification and characterization of the strains, their putative health benefits should be properly addressed in powered, well-designed, randomized clinical trials (RCTs). In the end, the strength of the evidence provided will determine conclusions on causality and its labelling as probiotic.

Diarrhea, inflammatory bowel diseases (IBD), irritable bowel syndrome (IBS) and, more recently, non-alcoholic fatty liver disease (NAFDL) and steatohepatitis (NASH) are among the clinical conditions for which the use of probiotics is recommended [45]. Obesity is not included in this list so far, but the evidence demonstrating the beneficial effects of probiotic supplementation in obesity management is growing (Table **1**).

In 2015, a meta-analysis on probiotics for weight loss pointed that probiotics have limited efficacy to decrease body weight and body mass index (BMI). Nevertheless, the number of RCTs available at that time was limited [46]. Recently, two well designed RCTs were published showing that *Lactobacillus rhamnosus* and probiotic mixtures containing *Lactobacillus* and *Bifidobacterium* species reduce body weight and abdominal obesity in a more effective way than dietary intervention alone (Table **1**) [47, 48]. Importantly, they look particularly effective in women.

Table **1** summarizes the studies evaluating the effects of probiotics or synbiotics (synergistic combination of prebiotics and probiotics) on obesity, in adults. The amount of colony-forming units (CFU) administered in these trials differed from 10^7 to 10^{11}. Health Canada has accepted several bacterial species as probiotics when delivered in food at a level of 1×10^9 CFU per serving [43]. In fact, it seems that when probiotic strains are administered in lower amounts, they do not exert effects on weight loss [49].

Except for some pilot studies in which the number of participants involved was too low [50, 51], most of the RCTs revealed that probiotic or synbiotic supplementation can enhance weight-loss. The effect does not seem to be strain specific, although most of the tested strains belong to the *Lactobacillus* or *Bifidobacterium* genera.

Table 1. Effects of probiotics and synbiotics supplementation in adult obesity management.

Population	Probiotics/Synbiotics	Study Design	Anthropometric Outcomes [a]	Ref.
Obese adults	LPR formulation (*Lactobacillus rhamnosus* CGMCC1.3724, oligofructose and inulin); 3.24 x 10^8 CFU/day	Randomized, double-blind, controlled trial. Intervention: *n* = 62 Control: *n* = 63 Follow-up: 24 weeks	↓Body weight in women	[59, 60]
Overweight and obese women	Probiotic mix (*Lactobacillus acidophilus* and *casei*; *Lactococcus lactis*; *Bifidobacterium bifidum* and *lactis*); 4 x 10^9 CFU of each strain/day	Randomized, double-blind, controlled trial. Intervention: *n* = 21 Control: *n* = 22 Follow-up: 8 weeks	↓Conicity index ↓Waist-height ratio ↓WC	[47]
Overweight and obese adults	*Bifidobacterium animalis* ssp. *lactis* 420; 1 x 10^{10} CFU/day	Randomized, double-blind, controlled trial. Intervention: *n* = 25 Control: *n* = 36 Follow-up: 24 weeks	↓Body fat mass ↓WC	[52]

(Table 1) cont.....

Population	Probiotics/Synbiotics	Study Design	Anthropometric Outcomes [a]	Ref.
Overweight and obese women	Yogurt enriched with *Lactobacillus acidophilus* LA5 and *Bifidobacterium lactis* BB12; 2 x 10^7 CFU/day.	Randomized, single-blind, controlled trial. Intervention: $n = 44$ Control: $n = 45$ Follow-up: 12 weeks	= BMI = Body weight = WC	[49]
NASH patients	Fiber Mais Flora® (*Lactobacillus reuteri*, partially hydrolyzed guar gum and inulin); 2 x 10^8 CFU/day	Randomized, open label, controlled trial. Intervention: $n = 27$ Control: $n = 23$ Follow-up: 12 weeks	[b] ↓BMI ↓Body weight ↓WC	[53]
MetS patients	Fermented milk containing *Bifidobacterium animalis* subsp. *lactis* subsp. nov. HN019; 2.72 x 10^{10} CFU/day	Randomized, open label, controlled trial. Intervention: n = 26 Control: n = 25 Follow-up: 45 days	↓BMI	[61]
Obese adults	*Lactobacillus reuteri* SD5865; 2 x 10^{10} CFU/day	Randomized, double-blind, controlled trial (pilot study). Intervention: $n = 5$ Control: $n = 5$ Follow-up: 4 weeks	= Body fat % = Body weight = Waist-to-hip ratio	[50]
Healthy, non-obese men	VSL#3; 9 x 10^{11} CFU/day	Randomized, double-blind, controlled trial. Intervention: $n = 9$ Control: $n = 11$ Follow-up: 4 weeks	↓Body weight increase after HF diet ↓Fat mass increase after HF diet	[62]
Obese postmenopausal women	*Lactobacillus paracasei* ssp. *paracasei* F19; 9.4 x 10^{10} CFU/day	Randomized, single-blind, controlled trial. Intervention: $n = 18$ Control: $n = 16$ Follow-up: 6 weeks	= BMI = WC	[63]

(Table 1) cont.....

Population	Probiotics/Synbiotics	Study Design	Anthropometric Outcomes [a]	Ref.
Overweight and obese adults	Yogurt enriched with *Lactobacillus acidophilus* La5, *Bifidobacterium* BB12, and *Lactobacillus casei* DN001; 2 x 10^{10} CFU/day	Randomized, double-blind, controlled trial. Intervention: $n = 25$ Control: $n = 25$ Follow-up: 8 weeks	↓Body fat %	[64]
Hypertriacylglycerolemic adults	Fermented milk containing *Lactobacillus gasseri* SBT2055; 1×10^{11} CFU/day	Within-subject, single-blind, controlled trial. $n = 20$ Follow-up: 4 weeks	= BMI = Body weight = WC	[48]
MetS patients	Cheese with *Lactobacillus plantarum* TENSIA; 1 x 10^{10} CFU/day	Randomized, double-blind, controlled trial (pilot study). Intervention: $n = 25$ Control: $n = 15$ Follow-up: 3 weeks	↓BMI ↓Waist-to-hip ratio	[65]
Obese adults	Fermented milk containing *Lactobacillus gasseri* SBT2055; 2×10^{8} CFU/day and 2×10^{10} CFU/day	Randomized, double-blind, controlled trial. Intervention: $n = 25$ Control: $n = 15$ Follow-up: 12 weeks	↓Abdominal fat area ↓BMI ↓WC	[66]
MetS patients	*Lactobacillus casei* Shirota; 2 x 10^{10} CFU/day	Randomized, open-label, controlled trial (pilot study). Intervention: $n = 13$ Control: $n = 15$ Follow-up: 12 weeks	= BMI = Body Weight	[51]

(Table 1) cont.....

Population	Probiotics/Synbiotics	Study Design	Anthropometric Outcomes [a]	Ref.
Obese adults	Fermented milk containing *Lactobacillus gasseri* SBT2055; 1×10^{11} CFU/day	Randomized, double-blind, controlled trial. Intervention: $n = 43$ Control: $n = 44$ Follow-up: 12 weeks	↓Abdominal fat area ↓BMI ↓Body weight ↓Waist- to-hip ratio ↓WC	[67]

[a] Differences between intervention and control groups ($p < 0.05$). [b] The study only reports differences from baseline values. Outcome variation (before and after intervention) is not compared between control and intervention groups. All studies included appropriate controls. Shade lines show studies where synbiotic products were tested. BMI, body mass index; CFU, colony-forming units; HF, high-fat; MetS, metabolic syndrome; NASH, non-alcoholic steatohepatitis; WC, waist circumference.

The mechanisms underlying these effects were not always addressed in the aforementioned trials. Only a few studies have evaluated the effect of probiotic supplementation on the gut microbiota composition and gut permeability [52 - 54]. Modulation of the gut microbiota, gut barrier reinforcement, stimulation of glucagon-like peptide 1 (GLP1) secretion are among the most probable mechanisms of action of these probiotics strains, as demonstrated in animal studies [55 - 58].

Apart from the anthropometric outcomes, these studies have included additional outcomes related with metabolic diseases often associated with obesity, *e.g.* type 2 diabetes. The effect of probiotic supplementation on these metabolic disorders is beyond the scope of this chapter but it is important to mention that probiotics may also have positive effects on lipid profiles and insulin sensitivity, independently of weight loss [49].

To sustain the claim that direct manipulation of gut microbiota with probiotics may contribute to weight loss, more RCTs are necessary. Additional trials that include a larger number of participants are needed to draw conclusions about the role of specific bacterial taxa in weight loss.

FECAL MICROBIOTA TRANSPLANT

Fecal microbiota transplantation (FMT) comprises the infusion of feces from a healthy donor into the gastrointestinal tract of a recipient patient, in order to treat a specific disease associated with alterations of the gut microbiota [68]. FMT has been shown highly effective in the treatment of recurrent *Clostridium difficile* infection (RCDI), presenting success rates of almost 90% [69]. Nevertheless, the use of FMT in the treatment of other diseases, especially obesity and metabolic diseases, is promising.

So far, the only study that have evaluated the efficacy of FMT in obese patients reported a greater diversity in the recipients' gut microbiota after 6 weeks, which was associated with improved insulin resistance [70]. Nevertheless, no weight loss was observed in these patients, 6 weeks after receiving the transplant [70].

FMT may have several associated risks (*e.g.,* infections) and undesirable outcomes (*e.g.,* increased risk of microbiota-associated diseases such as new-onset obesity), and the safety of these procedures (especially in the long-term) remains to be established [71].

The U.S. Food and Drug Administration (FDA) classified human stool as a biological agent and determined that its use in FMT should be regulated. Investigational new drug (IND) permit is required for FMT except for the treatment of *Clostridium difficile* infection not responding to standard therapies, provided that adequate informed consent is obtained from the patient [72]. This bureaucratic and lengthy approval process has discouraged researchers from exploring other potential applications of FMT.

In Europe, FMT is not considered a drug and implementation of FMT in clinical practice for the treatment of both mild and severe RCDI is strongly recommended [68].

FMT may have advantages over probiotics since not only microorganisms are transplanted but also bacterial metabolites (*e.g.,* SCFA) which, after absorption, may improve the disease state. Nonetheless, studies on FMT safety and long-terms effects are warranted.

CONCLUDING REMARKS

In obesity control, targeting the gut microbiota directly through probiotics and FMT or, indirectly, by dietary approaches and prebiotics seems to be a promising strategy that may improve weight loss. On the other hand, weight reducing strategies (dietary interventions, exercise, pharmacological therapy or surgical procedures) also induce changes in the gut microbiota composition, while they induce weight loss [73]. This demonstrates the central role of the gut microbiota in the regulation of energy homeostasis.

Another way to target the gut microbiota that was not entirely addressed in this chapter, but cannot be outside this discussion, is antibiotic therapy. Antibiotics strongly reduce bacterial diversity in the gut. Consequently, a large body of evidence has shown that their indiscriminate use, particularly in early life, may be one of the reasons for the obesity epidemic proportions we are facing today [74, 75]. Thus, cautious use of antibiotics is vital not only to minimize the dissemination of antibiotic-resistant organisms but also to reduce the potentially detrimental long-term metabolic consequences of early antibiotic exposure [76].

Lastly, revolutionizing approaches to target the gut microbiota in obesity and metabolic diseases are being developed. The inclusion of gut microbiota composition in algorithms used to predict the effects of diet on a variety of diseases will direct dietary interventions into a more successful treatment [77]. In addition, the development of microbiota-directed foods that could be, for example, food substrates to be transformed by the gut microbiota into different metabolites necessary for a healthy state [78], will also bring new tools for obesity control.

CONSENT FOR PUBLICATION

Not applicable.

CONFLICT OF INTEREST

The authors confirm that this chapter contents have no conflict of interest.

ACKNOWLEDGEMENTS

This chapter was supported by FEDER through the operation POCI-01-01-5-FEDER-007746 funded by the Programa Operacional Competitividade e Internacionalização – COMPETE2020 and by National Funds through FCT - Fundação para a Ciência e a Tecnologia within CINTESIS, R&D Unit (reference UID/IC/4255/2013). Cláudia Marques has a PhD scholarship from FCT: SFRH/BD/93073/2013.

REFERENCES

[1]   Grice EA, Segre JA. The skin microbiome. Nat Rev Microbiol 2011; 9(4): 244-53.
        [http://dx.doi.org/10.1038/nrmicro2537] [PMID: 21407241]

[2]   Man WH, de Steenhuijsen Piters WAA, Bogaert D. The microbiota of the respiratory tract: gatekeeper to respiratory health. Nat Rev Microbiol 2017; 15(5): 259-70.
        [http://dx.doi.org/10.1038/nrmicro.2017.14] [PMID: 28316330]

[3]   Mark Welch JL, Rossetti BJ, Rieken CW, Dewhirst FE, Borisy GG. Biogeography of a human oral microbiome at the micron scale. Proc Natl Acad Sci USA 2016; 113(6): E791-800.
        [http://dx.doi.org/10.1073/pnas.1522149113] [PMID: 26811460]

[4]   Sender R, Fuchs S, Milo R. Revised Estimates for the Number of Human and Bacteria Cells in the Body. PLoS Biol 2016; 14(8)e1002533
        [http://dx.doi.org/10.1371/journal.pbio.1002533] [PMID: 27541692]

[5]   Burcelin R. Gut microbiota and immune crosstalk in metabolic disease. Mol Metab 2016; 5(9): 771-81.
        [http://dx.doi.org/10.1016/j.molmet.2016.05.016] [PMID: 27617200]

[6]   Hill MJ. Intestinal flora and endogenous vitamin synthesis. Eur J Cancer Prev 1997; 6 (Suppl. 1): S43-5.
        [http://dx.doi.org/10.1097/00008469-199703001-00009] [PMID: 9167138]

[7]   Bäckhed F, Ding H, Wang T, *et al.* The gut microbiota as an environmental factor that regulates fat storage. Proc Natl Acad Sci USA 2004; 101(44): 15718-23.
        [http://dx.doi.org/10.1073/pnas.0407076101] [PMID: 15505215]

[8]   Ley RE, Bäckhed F, Turnbaugh P, Lozupone CA, Knight RD, Gordon JI. Obesity alters gut microbial ecology. Proc Natl Acad Sci USA 2005; 102(31): 11070-5.
        [http://dx.doi.org/10.1073/pnas.0504978102] [PMID: 16033867]

[9]   Turnbaugh PJ, Ley RE, Mahowald MA, Magrini V, Mardis ER, Gordon JI. An obesity-associated gut microbiome with increased capacity for energy harvest. Nature 2006; 444(7122): 1027-31.
        [http://dx.doi.org/10.1038/nature05414] [PMID: 17183312]

[10]   Turnbaugh PJ, Bäckhed F, Fulton L, Gordon JI. Diet-induced obesity is linked to marked but reversible alterations in the mouse distal gut microbiome. Cell Host Microbe 2008; 3(4): 213-23.
        [http://dx.doi.org/10.1016/j.chom.2008.02.015] [PMID: 18407065]

[11]   Ridaura VK, Faith JJ, Rey FE, *et al.* Gut microbiota from twins discordant for obesity modulate metabolism in mice. Science 2013; 341(6150)1241214
        [http://dx.doi.org/10.1126/science.1241214] [PMID: 24009397]

[12]   Bäckhed F, Manchester JK, Semenkovich CF, Gordon JI. Mechanisms underlying the resistance to diet-induced obesity in germ-free mice. Proc Natl Acad Sci USA 2007; 104(3): 979-84.
        [http://dx.doi.org/10.1073/pnas.0605374104] [PMID: 17210919]

[13]   Sukonina V, Lookene A, Olivecrona T, Olivecrona G. Angiopoietin-like protein 4 converts lipoprotein lipase to inactive monomers and modulates lipase activity in adipose tissue. Proc Natl Acad Sci USA 2006; 103(46): 17450-5.
        [http://dx.doi.org/10.1073/pnas.0604026103] [PMID: 17088546]

[14]   Medzhitov R, Horng T. Transcriptional control of the inflammatory response. Nat Rev Immunol 2009; 9(10): 692-703.
        [http://dx.doi.org/10.1038/nri2634] [PMID: 19859064]

[15]   Guerville M, Boudry G. Gastrointestinal and hepatic mechanisms limiting entry and dissemination of lipopolysaccharide into the systemic circulation. Am J Physiol Gastrointest Liver Physiol 2016; 311(1): G1-G15.
        [http://dx.doi.org/10.1152/ajpgi.00098.2016] [PMID: 27151941]

[16]   Cani PD, Bibiloni R, Knauf C, *et al.* Changes in gut microbiota control metabolic endotoxemia-induced inflammation in high-fat diet-induced obesity and diabetes in mice. Diabetes 2008; 57(6): 1470-81.
        [http://dx.doi.org/10.2337/db07-1403] [PMID: 18305141]

[17]   Brun P, Castagliuolo I, Di Leo V, *et al.* Increased intestinal permeability in obese mice: new evidence in the pathogenesis of nonalcoholic steatohepatitis. Am J Physiol Gastrointest Liver Physiol 2007; 292(2): G518-25.
        [http://dx.doi.org/10.1152/ajpgi.00024.2006] [PMID: 17023554]

[18]   Cani PD, Osto M, Geurts L, Everard A. Involvement of gut microbiota in the development of low-grade inflammation and type 2 diabetes associated with obesity. Gut Microbes 2012; 3(4): 279-88.
        [http://dx.doi.org/10.4161/gmic.19625] [PMID: 22572877]

[19]   Cani PD, Plovier H, Van Hul M, *et al.* Endocannabinoids--at the crossroads between the gut microbiota and host metabolism. Nat Rev Endocrinol 2016; 12(3): 133-43.
        [http://dx.doi.org/10.1038/nrendo.2015.211] [PMID: 26678807]

[20]   Bäckhed F, Fraser CM, Ringel Y, *et al.* Defining a healthy human gut microbiome: current concepts, future directions, and clinical applications. Cell Host Microbe 2012; 12(5): 611-22.

[http://dx.doi.org/10.1016/j.chom.2012.10.012] [PMID: 23159051]

[21]   Lloyd-Price J, Abu-Ali G, Huttenhower C. The healthy human microbiome. Genome Med 2016; 8(1): 51.
        [http://dx.doi.org/10.1186/s13073-016-0307-y] [PMID: 27122046]

[22]   Levy M, Kolodziejczyk AA, Thaiss CA, Elinav E. Dysbiosis and the immune system. Nat Rev Immunol 2017; 17(4): 219-32.
        [http://dx.doi.org/10.1038/nri.2017.7] [PMID: 28260787]

[23]   David LA, Maurice CF, Carmody RN, *et al.* Diet rapidly and reproducibly alters the human gut microbiome. Nature 2014; 505(7484): 559-63.
        [http://dx.doi.org/10.1038/nature12820] [PMID: 24336217]

[24]   Marques C, Meireles M, Norberto S, *et al.* High-fat diet-induced obesity Rat model: a comparison between Wistar and Sprague-Dawley Rat. Adipocyte 2015; 5(1): 11-21.
        [http://dx.doi.org/10.1080/21623945.2015.1061723] [PMID: 27144092]

[25]   Lau E, Marques C, Pestana D, *et al.* The role of I-FABP as a biomarker of intestinal barrier dysfunction driven by gut microbiota changes in obesity. Nutr Metab (Lond) 2016; 13: 31.
        [http://dx.doi.org/10.1186/s12986-016-0089-7] [PMID: 27134637]

[26]   Stenman LK, Holma R, Korpela R. High-fat-induced intestinal permeability dysfunction associated with altered fecal bile acids. World J Gastroenterol 2012; 18(9): 923-9.
        [http://dx.doi.org/10.3748/wjg.v18.i9.923] [PMID: 22408351]

[27]   Stenman LK, Holma R, Eggert A, Korpela R. A novel mechanism for gut barrier dysfunction by dietary fat: epithelial disruption by hydrophobic bile acids. Am J Physiol Gastrointest Liver Physiol 2013; 304(3): G227-34.
        [http://dx.doi.org/10.1152/ajpgi.00267.2012] [PMID: 23203158]

[28]   Fader KA, Nault R, Zhang C, Kumagai K, Harkema JR, Zacharewski TR. 2,3,7,8-Tetrachlorodibenz-
        -p-dioxin (TCDD)-elicited effects on bile acid homeostasis: Alterations in biosynthesis, enterohepatic circulation, and microbial metabolism. Sci Rep 2017; 7(1): 5921.
        [http://dx.doi.org/10.1038/s41598-017-05656-8] [PMID: 28725001]

[29]   Zhang L, Nichols RG, Correll J, *et al.* Persistent Organic Pollutants Modify Gut Microbiota-Host Metabolic Homeostasis in Mice Through Aryl Hydrocarbon Receptor Activation. Environ Health Perspect 2015; 123(7): 679-88.
        [http://dx.doi.org/10.1289/ehp.1409055] [PMID: 25768209]

[30]   Singh RK, Wheildon N, Ishikawa S. Food Additive P-80 Impacts Mouse Gut Microbiota Promoting Intestinal Inflammation, Obesity and Liver Dysfunction. SOJ Microbiol Infect Dis 2016; 4(1)
        [http://dx.doi.org/10.15226/sojmid/4/1/00148] [PMID: 27430014]

[31]   Chassaing B, Van de Wiele T, De Bodt J, Marzorati M, Gewirtz AT. Dietary emulsifiers directly alter human microbiota composition and gene expression ex vivo potentiating intestinal inflammation. Gut 2017; 66(8): 1414-27.
        [http://dx.doi.org/10.1136/gutjnl-2016-313099] [PMID: 28325746]

[32]   Chassaing B, Koren O, Goodrich JK, *et al.* Dietary emulsifiers impact the mouse gut microbiota promoting colitis and metabolic syndrome. Nature 2015; 519(7541): 92-6.
        [http://dx.doi.org/10.1038/nature14232] [PMID: 25731162]

[33]   Suez J, Korem T, Zilberman-Schapira G, Segal E, Elinav E. Non-caloric artificial sweeteners and the microbiome: findings and challenges. Gut Microbes 2015; 6(2): 149-55.
        [http://dx.doi.org/10.1080/19490976.2015.1017700] [PMID: 25831243]

[34]   Review A. Front Microbiol 2017; 8: 563. Dahiya DK, Renuka, Puniya M, et al. Gut Microbiota Modulation and Its Relationship with Obesity Using Prebiotic Fibers and Probiotics:
        [http://dx.doi.org/10.3389/fmicb.2017.00563] [PMID: 28421057]

[35]   Cani PD, Neyrinck AM, Fava F, *et al.* Selective increases of bifidobacteria in gut microflora improve

high-fat-diet-induced diabetes in mice through a mechanism associated with endotoxaemia. Diabetologia 2007; 50(11): 2374-83.
[http://dx.doi.org/10.1007/s00125-007-0791-0] [PMID: 17823788]

[36]   Cani PD, Possemiers S, Van de Wiele T, *et al.* Changes in gut microbiota control inflammation in obese mice through a mechanism involving GLP-2-driven improvement of gut permeability. Gut 2009; 58(8): 1091-103.
[http://dx.doi.org/10.1136/gut.2008.165886] [PMID: 19240062]

[37]   Parnell JA, Reimer RA. Weight loss during oligofructose supplementation is associated with decreased ghrelin and increased peptide YY in overweight and obese adults. Am J Clin Nutr 2009; 89(6): 1751-9.
[http://dx.doi.org/10.3945/ajcn.2009.27465] [PMID: 19386741]

[38]   Gibson GR, Probert HM, Loo JV, Rastall RA, Roberfroid MB. Dietary modulation of the human colonic microbiota: updating the concept of prebiotics. Nutr Res Rev 2004; 17(2): 259-75.
[http://dx.doi.org/10.1079/NRR200479] [PMID: 19079930]

[39]   Gibson GR, Hutkins R, Sanders ME, *et al.* Expert consensus document: The International Scientific Association for Probiotics and Prebiotics (ISAPP) consensus statement on the definition and scope of prebiotics. Nat Rev Gastroenterol Hepatol 2017; 14(8): 491-502.
[http://dx.doi.org/10.1038/nrgastro.2017.75] [PMID: 28611480]

[40]   Yu Y-J, Amorim M, Marques C, Calhau C, Pintado M. Effects of whey peptide extract on the growth of probiotics and gut microbiota. J Funct Foods 2016; 21: 507-16.
[http://dx.doi.org/10.1016/j.jff.2015.10.035]

[41]   Faria A, Fernandes I, Norberto S, Mateus N, Calhau C. Interplay between anthocyanins and gut microbiota. J Agric Food Chem 2014; 62(29): 6898-902.
[http://dx.doi.org/10.1021/jf501808a] [PMID: 24915058]

[42]   Moreira-Rosário A, Pinheiro H, Calhau C, Azevedo LF. Can wheat germ have a beneficial effect on human health? A study protocol for a randomised crossover controlled trial to evaluate its health effects. BMJ Open 2016; 6(11)e013098
[http://dx.doi.org/10.1136/bmjopen-2016-013098] [PMID: 28157671]

[43]   Hill C, Guarner F, Reid G, *et al.* Expert consensus document. The International Scientific Association for Probiotics and Prebiotics consensus statement on the scope and appropriate use of the term probiotic. Nat Rev Gastroenterol Hepatol 2014; 11(8): 506-14.
[http://dx.doi.org/10.1038/nrgastro.2014.66] [PMID: 24912386]

[44]   Fontana L, Bermudez-Brito M, Plaza-Diaz J, Muñoz-Quezada S, Gil A. Sources, isolation, characterisation and evaluation of probiotics. Br J Nutr 2013; 109 (Suppl. 2): S35-50.
[http://dx.doi.org/10.1017/S0007114512004011] [PMID: 23360880]

[45]   Recommendations for Probiotic Use-2015 Update: Proceedings and Consensus Opinion: Erratum. J Clin Gastroenterol 2016; 50(9): 800. [Erratum].
[http://dx.doi.org/10.1097/MCG.0000000000000700] [PMID: 27624459]

[46]   Park S, Bae JH. Probiotics for weight loss: a systematic review and meta-analysis. Nutr Res 2015; 35(7): 566-75.
[http://dx.doi.org/10.1016/j.nutres.2015.05.008] [PMID: 26032481]

[47]   Gomes AC, de Sousa RG, Botelho PB, Gomes TL, Prada PO, Mota JF. The additional effects of a probiotic mix on abdominal adiposity and antioxidant Status: A double-blind, randomized trial. Obesity (Silver Spring) 2017; 25(1): 30-8.
[http://dx.doi.org/10.1002/oby.21671] [PMID: 28008750]

[48]   Ogawa A, Kadooka Y, Kato K, Shirouchi B, Sato M. Lactobacillus gasseri SBT2055 reduces postprandial and fasting serum non-esterified fatty acid levels in Japanese hypertriacylglycerolemic subjects. Lipids Health Dis 2014; 13: 36.
[http://dx.doi.org/10.1186/1476-511X-13-36] [PMID: 24548293]

[49]   Madjd A, Taylor MA, Mousavi N, *et al.* Comparison of the effect of daily consumption of probiotic compared with low-fat conventional yogurt on weight loss in healthy obese women following an energy-restricted diet: a randomized controlled trial. Am J Clin Nutr 2016; 103(2): 323-9.
       [http://dx.doi.org/10.3945/ajcn.115.120170] [PMID: 26702123]

[50]   Simon MC, Strassburger K, Nowotny B, *et al.* Intake of Lactobacillus reuteri improves incretin and insulin secretion in glucose-tolerant humans: a proof of concept. Diabetes Care 2015; 38(10): 1827-34.
       [http://dx.doi.org/10.2337/dc14-2690] [PMID: 26084343]

[51]   Leber B, Tripolt NJ, Blattl D, *et al.* The influence of probiotic supplementation on gut permeability in patients with metabolic syndrome: an open label, randomized pilot study. Eur J Clin Nutr 2012; 66(10): 1110-5.
       [http://dx.doi.org/10.1038/ejcn.2012.103] [PMID: 22872030]

[52]   Stenman LK, Lehtinen MJ, Meland N, *et al.* Probiotic With or Without Fiber Controls Body Fat Mass, Associated With Serum Zonulin, in Overweight and Obese Adults-Randomized Controlled Trial. EBioMedicine 2016; 13: 190-200.
       [http://dx.doi.org/10.1016/j.ebiom.2016.10.036] [PMID: 27810310]

[53]   Ferolla SM, Couto CA, Costa-Silva L, *et al.* Beneficial Effect of Synbiotic Supplementation on Hepatic Steatosis and Anthropometric Parameters, But Not on Gut Permeability in a Population with Nonalcoholic Steatohepatitis. Nutrients 2016; 8(7)E397
       [http://dx.doi.org/10.3390/nu8070397] [PMID: 27367724]

[54]   Gøbel RJ, Larsen N, Jakobsen M, Mølgaard C, Michaelsen KF. Probiotics to adolescents with obesity: effects on inflammation and metabolic syndrome. J Pediatr Gastroenterol Nutr 2012; 55(6): 673-8.
       [http://dx.doi.org/10.1097/MPG.0b013e318263066c] [PMID: 22695039]

[55]   Yadav H, Lee JH, Lloyd J, Walter P, Rane SG. Beneficial metabolic effects of a probiotic via butyrate-induced GLP-1 hormone secretion. J Biol Chem 2013; 288(35): 25088-97.
       [http://dx.doi.org/10.1074/jbc.M113.452516] [PMID: 23836895]

[56]   Park DY, Ahn YT, Park SH, *et al.* Supplementation of Lactobacillus curvatus HY7601 and Lactobacillus plantarum KY1032 in diet-induced obese mice is associated with gut microbial changes and reduction in obesity. PLoS One 2013; 8(3)e59470
       [http://dx.doi.org/10.1371/journal.pone.0059470] [PMID: 23555678]

[57]   Rather SA, Pothuraju R, Sharma RK, *et al.* Anti-obesity effect of feeding probiotic dahi containing Lactobacillus casei NCDC 19 in high fat diet-induced obese mice. Int J Dairy Technol 2014; 67(4): 504-9.
       [http://dx.doi.org/10.1111/1471-0307.12154]

[58]   Alard J, Lehrter V, Rhimi M, *et al.* Beneficial metabolic effects of selected probiotics on diet-induced obesity and insulin resistance in mice are associated with improvement of dysbiotic gut microbiota. Environ Microbiol 2016; 18(5): 1484-97.
       [http://dx.doi.org/10.1111/1462-2920.13181] [PMID: 26689997]

[59]   Sanchez M, Darimont C, Panahi S, *et al.* Effects of a Diet-Based Weight-Reducing Program with Probiotic Supplementation on Satiety Efficiency, Eating Behaviour Traits, and Psychosocial Behaviours in Obese Individuals. Nutrients 2017; 9(3)E284
       [http://dx.doi.org/10.3390/nu9030284] [PMID: 28294985]

[60]   Sanchez M, Darimont C, Drapeau V, *et al.* Effect of Lactobacillus rhamnosus CGMCC1.3724 supplementation on weight loss and maintenance in obese men and women. Br J Nutr 2014; 111(8): 1507-19.
       [http://dx.doi.org/10.1017/S0007114513003875] [PMID: 24299712]

[61]   Bernini LJ, Simão AN, Alfieri DF, *et al.* Beneficial effects of Bifidobacterium lactis on lipid profile and cytokines in patients with metabolic syndrome: A randomized trial. Effects of probiotics on metabolic syndrome. Nutrition 2016; 32(6): 716-9.
       [http://dx.doi.org/10.1016/j.nut.2015.11.001] [PMID: 27126957]

[62]   Osterberg KL, Boutagy NE, McMillan RP, *et al.* Probiotic supplementation attenuates increases in body mass and fat mass during high-fat diet in healthy young adults. Obesity (Silver Spring) 2015; 23(12): 2364-70.
[http://dx.doi.org/10.1002/oby.21230] [PMID: 26466123]

[63]   Brahe LK, Le Chatelier E, Prifti E, *et al.* Dietary modulation of the gut microbiota--a randomised controlled trial in obese postmenopausal women. Br J Nutr 2015; 114(3): 406-17.
[http://dx.doi.org/10.1017/S0007114515001786] [PMID: 26134388]

[64]   Zarrati M, Salehi E, Nourijelyani K, *et al.* Effects of probiotic yogurt on fat distribution and gene expression of proinflammatory factors in peripheral blood mononuclear cells in overweight and obese people with or without weight-loss diet. J Am Coll Nutr 2014; 33(6): 417-25.
[http://dx.doi.org/10.1080/07315724.2013.874937] [PMID: 25079040]

[65]   Lee SJ, Bose S, Seo JG, Chung WS, Lim CY, Kim H. The effects of co-administration of probiotics with herbal medicine on obesity, metabolic endotoxemia and dysbiosis: a randomized double-blind controlled clinical trial. Clin Nutr 2014; 33(6): 973-81.
[http://dx.doi.org/10.1016/j.clnu.2013.12.006] [PMID: 24411490]

[66]   Kadooka Y, Sato M, Ogawa A, *et al.* Effect of Lactobacillus gasseri SBT2055 in fermented milk on abdominal adiposity in adults in a randomised controlled trial. Br J Nutr 2013; 110(9): 1696-703.
[http://dx.doi.org/10.1017/S0007114513001037] [PMID: 23614897]

[67]   Kadooka Y, Sato M, Imaizumi K, *et al.* Regulation of abdominal adiposity by probiotics (Lactobacillus gasseri SBT2055) in adults with obese tendencies in a randomized controlled trial. Eur J Clin Nutr 2010; 64(6): 636-43.
[http://dx.doi.org/10.1038/ejcn.2010.19] [PMID: 20216555]

[68]   Cammarota G, Ianiro G, Tilg H, *et al.* European FMT Working Group. European consensus conference on faecal microbiota transplantation in clinical practice. Gut 2017; 66(4): 569-80.
[http://dx.doi.org/10.1136/gutjnl-2016-313017] [PMID: 28087657]

[69]   Kassam Z, Lee CH, Yuan Y, Hunt RH. Fecal microbiota transplantation for Clostridium difficile infection: systematic review and meta-analysis. Am J Gastroenterol 2013; 108(4): 500-8.
[http://dx.doi.org/10.1038/ajg.2013.59] [PMID: 23511459]

[70]   Vrieze A, Van Nood E, Holleman F, *et al.* Transfer of intestinal microbiota from lean donors increases insulin sensitivity in individuals with metabolic syndrome. Gastroenterology 2012; 143(3): 913-6 e7..
[http://dx.doi.org/10.1053/j.gastro.2012.06.031]

[71]   de Groot PF, Frissen MN, de Clercq NC, Nieuwdorp M. Fecal microbiota transplantation in metabolic syndrome: History, present and future. Gut Microbes 2017; 8(3): 253-67.
[http://dx.doi.org/10.1080/19490976.2017.1293224] [PMID: 28609252]

[72]   U.S. Food and Drug Administration (FDA). Enforcement Policy Regarding Investigational New Drug Requirements for Use of Fecal Microbiota for Transplantation to Treat Clostridium difficile Infection Not Responsive to Standard Therapies 2016.

[73]   Seganfredo FB, Blume CA, Moehlecke M, *et al.* Weight-loss interventions and gut microbiota changes in overweight and obese patients: a systematic review. Obes Rev 2017; 18(8): 832-51.
[http://dx.doi.org/10.1111/obr.12541] [PMID: 28524627]

[74]   Ray K. Gut microbiota: adding weight to the microbiota's role in obesity--exposure to antibiotics early in life can lead to increased adiposity. Nat Rev Endocrinol 2012; 8(11): 623.
[http://dx.doi.org/10.1038/nrendo.2012.173] [PMID: 22965166]

[75]   Cox LM, Blaser MJ. Antibiotics in early life and obesity. Nat Rev Endocrinol 2015; 11(3): 182-90.
[http://dx.doi.org/10.1038/nrendo.2014.210] [PMID: 25488483]

[76]   Turta O, Rautava S. Antibiotics, obesity and the link to microbes - what are we doing to our children? BMC Med 2016; 14: 57.
[http://dx.doi.org/10.1186/s12916-016-0605-7] [PMID: 27090219]

[77]   Zeevi D, Korem T, Zmora N, *et al.* Personalized Nutrition by Prediction of Glycemic Responses. Cell 2015; 163(5): 1079-94.
[http://dx.doi.org/10.1016/j.cell.2015.11.001] [PMID: 26590418]

[78]   Green JM, Barratt MJ, Kinch M, Gordon JI. Food and microbiota in the FDA regulatory framework. Science 2017; 357(6346): 39-40.
[http://dx.doi.org/10.1126/science.aan0836] [PMID: 28684495]

CHAPTER 14

Modulatory Impact of Physical Exercise on the Morphological and Metabolic Features of White Adipose Tissue

Sílvia Rocha-Rodrigues[1,3,*], **Jorge Beleza**[1,2], **António Ascensão**[1,2] and **José Magalhães**[1,2]

[1] *CIAFEL - Research Center in Physical Activity, Health and Leisure, Faculty of Sport, University of Porto, Porto, Portugal*

[2] *LaMetEx - Laboratory of Metabolism and Exercise, Faculty of Sport, University of Porto, Porto, Portugal*

[3] *Escola Superior de Desporto e Lazer, Instituto Politécnico de Viana do Castelo, Viana do Castelo, Portugal*

Abstract: Regular physical exercise (PE) has been recognized as one of the most powerful lifestyle strategies used to mitigate overweight and obesity. In this context, white adipose tissue (WAT) plays a pivotal role as it is the largest site of storage and release of excess energy, thus participating in important metabolic, endocrine and inflammatory functions, which are intricately linked to the etiology and pathophysiology of obesity-associated chronic diseases. Moreover, current literature reports that PE, besides reducing visceral fat accumulation, also mitigates obesity-induced dysregulated adipokine synthesis and release, resulting in systemic metabolic improvements through beneficial dynamics changes in WAT. More recently, PE-induced hormone secretion by skeletal muscle has been described as a potential mechanism for inducing a brown fat-like phenotype in WAT. Thus, the modulatory impact of PE on WAT may also occur through the cross-talk between skeletal muscle and adipose organ axis. In this chapter, we focused on the overall impact of PE on WAT morphological, metabolic and inflammatory features, on the cross-talk between skeletal muscle and WAT as well as on the potential mediators of this process, providing an overview of the effects of PE on the obesity-related underlying pathways.

Keywords: Adipocyte turnover, Adiponectin, Angiogenesis, Apoptosis, Autophagy, Browning, Endurance training, Ghrelin, Inflammation, Interleukin 6,

---
* **Corresponding author Sílvia Rocha-Rodrigues:** CIAFEL - Research Centre in Physical Activity, Health and Leisure, Faculty of Sport, University of Porto, Porto, Portugal; LaMetEx - Laboratory of Metabolism and Exercise, Faculty of Sport, University of Porto, Porto, Portugal; Escola Superior de Desporto e Lazer, Instituto Politécnico de Viana do Castelo, Viana do Castelo, Portugal; Tel: +351 225074785; Fax: +351 225500689; E-mail: silviadarocharodrigues@gmail.com

Rosário Monteiro and Maria João Martins (Eds.)

Irisin, Leptin, Metabolism, Mitochondria, Myokines, Tumor necrosis factor α, Visceral adiposity.

INTRODUCTION

The alarming incidence of obesity worldwide and the rising costs of treating the associated diseases increased the urgency of developing preventive and therapeutic countermeasures to antagonize this phenomenon. Physical exercise (PE) is a mainstay of lifestyle modifications able to prevent and/or treat a variety of complications associated to overweight and obesity [1, 2]. PE represents an important fraction of the energy expenditure in active humans, stimulates fat mass loss and helps preserve lean mass, besides promoting important alterations in hormones and their physiological action. Accumulating evidence shows that distinct PE regimens, including endurance training (ET), resistance training (RT) and high-intensity interval training (HIIT), not only reduce visceral fat accumulation [3 - 6] but also have a profound impact against obesity-induced cellular disturbances, thus contributing to systemic metabolic improvements through favorable dynamic changes in white adipose tissue (WAT) [7 - 10]. Several studies have reported that PE regulates adipokine production and secretion, reduces adipogenesis, improves lipid and glucose metabolism, increases mitochondrial content and biogenesis as well as apoptotic signaling of WAT [11 - 19]. Mechanistically, contracting skeletal muscle induces local paracrine-mediated actions on several signaling pathways involved in its structure and metabolism and also produces and secretes bioactive molecules, designed as myokines, which act in an endocrine-like fashion on distant organs and tissues [20], including WAT [21]. Particularly, some myokines alter the metabolic phenotype of WAT by inducing browning, fatty acid oxidation and improving insulin sensitivity [22 - 26]. Therefore, myokines likely provide a conceptual basis to understand, at least in part, the modulatory impact of PE on WAT, *e.g.* the cross-talk between skeletal muscle and adipose organ axis, which is of particular interest in the context of obesity.

The present chapter highlights the prominent role of white adipose organ in whole-body adaptations induced by PE and contribute to a better understanding of the mechanisms by which PE possibly attenuates the adverse consequences of obesity, strengthening the relevance of this lifestyle-related strategy to prevent and/or treat obesity and related disorders.

THE EFFECTS OF PHYSICAL EXERCISE ON WHITE ADIPOSE TISSUE MORPHOLOGICAL FEATURES

Studies in both humans and animal models have shown that obesity-related metabolic dysfunction is more closely associated with visceral than with subcutaneous adipose tissue accumulation [27, 28]. Evidence suggests that intrinsic features of visceral and subcutaneous adipose tissue depots, rather than their anatomical position, play a key role regarding their distinct effects on metabolism and inflammation [28, 29]. Moreover, increased visceral adiposity during chronic high-fat diet (HFD) feeding was associated with hypertrophy rather than hyperplasia (*i.e.* adipogenesis) of adipose tissue [30], which provides a rationale for the distinct impact of specific adipose tissue depots in the context of obesity [30]. Therefore, we will mainly focus on the effects of PE on dynamic changes associated to the visceral adipose tissue depots.

Data from animal studies have clearly shown that distinct models of PE, including voluntary physical activity (VPA) and ET reduced the size of white adipocytes from diet-induced obesity (DIO) animals [18, 31 - 33]. Regarding adipogenesis, an interesting study from Zeve *et al* [34] demonstrated that 2 months of VPA modulated WAT homeostasis either through a decrease in progenitor activity or reduction in adipocyte turnover. Moreover, the authors showed that mice with higher percentage of type I (slow) myofibers were protected from HFD-induced weight gain possibly due to a decreased adipogenic potential of adipose progenitors [34]. Thus, it seems that skeletal muscle, in a non-autonomous manner, regulates adipose progenitor homeostasis, which supports a link between skeletal muscle and adipose progenitors and highlights a role for skeletal muscle-derived secreted factors in adipose stem cell function. From a molecular point of view, ET decreases the expression of adipocyte differentiation-related genes, such as *Glycerol-3-phosphate dehydrogenase*, regulators of G protein signaling-2, *β-catenin* and *Wtn10b* genes in epididymal stromal vascular fraction (SVF) cells [35], and increases delta-like 1/pre-adipocyte factor 1 (*Dlk1/Pref1*) gene expression [35 - 37], a gatekeeper of adipogenesis, in lean and DIO animals.

Angiogenesis

Angiogenesis, a process that ultimately results in the formation of new blood vessels, involves the participation of multiple angiogenic factors and plays an important role during adipogenesis [38]. An upregulation of vascular endothelial growth factor (VEGF) gene expression and its receptor has been reported in adipocytes and SVF cells after 11 days of VPA [11] as well as 6 and 8 weeks of ET [37, 39] in DIO mice. In addition, data from Hatano *et al* [40] suggested that angiogenesis in WAT might not be dependent on adipocyte size and/or number, as an increase of endothelial cell number *per* adipocyte and a decrease of adipocyte size and number were described after 9 weeks of ET. Altogether, these findings suggest that PE modulates adipocyte turnover, which results in decreased visceral adiposity through an inhibition of adipogenesis of adipocyte precursor cells, but without compromising angiogenesis.

Autophagy

This crucial process of response to various forms of stress, that intends to preserve the homeostatic balance between the synthesis, degradation and recycling of cellular proteins and organelles [41, 42], has been reported to be activated in the WAT of obese humans [43 - 45] and rodents [46, 47]. In this context, autophagy seems to be positively correlated with whole body adiposity, visceral adiposity as well as adipocyte hypertrophy [43, 48] and differentiation [49, 50]. Moreover, data suggest that the regulation of adipocyte autophagy may be a potential mechanism to attenuate and/or revert obesity-induced cellular abnormalities. In fact, a specific inhibition of autophagy mediated by decreased expression of *Atg5* or *Atg7* in WAT was associated with reduced adiposity and increased energy expenditure, thus conferring increased protection against obesity [50 - 52]. Regarding the effects of PE on WAT autophagy-related mechanisms, few studies have addressed this issue so far. In non-obese rats, Tanaka *et al* [14] demonstrated that 9 weeks of ET increased the accumulation of autophagosomes, but attenuated basal autophagy by increasing the protein expression of p62 in epididymal WAT (eWAT). Accordingly, data from our group in DIO animals also showed that 8 weeks of ET diminished basal autophagy in eWAT through p62 protein enhanced expression [19]. Together, data suggest that in response to ET, the increased autophagic adapter p62 might provide mechanistic positive influence on eWAT [53], as p62 inhibits extracellular signal-regulated kinase (ERK) activity and function through direct interaction [54]. Also, the phosphorylation of ERK, which is activated by oxidative stress and is involved in the expression of monocyte chemoattractant protein 1 (MCP1), was attenuated by PE [55, 56]. Of note, is that an increase in the expression of autophagy-related molecules in eWAT may not reflect an activation of autophagic clearance, but perhaps obesity-related changes in adipose tissue cells composition. These findings suggest that PE-induced autophagy may constitute a mechanism that positively potentiates adaptations in eWAT in order to regulate body lipid accumulation by controlling adipocyte differentiation in the context of obesity.

Apoptotic Signaling

As a consequence of increased adipocyte hypertrophy and/or hyperplasia, the pathological expansion of the WAT in obesity contributes to the formation of hypoxic areas, which result in the activation of death receptors (extrinsic) or mitochondrial (intrinsic) pathways, thus leading to the stimulation of effector caspases and adipocyte apoptotic signaling [57, 58]. Hence apoptosis, a programmed cell death mechanism related to damaged cell elimination [41], has been described to be augmented in both obese humans [59, 60] and animals [59, 61]. In contrast, some studies reported an increased anti-apoptotic Bcl-xl expression in mature epididymal adipocytes in response to high-intensity ET [62] and a reduced apoptotic signaling in WAT of lean rats after 12 weeks of ET [36]. In the same line of these results, data from our laboratory revealed that 8 weeks of ET were able to revert HFD-induced proapoptotic phenotype through stimulation of anti-apoptotic Bcl-2 expression in eWAT [19]. This might be related, at least in part, to a reduction on adipocyte size [18, 31 - 33] and number [34, 63] as well as to a decrease in hypoxia inducible factor 1α (HIF1α) expression in eWAT already described in DIO animals submitted to an ET program for 8 [37] and 12 weeks [64]. Altogether, the PE-induced reduction in visceral adiposity may lead to reduced local hypoxia, ameliorated oxygen flux to eWAT, thus attenuating autophagy and apoptotic pathway signaling, and ultimately improving morphological, metabolic and inflammatory eWAT features. However, further studies are yet needed to elucidate the molecular mechanisms involved in this process.

PHYSICAL EXERCISE-INDUCED ADAPTATIONS ON NON- AND ADIPOSE-DERIVED HORMONE SYNTHESIS AND SECRETION

As an important secretory organ, WAT synthesizes and secretes numerous hormones, cytokines and other factors, collectively designated as adipokines. These molecules play critical roles in several physiological processes, such as energy expenditure, insulin signaling, glucose and lipid metabolism, inflammation and immunity [65 - 67]. Therefore, a dysregulation in the expression of adipokines as a result of obesity is closely associated with the etiology and development of obesity-associated diseases [68]. Furthermore, the size of the white adipocytes affects adipokine expression in obesity [68]. Using isolated human adipocytes according to their volume, Skurk *et al* [69] showed that the secretion levels of tumor-necrosis factor α (TNFα), MCP1 and interleukin 6 (IL6) were positively correlated with cell size. In the present section, we will mainly focus on the modulatory impact of PE on adiponectin, leptin, and ghrelin variations due to their role on distinct processes related to obesity.

Adiponectin

Adiponectin is one of the key adipocyte-derived hormones that regulates systemic or tissue lipid and glucose metabolism [70]. In contrast to most other adipocyte-derived hormones, adiponectin increases insulin sensitivity in various tissues, including liver and skeletal muscle, apparently due to improved lipid and glucose metabolism [71]. Also, adiponectin has been shown to have anti-inflammatory properties [72]. In the context of obesity, reduced levels of circulating adiponectin were found in DIO mice [73, 74] and in obese subjects [75], which were inversely correlated with body mass index (BMI), visceral adiposity and indexes of insulin resistance (IR) [76]. Moreover, ET programs of 10 and 15 weeks increased gene expression of adiponectin in subcutaneous adipose tissue of obese individuals [77 - 79] and in retroperitoneal fat depot of Zucker rats [80]. However, no changes were reported in epididymal [80] and mesenteric WAT depots [81], suggesting that PE possibly modulates adiponectin synthesis and secretion by adipose tissue in a depot-dependent manner. A study with abdominally obese subjects reported an increase in plasma adiponectin concentrations 30 minutes after acute bouts of endurance exercise performed at high (75% VO_2 peak) and at low (50% VO_2 peak) intensities [82]. In contrast, 6 months of RT in obese subjects induced increased plasma adiponectin levels after moderate and high-intensity, but not after the low-intensity sessions [4]. Moreover, a recent meta-analysis found a statistically significant relationship between circulating adiponectin levels and change in body fat [83]. Accordingly, 1 year of combined RT and ET showed a significant increase in circulating adiponectin levels, possibly due to the significant reduction in body mass and body fat [84]. Additionally, 12 weeks of HIIT exercise induced a great increase on circulating adiponectin levels on obese female adolescents, highlighting the benefits of HIIT interventions in the obese population [85]. Other studies reported consistent elevated circulating adiponectin levels after 1 hour of daily ET for 4 weeks [86, 87] and after 2-3 hours *per* day for 15 weeks of ET [78] in overweight and obese individuals. Surprisingly, one study reported no alterations of plasma adiponectin concentrations despite improvements on insulin sensitivity on obese elderly individuals after 12 weeks of ET performed at 85% of maximal heart rate [88]. In an attempt to clarify this intriguing finding, other studies showed that the changes in the multimeric forms, particularly the high-molecular weight (HMW), of the protein may be more important than changes in total adiponectin itself [89, 90]. In fact, some authors have shown an increase of circulating HMW adiponectin levels after an acute moderate-intensity exercise bout in subjects with normal glucose tolerance [91], but others found no alterations in older insulin-resistant [92] or obese individuals [91]. In conclusion, being the positive impact of PE on adiponectin levels still not completely evident in some studies, more robust studies with measurement and control of dietary intake, visceral adiposity, WAT depot specificity, hormone and cytokine levels (such as insulin, cathecolamines [93, 94], IL6 [94] and TNFα [95]) and assessment of distal health outcomes are needed.

Leptin

Leptin is the key long-term satiety signaling peptide produced and secreted almost exclusively by differentiated adipocytes [96] and its circulating levels reflect the amount of adipose tissue and tend to decrease and increase in response to starvation and overfeeding, respectively [97]. Moreover, leptin functions as a signal on energy balance through metabolic-mediated effects on the endocrine and central nervous system [98]. Therefore, an increase of circulating leptin levels is commonly observed in obesity [31, 64], these levels being positively correlated with body fat and adipocyte size [76]. Moreover, chronic conditions seem to promote a hypothalamic leptin resistance that aggravates the obesity *status* through the inhibition of the appetite control and lipid oxidation [99]. Surprisingly, data are not consistent regarding the impact of PE on leptin secretion levels. Data from some animal studies revealed that both VPA and ET interventions decreased leptin levels in plasma and in WAT of distinct obese models [31, 64, 100 - 104]; while other studies reported no changes [39, 80, 101, 105, 106]. Accordingly, acute and short-term bouts of PE do not appear to affect leptin levels. For example, single short-term bouts of PE (between 45 and 60 minutes) do not alter leptin concentration in plasma [87, 88, 107] and in subcutaneous adipose tissue [108] of obese females and males. In contrast, long-term periods (>3 months) of ET [109, 110] and RT [4] programs seem to result in reduced fat mass accompanied by lower leptin concentrations in healthy individuals. In addition, reduced leptin levels have been associated to fat mass loss after 1 year of ET programs [111, 112]; however, other studies demonstrated that lower plasma leptin levels were independent of body weight, fat mass or adipose tissue mRNA expression of leptin after a RT intervention of 12 weeks [5, 113], which suggest a direct impact of PE on leptin secretion and/or protein turnover. Moreover, in obese individuals, a 6-month program of RT decreased plasma leptin levels in all PE sessions compared to pre-training levels, the magnitude of the decrease being dependent on PE intensity [4]. These findings suggest that the duration of the intervention and the intensity of the PE sessions are negatively related to leptin levels [83].

Ghrelin

Ghrelin, an appetite-stimulating hormone, is predominately synthesized and secreted from the stomach and small intestine. Although ghrelin was initially identified because of its potent growth hormone (GH)-secreting actions, a number of other potential functions for ghrelin have since been described, including roles in food intake, energy expenditure, body weight regulation and visceral adiposity [76, 114, 115]. In obesity conditions, ghrelin production has been reported to be markedly suppressed in obese individuals [116, 117] and in animals submitted to DIO [118]. Regarding the impact of PE on ghrelin levels, conflicting data has been published. We have previously demonstrated that 8 weeks of ET increased plasma ghrelin levels concomitantly with a decrease in body weight and visceral adiposity in DIO rats [37]. Human-based studies observed reduction [119 - 122], increment [123 - 125] or no alterations [126] in plasma total ghrelin concentrations following an acute bout of PE. A recent study demonstrated that 12 weeks of HIIT had no impact on plasma acylated ghrelin, the active form of ghrelin [127], suggesting that this model of exercise training has no effect on appetite when compared with an isocaloric program of moderate-intensity continuous program in obese individuals. In addition, a 3-month and 12-month energy deficit-imposing diet and exercise interventions produced weight loss which was associated with increased total ghrelin concentration in normal-weight women [128] and in overweight or obese postmenopausal women [129]. Moreover, effects of ghrelin on GH release and appetite are mediated through its receptor, the GH secretagogue receptor (GHS-R), mainly GSH-R1a [130]. GHS-R1a is expressed in WAT and has been described to have implications on glucose and lipid metabolism as well as on the inflammatory response [130]. Therefore, the pleiotropic effects of the ghrelin/GHS-R system suggest its implication in the prevention and treatment of obesity and associated diseases. We have previously demonstrated that two distinct models of PE (VPA and ET) increased GHS-R1a protein content in WAT from DIO animals concomitantly with reduced visceral adiposity, but not with body weight [37]. Additional studies are clearly needed to further understand the mechanistic involvement of GHS-R1a in PE-induced modulation of obesity-related constraints. Considering the inconsistent findings, future studies should take into account important variables that could interfere with ghrelin variations, such as exercise intensity, degree of obesity and gender differences as well as the time points of plasma and tissue collection, as humans' plasma ghrelin concentration increases before meals and decreases in the postprandial state [131].

PE-induced alterations in adipokines and ghrelin in obesity may also be dependent on changes in fat-free mass and on some specific hormones/factors, such as cathecolamines and insulin. In fact, several studies reported small increases in fat-free mass following ET programs [132], which may be sufficient to influence metabolic activity and overall energy balance with positive metabolic consequences, ultimately compromising some adipokines and ghrelin expression [4]. For instance, an HIIT program resulted in significant increases in plasma glucose and in peak insulin concentrations immediately post-exercise [133, 134], which may have different effects on adipokine and ghrelin secretion. In addition, lactate production from skeletal muscle during high-intensity PE, and its consequent accumulation in plasma, also seems to have an important impact on the secretion of appetite-regulating hormones [135, 136]. Nevertheless, being the mechanisms responsible for altering adipokine and ghrelin secretion in response to PE still very unclear, additional studies are needed.

PHYSICAL EXERCISE-INDUCED ADAPTATIONS ON INFLAMMA-TORY-RELATED MECHANISMS

Obesity is often linked to a chronic low-grade inflammatory state [137, 138].

Moreover, it has been described that the expression of several critical factors involved in energy metabolism, such as peroxisome proliferator-activated receptors (PPAR), toll-like receptors (TLR) and fatty acid-binding proteins also act as cross-linking agents between metabolic regulation and inflammatory signaling pathways [139]. In fact, the increased plasma non-esterified fatty acids (NEFA) reported in obesity may be involved in the inflammatory response [139, 140]. Some authors reported that the NEFA-mediated activation of IκB kinase β (IKKβ) induces the translocation of nuclear factor kappa B (NFκB) to the nucleus and the posterior transcription of target genes that result in an increase of proinflammatory cytokines and other factors, such as TNFα and MCP1 [28]. Furthermore, the IKKβ/NFκB pathway seems to be activated in obese humans [141] and animals [142, 143], being therefore considered a key pathogenic mechanism in obesity-associated inflammation [144, 145]. Distinct PE interventions have been described to reduce the risk of inflammation in DIO animals [64, 146 - 149] and in individuals with overweight and obesity [150 - 152]; however, it remains unknown how PE exerts its anti-inflammatory effects under these conditions. An attenuating effect of PE on IKKβ/NFkB pathway in DIO rats submitted to acute exercise [142] or 8 weeks of ET [143] has been reported. This effect may be linked to the PE-induced adipokine secretion alterations, namely adiponectin, since this adipokine exerts several anti-inflammatory effects, including not only the inhibition of NFkB, suppression of phagocytic activity and TNFα production in macrophages [71], but also the increased production of anti-inflammatory cytokines, such as IL10 [72]. Moreover, both acute and long-term swimming exercise mitigated obesity-induced adipose tissue activation of TLR4 [142], which is an activator of both IKKβ and c-Jun N-terminal kinase (JNK) [153]. Thus, it seems that the reduced TLR4 expression in adipose tissue may also be a consequence of the PE-induced suppression of M1 macrophage infiltration [55] and/or induction of the phenotype switching from proinflammatory M1 macrophages to anti-inflammatory M2 macrophages [64, 77, 102, 105, 106, 146, 154 - 156]. In fact, studies suggested that, under obesity conditions, a shift of the activation state of adipose tissue macrophages from an M2-polarized state to an M1 proinflammatory state occurs [105, 146, 155]. Moreover, the majority of macrophages in obese adipose tissue aggregate in "crown-like structures" completely surrounding dead (necrotic-like) adipocytes and scavenging adipocyte debris [157], which seem to be reverted by VPA in obese mice [155, 156]. Kawanishi *et al* [147] found that CD8[+] T cells, which have a critical role in adipose tissue inflammation and are abundant in adipose tissue of obese animals, were suppressed after 12 weeks of ET. In individuals with obesity, distinct PE regimens reduced both RANTES and C-C chemokine receptor type 5 in the subcutaneous adipose tissue [158] and decreased circulating proinflammatory markers, such as IL6 [9, 78, 151, 158 - 160] and

TNFα [78, 151, 159, 161].

Interleukin 6

In the context of obesity, an excessive production of IL6 by adipose tissue has an adverse effect on glucose metabolism and insulin sensitivity [162] and has been reported to be a secondary response to the elevated amount of TNFα [162]. Conflicting data exist in literature, with studies reporting decreased circulating IL6 levels in response to an acute HIIT session [9] and long-term ET [78, 151, 158 - 160], while others showed that the circulating IL6 levels remain unchanged [5, 108, 163, 164] in overweight or obese individuals engaged in distinct PE routines.

Tumor Necrosis Factor α

Regarding the impact of PE on TNFα concentrations, an important pathophysiological player in obesity [138], studies also report conflicting data. Some reported that the increased TNFα expression in WAT from DIO animals was suppressed after 8 weeks of climbing PE [18], VPA [102, 104] and ET [18, 64, 146, 154] interventions, whereas others reported no changes [10, 39, 80, 81, 165, 166] after distinct PE regimens. Likewise, some studies with humans with overweight/obesity engaged in programs of ET reported a decrease [151, 159, 161, 167], while others reported no changes in the levels of TNFα [9, 88, 108, 164]. Moreover, a study showed that 12 weeks of ET did not change TNFα mRNA expression in subcutaneous adipose tissue of obese individuals, despite a reduction in body weight and body fat [77].

In obesity, an increased production of reactive oxygen species in adipocytes may also be associated with the dysregulated expression of inflammatory-related cytokines [168]. As an acute bout of PE immediately elevates oxidative stress, the chronic adaptation of WAT against PE-induced oxidative stress may be mediated by increases in antioxidant system via an increase in the enzyme manganese superoxide dismutase (Mn-SOD) and possibly a decrease in the proinflammatory adipokines [62]. In fact, ET significantly lowered the levels of lipid peroxidation and elevated protein expression of Mn-SOD in eWAT from DIO rats [169]. Moreover, the eWAT protein contents of TNFα, MCP1 and phosphorylated ERK, activated by reactive oxygen species and important for MCP1 expression, were significantly reduced after 8 weeks of ET [53]. Nevertheless, the molecular mechanisms and consequences underpinning the role of the different PE approaches on IL6, TNFα and other important inflammatory markers in the context of obesity are clearly elusive and further studies are needed to clarify the misunderstandings and conflicting results.

THE EFFECTS OF PHYSICAL EXERCISE ON BROWN ADIPOCYTE-LIKE PHENOTYPE

Although structural and functional differences between white and brown adipose tissues exist, they have a remarkable plasticity and can share features under specific physiological conditions and stimuli [25], such as chronic cold exposure [170], PE [22, 25, 26, 171], PPARγ agonists or β-adrenergic stimulation [172], and therefore a brown adipocyte-like phenotype may be aroused in classical white adipocytes. Data from animal studies showed that browning-associated genes, such as uncoupling protein 1 (*Ucp1*) and PR domain containing 16 *(Prdm16)*, are overexpressed in both subcutaneous and visceral adipose tissues in response to an acute bout of ET [22], chronic ET [25, 26, 33] or VPA [26, 155, 173]. Moreover, morphologic alterations in subcutaneous adipose tissue, such as increased UCP1 immunofluorescence in multilocular cells, were also observed after 11 days of VPA in DIO mice [11]. Accordingly, a human-based study found that the combination of ET and RT over 12 weeks promoted a mild increased expression of the "beige"- and "brown"-associated genes, transmembrane protein 26 *(Tmem26)* and *Ucp1*, respectively, in subcutaneous adipose tissue [174]. However, so far, most studies performed in humans [174 - 176] failed to clearly demonstrate "browning" in response to PE. Distinct important factors, such as type, duration and intensity of the PE programs, ambient temperature, genetic factors, age, the pre-training BMI, and the initial cardiorespiratory fitness levels of the individuals could, at least in part, explain the discrepant data between animal and human studies.

As an important transcriptional coactivator involved in energy metabolism [177], the PPAR gamma coactivator 1α (PGC1α) has been associated with the increased mitochondrial content and fatty acid oxidation in WAT as well as with browning, therefore preventing body weight gain and improving glucose tolerance in HFD-fed mice [11, 26]. Moreover, sirtuin 1 (SIRT1), a NAD^+-dependent type III metabolic sensor, also seems to be closely involved in the regulation of this process [177]. SIRT1 activates PGC1α and deacetylates two critical lysine residues on PPARγ in adipocytes, which contributes to increased energy expenditure and seems to promote brown adipocyte-like phenotype in WAT [178]. Data from our group showed that ET-induced increases in PGC1α and SIRT1 protein content in eWAT were associated with the increased expression of "browning" markers and their regulators, such as bone morphogenetic protein 7 (BMP7) in conditions of pre-exiting obesity [33]. BMP7 activates a full program of brown-related adipogenesis, including the induction of mitochondrial biogenesis via p38 mitogen-activated protein kinase (p38 MAPK) and PGC1α-dependent pathways, increases the expression of the early regulator of brown fat fate PRDM16, brown-specific marker UCP1, and of the adipogenic transcription factors PPARγ and CCAAT/enhancer-binding proteins [28].

Taken together, data clearly suggest that more studies are still needed to unravel the inconsistencies found in literature as well as the precise regulatory mechanisms regarding the potential impact of PE in human's white adipose tissue "brown" signaling.

Mitochondrial Activity

Some data suggest that white adipose cells initiate adaptive responses to PE and acquire a brown adipocyte-like phenotype [22, 25, 179], being this process related to an increase in mitochondrial density and function [17, 180, 181], and to an uncoupling of the oxidative phosphorylation (OXPHOS) caused by the increase of UCP1 expression. Moreover, the expression of the *Pgc1α*, a critical player in mitochondrial biogenesis regulation [182], and the expression of mitochondrial transcription factor (*Tfam*) are upregulated in WAT after both an acute bout of exercise [17] and chronic ET [17, 183]. Regarding the impact of PE in the context of obesity, the information provided by the literature is still scarce. Nevertheless, oxidative phosphorylation (OXPHOS) subunit genes, such as *mt-Nd5* and *mt-Cytb*, are overexpressed after 16 weeks of VPA in adipocytes of DIO mice [184]. Furthermore, few studies demonstrated that PE induced positive mitochondrial alterations, including the gene expression of subunit IV of cytochrome C oxidase and *Pgc1α* in DIO mice [180] and in hyperphagic, obese rats [181]. These findings suggest that PE has a significant impact on WAT mitochondrial function, which may contribute to a brown adipocyte-like phenotype in WAT; however further studies are still needed to better understand the mechanisms underlying the impact of PE on WAT mitochondrial activity in the context of obesity.

Myokines

Notwithstanding the gaps regarding the effects of PE on brown adipocyte-like phenotype response, some hypotheses have been proposed for the underlying molecular mechanisms. An increased number of studies suggest that besides some PE-induced myokines that act locally in the muscle through autocrine/paracrine mechanisms, other myokines, such as brain-derived neurotrophic factor (BDNF) [173], IL6 [185], meteorin-like [186] or irisin [22] are released into circulation as endocrine factors and may drive important stimuli ultimately leading to a brown adipocyte-like phenotype in WAT. In fact, an overexpression of the *Il6* gene mediated by PE increased the *Ucp1* gene and protein expression in rat brown adipose tissue [187] and subcutaneous adipose tissue [185]. Moreover, the ET-induced increase in skeletal muscle IL6 levels was strongly correlated with brown adipocyte-like phenotype markers expression and regulators in HFD-fed rats [33].

Meteorin-like is a myokine mainly induced in response to RT and PGC1α4 overexpression, which promotes activation of M2 macrophages and catecholamines production from these cells to induce browning effects [186] and sustain adaptive thermogenesis [188]. Nevertheless, among all the myokines that potentially regulate the browning adipocyte-like phenotype, the fibronectin type III domain-containing protein 5 (FNDC5) is the one that has received more attention in literature.

The FNDC5 is produced by skeletal muscle, proteolytically cleaved and released into circulation as irisin. It has been proposed that irisin is elevated after VPA [22, 24], an acute bout of exercise [189, 190] as well as chronic ET and RT programs [25, 26, 33, 191, 192]. In fact, studies with rodents revealed that circulating irisin levels were acutely increased immediately after one bout of strenuous exercise [189], and were associated with the commonly described exercise-induced oxidative stress. On the other hand, oxidative stress is known to stimulate p38 MAPK and ERK [193, 194], which in turn activates PGC1α in skeletal muscle, an important regulator of FNDC5, but also of the browning signaling process [22]. In exercised animals, skeletal muscle FNDC5 and circulating irisin levels were positively associated with the upregulation of browning-related markers, including *Pgc1α* and its downstream target *Ucp1*, *Cidea* and *Dio2* genes, and *Prdm16*, a transcriptional regulator of brown adipose tissue differentiation, among others [11, 15, 17, 22, 25, 26, 180]. Accordingly, this augmented signaling was also coupled with reductions in adipocyte hypertrophy, visceral adiposity as well as with improvements in glucose tolerance in DIO animals [33, 195].

Nevertheless, data from studies performed with humans are not so consistent. Some studies showed that chronic ET, RT or the combination of both PE models did not affect skeletal muscle FNDC5 [196, 197] or circulating irisin [197 - 199] levels in sedentary healthy individuals or in children with obesity [200]. In contrast, other studies revealed an increased FNDC5 and PGC1α expression in response to an acute bout of high-intensity exercise [196] and to 12 weeks of combined ET and RT [174]. In fact, although increased muscle FNDC5 has been detected without any changes in circulating irisin levels after chronic PE [197, 201], acute increases in irisin levels have been reported during exercise in sedentary individuals [22, 174, 202 - 207]. Kraemer *et al* [206] found that plasma irisin levels increased during the course of a 90-min (60% of VO_2 max) treadmill running, reaching the peak values at 54 min; however, returned to baseline levels immediately post-exercise. Moreover, Norheim *et al* [174] reported a peak concentration of irisin after 45 min cycling without a concomitant increase in *Fndc5* gene expression, which suggests that increases in irisin levels during acute exercise may be associated with protein *post-translational* modifications.

Actually, the type, duration and particularly the intensity of the PE sessions also seem to influence the expression of circulating irisin. High-intensity exercise (80% VO_2max for 20 min) promoted greater irisin response compared with low-intensity exercise (40% VO_2max for 40 min) under similar energy consumption conditions [202]. In accordance, it has been demonstrated that circulating irisin levels increase when the muscle adenosine triphosphate (ATP) levels acutely drop, but remain unchanged when muscle ATP content is restored, suggesting that irisin may contribute to ATP homeostasis [208]. Based on this hypothesis, the lack of irisin changes in some studies may be explained by the PE intensity, as short-term low-to-moderate intensity PE induces low ATP depletion [208]. Of note, plasma irisin levels seem to be progressively elevated in response to increasing PE workloads. In fact, physically active individuals with higher VO_2max showed greater concentrations of irisin during maximal workload PE [202, 205, 207]. Furthermore, irisin levels were positively correlated with skeletal muscle volume, fat-free mass, glucose, ghrelin and insulin-like growth factor 1 (IGF1) levels [209 - 212].

Collectively, data suggest that circulating irisin levels seem to be increased in response to acute intense PE in humans; however new insights into irisin regulation during PE are clearly needed. Of note is that some inconsistencies may be related to interactions between irisin and other cytokines and hormones, such as IL6, BDNF and adiponectin [213 - 215]. Moreover, other cells, such as cardiomyocytes and Purkinje cells of cerebellum [24, 214, 216], have been described to interfere with irisin metabolism/regulation and should also be considered in future studies.

CONCLUDING REMARKS

In summary, the pathological increase of visceral adiposity has been associated with systemic and adipose tissue morphological, inflammatory and metabolic alterations, which likely contribute to WAT dysfunction in the context of obesity. In contrast, PE seems to have a significant modulatory impact on a large number of molecules/factors involved in the improvement of adipokine profile secretion, metabolic and inflammatory response at both systemic and local levels. It also influences WAT browning, and mitochondrial biogenesis and activity, which are determinant for improving metabolic function and energy expenditure, likely preventing and/or counteracting overweight/obesity and visceral adiposity in obesity. As illustrated in Fig. (**1**), these effects may be due to the novel PE-induced adipokines/myokines secreted by "trained" adipose tissue and skeletal muscle; nevertheless the understanding of putative adipokines/myokines and their role in the function of tissues need further research. In fact, future studies are needed to better understand whether the benefits of PE on adipose tissue, primarily described in rodent models, also really occur in human subjects, thus contributing for counteracting lifestyle-related diseases.

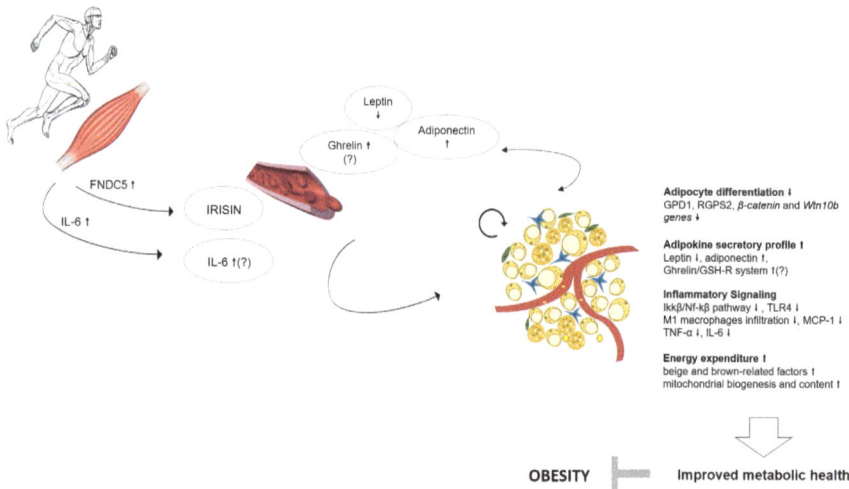

Fig. (1).   Schematic view of hypothetical mechanisms underlying PE impact on white adipose tissue morphological, metabolic and inflammatory features in the context of obesity. FNDC5, fibronectin type III domain-containing protein 5; GHS-R, growth hormone secretagogue receptor; G3PD, glycerol-3-phosphate dehydrogenase; IκKβ, IκB kinase β; IL6, interleukin- 6; MCP1, macrophage/monocyte chemotactic protein; NFkβ, nuclear factor β; RGPS2, regulators of G protein signaling-2; TLR4, toll-like receptor 4; TNFα, tumor necrosis factor α; ?, conflicting data.

CONSENT FOR PUBLICATION

Not applicable.

CONFLICT OF INTEREST

The authors confirm that this chapter contents have no conflict of interest.

ACKNOWLEDGEMENTS

Declared none.

REFERENCES

[1]   Fiuza-Luces C, Garatachea N, Berger NA, Lucia A. Exercise is the real polypill. Physiology (Bethesda) 2013; 28(5): 330-58.
[http://dx.doi.org/10.1152/physiol.00019.2013] [PMID: 23997192]

[2]   Allen J, Sun Y, Woods JA. Exercise and the Regulation of Inflammatory Responses. Prog Mol Biol Transl Sci 2015; 135: 337-54.
[http://dx.doi.org/10.1016/bs.pmbts.2015.07.003] [PMID: 26477921]

[3]   Zhang H, Tong TK, Qiu W, *et al.* Comparable Effects of High-Intensity Interval Training and Prolonged Continuous Exercise Training on Abdominal Visceral Fat Reduction in Obese Young Women. J Diabetes Res 2017; 20175071740
[http://dx.doi.org/10.1155/2017/5071740] [PMID: 28116314]

[4]   Fatouros IG, Tournis S, Leontsini D, *et al.* Leptin and adiponectin responses in overweight inactive elderly following resistance training and detraining are intensity related. J Clin Endocrinol Metab 2005; 90(11): 5970-7.
[http://dx.doi.org/10.1210/jc.2005-0261] [PMID: 16091494]

[5]   Klimcakova E, Polak J, Moro C, *et al.* Dynamic strength training improves insulin sensitivity without altering plasma levels and gene expression of adipokines in subcutaneous adipose tissue in obese men. J Clin Endocrinol Metab 2006; 91(12): 5107-12.
[http://dx.doi.org/10.1210/jc.2006-0382] [PMID: 16968804]

[6]   Maillard F, Rousset S, Pereira B, *et al.* High-intensity interval training reduces abdominal fat mass in postmenopausal women with type 2 diabetes. Diabetes Metab 2016; 42(6): 433-41.
[http://dx.doi.org/10.1016/j.diabet.2016.07.031] [PMID: 27567125]

[7]   Dietz P, Hoffmann S, Lachtermann E, Simon P. Influence of exclusive resistance training on body composition and cardiovascular risk factors in overweight or obese children: a systematic review. Obes Facts 2012; 5(4): 546-60.
[http://dx.doi.org/10.1159/000341560] [PMID: 22854678]

[8]   Bajer B, Vlcek M, Galusova A, Imrich R, Penesova A. Exercise associated hormonal signals as powerful determinants of an effective fat mass loss. Endocr Regul 2015; 49(3): 151-63.
[http://dx.doi.org/10.4149/endo_2015_03_151] [PMID: 26238498]

[9]   Leggate M, Carter WG, Evans MJ, *et al.* Determination of inflammatory and prominent proteomic changes in plasma and adipose tissue after high-intensity intermittent training in overweight and obese males J Appl Physiol (1985) 2012; 112(8): 1353-60.

[10]   Marcinko K, Sikkema SR, Samaan MC, Kemp BE, Fullerton MD, Steinberg GR. High intensity interval training improves liver and adipose tissue insulin sensitivity. Mol Metab 2015; 4(12): 903-15.
[http://dx.doi.org/10.1016/j.molmet.2015.09.006] [PMID: 26909307]

[11]   Stanford KI, Middelbeek RJ, Townsend KL, *et al.* A novel role for subcutaneous adipose tissue in exercise-induced improvements in glucose homeostasis. Diabetes 2015; 64(6): 2002-14.
[http://dx.doi.org/10.2337/db14-0704] [PMID: 25605808]

[12]   Giles ED, Steig AJ, Jackman MR, *et al.* Exercise Decreases Lipogenic Gene Expression in Adipose Tissue and Alters Adipocyte Cellularity during Weight Regain After Weight Loss. Front Physiol 2016; 7: 32.
[http://dx.doi.org/10.3389/fphys.2016.00032] [PMID: 26903882]

[13]   Holland AM, Kephart WC, Mumford PW, *et al.* Effects of a ketogenic diet on adipose tissue, liver, and serum biomarkers in sedentary rats and rats that exercised via resisted voluntary wheel running. Am J Physiol Regul Integr Comp Physiol 2016; 311(2): R337-51.
[http://dx.doi.org/10.1152/ajpregu.00156.2016] [PMID: 27357802]

[14]   Tanaka G, Kato H, Izawa T. Endurance exercise training induces fat depot-specific differences in basal autophagic activity. Biochem Biophys Res Commun 2015; 466(3): 512-7.
[http://dx.doi.org/10.1016/j.bbrc.2015.09.061] [PMID: 26381175]

[15]   De Matteis R, Lucertini F, Guescini M, *et al.* Exercise as a new physiological stimulus for brown adipose tissue activity. Nutr Metab Cardiovasc Dis 2013; 23(6): 582-90.
[http://dx.doi.org/10.1016/j.numecd.2012.01.013] [PMID: 22633794]

[16]   Rocha-Rodrigues S, Rodriguez A, Becerril S, *et al.* Physical exercise remodels visceral adipose tissue and mitochondrial lipid metabolism in rats fed a high-fat diet. Clin Exp Pharmacol Physiol 2016.
[PMID: 27873387]

[17]　Sutherland LN, Bomhof MR, Capozzi LC, Basaraba SA, Wright DC. Exercise and adrenaline increase PGC-1alpha mRNA expression in rat adipose tissue. J Physiol 2009; 587(Pt 7): 1607-17.
　　　[http://dx.doi.org/10.1113/jphysiol.2008.165464] [PMID: 19221126]

[18]　Speretta GF, Rosante MC, Duarte FO, *et al.* The effects of exercise modalities on adiposity in obese rats. Clinics (São Paulo) 2012; 67(12): 1469-77.
　　　[http://dx.doi.org/10.6061/clinics/2012(12)19] [PMID: 23295603]

[19]　Rocha-Rodrigues S, Gonçalves IO, Beleza J, Ascensão A, Magalhães J. Effects of endurance training on autophagy and apoptotic signaling in visceral adipose tissue of prolonged high fat diet-fed rats. Eur J Nutr 2018; 57(6): 2237-47.
　　　[http://dx.doi.org/10.1007/s00394-017-1500-5] [PMID: 28699087]

[20]　Pedersen BK. Muscles and their myokines. J Exp Biol 2011; 214(Pt 2): 337-46.
　　　[http://dx.doi.org/10.1242/jeb.048074] [PMID: 21177953]

[21]　Rodríguez A, Becerril S, Ezquerro S, Mendez-Gimenez L, Frühbeck G. Cross-talk between adipokines and myokines in fat browning. Acta Physiol (Oxf) 2016.
　　　[PMID: 27040995]

[22]　Boström P, Wu J, Jedrychowski MP, *et al.* A PGC1-α-dependent myokine that drives brown-fat-like development of white fat and thermogenesis. Nature 2012; 481(7382): 463-8.
　　　[http://dx.doi.org/10.1038/nature10777] [PMID: 22237023]

[23]　Lee P, Linderman JD, Smith S, *et al.* Irisin and FGF21 are cold-induced endocrine activators of brown fat function in humans. Cell Metab 2014; 19(2): 302-9.
　　　[http://dx.doi.org/10.1016/j.cmet.2013.12.017] [PMID: 24506871]

[24]　Roca-Rivada A, Castelao C, Senin LL, *et al.* FNDC5/irisin is not only a myokine but also an adipokine. PLoS One 2013; 8(4)e60563
　　　[http://dx.doi.org/10.1371/journal.pone.0060563] [PMID: 23593248]

[25]　Wu MV, Bikopoulos G, Hung S, Ceddia RB. Thermogenic capacity is antagonistically regulated in classical brown and white subcutaneous fat depots by high fat diet and endurance training in rats: impact on whole-body energy expenditure. J Biol Chem 2014; 289(49): 34129-40.
　　　[http://dx.doi.org/10.1074/jbc.M114.591008] [PMID: 25344623]

[26]　Tiano JP, Springer DA, Rane SG. SMAD3 negatively regulates serum irisin and skeletal muscle FNDC5 and peroxisome proliferator-activated receptor γ coactivator 1-α (PGC-1α) during exercise. J Biol Chem 2015; 290(12): 7671-84.
　　　[http://dx.doi.org/10.1074/jbc.M114.617399] [PMID: 25648888]

[27]　Björntorp P. "Portal" adipose tissue as a generator of risk factors for cardiovascular disease and diabetes. Arteriosclerosis 1990; 10(4): 493-6.
　　　[http://dx.doi.org/10.1161/01.ATV.10.4.493] [PMID: 2196039]

[28]　Rodríguez A, Gena P, Méndez-Giménez L, *et al.* Reduced hepatic aquaporin-9 and glycerol permeability are related to insulin resistance in non-alcoholic fatty liver disease. Int J Obes 2014; 38(9): 1213-20.
　　　[http://dx.doi.org/10.1038/ijo.2013.234] [PMID: 24418844]

[29]　Foster MT, Pagliassotti MJ. Metabolic alterations following visceral fat removal and expansion: Beyond anatomic location. Adipocyte 2012; 1(4): 192-9.
　　　[http://dx.doi.org/10.4161/adip.21756] [PMID: 23700533]

[30]　Joe AW, Yi L, Even Y, Vogl AW, Rossi FM. Depot-specific differences in adipogenic progenitor abundance and proliferative response to high-fat diet. Stem Cells 2009; 27(10): 2563-70.
　　　[http://dx.doi.org/10.1002/stem.190] [PMID: 19658193]

[31]　Gollisch KS, Brandauer J, Jessen N, *et al.* Effects of exercise training on subcutaneous and visceral adipose tissue in normal- and high-fat diet-fed rats. Am J Physiol Endocrinol Metab 2009; 297(2): E495-504.

[http://dx.doi.org/10.1152/ajpendo.90424.2008] [PMID: 19491293]

[32] Guerra RL, Prado WL, Cheik NC, *et al.* Effects of 2 or 5 consecutive exercise days on adipocyte area and lipid parameters in Wistar rats. Lipids Health Dis 2007; 6: 16.
[http://dx.doi.org/10.1186/1476-511X-6-16] [PMID: 17605802]

[33] Rocha-Rodrigues S, Rodríguez A, Gouveia AM, *et al.* Effects of physical exercise on myokines expression and brown adipose-like phenotype modulation in rats fed a high-fat diet. Life Sci 2016; 165: 100-8.
[http://dx.doi.org/10.1016/j.lfs.2016.09.023] [PMID: 27693382]

[34] Zeve D, Millay DP, Seo J, Graff JM. Exercise-Induced Skeletal Muscle Adaptations Alter the Activity of Adipose Progenitor Cells. PLoS One 2016; 11(3)e0152129
[http://dx.doi.org/10.1371/journal.pone.0152129] [PMID: 27015423]

[35] Sakurai T, Endo S, Hatano D, *et al.* Effects of exercise training on adipogenesis of stromal-vascular fraction cells in rat epididymal white adipose tissue. Acta Physiol (Oxf) 2010; 200(4): 325-38.
[http://dx.doi.org/10.1111/j.1748-1716.2010.02159.x] [PMID: 20590530]

[36] Sertie RA, Andreotti S, Proenca AR, *et al.* Cessation of physical exercise changes metabolism and modifies the adipocyte cellularity of the periepididymal white adipose tissue in rats J Appl Physiol (1985) 2013; 115(3): 394-402.

[37] Rocha-Rodrigues S, Gonçalves IO, Beleza J, Ascensão A, Magalhães J. Physical exercise mitigates high-fat diet-induced adiposopathy and related endocrine alterations in an animal model of obesity. J Physiol Biochem 2018; 74(2): 235-46.
[http://dx.doi.org/10.1007/s13105-018-0609-1] [PMID: 29478123]

[38] Corvera S, Gealekman O. Adipose tissue angiogenesis: impact on obesity and type-2 diabetes. Biochim Biophys Acta 2014; 1842(3): 463-72.
[http://dx.doi.org/10.1016/j.bbadis.2013.06.003] [PMID: 23770388]

[39] Baynard T, Vieira-Potter VJ, Valentine RJ, Woods JA. Exercise training effects on inflammatory gene expression in white adipose tissue of young mice. Mediators Inflamm 2012; 2012767953
[http://dx.doi.org/10.1155/2012/767953] [PMID: 23319832]

[40] Hatano D, Ogasawara J, Endoh S, *et al.* Effect of exercise training on the density of endothelial cells in the white adipose tissue of rats. Scand J Med Sci Sports 2011; 21(6): e115-21.
[http://dx.doi.org/10.1111/j.1600-0838.2010.01176.x] [PMID: 20807385]

[41] Benbrook DM, Long A. Integration of autophagy, proteasomal degradation, unfolded protein response and apoptosis. Exp Oncol 2012; 34(3): 286-97.
[PMID: 23070014]

[42] Sarparanta J, Garcia-Macia M, Singh R. Autophagy and mitochondria in obesity and type 2 diabetes. Curr Diabetes Rev 2016.

[43] Kovsan J, Blüher M, Tarnovscki T, *et al.* Altered autophagy in human adipose tissues in obesity. J Clin Endocrinol Metab 2011; 96(2): E268-77.
[http://dx.doi.org/10.1210/jc.2010-1681] [PMID: 21047928]

[44] Haim Y, Blüher M, Slutsky N, *et al.* Elevated autophagy gene expression in adipose tissue of obese humans: A potential non-cell-cycle-dependent function of E2F1. Autophagy 2015; 11(11): 2074-88.
[http://dx.doi.org/10.1080/15548627.2015.1094597] [PMID: 26391754]

[45] Kosacka J, Kern M, Klöting N, *et al.* Autophagy in adipose tissue of patients with obesity and type 2 diabetes. Mol Cell Endocrinol 2015; 409: 21-32.
[http://dx.doi.org/10.1016/j.mce.2015.03.015] [PMID: 25818883]

[46] Cummins TD, Holden CR, Sansbury BE, *et al.* Metabolic remodeling of white adipose tissue in obesity. Am J Physiol Endocrinol Metab 2014; 307(3): E262-77.
[http://dx.doi.org/10.1152/ajpendo.00271.2013] [PMID: 24918202]

[47]　Mizunoe Y, Sudo Y, Okita N, *et al.* Involvement of lysosomal dysfunction in autophagosome accumulation and early pathologies in adipose tissue of obese mice. Autophagy 2017; 13(4): 642-53.
[http://dx.doi.org/10.1080/15548627.2016.1274850] [PMID: 28121218]

[48]　Rodríguez A, Gómez-Ambrosi J, Catalán V, *et al.* The ghrelin O-acyltransferase-ghrelin system reduces TNF-α-induced apoptosis and autophagy in human visceral adipocytes. Diabetologia 2012; 55(11): 3038-50.
[http://dx.doi.org/10.1007/s00125-012-2671-5] [PMID: 22869322]

[49]　Zhang C, He Y, Okutsu M, *et al.* Autophagy is involved in adipogenic differentiation by repressesing proteasome-dependent PPARγ2 degradation. Am J Physiol Endocrinol Metab 2013; 305(4): E530-9.
[http://dx.doi.org/10.1152/ajpendo.00640.2012] [PMID: 23800883]

[50]　Singh R, Xiang Y, Wang Y, *et al.* Autophagy regulates adipose mass and differentiation in mice. J Clin Invest 2009; 119(11): 3329-39.
[http://dx.doi.org/10.1172/JCI39228] [PMID: 19855132]

[51]　Baerga R, Zhang Y, Chen PH, Goldman S, Jin S. Targeted deletion of autophagy-related 5 (atg5) impairs adipogenesis in a cellular model and in mice. Autophagy 2009; 5(8): 1118-30.
[http://dx.doi.org/10.4161/auto.5.8.9991] [PMID: 19844159]

[52]　Parray HA, Yun JW. Combined inhibition of autophagy protein 5 and galectin-1 by thiodigalactoside reduces diet-induced obesity through induction of white fat browning. IUBMB Life 2017; 69(7): 510-21.
[http://dx.doi.org/10.1002/iub.1634] [PMID: 28444942]

[53]　Ahn N, Kim K. Combined influence of dietary restriction and treadmill running on MCP-1 and the expression of oxidative stress-related mRNA in the adipose tissue in obese mice. J Exerc Nutrition Biochem 2014; 18(3): 311-8.
[http://dx.doi.org/10.5717/jenb.2014.18.3.311] [PMID: 25566468]

[54]　Rodríguez A, Durán A, Selloum M, *et al.* Mature-onset obesity and insulin resistance in mice deficient in the signaling adapter p62. Cell Metab 2006; 3(3): 211-22.
[http://dx.doi.org/10.1016/j.cmet.2006.01.011] [PMID: 16517408]

[55]　Ito A, Suganami T, Yamauchi A, *et al.* Role of CC chemokine receptor 2 in bone marrow cells in the recruitment of macrophages into obese adipose tissue. J Biol Chem 2008; 283(51): 35715-23.
[http://dx.doi.org/10.1074/jbc.M804220200] [PMID: 18977759]

[56]　Sakurai T, Izawa T, Kizaki T, *et al.* Exercise training decreases expression of inflammation-related adipokines through reduction of oxidative stress in rat white adipose tissue. Biochem Biophys Res Commun 2009; 379(2): 605-9.
[http://dx.doi.org/10.1016/j.bbrc.2008.12.127] [PMID: 19121629]

[57]　Sun K, Kusminski CM, Scherer PE. Adipose tissue remodeling and obesity. J Clin Invest 2011; 121(6): 2094-101.
[http://dx.doi.org/10.1172/JCI45887] [PMID: 21633177]

[58]　Yin J, Gao Z, He Q, Zhou D, Guo Z, Ye J. Role of hypoxia in obesity-induced disorders of glucose and lipid metabolism in adipose tissue. Am J Physiol Endocrinol Metab 2009; 296(2): E333-42.
[http://dx.doi.org/10.1152/ajpendo.90760.2008] [PMID: 19066318]

[59]　Alkhouri N, Gornicka A, Berk MP, *et al.* Adipocyte apoptosis, a link between obesity, insulin resistance, and hepatic steatosis. J Biol Chem 2010; 285(5): 3428-38.
[http://dx.doi.org/10.1074/jbc.M109.074252] [PMID: 19940134]

[60]　Camargo A, Rangel-Zuniga OA, Alcala-Diaz J, *et al.* Dietary fat may modulate adipose tissue homeostasis through the processes of autophagy and apoptosis. Eur J Nutr 2016.
[PMID: 27029919]

[61]　Feng D, Tang Y, Kwon H, *et al.* High-fat diet-induced adipocyte cell death occurs through a cyclophilin D intrinsic signaling pathway independent of adipose tissue inflammation. Diabetes 2011;

60(8): 2134-43.
[http://dx.doi.org/10.2337/db10-1411] [PMID: 21734017]

[62]   Sakurai T, Takei M, Ogasawara J, *et al.* Exercise training enhances tumor necrosis factor-alph-
       -induced expressions of anti-apoptotic genes without alterations in caspase-3 activity in rat epididymal
       adipocytes. Jpn J Physiol 2005; 55(3): 181-9.
       [http://dx.doi.org/10.2170/jjphysiol.R2096] [PMID: 16129069]

[63]   Morris RT, Laye MJ, Lees SJ, *et al.* Exercise-induced attenuation of obesity, hyperinsulinemia, and
       skeletal muscle lipid peroxidation in the OLETF rat J Appl Physiol (1985) 2008; 104(3): 708-15.

[64]   Linden MA, Pincu Y, Martin SA, Woods JA, Baynard T. Moderate exercise training provides modest
       protection against adipose tissue inflammatory gene expression in response to high-fat feeding.
       Physiol Rep 2014; 2(7)e12071
       [http://dx.doi.org/10.14814/phy2.12071] [PMID: 25347855]

[65]   Harms M, Seale P. Brown and beige fat: development, function and therapeutic potential. Nat Med
       2013; 19(10): 1252-63.
       [http://dx.doi.org/10.1038/nm.3361] [PMID: 24100998]

[66]   Rodríguez A, Becerril S, Méndez-Giménez L, *et al.* Leptin administration activates irisin-induced
       myogenesis via nitric oxide-dependent mechanisms, but reduces its effect on subcutaneous fat
       browning in mice. Int J Obes 2015; 39(3): 397-407.
       [http://dx.doi.org/10.1038/ijo.2014.166] [PMID: 25199621]

[67]   Mather KJ, Funahashi T, Matsuzawa Y, *et al.* Adiponectin, change in adiponectin, and progression to
       diabetes in the Diabetes Prevention Program. Diabetes 2008; 57(4): 980-6.
       [http://dx.doi.org/10.2337/db07-1419] [PMID: 18192541]

[68]   Lumeng CN, Deyoung SM, Bodzin JL, Saltiel AR. Increased inflammatory properties of adipose
       tissue macrophages recruited during diet-induced obesity. Diabetes 2007; 56(1): 16-23.
       [http://dx.doi.org/10.2337/db06-1076] [PMID: 17192460]

[69]   Skurk T, Alberti-Huber C, Herder C, Hauner H. Relationship between adipocyte size and adipokine
       expression and secretion. J Clin Endocrinol Metab 2007; 92(3): 1023-33.
       [http://dx.doi.org/10.1210/jc.2006-1055] [PMID: 17164304]

[70]   Yamauchi T, Kamon J, Ito Y, *et al.* Cloning of adiponectin receptors that mediate antidiabetic
       metabolic effects. Nature 2003; 423(6941): 762-9.
       [http://dx.doi.org/10.1038/nature01705] [PMID: 12802337]

[71]   Lim S, Quon MJ, Koh KK. Modulation of adiponectin as a potential therapeutic strategy.
       Atherosclerosis 2014; 233(2): 721-8.
       [http://dx.doi.org/10.1016/j.atherosclerosis.2014.01.051] [PMID: 24603219]

[72]   Wolf AM, Wolf D, Rumpold H, Enrich B, Tilg H. Adiponectin induces the anti-inflammatory
       cytokines IL-10 and IL-1RA in human leukocytes. Biochem Biophys Res Commun 2004; 323(2):
       630-5.
       [http://dx.doi.org/10.1016/j.bbrc.2004.08.145] [PMID: 15369797]

[73]   Fukao K, Shimada K, Naito H, *et al.* Voluntary exercise ameliorates the progression of atherosclerotic
       lesion formation via anti-inflammatory effects in apolipoprotein E-deficient mice. J Atheroscler
       Thromb 2010; 17(12): 1226-36.
       [http://dx.doi.org/10.5551/jat.4788] [PMID: 20808053]

[74]   Ansar H, Zamaninour N, Djazayery A, *et al.* Weight Changes and Metabolic Outcomes in Calorie-
       Restricted Obese Mice Fed High-Fat Diets Containing Corn or Flaxseed Oil: Physiological Role of
       Sugar Replacement with Polyphenol-Rich Grape. J Am Coll Nutr 2017; 36(6): 422-33.
       [http://dx.doi.org/10.1080/07315724.2017.1318315] [PMID: 28665260]

[75]   Lara-Castro C, Luo N, Wallace P, Klein RL, Garvey WT. Adiponectin multimeric complexes and the
       metabolic syndrome trait cluster. Diabetes 2006; 55(1): 249-59.

[http://dx.doi.org/10.2337/diabetes.55.01.06.db05-1105] [PMID: 16380500]

[76]   Choe SS, Huh JY, Hwang IJ, Kim JI, Kim JB. Adipose Tissue Remodeling: Its Role in Energy Metabolism and Metabolic Disorders. Front Endocrinol (Lausanne) 2016; 7: 30.
[http://dx.doi.org/10.3389/fendo.2016.00030] [PMID: 27148161]

[77]   Christiansen T, Paulsen SK, Bruun JM, Pedersen SB, Richelsen B. Exercise training versus diet-induced weight-loss on metabolic risk factors and inflammatory markers in obese subjects: a 12-week randomized intervention study. Am J Physiol Endocrinol Metab 2010; 298(4): E824-31.
[http://dx.doi.org/10.1152/ajpendo.00574.2009] [PMID: 20086201]

[78]   Bruun JM, Helge JW, Richelsen B, Stallknecht B. Diet and exercise reduce low-grade inflammation and macrophage infiltration in adipose tissue but not in skeletal muscle in severely obese subjects. Am J Physiol Endocrinol Metab 2006; 290(5): E961-7.
[http://dx.doi.org/10.1152/ajpendo.00506.2005] [PMID: 16352667]

[79]   Moghadasi M, Mohebbi H, Rahmani-Nia F, Hassan-Nia S, Noroozi H. Effects of short-term lifestyle activity modification on adiponectin mRNA expression and plasma concentrations. Eur J Sport Sci 2013; 13(4): 378-85.
[http://dx.doi.org/10.1080/17461391.2011.635701] [PMID: 23834543]

[80]   Krskova K, Eckertova M, Kukan M, *et al.* Aerobic training lasting for 10 weeks elevates the adipose tissue FABP4, Giα, and adiponectin expression associated by a reduced protein oxidation. Endocr Regul 2012; 46(3): 137-46.
[http://dx.doi.org/10.4149/endo_2012_03_137] [PMID: 22808905]

[81]   Svidnicki PV, Leite NC, Vicari MR, *et al.* Swim training and the genetic expression of adipokines in monosodium glutamate-treated obese rats. Arch Endocrinol Metab 2015; 59(3): 210-4.
[http://dx.doi.org/10.1590/2359-3997000000039] [PMID: 26154087]

[82]   Saunders TJ, Palombella A, McGuire KA, Janiszewski PM, Després JP, Ross R. Acute exercise increases adiponectin levels in abdominally obese men. J Nutr Metab 2012; 2012148729
[http://dx.doi.org/10.1155/2012/148729] [PMID: 22701167]

[83]   García-Hermoso A, Ceballos-Ceballos RJ, Poblete-Aro CE, Hackney AC, Mota J, Ramírez-Vélez R. Exercise, adipokines and pediatric obesity: a meta-analysis of randomized controlled trials. Int J Obes 2017; 41(4): 475-82.
[http://dx.doi.org/10.1038/ijo.2016.230] [PMID: 28017965]

[84]   Dâmaso AR, da Silveira Campos RM, Caranti DA, *et al.* Aerobic plus resistance training was more effective in improving the visceral adiposity, metabolic profile and inflammatory markers than aerobic training in obese adolescents. J Sports Sci 2014; 32(15): 1435-45.
[http://dx.doi.org/10.1080/02640414.2014.900692] [PMID: 24730354]

[85]   Racil G, Ben Ounis O, Hammouda O, *et al.* Effects of high vs. moderate exercise intensity during interval training on lipids and adiponectin levels in obese young females. Eur J Appl Physiol 2013; 113(10): 2531-40.
[http://dx.doi.org/10.1007/s00421-013-2689-5] [PMID: 23824463]

[86]   Blüher M, Williams CJ, Klöting N, *et al.* Gene expression of adiponectin receptors in human visceral and subcutaneous adipose tissue is related to insulin resistance and metabolic parameters and is altered in response to physical training. Diabetes Care 2007; 30(12): 3110-5.
[http://dx.doi.org/10.2337/dc07-1257] [PMID: 17878241]

[87]   Oberbach A, Tönjes A, Klöting N, *et al.* Effect of a 4 week physical training program on plasma concentrations of inflammatory markers in patients with abnormal glucose tolerance. Eur J Endocrinol 2006; 154(4): 577-85.
[http://dx.doi.org/10.1530/eje.1.02127] [PMID: 16556721]

[88]   O'Leary VB, Marchetti CM, Krishnan RK, *et al.* Exercise-induced reversal of insulin resistance in obese elderly is associated with reduced visceral fat J Appl Physiol (1985) 2006; 100(5): 1584-9.

[89]   Waki H, Yamauchi T, Kamon J, *et al.* Impaired multimerization of human adiponectin mutants associated with diabetes. Molecular structure and multimer formation of adiponectin. J Biol Chem 2003; 278(41): 40352-63.
[http://dx.doi.org/10.1074/jbc.M300365200] [PMID: 12878598]

[90]   Hada Y, Yamauchi T, Waki H, *et al.* Selective purification and characterization of adiponectin multimer species from human plasma. Biochem Biophys Res Commun 2007; 356(2): 487-93.
[http://dx.doi.org/10.1016/j.bbrc.2007.03.004] [PMID: 17368570]

[91]   Numao S, Katayama Y, Hayashi Y, Matsuo T, Tanaka K. Influence of acute aerobic exercise on adiponectin oligomer concentrations in middle-aged abdominally obese men. Metabolism 2011; 60(2): 186-94.
[http://dx.doi.org/10.1016/j.metabol.2009.12.011] [PMID: 20102772]

[92]   O'Leary VB, Jorett AE, Marchetti CM, *et al.* Enhanced adiponectin multimer ratio and skeletal muscle adiponectin receptor expression following exercise training and diet in older insulin-resistant adults. Am J Physiol Endocrinol Metab 2007; 293(1): E421-7.
[http://dx.doi.org/10.1152/ajpendo.00123.2007] [PMID: 17488807]

[93]   Blümer RM, van der Crabben SN, Stegenga ME, *et al.* Hyperglycemia prevents the suppressive effect of hyperinsulinemia on plasma adiponectin levels in healthy humans. Am J Physiol Endocrinol Metab 2008; 295(3): E613-7.
[http://dx.doi.org/10.1152/ajpendo.90288.2008] [PMID: 18577692]

[94]   Fasshauer M, Kralisch S, Klier M, *et al.* Adiponectin gene expression and secretion is inhibited by interleukin-6 in 3T3-L1 adipocytes. Biochem Biophys Res Commun 2003; 301(4): 1045-50.
[http://dx.doi.org/10.1016/S0006-291X(03)00090-1] [PMID: 12589818]

[95]   Bruun JM, Lihn AS, Verdich C, *et al.* Regulation of adiponectin by adipose tissue-derived cytokines: in vivo and in vitro investigations in humans. Am J Physiol Endocrinol Metab 2003; 285(3): E527-33.
[http://dx.doi.org/10.1152/ajpendo.00110.2003] [PMID: 12736161]

[96]   Saad MF, Khan A, Sharma A, *et al.* Physiological insulinemia acutely modulates plasma leptin. Diabetes 1998; 47(4): 544-9.
[http://dx.doi.org/10.2337/diabetes.47.4.544] [PMID: 9568685]

[97]   Chan JL, Heist K, DePaoli AM, Veldhuis JD, Mantzoros CS. The role of falling leptin levels in the neuroendocrine and metabolic adaptation to short-term starvation in healthy men. J Clin Invest 2003; 111(9): 1409-21.
[http://dx.doi.org/10.1172/JCI200317490] [PMID: 12727933]

[98]   Nogueiras R, Tschöp MH, Zigman JM. Central nervous system regulation of energy metabolism: ghrelin versus leptin. Ann N Y Acad Sci 2008; 1126: 14-9.
[http://dx.doi.org/10.1196/annals.1433.054] [PMID: 18448790]

[99]   Münzberg H, Flier JS, Bjørbaek C. Region-specific leptin resistance within the hypothalamus of diet-induced obese mice. Endocrinology 2004; 145(11): 4880-9.
[http://dx.doi.org/10.1210/en.2004-0726] [PMID: 15271881]

[100]   Zachwieja JJ, Hendry SL, Smith SR, Harris RB. Voluntary wheel running decreases adipose tissue mass and expression of leptin mRNA in Osborne-Mendel rats. Diabetes 1997; 46(7): 1159-66.
[http://dx.doi.org/10.2337/diab.46.7.1159] [PMID: 9200651]

[101]   Jenkins NT, Padilla J, Arce-Esquivel AA, *et al.* Effects of endurance exercise training, metformin, and their combination on adipose tissue leptin and IL-10 secretion in OLETF rats J Appl Physiol (1985) 2012; 113(12): 1873-83.

[102]   Bradley RL, Jeon JY, Liu FF, Maratos-Flier E. Voluntary exercise improves insulin sensitivity and adipose tissue inflammation in diet-induced obese mice. Am J Physiol Endocrinol Metab 2008; 295(3): E586-94.
[http://dx.doi.org/10.1152/ajpendo.00309.2007] [PMID: 18577694]

[103] Chapados N, Collin P, Imbeault P, Corriveau P, Lavoie JM. Exercise training decreases in vitro stimulated lipolysis in a visceral (mesenteric) but not in the retroperitoneal fat depot of high-fat-fed rats. Br J Nutr 2008; 100(3): 518-25.
[http://dx.doi.org/10.1017/S0007114508921735] [PMID: 18284712]

[104] Huang P, Li S, Shao M, *et al.* Calorie restriction and endurance exercise share potent anti-inflammatory function in adipose tissues in ameliorating diet-induced obesity and insulin resistance in mice. Nutr Metab (Lond) 2010; 7: 59.
[http://dx.doi.org/10.1186/1743-7075-7-59] [PMID: 20633301]

[105] Vieira VJ, Valentine RJ, Wilund KR, Antao N, Baynard T, Woods JA. Effects of exercise and low-fat diet on adipose tissue inflammation and metabolic complications in obese mice. Am J Physiol Endocrinol Metab 2009; 296(5): E1164-71.
[http://dx.doi.org/10.1152/ajpendo.00054.2009] [PMID: 19276393]

[106] Vieira VJ, Valentine RJ, Wilund KR, Woods JA. Effects of diet and exercise on metabolic disturbances in high-fat diet-fed mice. Cytokine 2009; 46(3): 339-45.
[http://dx.doi.org/10.1016/j.cyto.2009.03.006] [PMID: 19362852]

[107] Ozcelik O, Celik H, Ayar A, Serhatlioglu S, Kelestimur H. Investigation of the influence of training status on the relationship between the acute exercise and serum leptin levels in obese females. Neuroendocrinol Lett 2004; 25(5): 381-5.
[PMID: 15580174]

[108] Polak J, Klimcakova E, Moro C, *et al.* Effect of aerobic training on plasma levels and subcutaneous abdominal adipose tissue gene expression of adiponectin, leptin, interleukin 6, and tumor necrosis factor alpha in obese women. Metabolism 2006; 55(10): 1375-81.
[http://dx.doi.org/10.1016/j.metabol.2006.06.008] [PMID: 16979409]

[109] Hickey MS, Houmard JA, Considine RV, *et al.* Gender-dependent effects of exercise training on serum leptin levels in humans. Am J Physiol 1997; 272(4 Pt 1): E562-6.
[PMID: 9142875]

[110] Perusse L, Collier G, Gagnon J, *et al.* Acute and chronic effects of exercise on leptin levels in humans J Appl Physiol (1985) 1997; 83(1): 5-10.

[111] Miyatake N, Takahashi K, Wada J, *et al.* Changes in serum leptin concentrations in overweight Japanese men after exercise. Diabetes Obes Metab 2004; 6(5): 332-7.
[http://dx.doi.org/10.1111/j.1462-8902.2004.00351.x] [PMID: 15287925]

[112] Reseland JE, Anderssen SA, Solvoll K, *et al.* Effect of long-term changes in diet and exercise on plasma leptin concentrations. Am J Clin Nutr 2001; 73(2): 240-5.
[http://dx.doi.org/10.1093/ajcn/73.2.240] [PMID: 11157319]

[113] Phillips MD, Patrizi RM, Cheek DJ, Wooten JS, Barbee JJ, Mitchell JB. Resistance training reduces subclinical inflammation in obese, postmenopausal women. Med Sci Sports Exerc 2012; 44(11): 2099-110.
[http://dx.doi.org/10.1249/MSS.0b013e3182644984] [PMID: 22874536]

[114] Delporte C. Structure and physiological actions of ghrelin. Scientifica (Cairo) 2013; 2013518909
[http://dx.doi.org/10.1155/2013/518909] [PMID: 24381790]

[115] Sondergaard E, Gormsen LC, Nellemann B, Vestergaard ET, Christiansen JS, Nielsen S. Visceral fat mass is a strong predictor of circulating ghrelin levels in premenopausal women. Eur J Endocrinol 2009; 160(3): 375-9.
[http://dx.doi.org/10.1530/EJE-08-0735] [PMID: 19106245]

[116] Tschöp M, Weyer C, Tataranni PA, Devanarayan V, Ravussin E, Heiman ML. Circulating ghrelin levels are decreased in human obesity. Diabetes 2001; 50(4): 707-9.
[http://dx.doi.org/10.2337/diabetes.50.4.707] [PMID: 11289032]

[117] Oner-Iyidoğan Y, Koçak H, Gürdöl F, Oner P, Issever H, Esin D. Circulating ghrelin levels in obese

women: a possible association with hypertension. Scand J Clin Lab Invest 2007; 67(5): 568-76.
[http://dx.doi.org/10.1080/00365510701210186] [PMID: 17763194]

[118] Handjieva-Darlenska T, Boyadjieva N. The effect of high-fat diet on plasma ghrelin and leptin levels in rats. J Physiol Biochem 2009; 65(2): 157-64.
[http://dx.doi.org/10.1007/BF03179066] [PMID: 19886394]

[119] Broom DR, Stensel DJ, Bishop NC, Burns SF, Miyashita M. Exercise-induced suppression of acylated ghrelin in humans J Appl Physiol (1985) 2007; 102(6): 2165-71.

[120] Broom DR, Batterham RL, King JA, Stensel DJ. Influence of resistance and aerobic exercise on hunger, circulating levels of acylated ghrelin, and peptide YY in healthy males. Am J Physiol Regul Integr Comp Physiol 2009; 296(1): R29-35.
[http://dx.doi.org/10.1152/ajpregu.90706.2008] [PMID: 18987287]

[121] King JA, Wasse LK, Stensel DJ. The acute effects of swimming on appetite, food intake, and plasma acylated ghrelin J Obes 2011; 2011

[122] Ghanbari-Niaki A, Jafari A, Moradi M, Kraemer RR. Short-,moderate-, and long-term treadmill training protocols reduce plasma, fundus, but not small intestine ghrelin concentrations in male rats. J Endocrinol Invest 2011; 34(6): 439-43.
[http://dx.doi.org/10.1007/BF03346710] [PMID: 21183796]

[123] Larson-Meyer DE, Palm S, Bansal A, Austin KJ, Hart AM, Alexander BM. Influence of running and walking on hormonal regulators of appetite in women. J Obes 2012; 2012730409
[http://dx.doi.org/10.1155/2012/730409] [PMID: 22619704]

[124] Christ ER, Zehnder M, Boesch C, *et al.* The effect of increased lipid intake on hormonal responses during aerobic exercise in endurance-trained men. Eur J Endocrinol 2006; 154(3): 397-403.
[http://dx.doi.org/10.1530/eje.1.02106] [PMID: 16498052]

[125] Russell M, Misra M. Influence of ghrelin and adipocytokines on bone mineral density in adolescent female athletes with amenorrhea and eumenorrheic athletes. Med Sport Sci 2010; 55: 103-13.
[http://dx.doi.org/10.1159/000321975] [PMID: 20956863]

[126] King JA, Wasse LK, Broom DR, Stensel DJ. Influence of brisk walking on appetite, energy intake, and plasma acylated ghrelin. Med Sci Sports Exerc 2010; 42(3): 485-92.
[http://dx.doi.org/10.1249/MSS.0b013e3181ba10c4] [PMID: 19952806]

[127] Martins C, Aschehoug I, Ludviksen M, *et al.* High-Intensity Interval Training, Appetite, and Reward Value of Food in the Obese. Med Sci Sports Exerc 2017; 49(9): 1851-8.
[http://dx.doi.org/10.1249/MSS.0000000000001296] [PMID: 28398946]

[128] Leidy HJ, Gardner JK, Frye BR, *et al.* Circulating ghrelin is sensitive to changes in body weight during a diet and exercise program in normal-weight young women. J Clin Endocrinol Metab 2004; 89(6): 2659-64.
[http://dx.doi.org/10.1210/jc.2003-031471] [PMID: 15181038]

[129] Mason C, Xiao L, Imayama I, *et al.* The effects of separate and combined dietary weight loss and exercise on fasting ghrelin concentrations in overweight and obese women: a randomized controlled trial. Clin Endocrinol (Oxf) 2015; 82(3): 369-76.
[http://dx.doi.org/10.1111/cen.12483] [PMID: 24796864]

[130] Mihalache L, Gherasim A, Niță O, *et al.* Effects of ghrelin in energy balance and body weight homeostasis. Hormones (Athens) 2016; 15(2): 186-96.
[http://dx.doi.org/10.14310/horm.2002.1672] [PMID: 27376422]

[131] Fathi R, Ghanbari-Niaki A, Kraemer RR, Talebi-Garakani E, Saghebjoo M. The effect of exercise intensity on plasma and tissue acyl ghrelin concentrations in fasted rats. Regul Pept 2010; 165(2-3): 133-7.
[http://dx.doi.org/10.1016/j.regpep.2010.05.013] [PMID: 20542063]

[132] Markofski MM, Carrillo AE, Timmerman KL, *et al.* Exercise training modifies ghrelin and

adiponectin concentrations and is related to inflammation in older adults. J Gerontol A Biol Sci Med Sci 2014; 69(6): 675-81.
[http://dx.doi.org/10.1093/gerona/glt132] [PMID: 24013674]

[133] Hazell TJ, Islam H, Townsend LK, Schmale MS, Copeland JL. Effects of exercise intensity on plasma concentrations of appetite-regulating hormones: Potential mechanisms. Appetite 2016; 98: 80-8.
[http://dx.doi.org/10.1016/j.appet.2015.12.016] [PMID: 26721721]

[134] Adams OP. The impact of brief high-intensity exercise on blood glucose levels. Diabetes Metab Syndr Obes 2013; 6: 113-22.
[http://dx.doi.org/10.2147/DMSO.S29222] [PMID: 23467903]

[135] Hsu YW, Pan YJ, Cho YM, Liou TH, Chou P, Wang PS. Aging effects on exercise-induced alternations in plasma acylated ghrelin and leptin in male rats. Eur J Appl Physiol 2011; 111(5): 809-17.
[http://dx.doi.org/10.1007/s00421-010-1704-3] [PMID: 21046141]

[136] Erdmann J, Tahbaz R, Lippl F, Wagenpfeil S, Schusdziarra V. Plasma ghrelin levels during exercise - effects of intensity and duration. Regul Pept 2007; 143(1-3): 127-35.
[http://dx.doi.org/10.1016/j.regpep.2007.05.002] [PMID: 17570540]

[137] Saltiel AR, Olefsky JM. Inflammatory mechanisms linking obesity and metabolic disease. J Clin Invest 2017; 127(1): 1-4.
[http://dx.doi.org/10.1172/JCI92035] [PMID: 28045402]

[138] Hotamisligil GS. Inflammation and metabolic disorders. Nature 2006; 444(7121): 860-7.
[http://dx.doi.org/10.1038/nature05485] [PMID: 17167474]

[139] Johnson AR, Milner JJ, Makowski L. The inflammation highway: metabolism accelerates inflammatory traffic in obesity. Immunol Rev 2012; 249(1): 218-38.
[http://dx.doi.org/10.1111/j.1600-065X.2012.01151.x] [PMID: 22889225]

[140] Frühbeck G, Méndez-Giménez L, Fernández-Formoso JA, Fernández S, Rodríguez A. Regulation of adipocyte lipolysis. Nutr Res Rev 2014; 27(1): 63-93.
[http://dx.doi.org/10.1017/S095442241400002X] [PMID: 24872083]

[141] Tantiwong P, Shanmugasundaram K, Monroy A, *et al.* NF-κB activity in muscle from obese and type 2 diabetic subjects under basal and exercise-stimulated conditions. Am J Physiol Endocrinol Metab 2010; 299(5): E794-801.
[http://dx.doi.org/10.1152/ajpendo.00776.2009] [PMID: 20739506]

[142] Oliveira AG, Carvalho BM, Tobar N, *et al.* Physical exercise reduces circulating lipopolysaccharide and TLR4 activation and improves insulin signaling in tissues of DIO rats. Diabetes 2011; 60(3): 784-96.
[http://dx.doi.org/10.2337/db09-1907] [PMID: 21282367]

[143] da Luz G, Frederico MJ, da Silva S, *et al.* Endurance exercise training ameliorates insulin resistance and reticulum stress in adipose and hepatic tissue in obese rats. Eur J Appl Physiol 2011; 111(9): 2015-23.
[http://dx.doi.org/10.1007/s00421-010-1802-2] [PMID: 21249392]

[144] Guilherme A, Virbasius JV, Puri V, Czech MP. Adipocyte dysfunctions linking obesity to insulin resistance and type 2 diabetes. Nat Rev Mol Cell Biol 2008; 9(5): 367-77.
[http://dx.doi.org/10.1038/nrm2391] [PMID: 18401346]

[145] van der Poorten D, Milner KL, Hui J, *et al.* Visceral fat: a key mediator of steatohepatitis in metabolic liver disease. Hepatology 2008; 48(2): 449-57.
[http://dx.doi.org/10.1002/hep.22350] [PMID: 18627003]

[146] Kawanishi N, Niihara H, Mizokami T, Yada K, Suzuki K. Exercise training attenuates neutrophil infiltration and elastase expression in adipose tissue of high-fat-diet-induced obese mice. Physiol Rep 2015; 3(9)e12534

[http://dx.doi.org/10.14814/phy2.12534] [PMID: 26341995]

[147] Kawanishi N, Mizokami T, Yano H, Suzuki K. Exercise attenuates M1 macrophages and CD8+ T cells in the adipose tissue of obese mice. Med Sci Sports Exerc 2013; 45(9): 1684-93.
[http://dx.doi.org/10.1249/MSS.0b013e31828ff9c6] [PMID: 23954991]

[148] Mazur-Bialy AI, Bilski J, Pochec E, Brzozowski T. New insight into the direct anti-inflammatory activity of a myokine irisin against proinflammatory activation of adipocytes. Implication for exercise in obesity. J Physiol Pharmacol 2017; 68(2): 243-51.
[PMID: 28614774]

[149] Rocha-Rodrigues S, Rodríguez A, Gonçalves IO, *et al.* Impact of physical exercise on visceral adipose tissue fatty acid profile and inflammation in response to a high-fat diet regimen. Int J Biochem Cell Biol 2017; 87: 114-24.
[http://dx.doi.org/10.1016/j.biocel.2017.04.008] [PMID: 28438715]

[150] Barry JC, Simtchouk S, Durrer C, Jung ME, Little JP. Short-Term Exercise Training Alters Leukocyte Chemokine Receptors in Obese Adults. Med Sci Sports Exerc 2017; 49(8): 1631-40.
[http://dx.doi.org/10.1249/MSS.0000000000001261] [PMID: 28319586]

[151] Donges CE, Duffield R, Guelfi KJ, Smith GC, Adams DR, Edge JA. Comparative effects of single-mode vs. duration-matched concurrent exercise training on body composition, low-grade inflammation, and glucose regulation in sedentary, overweight, middle-aged men. Appl Physiol Nutr Metab 2013; 38(7): 779-88.
[http://dx.doi.org/10.1139/apnm-2012-0443] [PMID: 23980737]

[152] Dorneles GP, Haddad DO, Fagundes VO, *et al.* High intensity interval exercise decreases IL-8 and enhances the immunomodulatory cytokine interleukin-10 in lean and overweight-obese individuals. Cytokine 2016; 77: 1-9.
[http://dx.doi.org/10.1016/j.cyto.2015.10.003] [PMID: 26476404]

[153] Sriwijitkamol A, Christ-Roberts C, Berria R, *et al.* Reduced skeletal muscle inhibitor of kappaB beta content is associated with insulin resistance in subjects with type 2 diabetes: reversal by exercise training. Diabetes 2006; 55(3): 760-7.
[http://dx.doi.org/10.2337/diabetes.55.03.06.db05-0677] [PMID: 16505240]

[154] Kawanishi N, Yano H, Yokogawa Y, Suzuki K. Exercise training inhibits inflammation in adipose tissue via both suppression of macrophage infiltration and acceleration of phenotypic switching from M1 to M2 macrophages in high-fat-diet-induced obese mice. Exerc Immunol Rev 2010; 16: 105-18.
[PMID: 20839495]

[155] Haczeyni F, Barn V, Mridha AR, *et al.* Exercise improves adipose function and inflammation and ameliorates fatty liver disease in obese diabetic mice. Obesity (Silver Spring) 2015; 23(9): 1845-55.
[http://dx.doi.org/10.1002/oby.21170] [PMID: 26250514]

[156] Wainright KS, Fleming NJ, Rowles JL, *et al.* Retention of sedentary obese visceral white adipose tissue phenotype with intermittent physical activity despite reduced adiposity. Am J Physiol Regul Integr Comp Physiol 2015; 309(5): R594-602.
[http://dx.doi.org/10.1152/ajpregu.00042.2015] [PMID: 26180183]

[157] Weisberg SP, McCann D, Desai M, Rosenbaum M, Leibel RL, Ferrante AW Jr. Obesity is associated with macrophage accumulation in adipose tissue. J Clin Invest 2003; 112(12): 1796-808.
[http://dx.doi.org/10.1172/JCI200319246] [PMID: 14679176]

[158] Baturcam E, Abubaker J, Tiss A, *et al.* Physical exercise reduces the expression of RANTES and its CCR5 receptor in the adipose tissue of obese humans. Mediators Inflamm 2014; 2014627150
[http://dx.doi.org/10.1155/2014/627150] [PMID: 24895488]

[159] Kohut ML, McCann DA, Russell DW, *et al.* Aerobic exercise, but not flexibility/resistance exercise, reduces serum IL-18, CRP, and IL-6 independent of beta-blockers, BMI, and psychosocial factors in older adults. Brain Behav Immun 2006; 20(3): 201-9.
[http://dx.doi.org/10.1016/j.bbi.2005.12.002] [PMID: 16504463]

[160] Oberbach A, Lehmann S, Kirsch K, *et al.* Long-term exercise training decreases interleukin-6 (IL-6) serum levels in subjects with impaired glucose tolerance: effect of the -174G/C variant in IL-6 gene. Eur J Endocrinol 2008; 159(2): 129-36.
[http://dx.doi.org/10.1530/EJE-08-0220] [PMID: 18469018]

[161] Straczkowski M, Kowalska I, Dzienis-Straczkowska S, *et al.* Changes in tumor necrosis factor-alpha system and insulin sensitivity during an exercise training program in obese women with normal and impaired glucose tolerance. Eur J Endocrinol 2001; 145(3): 273-80.
[http://dx.doi.org/10.1530/eje.0.1450273] [PMID: 11517007]

[162] Golbidi S, Laher I. Exercise induced adipokine changes and the metabolic syndrome. J Diabetes Res 2014; 2014726861
[http://dx.doi.org/10.1155/2014/726861] [PMID: 24563869]

[163] Nassis GP, Papantakou K, Skenderi K, *et al.* Aerobic exercise training improves insulin sensitivity without changes in body weight, body fat, adiponectin, and inflammatory markers in overweight and obese girls. Metabolism 2005; 54(11): 1472-9.
[http://dx.doi.org/10.1016/j.metabol.2005.05.013] [PMID: 16253636]

[164] Nicklas BJ, Ambrosius W, Messier SP, *et al.* Diet-induced weight loss, exercise, and chronic inflammation in older, obese adults: a randomized controlled clinical trial. Am J Clin Nutr 2004; 79(4): 544-51.
[http://dx.doi.org/10.1093/ajcn/79.4.544] [PMID: 15051595]

[165] Shen W, Baldwin J, Collins B, *et al.* Low level of trans-10, cis-12 conjugated linoleic acid decreases adiposity and increases browning independent of inflammatory signaling in overweight Sv129 mice. J Nutr Biochem 2015; 26(6): 616-25.
[http://dx.doi.org/10.1016/j.jnutbio.2014.12.016] [PMID: 25801353]

[166] Mardare C, Krüger K, Liebisch G, *et al.* Endurance and Resistance Training Affect High Fat Diet-Induced Increase of Ceramides, Inflammasome Expression, and Systemic Inflammation in Mice. J Diabetes Res 2016; 20164536470
[http://dx.doi.org/10.1155/2016/4536470] [PMID: 26788518]

[167] Kondo T, Kobayashi I, Murakami M. Effect of exercise on circulating adipokine levels in obese young women. Endocr J 2006; 53(2): 189-95.
[http://dx.doi.org/10.1507/endocrj.53.189] [PMID: 16618976]

[168] Sakurai T, Ogasawara J, Kizaki T, *et al.* The effects of exercise training on obesity-induced dysregulated expression of adipokines in white adipose tissue. Int J Endocrinol 2013; 2013801743
[http://dx.doi.org/10.1155/2013/801743] [PMID: 24369466]

[169] Farias JM, Maggi RM, Tromm CB, *et al.* Exercise training performed simultaneously to a high-fat diet reduces the degree of insulin resistance and improves adipoR1-2/APPL1 protein levels in mice. Lipids Health Dis 2012; 11: 134.
[http://dx.doi.org/10.1186/1476-511X-11-134] [PMID: 23046739]

[170] Petrovic N, Walden TB, Shabalina IG, Timmons JA, Cannon B, Nedergaard J. Chronic peroxisome proliferator-activated receptor gamma (PPARgamma) activation of epididymally derived white adipocyte cultures reveals a population of thermogenically competent, UCP1-containing adipocytes molecularly distinct from classic brown adipocytes. J Biol Chem 2010; 285(10): 7153-64.
[http://dx.doi.org/10.1074/jbc.M109.053942] [PMID: 20028987]

[171] Fain JN, Company JM, Booth FW, *et al.* Exercise training does not increase muscle FNDC5 protein or mRNA expression in pigs. Metabolism 2013; 62(10): 1503-11.
[http://dx.doi.org/10.1016/j.metabol.2013.05.021] [PMID: 23831442]

[172] Ishibashi J, Seale P. Medicine. Beige can be slimming. Science 2010; 328(5982): 1113-4.
[http://dx.doi.org/10.1126/science.1190816] [PMID: 20448151]

[173] Cao L, Choi EY, Liu X, *et al.* White to brown fat phenotypic switch induced by genetic and

environmental activation of a hypothalamic-adipocyte axis. Cell Metab 2011; 14(3): 324-38.
[http://dx.doi.org/10.1016/j.cmet.2011.06.020] [PMID: 21907139]

[174]   Norheim F, Langleite TM, Hjorth M, *et al.* The effects of acute and chronic exercise on PGC-1α, irisin and browning of subcutaneous adipose tissue in humans. FEBS J 2014; 281(3): 739-49.
[http://dx.doi.org/10.1111/febs.12619] [PMID: 24237962]

[175]   Besse-Patin A, Montastier E, Vinel C, *et al.* Effect of endurance training on skeletal muscle myokine expression in obese men: identification of apelin as a novel myokine. Int J Obes 2014; 38(5): 707-13.
[http://dx.doi.org/10.1038/ijo.2013.158] [PMID: 23979219]

[176]   Rönn T, Volkov P, Tornberg A, *et al.* Extensive changes in the transcriptional profile of human adipose tissue including genes involved in oxidative phosphorylation after a 6-month exercise intervention. Acta Physiol (Oxf) 2014; 211(1): 188-200.
[http://dx.doi.org/10.1111/apha.12247] [PMID: 24495239]

[177]   Cantó C, Auwerx J. PGC-1alpha, SIRT1 and AMPK, an energy sensing network that controls energy expenditure. Curr Opin Lipidol 2009; 20(2): 98-105.
[http://dx.doi.org/10.1097/MOL.0b013e328328d0a4] [PMID: 19276888]

[178]   Qiang L, Wang L, Kon N, *et al.* Brown remodeling of white adipose tissue by SirT1-dependent deacetylation of Ppary. Cell 2012; 150(3): 620-32.
[http://dx.doi.org/10.1016/j.cell.2012.06.027] [PMID: 22863012]

[179]   Nakhuda A, Josse AR, Gburcik V, *et al.* Biomarkers of browning of white adipose tissue and their regulation during exercise- and diet-induced weight loss. Am J Clin Nutr 2016; 104(3): 557-65.
[http://dx.doi.org/10.3945/ajcn.116.132563] [PMID: 27488235]

[180]   Xu X, Ying Z, Cai M, *et al.* Exercise ameliorates high-fat diet-induced metabolic and vascular dysfunction, and increases adipocyte progenitor cell population in brown adipose tissue. Am J Physiol Regul Integr Comp Physiol 2011; 300(5): R1115-25.
[http://dx.doi.org/10.1152/ajpregu.00806.2010] [PMID: 21368268]

[181]   Laye MJ, Rector RS, Warner SO, *et al.* Changes in visceral adipose tissue mitochondrial content with type 2 diabetes and daily voluntary wheel running in OLETF rats. J Physiol 2009; 587(Pt 14): 3729-39.
[http://dx.doi.org/10.1113/jphysiol.2009.172601] [PMID: 19491243]

[182]   Conley KE. Mitochondria to motion: optimizing oxidative phosphorylation to improve exercise performance. J Exp Biol 2016; 219(Pt 2): 243-9.
[http://dx.doi.org/10.1242/jeb.126623] [PMID: 26792336]

[183]   Castellani L, Root-Mccaig J, Frendo-Cumbo S, Beaudoin MS, Wright DC. Exercise training protects against an acute inflammatory insult in mouse epididymal adipose tissue J Appl Physiol (1985) 2014; 116(10): 1272-80.

[184]   Sae-Tan S, Rogers CJ, Lambert JD. Decaffeinated Green Tea and Voluntary Exercise Induce Gene Changes Related to Beige Adipocyte Formation in High Fat-Fed Obese Mice. J Funct Foods 2015; 14: 210-4.
[http://dx.doi.org/10.1016/j.jff.2015.01.036] [PMID: 25844091]

[185]   Knudsen JG, Murholm M, Carey AL, *et al.* Role of IL-6 in exercise training- and cold-induced UCP1 expression in subcutaneous white adipose tissue. PLoS One 2014; 9(1)e84910
[http://dx.doi.org/10.1371/journal.pone.0084910] [PMID: 24416310]

[186]   Rao RR, Long JZ, White JP, *et al.* Meteorin-like is a hormone that regulates immune-adipose interactions to increase beige fat thermogenesis. Cell 2014; 157(6): 1279-91.
[http://dx.doi.org/10.1016/j.cell.2014.03.065] [PMID: 24906147]

[187]   Li G, Klein RL, Matheny M, King MA, Meyer EM, Scarpace PJ. Induction of uncoupling protein 1 by central interleukin-6 gene delivery is dependent on sympathetic innervation of brown adipose tissue and underlies one mechanism of body weight reduction in rats. Neuroscience 2002; 115(3): 879-89.

[http://dx.doi.org/10.1016/S0306-4522(02)00447-5] [PMID: 12435426]

[188] Nguyen KD, Qiu Y, Cui X, *et al.* Alternatively activated macrophages produce catecholamines to sustain adaptive thermogenesis. Nature 2011; 480(7375): 104-8.
[http://dx.doi.org/10.1038/nature10653] [PMID: 22101429]

[189] Brenmoehl J, Albrecht E, Komolka K, *et al.* Irisin is elevated in skeletal muscle and serum of mice immediately after acute exercise. Int J Biol Sci 2014; 10(3): 338-49.
[http://dx.doi.org/10.7150/ijbs.7972] [PMID: 24644429]

[190] Liu J, Cui XY, Yang YQ, *et al.* Effects of high-intensity treadmill training on timeliness and plasticity expression of irisin in mice. Eur Rev Med Pharmacol Sci 2015; 19(12): 2168-73.
[PMID: 26166638]

[191] Kim HJ, So B, Choi M, Kang D, Song W. Resistance exercise training increases the expression of irisin concomitant with improvement of muscle function in aging mice and humans. Exp Gerontol 2015; 70: 11-7.
[http://dx.doi.org/10.1016/j.exger.2015.07.006] [PMID: 26183690]

[192] Zhou Q, Chen K, Liu P, *et al.* Dihydromyricetin stimulates irisin secretion partially via the PGC-1α pathway. Mol Cell Endocrinol 2015; 412: 349-57.
[http://dx.doi.org/10.1016/j.mce.2015.05.036] [PMID: 26054747]

[193] Sanchis-Gomar F, Perez-Quilis C. The p38-PGC-1α-irisin-betatrophin axis: Exploring new pathways in insulin resistance. Adipocyte 2014; 3(1): 67-8.
[http://dx.doi.org/10.4161/adip.27370] [PMID: 24575373]

[194] Zhang Y, Li R, Meng Y, *et al.* Irisin stimulates browning of white adipocytes through mitogen-activated protein kinase p38 MAP kinase and ERK MAP kinase signaling. Diabetes 2014; 63(2): 514-25.
[http://dx.doi.org/10.2337/db13-1106] [PMID: 24150604]

[195] Wu J, Spiegelman BM. Irisin ERKs the fat. Diabetes 2014; 63(2): 381-3.
[http://dx.doi.org/10.2337/db13-1586] [PMID: 24464712]

[196] Nygaard H, Slettaløkken G, Vegge G, *et al.* Irisin in blood increases transiently after single sessions of intense endurance exercise and heavy strength training. PLoS One 2015; 10(3)e0121367
[http://dx.doi.org/10.1371/journal.pone.0121367] [PMID: 25781950]

[197] Pekkala S, Wiklund PK, Hulmi JJ, *et al.* Are skeletal muscle FNDC5 gene expression and irisin release regulated by exercise and related to health? J Physiol 2013; 591(21): 5393-400.
[http://dx.doi.org/10.1113/jphysiol.2013.263707] [PMID: 24000180]

[198] Hecksteden A, Wegmann M, Steffen A, *et al.* Irisin and exercise training in humans - results from a randomized controlled training trial. BMC Med 2013; 11: 235.
[http://dx.doi.org/10.1186/1741-7015-11-235] [PMID: 24191966]

[199] Timmons JA, Baar K, Davidsen PK, Atherton PJ. Is irisin a human exercise gene? Nature 2012; 488(7413): E9-E10.
[http://dx.doi.org/10.1038/nature11364] [PMID: 22932392]

[200] Palacios-González B, Vadillo-Ortega F, Polo-Oteyza E, *et al.* Irisin levels before and after physical activity among school-age children with different BMI: a direct relation with leptin. Obesity (Silver Spring) 2015; 23(4): 729-32.
[http://dx.doi.org/10.1002/oby.21029] [PMID: 25820255]

[201] Vosselman MJ, Hoeks J, Brans B, *et al.* Low brown adipose tissue activity in endurance-trained compared with lean sedentary men. Int J Obes 2015; 39(12): 1696-702.
[http://dx.doi.org/10.1038/ijo.2015.130] [PMID: 26189600]

[202] Tsuchiya Y, Ando D, Goto K, Kiuchi M, Yamakita M, Koyama K. High-intensity exercise causes greater irisin response compared with low-intensity exercise under similar energy consumption. Tohoku J Exp Med 2014; 233(2): 135-40.

[http://dx.doi.org/10.1620/tjem.233.135] [PMID: 24910199]

[203] Miyamoto-Mikami E, Sato K, Kurihara T, *et al*. Endurance training-induced increase in circulating irisin levels is associated with reduction of abdominal visceral fat in middle-aged and older adults. PLoS One 2015; 10(3)e0120354
[http://dx.doi.org/10.1371/journal.pone.0120354] [PMID: 25793753]

[204] Jedrychowski MP, Wrann CD, Paulo JA, *et al*. Detection and Quantitation of Circulating Human Irisin by Tandem Mass Spectrometry. Cell Metab 2015; 22(4): 734-40.
[http://dx.doi.org/10.1016/j.cmet.2015.08.001] [PMID: 26278051]

[205] Huh JY, Mougios V, Kabasakalis A, *et al*. Exercise-induced irisin secretion is independent of age or fitness level and increased irisin may directly modulate muscle metabolism through AMPK activation. J Clin Endocrinol Metab 2014; 99(11): E2154-61.
[http://dx.doi.org/10.1210/jc.2014-1437] [PMID: 25119310]

[206] Kraemer RR, Shockett P, Webb ND, Shah U, Castracane VD. A transient elevated irisin blood concentration in response to prolonged, moderate aerobic exercise in young men and women. Horm Metab Res 2014; 46(2): 150-4.
[PMID: 24062088]

[207] Daskalopoulou SS, Cooke AB, Gomez YH, *et al*. Plasma irisin levels progressively increase in response to increasing exercise workloads in young, healthy, active subjects. Eur J Endocrinol 2014; 171(3): 343-52.
[http://dx.doi.org/10.1530/EJE-14-0204] [PMID: 24920292]

[208] Egan B, Zierath JR. Exercise metabolism and the molecular regulation of skeletal muscle adaptation. Cell Metab 2013; 17(2): 162-84.
[http://dx.doi.org/10.1016/j.cmet.2012.12.012] [PMID: 23395166]

[209] Huh JY, Panagiotou G, Mougios V, *et al*. FNDC5 and irisin in humans: I. Predictors of circulating concentrations in serum and plasma and II. mRNA expression and circulating concentrations in response to weight loss and exercise. Metabolism 2012; 61(12): 1725-38.
[http://dx.doi.org/10.1016/j.metabol.2012.09.002] [PMID: 23018146]

[210] Ellefsen S, Vikmoen O, Slettaløkken G, *et al*. Irisin and FNDC5: effects of 12-week strength training, and relations to muscle phenotype and body mass composition in untrained women. Eur J Appl Physiol 2014; 114(9): 1875-88.
[http://dx.doi.org/10.1007/s00421-014-2922-x] [PMID: 24906447]

[211] Kurdiova T, Balaz M, Vician M, *et al*. Effects of obesity, diabetes and exercise on Fndc5 gene expression and irisin release in human skeletal muscle and adipose tissue: in vivo and in vitro studies. J Physiol 2014; 592(5): 1091-107.
[http://dx.doi.org/10.1113/jphysiol.2013.264655] [PMID: 24297848]

[212] Anastasilakis AD, Polyzos SA, Saridakis ZG, *et al*. Circulating irisin in healthy, young individuals: day-night rhythm, effects of food intake and exercise, and associations with gender, physical activity, diet, and body composition. J Clin Endocrinol Metab 2014; 99(9): 3247-55.
[http://dx.doi.org/10.1210/jc.2014-1367] [PMID: 24915120]

[213] Pedersen BK, Febbraio MA. Muscles, exercise and obesity: skeletal muscle as a secretory organ. Nat Rev Endocrinol 2012; 8(8): 457-65.
[http://dx.doi.org/10.1038/nrendo.2012.49] [PMID: 22473333]

[214] Wrann CD, White JP, Salogiannnis J, *et al*. Exercise induces hippocampal BDNF through a PGC-1α/FNDC5 pathway. Cell Metab 2013; 18(5): 649-59.
[http://dx.doi.org/10.1016/j.cmet.2013.09.008] [PMID: 24120943]

[215] Comassi M, Vitolo E, Pratali L, *et al*. Acute effects of different degrees of ultra-endurance exercise on systemic inflammatory responses. Intern Med J 2015; 45(1): 74-9.
[http://dx.doi.org/10.1111/imj.12625] [PMID: 25371101]

[216] Raschke S, Eckel J. Adipo-myokines: two sides of the same coin--mediators of inflammation and mediators of exercise. Mediators Inflamm 2013; 2013320724
[http://dx.doi.org/10.1155/2013/320724] [PMID: 23861558]

CHAPTER 15

Stress and Obesity

Isabel Azevedo[*]

Department of Biomedicine, Biochemistry Unit, Faculty of Medicine, University of Porto, Porto, Portugal

Abstract: Central obesity associates with cardiovascular pathology and death. Although it constitutes a component of the metabolic syndrome, there are obese people without other cardiometabolic risk factors and there are normal weight people with cardiometabolic risk factor clustering, indicating that the problem may be another rather than obesity itself. It appears that more than the amount of accumulated fat, large adipocytes and fat deposition in other tissues, such as the liver, indicate metabolic disease. There is an impressive overlap between Cushing's syndrome and metabolic syndrome. Stress reactions appear in a variety of forms, one of them particularly serious in its consequences, the defeat reaction, in which there is a marked activation of the hypothalamus-pituitary-adrenal axis with the production of cortisol. Psychosocial chronic stress, particularly subordinate stress, promotes an increase of cortisol production. This excess of cortisol, with time, leads to a clinical status of metabolic syndrome (central obesity, hypertension, dyslipidemia and insulin resistance). This chain of reactions and events appears to be an important factor in the association between social-economic status and health, as unemployed, refugees, ethnic minorities, homeless people, humiliated workers and a huge proportion of women across countries, small areas, social classes and income distribution, suffer from this type of chronic stress and have poor health, namely cardiometabolic diseases and depression. Adverse effects of central obesity are partly directly attributable to obesity itself, but a large part of those effects is probably due to cortisol. More important than to reduce obesity will be, therefore, to prevent stress and cortisol excess.

Keywords: Adipocyte, Adrenaline, Benign obesity, 11beta-hydroxysteroid dehydrogenase type 1, Cardiovascular diseases, Catecholamines, Catechol-O-methyltransferase, Central obesity, Cortisol, Cushing' syndrome, Defeat reaction, Defense reaction, Hypertrophic adipocytes, Metabolic syndrome, Metanephrine, Noradrenaline, Obesity, Socio-economic status, Stress, Subordinate stress, Vigilance reaction.

---

[*] **Corresponding author Isabel Azevedo:** Department of Biomedicine, Biochemistry Unit, Faculty of Medicine, University of Porto, 4200-319 Porto, Portugal; Tel/Fax: +351225513624; E-mail: isabelazeve@gmail.com

INTRODUCTION

Obesity and overweight are global health concerns, with about half a billion adults and nearly 40 million children considered obese or overweight around the globe [1]. Obesity prevalence has been calculated to be even higher in a very recent publication [2], in good agreement with its incidence and prevalence tendency to rise, with a twofold increase in overweight and a threefold increase in obese individuals over the past 50 years [3].

Obesity is measured by means of various indices, mainly body mass index (BMI), waist circumference (WC), waist-to-hip ratio (WHR) and waist-to-height ratio. Regardless of the index used to define obesity, a lot of studies indicate a greater risk of cardiovascular disease in obese individuals [4].

Cardiovascular diseases constitute the leading cause of death worldwide, accounting for half of all deaths in middle age and one-third of all deaths in old age in most developed countries [5]. And although cardiovascular mortality has decreased progressively through the last five decades in the rich world [6], a deceleration of that reduction has been observed since the last years of the past century, in pair with an increment of physical inactivity, overweight, obesity and metabolic disturbances [7]. Beyond cardiovascular risk increase, obesity associates with many other comorbidities and increased mortality from certain cancers and all-cause mortality [8].

No wonder, then, that so many scientific and medical communities are devoting their attention and work-force to the putative solving of this health problem. Inefficacy of those efforts, however, indicates that important variables and causes of obesity are being ignored, in a situation that has emerged as a highly complex etiopathogenic reality.

In this chapter we will address the putative role of stress pathophysiology, in the context of both biological and social determinants of health, in the appearance and evolution of the obesity epidemic.

LESS TRAVELED ROADS

More than ten years ago Keith *et al* [9] published a paper, containing this heading in the title, calling attention to other putative causes/mechanisms of obesity beyond the big two (lack of physical exercise and marketing practices of energy-dense foods). This team went on insisting on that point, reviewing evidence for the involvement of microorganisms, epigenetics, increase in maternal age, greater fecundity among people with higher adiposity, assortative mating, sleep debt, endocrine disruptors, pharmaceutical iatrogenesis, reduction in variability of ambient temperatures and intrauterine and intergenerational effects as contributing factors to the obesity epidemic [10]. While they gathered evidence for some contributors, such as pharmaceutical-induced weight gain, evidence was not so strong for other reviewed factors. Furthermore, some important candidates had not been considered: chronobiology disruption beyond sleep debt (subjective time acceleration, lack of discipline in meal time), lack of meal management (no one in charge of meal programming, shopping and cooking), psychological and social changes (individualism/hedonism, devaluation of symbolic and affective character of food, loss of control through social circumstances at the table), and changes in stress environment/characteristics.

Stress

One important characteristic of modern social environment is the level of chronic psychological stress [11]. Stress may be defined as any event, such as an adverse experience or perceived threat, which challenges the individual's homeostasis, resulting in physiological alterations of two important neurohumoral systems, the sympatho-adrenomedullary axis and the hypothalamus-pituitary-adrenal cortex (HPA) axis, among others.

The survival value of the stress response has been paramount along evolution. However, the effect of modern life strains upon the neurohumoral stress systems, mostly when they act in a chronic way, are no more adaptive, leading instead to dysregulation, allostasis and disease. These ill aspects of modern life are clearly demonstrated in the work of James Henry, collaborators and followers, either with animal or human communities [12 - 15]. They show how the repeated stress reaction, which acutely prepares for attack or flight, when not followed by the naturally subsequent intense physical activity, leads to arterial hypertension.

Sympatho-Adrenomedullary System and Catecholamines

The sympathoadrenomedullary system is activated in stress situations, responding also to psychological stimuli, and plays an essential role in the regulation of metabolic and cardiovascular homeostasis. It exerts an excitatory action on smooth muscle in blood vessels supplying skin, kidney, mucous membranes and gland cells; an inhibitory action on smooth muscle of the gut, bronchial tree and blood vessels supplying skeletal muscle; and a cardiac excitatory action, leading to an increase in heart rate and force of contraction. Sympathetic stimulation increases the rate of glycogenolysis and lipolysis, and modulates the secretion of insulin, renin and pituitary hormones. It stimulates respiratory activity, wakefulness and psychomotor activity and may reduce appetite.

The primary neurotransmitter released from sympathetic nerves was identified as noradrenaline [16], this amine receiving the largest part of attention in a system which has many more agents to be considered, namely adrenaline, ATP and several peptides. Although the two catecholamines, adrenaline and noradrenaline, have different actions at some sites, their actions are very similar at other sites, and it is rather common to see them addressed, in the literature, simply as catecholamines as if they were alike. However, the role of these amines in the pathophysiology of obesity seems to be very different: whereas the levels of noradrenaline associate positively with obesity and cardiovascular risk, adrenaline shows an inverse association with cardiovascular and overall mortality [17]. In a very interesting long-term prospective study, in Norway, it has been shown that the adrenaline response to a mental stress is a negative predictor of future BMI, WC and triceps skinfold thickness after 18 years of follow-up [18].

Noradrenaline is mainly released from the sympathetic nerve terminals, evoked by central sympathetic outflow. Adrenaline is mainly released from the adrenal medulla, which responds to central sympathetic command according to a large range of local and historical factors. To begin with, the proportion of adrenaline and noradrenaline cells in adrenal medulla is highly variable, probably in relation with genetic and developmental factors. Local, paracrine agents, such as cortisol, somatostatin and others, determine the level of expression of the phenylethanolamine-N-methyl transferase (PNMT, the enzyme which converts noradrenaline into adrenaline), the release of adrenaline or the differential release of adrenaline and noradrenaline [19].

The impact of catechol-O-methyltransferase (COMT) polymorphisms on cardiovascular health is also gathering attention. One of the COMT gene polymorphisms, Val158Met, has a significant impact on the activity of the enzyme [20] and is related with cardiovascular risk [21, 22]. COMT plays a most important role in the metabolism of catecholamines, much more of adrenaline than of noradrenaline. Released noradrenaline is, for the most part, taken up into the nerve terminals, where metabolism occurs primarily through monoaminoxidase (MAO). As to adrenaline, mostly released from the adrenals into the circulation, it is taken up through extraneuronal uptake system (EMT) and metabolised by COMT [23, 24]. The inverse relation between cardiovascular risk and both adrenaline levels (more adrenaline – lower risk) and COMT gene polymorphism (higher activity – lower risk) seemed incongruent, pointing to the possibility of further intervenients in that relationship. Metanephrine, the product of COMT action upon adrenaline, appeared as an interesting candidate. The primordial work of Eisenhofer *et al* [25] had already shown that 91% of plasma metanephrine was directly produced and released from the adrenal gland. Moreover, metanephrine outflow of all inquired organs except adrenals (heart, forearm, lungs, kidneys, mesenteric organs and liver) was always of a lesser magnitude than metanephrine inflow, indicating a net removal of metanephrine by the organs, instead of a net production were it only a metabolic product. We thus proposed that metanephrine should be considered a hormone, not only an adrenaline metabolite, and its physiological effects looked after [11]. An inhibitory effect on platelet aggregation had already been described, suggesting an alpha 2-adrenoceptor antagonist effect [26]. Metanephrine may also inhibit nucleoside transport, what may be of physiological relevance in the putative potentiation of adenosine effects [27].

Corticosteroids are classic inhibitors of extraneuronal uptake of catecholamines. We showed that the pharmacological blockade of COMT activity in the presence of corticosterone leads to a marked accumulation of a catecholamine taken up from the extracellular space into the sympathetic nerve terminals [28]. Under circumstances of a low activity COMT polymorphism (genetic factor) and chronic stress with high cortisol levels (environmental factor), adrenaline may accumulate in the sympathetic nerve terminals. Upon nerve stimulation, this amine will be released and may reinforce neurotransmitter release through action upon presynaptic facilitatory beta 2-adrenoceptors [29], what may amplify cardiovascular responses to stress.

Considering adrenaline protective effects upon metabolic and cardiovascular health, it is interesting to remember that stimuli known to favor adrenaline release – physical exercise, hypoxia and hypoglycemia, are known to associate with protective lifestyles.

Hypothalamus-Pituitary-Adrenal Cortex and Corticoids

The HPA system, which has cortisol as its main effector, is activated in stress situations, responding also to psychological stimuli, and plays an essential role in the regulation of metabolic and cardiovascular homeostasis.

Hypothalamic corticotropin-releasing hormone (CRH) neurons drive both basal and stress-induced HPA activation. Stimuli that challenge homeostasis are communicated to the central nervous system by neurochemical pathways and integrated at the hypothalamic level where they reach paraventricular neurons controlling CRH secretion to the hypophysial portal vessels that access the anterior pituitary gland. The binding of CRH to its receptors activates adrenocorticotropic hormone (ACTH) release from pituitary corticotrophs. ACTH stimulates the synthesis and release of glucocorticoids from the zona fasciculata of the adrenal cortex. The biological effects of glucocorticoids support the adaptation to stress-induced demands by controlling energy metabolism [30, 31].

Corticosteroids are released in a pulsatile circadian pattern that may vary in amplitude and frequency under stressful conditions. The adaptive function of the HPA system depends on the negative feedback mechanisms that bring the HPA to baseline levels [32].

The effects of cortisol are numerous and widespread. It exerts catabolic and anti-anabolic actions, with alterations in carbohydrate, protein and lipid metabolism; maintains fluid and electrolyte balance; and preserves the normal function of the cardiovascular and immune systems, kidney, skeletal muscle, endocrine and nervous systems.

There is a strong relationship between the HPA system and metabolism [33]. This relationship includes expression of the enzyme 11beta-hydroxysteroid dehydrogenase type 1 (11beta-HSD1), which can generate active cortisol from inactive cortisone, and which increases in adipose tissue with age [34] and in obesity [35]. Furthermore, 11beta-HSD1 expression increases after exposure to cortisol and insulin [36]. Bujalska *et al* showed that 11beta-HSD1 gene was one of the most upregulated genes in omental but not subcutaneous preadipocytes after exposure to cortisol [37], in agreement with the results of Veilleux *et al* [38] showing relatively higher 11beta-HSD1 activity in omental *vs.* subcutaneous adipose tissue, in association with preferential visceral fat accumulation and concomitant metabolic alterations. In Bujalska *et al* study [37], glucocorticoid receptor expression was shown to be similar among omental and subcutaneous adipocytes, and not regulated by glucocorticoids. Cortisol produced by omental adipocytes acts locally, as splanchnic cortisol production is not altered by obesity [39]. Probably of utmost importance is the finding that omental 11beta-HSD1 correlates with fat cell size independently of obesity [40].

AMP-activated protein kinase (AMPK), a central enzyme in the control of metabolism, seems to mediate glucocorticoid metabolic effects [41]. On the other hand, mineralocorticoid receptors, which also bind glucocorticoids, seem to be involved in adipogenesis, obesity and other metabolic syndrome features [42 - 45]. And adipocytes secrete factors that stimulate adrenal mineralocorticoid release and sensitize the adrenal cortex to angiotensin II [46]. In conclusion, besides causing direct metabolic effects as known for a long time in the context of the stress response, corticosteroids influence the expression of 11beta-HSD1 in omental adipocytes, more so when these adipocytes are hypertrophic. Metabolic alterations reactive to cortisol tend, thus, to be feed-forward and may end in an endless spiral.

Stress is Not All Alike

Each person reacts to stressors in her own way, dependent on genes [47, 48], early life stress history [49 - 52], position in social hierarchy [53, 54] and cognitive/cultural characteristics, including coping strategies [55]. The brain, including its higher cognitive centers, is the key organ of the response to stressors, both in terms of perception of what is stressful and for its ability to determine the consequences of stress for both brain and body via the neuroendocrine, autonomic, immune and metabolic systems [55, 56]. Folkow *et al* [13, 15, 57] propose a most useful simplification of neurohormonal adjustments in the different kinds of stress reactions. In the vigilance reaction, the state of hyperarousal in which most of urban people live nowadays [58], there is mainly involvement of the sympathetic nervous system, with a rise in blood pressure as the more common consequence. No wonder that around half of adult population present arterial hypertension [59, 60], masked hypertension [61] or prehypertension [62] over different parts of the world. The defense reaction (Table **1**), the best studied and known among the stress response patterns, corresponds to the classic description of the flight/fight reaction: there is an intense engagement of the sympathetic nervous system, combined with inhibition of parasympathetic activity. The systemic vasculature is adjusted to increase blood supply to skeletal muscles, myocardium and brain, while blood flow to the kidneys, gastrointestinal tract, most skin regions and others is reduced. An increase of venous return to the heart, where rate and contractility are stimulated, contribute to increase cardiac output. Metabolic and fluid-electrolyte effects of sympathetic stimulation also contribute to the success of the fight/flight reaction. Maintenance of control is crucial for a positive outcome: leaders have lower levels of the stress hormone cortisol and lower reports of anxiety than subordinate workers [63].

On the other hand, in the defeat-submission reaction (Table **1**), when there is loss of control and social support, the most salient neurohormonal response consists in an increase of the HPA activation, with the correspondent production of cortisol. In the long-term, this disruption of cortisol physiology leads to marked metabolic alterations, reminiscent of the metabolic syndrome. Social determinants of health, or the effect of social organization on stress and health [53] have been carefully analysed and should be taken into consideration in any effort to understand the metabolic syndrome [64 - 69].

Obesity

Obesity is the state of having excess body fat. In general terms, it can be said that obesity increases the risk of diseases. It is considered an extremely important risk factor in the development of metabolic syndrome and the respective accompanying problems of insulin resistance, hypertension, dyslipidemia, blood coagulation problems and cardiovascular disease. However, even if obesity *per se* may bring deleterious consequences of excess volume/weight, such as mechanical constraints, arthritis, cosmetic, psychological problems and social inconveniences, there are now doubts about its direct/obligatory relationship with cardiometabolic pathology.

Table 1. A simplified illustration of the drastically different neurohormonal adjustments in the defeat reaction *vs.* defense reaction in stress situations. The arrows indicate increase or decrease; their size, extent. Two arrows in opposite directions indicate differentiated nervous discharge (Adapted from [15]).

	Defense Reaction	Defeat Reaction
Sympathetic system	↑	↑ ↓
Parasympathetic system	↓	↑
ACTH-glucocorticoid axis	↑	↑
Blood pressure	↑	↑
Immune system	↑	↓

ACTH: adrenocorticotropic hormone.

Obesity is Not All Alike

Although the negative health effects associated with obesity in the general population are well supported by available evidence [70], health outcomes in certain subgroups seem to be improved at an increased BMI, a phenomenon known as the obesity paradox [71 - 73]. Furthermore, there is a high prevalence of clustering of cardiometabolic abnormalities among normal-weight individuals and a high prevalence of overweight/obese individuals who are metabolically healthy [74]. Consequently, "metabolically benign obesity" which is not accompanied by insulin resistance and early atherosclerosis has recently been postulated to exist in humans [75].

Visceral Obesity and the Metabolic Syndrome

In 1947, Vague suggested that a particular obesity phenotype, which he called android or male-type obesity, was associated with the metabolic disturbances seen with diabetes and cardiovascular diseases [76].

The metabolic syndrome (disturbed glucose and insulin metabolism, overweight and predominant abdominal fat distribution, dyslipidemia and/or high blood pressure), now recognized as a major cause of type 2 diabetes and cardiovascular disease, has become one of the major public health challenges worldwide [77 - 79]. The diversity of features associated with this condition and the study of the problem by different associations led to a variety of definitions, with differences in details and criteria. A consensus group of the International Diabetes Federation (IDF) [80] recognized central obesity as the core and necessary feature of the metabolic syndrome. Central obesity is, thus, considered as a determinant in the causative pathway of the syndrome, impacting on the other components of the syndrome and on the cardiovascular disease. As a matter of fact, it seems to be the major predictor of incident metabolic syndrome, even when compared to insulin resistance [81 - 83].

The pathogenesis of the metabolic syndrome is complex and still poorly understood, and no single factor has yet been identified as an underlying causative factor [84]. It has been proposed that obesity, particularly visceral obesity, may play an important role in the development of the syndrome. Visceral adiposity seems to be an independent predictor of insulin sensitivity [85 - 87], impaired glucose tolerance [88], elevated blood pressure [89, 90] and dyslipidemia [86, 91].

Intraabdominal fat is a strongly metabolically active tissue. It seems more susceptible to lipolysis as compared with subcutaneous adipose tissue [92]. Furthermore, it produces various adipokines, such as tumor necrosis factor alpha [93], plasminogen activator inhibitor 1 [94], interleukin 6 and C-reactive protein

[95], being a feebler producer of adiponectin, more strongly correlated with subcutaneous fat [96].

Amount of Fat/Storing Capacity

As long as adipose tissue has available adipose cells and space to store the energy surplus, the organism may handle it healthily.

When fat is too much for the amount of adipocytes, these will increase their size up to big dimensions giving origin to various problems, and, on the other hand, fat starts to accumulate in various other tissues, particularly in the liver [97]. Bahceci *et al* [98] found a positive correlation between adipocyte size and tumor necrosis factor alpha, interleukin 6 and high-sensitivity C-reactive protein. On the other hand, adiponectin was found to be negatively correlated with adipocyte size.

As referred above, visceral obesity seems to play a central role in the development of the metabolic syndrome. However, some individuals with central obesity do not present the syndrome, in some way contradicting that primordial role. Perhaps more important than the amount of accumulated fat in the abdominal cavity is the size of abdominal adipocytes. We have shown that big adipocytes are prone to rupture [99], and cell rupture will obviously constitute a focus of inflammation. Macrophage crowns surrounding dead adipocytes have been shown by Cinti *et al* [100].

Subcutaneous adipocytes can also become hypertrophic, and most probably do also rupture. But abdominal adipocytes are probably more prone to rupture. They are supported by a much less dense connective tissue, when compared to adipocytes in subcutaneous adipose tissue, and are subject to sudden pressure variations associated with cough, physical exercise [101] or sleep apnoea [102]. Furthermore, intraabdominal pressure is higher in obese patients [103].

Preadipocytes of upper-body-obese women exhibit reduced differentiation and are more prone to apoptosis than pre-adipocytes isolated from adipose tissue of lower-body-obese or lean women [104]. The factors involved in this preadipocyte behaviour deserve investigation [105].

Another characteristic of abdominal adipose tissue is its high metabolic activity and dense vascularisation. This high vascularisation is most probably due to the action of angiogenic/proinflammatory factors, of which leptin constitutes an example [106 - 108]. On the other hand, increased intra-abdominal pressure, as well as pressure variations, may easily create periods/zones of hypoxia, contributing to the production of hypoxia-inducible factors. Vascular endothelial growth factor (VEGF), leptin, adenosine, and substance P, among others, will impact on other features of the metabolic syndrome. Furthermore, hypoxia by itself inactivates the adiponectin promoter [109, 110].

Beyond the number of adipocytes, the existence of space/low pressure in organism sectors may facilitate fat deposition. This explains the frequent occurrence of benign visceral adiposity in parous women, in comparison with nulliparous women [111 - 113].

Chronic Defeat Stress Reaction, Cortisol, Visceral Obesity and the Metabolic Syndrome

Let us consider now the importance of chronic stress imposed by the present socio-economic/cultural environment upon a large fraction of the human population, and its role in the development of the metabolic syndrome.

There are impressive similarities in presentation of cortisol excess and metabolic syndrome (Fig. **1**), suggesting that abnormalities of that endocrine hormone may play a causal role in the development of this syndrome. Chanson and Salenave [114] had already considered Cushing's syndrome an archetype of metabolic syndrome, as high glucocorticoid levels lead to muscle, liver and adipocyte insulin resistance, almost all patients with Cushing's syndrome being obese or overweight, and having visceral adiposity. Many also have glucose metabolism abnormalities, hypertension and elevated triglyceride levels. More recently, it has been verified that chronic exposure to elevated cortisol concentrations, assessed in hair, is associated with markers of adiposity and with the persistence of obesity over time [115]. Yener *et al* showed that autonomous cortisol secretion is associated with increased visceral fat accumulation after a follow-up duration of around three years [116]. There is, also, evidence for cortisol dysregulation in obesity-related metabolic disorders [45, 117]. Moreover, the presence of subclinical Cushing's syndrome has been found in a notable number of type 2 diabetic patients with poor metabolic control [118]. As a matter of fact, endocrinologists are reporting difficulties in distinguishing pathologic/neoplastic hypercortisolism (true Cushing's syndrome) from physiologic/non-neoplastic hypercortisolism (formerly known as pseudo-Cushing's syndrome), nowadays a highly common finding among the highly prevalent metabolic syndrome [119 - 121].

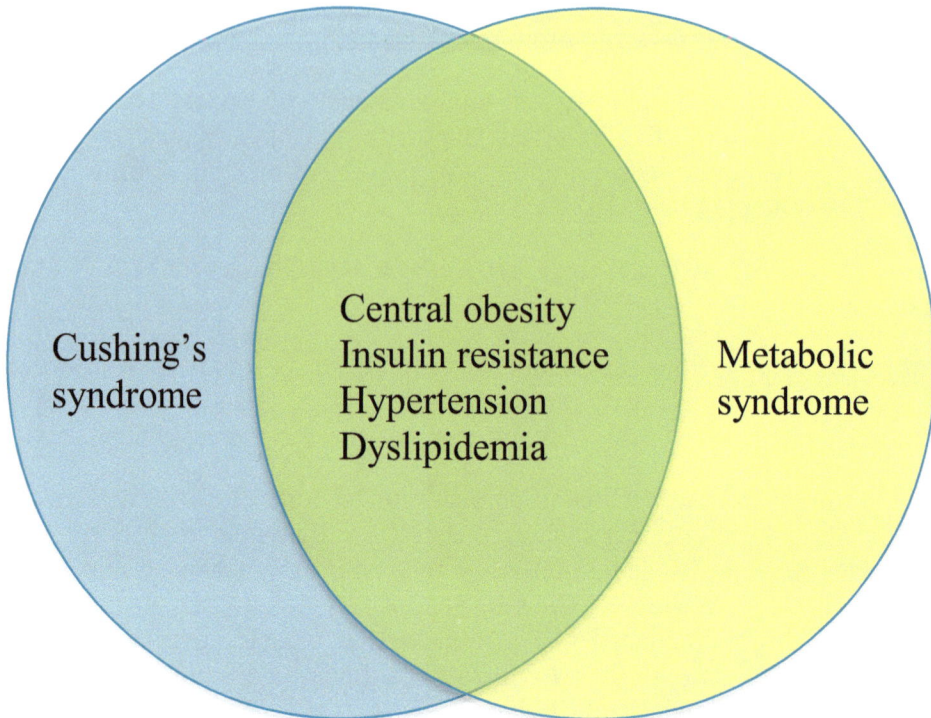

Fig. (1). Cushing's syndrome and metabolic syndrome overlapping signs and symptoms.

Cortisol concentrations increase in response to stressful situations [122, 123]. Under conditions of chronic stress, prolonged increased cortisol concentrations can have detrimental downstream physiological effects. Several population-based studies have linked daily cortisol patterns to health outcomes, including elevated blood pressure, abdominal obesity and coronary calcification [124, 125] or the metabolic syndrome [126 - 128]. Cortisol is synthesized on demand, and there is an obligatory role for cholesterol in steroidogenesis [129, 130]. Hypercortisolemia or chronic stress stimulate, therefore, the processes of cholesterol synthesis [130] and may contribute to the correspondent dyslipidemia.

Obesity and the metabolic syndrome are strongly associated with individual income and education. Other socio-economic variables, such as geographic localization (disparities in obesity rates by ZIP code area are greater than disparities associated with individual income or race/ethnicity) or house value, do also constitute predictors of the area-based obesity prevalence [131]. Analysis of the huge data in the study by Chetty *et al* [132] (1.4 billion tax records and mortality data between 1999 and 2014, in the USA) showed that higher income is associated with greater longevity throughout the income distribution, the gap in life expectancy between the 1% richest and 1% poorest of individuals being 14.6 years for men and 10.1 years for women. This work confirms, with much more precision and detail, what has been described since the nineteenth-century ([133 - 135], as quoted by Deaton [136]). After that, we have the tremendous work by Marmot *et al*, which started with the Whitehall study of British civil servants and extended well beyond [137], and a growing number of new studies with the same kind of results [138].

But more important than absolute income seems to be the social rank position [139 - 142]. Various experimental studies with animal communities give strong support to this hypothesis [13, 143, 144]. Perception of oneself as low-rank, subordinate, without control, leads to a chronic situation of defeat stress reaction, with an increase in cortisol production [15, 122, 123, 145, 146]. Chronic stress and hypercortisolism progressively evolve toward the various components of the metabolic syndrome, with an important negative influence on health-related quality of life [147], including obesity [117, 148 - 151] and depression [152, 153]. Subordination stress was shown to be a potent stimulus for the downregulation of the insulin signaling pathway in liver and muscle and a major risk factor for the development of obesity, insulin resistance and type 2 diabetes *mellitus* [154].

Clustering and accumulation of psychosocial disadvantage create health problems down the social strata in industrialized countries [52, 53, 155]. Social exclusion, with detrimental effects on health for particular minority groups (the unemployed, refugees, poorer migrants, ethnic minorities and homeless people), tends to receive primordial attention from social workers and researchers [156]. But there are many more people living under chronic stress conditions, the "insulted and humiliated" of Dostoyevsky, or the "tired and oppressed" of the Bible.

Women across the countries, small areas, social classes and income distribution constitute an important group suffering from subordinate conditions, lack of control, chronic stress and hypercortisolism. They tend to react with greater overall secretion of cortisol [153, 157], and present a higher prevalence of obesity [158] and metabolic syndrome [159, 160]. Furthermore, women seem to be more strongly affected by psychosocial stressors related to cardiovascular disease and depression as well as by chronic stress [161, 162]. They are well-known to frequently suffer from cumulative and specific forms of domestic violence, particularly emotional violence and controling behavior [163]. In a population-based cross-sectional survey among 1100 adult Jewish and Arab Israelis, the prevalence of diabetes was higher among Arab participants than among Jewish participants, but Arab females had a much higher prevalence of diabetes than Arab males, differently from Jewish gender groups [164]. Another sign of the importance of subordinate and controlled behavior of women on their health may be the observed minor effect of income on women mortality in Chetty *et al* study [132] as compared with the income effect on men. This difference may denote the superimposition of inequality over the income effect, as inequality and domestic violence pervade across all social classes, albeit more markedly among poor and uneducated populations.

Abdominal obesity is a sign of health risk, but so is hypercortisolism. Hypercortisolism leads to abdominal obesity and other metabolic alterations, and may be the main causative factor of cardiometabolic complications of the metabolic syndrome. A recent publication indicates that "abdominal fat reduction alone is not directly linked to improvement in obesity-related health risk factors, abdominal fat being probably not a causal factor but simply a symptom of obesity-related health risk" [165]. Notwithstanding the direct adverse effects of central obesity, excess cortisol associated with chronic defeat stress reaction is probably an important causative agent of the metabolic syndrome, obesity included.

CONCLUDING REMARKS

Psychosocial chronic stress is highly prevalent. The typical stress reaction for this kind of situation is a defeat stress reaction, with increased production of cortisol, more so in women. Cortisol excess leads to a number of physiological alterations that, with time, configurate a pathological condition reminiscent of Cushing's syndrome, including central obesity. Adverse effects of central obesity are partly directly attributable to obesity itself, but a large part of those effects is probably due to cortisol. More important than to reduce obesity will be, therefore, to prevent cortisol excess. This is not an easy task, although it had already been expressed in Virchow's statement that "medicine is a social science, and politics is nothing but medicine at a larger scale" ([135], quoted by Mackenbach [166]).

CONSENT FOR PUBLICATION

Not applicable.

CONFLICT OF INTEREST

The authors confirm that this chapter contents have no conflict of interest.

ACKNOWLEDGEMENTS

Declared none.

REFERENCES

[1]   World Health Organization [homepage on the internet]. Geneva: Obesity and Overweight (Factsheet no 311) [updated: 11th August 2015; cited: 25th July 2017]. http://www.who.int/mediacentre/factsheets/fs311/en/index.html

[2]   Afshin A, Forouzanfar MH, Reitsma MB, *et al.* Health Effects of Overweight and Obesity in 195 Countries over 25 Years. N Engl J Med 2017; 377(1): 13-27.
[http://dx.doi.org/10.1056/NEJMoa1614362] [PMID: 28604169]

[3]   Finucane MM, Stevens GA, Cowan MJ, *et al.* National, regional, and global trends in body-mass index since 1980: systematic analysis of health examination surveys and epidemiological studies with 960 country-years and 9·1 million participants. Lancet 2011; 377(9765): 557-67.
[http://dx.doi.org/10.1016/S0140-6736(10)62037-5] [PMID: 21295846]

[4]   Hamzeh N, Ghadimi F, Farzaneh R, Hosseini SK. Obesity, Heart Failure, and Obesity Paradox. J Tehran Heart Cent 2017; 12(1): 1-5.
[PMID: 28469684]

[5]   World Health Organization. World health statistics 2007. Geneva: World Health Organization 2007.

[6]   Roth GA, Dwyer-Lindgren L, Bertozzi-Villa A, *et al.* Trends and Patterns of Geographic Variation in Cardiovascular Mortality Among US Counties, 1980-2014. JAMA 2017; 317(19): 1976-92.
[http://dx.doi.org/10.1001/jama.2017.4150] [PMID: 28510678]

[7]   Gaziano JM. Global burden of Cardiovascular Disease.Braunwald's Heart Disease. 8th ed. Philadelphia: Saunders-Elsevier 2008; pp. 1-22.

[8]   Berrington de Gonzalez A, Hartge P, Cerhan JR, *et al.* Body-mass index and mortality among 1.46 million white adults. N Engl J Med 2010; 363(23): 2211-9.
[http://dx.doi.org/10.1056/NEJMoa1000367] [PMID: 21121834]

[9]   Keith SW, Redden DT, Katzmarzyk PT, *et al.* Putative contributors to the secular increase in obesity: exploring the roads less traveled. Int J Obes 2006; 30(11): 1585-94.
[http://dx.doi.org/10.1038/sj.ijo.0803326] [PMID: 16801930]

[10]   McAllister EJ, Dhurandhar NV, Keith SW, *et al.* Ten putative contributors to the obesity epidemic. Crit Rev Food Sci Nutr 2009; 49(10): 868-913.
[http://dx.doi.org/10.1080/10408390903372599] [PMID: 19960394]

[11]   Azevedo A, Santos AC, Azevedo I. The metabolic syndrome.Oxidative stress, inflammation and angiogenesis: joint partners in the metabolic syndrome. Milton Keynes: Springer 2009; pp. 1-19.
[http://dx.doi.org/10.1007/978-1-4020-9701-0_1]

[12]   Henry JP, Stephens PM, Eds. Stress, health and the psychosocial environment.A sociobiological approach to medicine. New York: Springer Verlag 1977.
[http://dx.doi.org/10.1007/978-1-4612-6363-0]

[13]   Folkow B, Schmidt T, Uvnäs-Moberg K. Stress, health and the social environment. James P Henry's ethological approach to medicine, reflected by recent research in animals and man. Acta Physiol Scand Suppl 1997; 640: 1-179.
[PMID: 9454507]

[14]   Henry JP, Grim CE. Psychosocial mechanisms of primary hypertension. J Hypertens 1990; 8(9): 783-93.
[http://dx.doi.org/10.1097/00004872-199009000-00001] [PMID: 2172367]

[15]   Folkow B. Evolutionary aspects of stress.Stress in health and disease. Indianapolis: Wiley-VCH 2006; pp. 20-45.
[http://dx.doi.org/10.1002/3527609156.ch2]

[16]   von Euler U. Identification of the sympathomimetic ergone in adrenergic nerves of cattle (sympathin N) with laevo-nor-adrenaline. Acta Physiol Scand 1948; 16: 63-74.

[http://dx.doi.org/10.1111/j.1748-1716.1948.tb00526.x]

[17] Christensen NJ, Schultz-Larsen K. Resting venous plasma adrenalin in 70-year-old men correlated positively to survival in a population study: the significance of the physical working capacity. J Intern Med 1994; 235(3): 229-32.
[http://dx.doi.org/10.1111/j.1365-2796.1994.tb01064.x] [PMID: 8120517]

[18] Flaa A, Sandvik L, Kjeldsen SE, Eide IK, Rostrup M. Does sympathoadrenal activity predict changes in body fat? An 18-y follow-up study. Am J Clin Nutr 2008; 87(6): 1596-601.
[http://dx.doi.org/10.1093/ajcn/87.6.1596] [PMID: 18541545]

[19] Ribeiro L, Martel F, Azevedo I. Effect of somatostatin on the release of adrenaline and noradrenaline from bovine adrenal chromaffin cells.Cell Biology of the chromaffin cell. Madrid: Instituto Teófilo Hernando 2004; pp. 1-4.

[20] Lachman HM, Papolos DF, Saito T, Yu YM, Szumlanski CL, Weinshilboum RM. Human catechol-O-methyltransferase pharmacogenetics: description of a functional polymorphism and its potential application to neuropsychiatric disorders. Pharmacogenetics 1996; 6(3): 243-50.
[http://dx.doi.org/10.1097/00008571-199606000-00007] [PMID: 8807664]

[21] Voutilainen S, Tuomainen TP, Korhonen M, *et al.* Functional COMT Val158Met polymorphism, risk of acute coronary events and serum homocysteine: the Kuopio ischaemic heart disease risk factor study. PLoS One 2007; 2(1)e181
[http://dx.doi.org/10.1371/journal.pone.0000181] [PMID: 17264883]

[22] Annerbrink K, Westberg L, Nilsson S, Rosmond R, Holm G, Eriksson E. Catechol O-methyltransferase val158-met polymorphism is associated with abdominal obesity and blood pressure in men. Metabolism 2008; 57(5): 708-11.
[http://dx.doi.org/10.1016/j.metabol.2008.01.012] [PMID: 18442637]

[23] Trendelenburg U. A kinetic analysis of the extraneuronal uptake and metabolism of catecholamines. Rev Physiol Biochem Pharmacol 1980; 87: 33-115.
[http://dx.doi.org/10.1007/BFb0030896] [PMID: 6999585]

[24] Martel F, Ribeiro L, Calhau C, Azevedo I. Comparison between uptake$_2$ and rOCT1: effects of catecholamines, metanephrines and corticosterone. Naunyn Schmiedebergs Arch Pharmacol 1999; 359(4): 303-9.
[http://dx.doi.org/10.1007/PL00005356] [PMID: 10344529]

[25] Eisenhofer G, Rundquist B, Aneman A, *et al.* Regional release and removal of catecholamines and extraneuronal metabolism to metanephrines. J Clin Endocrinol Metab 1995; 80(10): 3009-17.
[PMID: 7559889]

[26] Lenz T, Werle E, Strobel G, Weicker H. O-Methylated and sulfoconjugated catecholamines: differential activities at human platelet alpha 2-adrenoceptors. Can J Physiol Pharmacol 1991; 69(7): 929-37.
[http://dx.doi.org/10.1139/y91-141] [PMID: 1683267]

[27] Sarmento A, Albino Teixeira A, Azevedo I. Decrease of 3H-uridine incorporation in the dog saphenous smooth muscle by isoprenaline or noradrenaline. Arq Inst Farm Terap Exp Coimbra 1984; 22: 145-6.

[28] Azevedo I, Osswald W. Uptake, distribution and metabolism of isoprenaline in the dog saphenous vein. Naunyn Schmiedebergs Arch Pharmacol 1976; 295(2): 141-7.
[http://dx.doi.org/10.1007/BF00499446] [PMID: 995209]

[29] Guimarães S, Moura D. Vascular adrenoceptors: an update. Pharmacol Rev 2001; 53(2): 319-56.
[PMID: 11356987]

[30] Sapolsky RM, Romero LM, Munck AU. How do glucocorticoids influence stress responses? Integrating permissive, suppressive, stimulatory, and preparative actions. Endocr Rev 2000; 21(1): 55-89.

[PMID: 10696570]

[31] Herman JP, Figueiredo H, Mueller NK, *et al.* Central mechanisms of stress integration: hierarchical circuitry controlling hypothalamo-pituitary-adrenocortical responsiveness. Front Neuroendocrinol 2003; 24(3): 151-80.
[http://dx.doi.org/10.1016/j.yfrne.2003.07.001] [PMID: 14596810]

[32] Quax RA, Manenschijn L, Koper JW, *et al.* Glucocorticoid sensitivity in health and disease. Nat Rev Endocrinol 2013; 9(11): 670-86.
[http://dx.doi.org/10.1038/nrendo.2013.183] [PMID: 24080732]

[33] Nieuwenhuizen AG, Rutters F. The hypothalamic-pituitary-adrenal-axis in the regulation of energy balance. Physiol Behav 2008; 94(2): 169-77.
[http://dx.doi.org/10.1016/j.physbeh.2007.12.011] [PMID: 18275977]

[34] Li X, Lindquist S, Chen R, *et al.* Depot-specific messenger RNA expression of 11 beta-hydroxysteroid dehydrogenase type 1 and leptin in adipose tissue of children and adults. Int J Obes 2007; 31(5): 820-8.
[http://dx.doi.org/10.1038/sj.ijo.0803470] [PMID: 17060929]

[35] Desbriere R, Vuaroqueaux V, Achard V, *et al.* 11beta-hydroxysteroid dehydrogenase type 1 mRNA is increased in both visceral and subcutaneous adipose tissue of obese patients. Obesity (Silver Spring) 2006; 14(5): 794-8.
[http://dx.doi.org/10.1038/oby.2006.92] [PMID: 16855188]

[36] Bujalska IJ, Kumar S, Stewart PM. Does central obesity reflect "Cushing's disease of the omentum"? Lancet 1997; 349(9060): 1210-3.
[http://dx.doi.org/10.1016/S0140-6736(96)11222-8] [PMID: 9130942]

[37] Bujalska IJ, Quinkler M, Tomlinson JW, Montague CT, Smith DM, Stewart PM. Expression profiling of 11β-hydroxysteroid dehydrogenase type-1 and glucocorticoid-target genes in subcutaneous and omental human preadipocytes. J Mol Endocrinol 2006; 37(2): 327-40.
[http://dx.doi.org/10.1677/jme.1.02048] [PMID: 17032748]

[38] Veilleux A, Rhéaume C, Daris M, Luu-The V, Tchernof A. Omental adipose tissue 11{beta}-HSD1 oxoreductase activity, body fat distribution and metabolic alterations in women. J Clin Endocrinol Metab 2009; 94(9): 3550-7.
[http://dx.doi.org/10.1210/jc.2008-2011] [PMID: 19567539]

[39] Basu R, Singh RJ, Basu A, *et al.* Obesity and type 2 diabetes do not alter splanchnic cortisol production in humans. J Clin Endocrinol Metab 2005; 90(7): 3919-26.
[http://dx.doi.org/10.1210/jc.2004-2390] [PMID: 15811928]

[40] Michailidou Z, Jensen MD, Dumesic DA, *et al.* Omental 11beta-hydroxysteroid dehydrogenase 1 correlates with fat cell size independently of obesity. Obesity (Silver Spring) 2007; 15(5): 1155-63.
[http://dx.doi.org/10.1038/oby.2007.618] [PMID: 17495191]

[41] Christ-Crain M, Kola B, Lolli F, *et al.* AMP-activated protein kinase mediates glucocorticoid-induced metabolic changes: a novel mechanism in Cushing's syndrome. FASEB J 2008; 22(6): 1672-83.
[http://dx.doi.org/10.1096/fj.07-094144] [PMID: 18198220]

[42] de Paula RB, da Silva AA, Hall JE. Aldosterone antagonism attenuates obesity-induced hypertension and glomerular hyperfiltration. Hypertension 2004; 43(1): 41-7.
[http://dx.doi.org/10.1161/01.HYP.0000105624.68174.00] [PMID: 14638627]

[43] Caprio M, Fève B, Claës A, Viengchareun S, Lombès M, Zennaro MC. Pivotal role of the mineralocorticoid receptor in corticosteroid-induced adipogenesis. FASEB J 2007; 21(9): 2185-94.
[http://dx.doi.org/10.1096/fj.06-7970com] [PMID: 17384139]

[44] Guo C, Ricchiuti V, Lian BQ, *et al.* Mineralocorticoid receptor blockade reverses obesity-related changes in expression of adiponectin, peroxisome proliferator-activated receptor-gamma, and proinflammatory adipokines. Circulation 2008; 117(17): 2253-61.

[http://dx.doi.org/10.1161/CIRCULATIONAHA.107.748640] [PMID: 18427128]

[45]   Baudrand R, Vaidya A. Cortisol dysregulation in obesity-related metabolic disorders. Curr Opin Endocrinol Diabetes Obes 2015; 22(3): 143-9.
[http://dx.doi.org/10.1097/MED.0000000000000152] [PMID: 25871955]

[46]   Krug AW, Ehrhart-Bornstein M. Adrenocortical dysfunction in obesity and the metabolic syndrome. Horm Metab Res 2008; 40(8): 515-7.
[http://dx.doi.org/10.1055/s-2008-1073154] [PMID: 18446685]

[47]   Lesch KP, Bengel D, Heils A, *et al*. Association of anxiety-related traits with a polymorphism in the serotonin transporter gene regulatory region. Science 1996; 274(5292): 1527-31.
[http://dx.doi.org/10.1126/science.274.5292.1527] [PMID: 8929413]

[48]   Furmark T, Tillfors M, Garpenstrand H, *et al*. Serotonin transporter polymorphism related to amygdala excitability and symptom severity in patients with social phobia. Neurosci Lett 2004; 362(3): 189-92.
[http://dx.doi.org/10.1016/j.neulet.2004.02.070] [PMID: 15158011]

[49]   Wadsworth M, Butterworth S. Early life.Social determinants of health. 2nd ed. Oxford: University Press 2006; pp. 31-53.

[50]   Harris A, Seckl J. Glucocorticoids, prenatal stress and the programming of disease. Horm Behav 2011; 59(3): 279-89.
[http://dx.doi.org/10.1016/j.yhbeh.2010.06.007] [PMID: 20591431]

[51]   Maniam J, Antoniadis C, Morris MJ. Early-Life Stress, HPA Axis Adaptation, and Mechanisms Contributing to Later Health Outcomes. Front Endocrinol (Lausanne) 2014; 5: 73.
[http://dx.doi.org/10.3389/fendo.2014.00073] [PMID: 24860550]

[52]   Liu H, Umberson D. Gender, stress in childhood and adulthood, and trajectories of change in body mass. Soc Sci Med 2015; 139: 61-9.
[http://dx.doi.org/10.1016/j.socscimed.2015.06.026] [PMID: 26151391]

[53]   Brunner E, Marmot M. Social organization, stress, and health.Social determinants of health. 2nd ed. Oxford: University Press 2006; pp. 6-30.

[54]   Steptoe A, Kunz-Ebrecht S, Owen N, *et al*. Socioeconomic status and stress-related biological responses over the working day. Psychosom Med 2003; 65(3): 461-70.
[http://dx.doi.org/10.1097/01.PSY.0000035717.78650.A1] [PMID: 12764220]

[55]   Eriksen HR, Ursin H. Stress – It is all in the brain.Stress in health and disease. Indianapolis: Wiley-VCH 2006; pp. 46-68.
[http://dx.doi.org/10.1002/3527609156.ch3]

[56]   McEwen BS. The Brain on Stress: Toward an Integrative Approach to Brain, Body, and Behavior. Perspect Psychol Sci 2013; 8(6): 673-5.
[http://dx.doi.org/10.1177/1745691613506907] [PMID: 25221612]

[57]   Folkow B. Physiological organization of neurohormonal responses to psychosocial stimuli: implications for health and disease. Ann Behav Med 1993; 15(4): 236-44.

[58]   Bettencourt LM, Lobo J, Helbing D, Kühnert C, West GB. Growth, innovation, scaling, and the pace of life in cities. Proc Natl Acad Sci USA 2007; 104(17): 7301-6.
[http://dx.doi.org/10.1073/pnas.0610172104] [PMID: 17438298]

[59]   Vital signs: prevalence, treatment, and control of hypertension--United States, 1999-2002 and 2005-2008. MMWR Morb Mortal Wkly Rep 2011; 60(4): 103-8.
[PMID: 21293325]

[60]   Roy A, Praveen PA, Amarchand R, *et al*. Changes in hypertension prevalence, awareness, treatment and control rates over 20 years in National Capital Region of India: results from a repeat cross-sectional study. BMJ Open 2017; 7(7)e015639
[http://dx.doi.org/10.1136/bmjopen-2016-015639] [PMID: 28706098]

[61]   Anstey DE, Booth JN III, Abdalla M, *et al.* Predicted Atherosclerotic Cardiovascular Disease Risk and Masked Hypertension Among Blacks in the Jackson Heart Study. Circ Cardiovasc Qual Outcomes 2017; 10(7)e003421
[http://dx.doi.org/10.1161/CIRCOUTCOMES.116.003421] [PMID: 28698190]

[62]   Zhang R, Deng R, Shen P, *et al.* Prehypertension and socioeconomic status: A cross-sectional study in Chongqing, China. Clin Exp Hypertens 2017; 39(8): 774-80.
[http://dx.doi.org/10.1080/10641963.2017.1334794] [PMID: 28692313]

[63]   Sherman GD, Lee JJ, Cuddy AJ, *et al.* Leadership is associated with lower levels of stress. Proc Natl Acad Sci USA 2012; 109(44): 17903-7.
[http://dx.doi.org/10.1073/pnas.1207042109] [PMID: 23012416]

[64]   Björntorp P. Visceral fat accumulation: the missing link between psychosocial factors and cardiovascular disease? J Intern Med 1991; 230(3): 195-201.
[http://dx.doi.org/10.1111/j.1365-2796.1991.tb00431.x] [PMID: 1895041]

[65]   Bosma H, Marmot MG, Hemingway H, Nicholson AC, Brunner E, Stansfeld SA. Low job control and risk of coronary heart disease in Whitehall II (prospective cohort) study. BMJ 1997; 314(7080): 558-65.
[http://dx.doi.org/10.1136/bmj.314.7080.558] [PMID: 9055714]

[66]   Brunner E. Stress and the biology of inequality. BMJ 1997; 314(7092): 1472-6.
[http://dx.doi.org/10.1136/bmj.314.7092.1472] [PMID: 9167568]

[67]   Brydon L, Edwards S, Mohamed-Ali V, Steptoe A. Socioeconomic status and stress-induced increases in interleukin-6. Brain Behav Immun 2004; 18(3): 281-90.
[http://dx.doi.org/10.1016/j.bbi.2003.09.011] [PMID: 15050655]

[68]   Siegrist J. Adverse health effects of high-effort/low-reward conditions. J Occup Health Psychol 1996; 1(1): 27-41.
[http://dx.doi.org/10.1037/1076-8998.1.1.27] [PMID: 9547031]

[69]   Steptoe A, Marmot M. The role of psychobiological pathways in socio-economic inequalities in cardiovascular disease risk. Eur Heart J 2002; 23(1): 13-25.
[http://dx.doi.org/10.1053/euhj.2001.2611] [PMID: 11741358]

[70]   Zheng Y, Manson JE, Yuan C, *et al.* Associations of Weight Gain From Early to Middle Adulthood With Major Health Outcomes Later in Life. JAMA 2017; 318(3): 255-69.
[http://dx.doi.org/10.1001/jama.2017.7092] [PMID: 28719691]

[71]   Gruberg L, Weissman NJ, Waksman R, *et al.* The impact of obesity on the short-term and long-term outcomes after percutaneous coronary intervention: the obesity paradox? J Am Coll Cardiol 2002; 39(4): 578-84.
[http://dx.doi.org/10.1016/S0735-1097(01)01802-2] [PMID: 11849854]

[72]   Shubair MM, Prabhakaran P, Pavlova V, Velianou JL, Sharma AM, Natarajan MK. The relationship of body mass index to outcomes after percutaneous coronary intervention. J Interv Cardiol 2006; 19(5): 388-95.
[http://dx.doi.org/10.1111/j.1540-8183.2006.00189.x] [PMID: 17020562]

[73]   Uretsky S, Messerli FH, Bangalore S, *et al.* Obesity paradox in patients with hypertension and coronary artery disease. Am J Med 2007; 120(10): 863-70.
[http://dx.doi.org/10.1016/j.amjmed.2007.05.011] [PMID: 17904457]

[74]   Wildman RP, Muntner P, Reynolds K, *et al.* The obese without cardiometabolic risk factor clustering and the normal weight with cardiometabolic risk factor clustering: prevalence and correlates of 2 phenotypes among the US population (NHANES 1999-2004). Arch Intern Med 2008; 168(15): 1617-24.
[http://dx.doi.org/10.1001/archinte.168.15.1617] [PMID: 18695075]

[75]   Stefan N, Kantartzis K, Machann J, *et al.* Identification and characterization of metabolically benign

obesity in humans. Arch Intern Med 2008; 168(15): 1609-16.
[http://dx.doi.org/10.1001/archinte.168.15.1609] [PMID: 18695074]

[76]　Vague J. La différenciation sexuelle; facteur déterminant des formes de l'obésité. Presse Med 1947; 55(30): 339.
[PMID: 18918084]

[77]　Caterson ID, Hubbard V, Bray GA, *et al.* Prevention Conference VII: Obesity, a worldwide epidemic related to heart disease and stroke: Group III: worldwide comorbidities of obesity. Circulation 2004; 110(18): e476-83.
[http://dx.doi.org/10.1161/01.CIR.0000140114.83145.59] [PMID: 15520332]

[78]　Eckel RH, Grundy SM, Zimmet PZ. The metabolic syndrome. Lancet 2005; 365(9468): 1415-28.
[http://dx.doi.org/10.1016/S0140-6736(05)66378-7] [PMID: 15836891]

[79]　Galassi A, Reynolds K, He J. Metabolic syndrome and risk of cardiovascular disease: a meta-analysis. Am J Med 2006; 119(10): 812-9.
[http://dx.doi.org/10.1016/j.amjmed.2006.02.031] [PMID: 17000207]

[80]　Alberti KG, Zimmet P, Shaw J. Metabolic syndrome – a new world-wide definition. A consensus Statement from the International Diabetes Federation. Diabet Med 2006; 23(5): 469-80.
[http://dx.doi.org/10.1111/j.1464-5491.2006.01858.x] [PMID: 16681555]

[81]　Srinivasan SR, Myers L, Berenson GS. Predictability of childhood adiposity and insulin for developing insulin resistance syndrome (syndrome X) in young adulthood: the Bogalusa Heart Study. Diabetes 2002; 51(1): 204-9.
[http://dx.doi.org/10.2337/diabetes.51.1.204] [PMID: 11756342]

[82]　Palaniappan L, Carnethon MR, Wang Y, *et al.* Predictors of the incident metabolic syndrome in adults: the Insulin Resistance Atherosclerosis Study. Diabetes Care 2004; 27(3): 788-93.
[http://dx.doi.org/10.2337/diacare.27.3.788] [PMID: 14988303]

[83]　Tong J, Boyko EJ, Utzschneider KM, *et al.* Intra-abdominal fat accumulation predicts the development of the metabolic syndrome in non-diabetic Japanese-Americans. Diabetologia 2007; 50(6): 1156-60.
[http://dx.doi.org/10.1007/s00125-007-0651-y] [PMID: 17387445]

[84]　Grundy SM, Cleeman JI, Daniels SR, *et al.* Diagnosis and management of the metabolic syndrome: an American Heart Association/National Heart, Lung, and Blood Institute scientific statement. Circulation 2005; 112(17): 2735-52.
[http://dx.doi.org/10.1161/CIRCULATIONAHA.105.169404] [PMID: 16157765]

[85]　Cnop M, Landchild MJ, Vidal J, *et al.* The concurrent accumulation of intra-abdominal and subcutaneous fat explains the association between insulin resistance and plasma leptin concentrations : distinct metabolic effects of two fat compartments. Diabetes 2002; 51(4): 1005-15.
[http://dx.doi.org/10.2337/diabetes.51.4.1005] [PMID: 11916919]

[86]　Katsuki A, Sumida Y, Urakawa H, *et al.* Increased visceral fat and serum levels of triglyceride are associated with insulin resistance in Japanese metabolically obese, normal weight subjects with normal glucose tolerance. Diabetes Care 2003; 26(8): 2341-4.
[http://dx.doi.org/10.2337/diacare.26.8.2341] [PMID: 12882859]

[87]　Wagenknecht LE, Langefeld CD, Scherzinger AL, *et al.* Insulin sensitivity, insulin secretion, and abdominal fat: the Insulin Resistance Atherosclerosis Study (IRAS) Family Study. Diabetes 2003; 52(10): 2490-6.
[http://dx.doi.org/10.2337/diabetes.52.10.2490] [PMID: 14514631]

[88]　Hayashi T, Boyko EJ, Leonetti DL, *et al.* Visceral adiposity and the risk of impaired glucose tolerance: a prospective study among Japanese Americans. Diabetes Care 2003; 26(3): 650-5.
[http://dx.doi.org/10.2337/diacare.26.3.650] [PMID: 12610016]

[89]　Bacha F, Saad R, Gungor N, Janosky J, Arslanian SA. Obesity, regional fat distribution, and syndrome X in obese black *versus* white adolescents: race differential in diabetogenic and atherogenic risk

factors. J Clin Endocrinol Metab 2003; 88(6): 2534-40.
[http://dx.doi.org/10.1210/jc.2002-021267] [PMID: 12788850]

[90] Rattarasarn C, Leelawattana R, Soonthornpun S, *et al.* Regional abdominal fat distribution in lean and obese Thai type 2 diabetic women: relationships with insulin sensitivity and cardiovascular risk factors. Metabolism 2003; 52(11): 1444-7.
[http://dx.doi.org/10.1016/S0026-0495(03)00257-9] [PMID: 14624404]

[91] Nieves DJ, Cnop M, Retzlaff B, *et al.* The atherogenic lipoprotein profile associated with obesity and insulin resistance is largely attributable to intra-abdominal fat. Diabetes 2003; 52(1): 172-9.
[http://dx.doi.org/10.2337/diabetes.52.1.172] [PMID: 12502509]

[92] van Harmelen V, Dicker A, Rydén M, *et al.* Increased lipolysis and decreased leptin production by human omental as compared with subcutaneous preadipocytes. Diabetes 2002; 51(7): 2029-36.
[http://dx.doi.org/10.2337/diabetes.51.7.2029] [PMID: 12086930]

[93] Bertin E, Nguyen P, Guenounou M, Durlach V, Potron G, Leutenegger M. Plasma levels of tumor necrosis factor-alpha (TNF-alpha) are essentially dependent on visceral fat amount in type 2 diabetic patients. Diabetes Metab 2000; 26(3): 178-82.
[PMID: 10880890]

[94] Alessi MC, Peiretti F, Morange P, Henry M, Nalbone G, Juhan-Vague I. Production of plasminogen activator inhibitor 1 by human adipose tissue: possible link between visceral fat accumulation and vascular disease. Diabetes 1997; 46(5): 860-7.
[http://dx.doi.org/10.2337/diab.46.5.860] [PMID: 9133556]

[94] You T, Nicklas BJ, Ding J, *et al.* The metabolic syndrome is associated with circulating adipokines in older adults across a wide range of adiposity. J Gerontol A Biol Sci Med Sci 2008; 63(4): 414-9.
[http://dx.doi.org/10.1093/gerona/63.4.414] [PMID: 18426966]

[96] Cnop M, Havel PJ, Utzschneider KM, *et al.* Relationship of adiponectin to body fat distribution, insulin sensitivity and plasma lipoproteins: evidence for independent roles of age and sex. Diabetologia 2003; 46(4): 459-69.
[http://dx.doi.org/10.1007/s00125-003-1074-z] [PMID: 12687327]

[97] Tarantino G, Pizza G, Colao A, *et al.* Hepatic steatosis in overweight/obese females: new screening method for those at risk. World J Gastroenterol 2009; 15(45): 5693-9.
[http://dx.doi.org/10.3748/wjg.15.5693] [PMID: 19960566]

[98] Bahceci M, Gokalp D, Bahceci S, Tuzcu A, Atmaca S, Arikan S. The correlation between adiposity and adiponectin, tumor necrosis factor alpha, interleukin-6 and high sensitivity C-reactive protein levels. Is adipocyte size associated with inflammation in adults? J Endocrinol Invest 2007; 30(3): 210-4.
[http://dx.doi.org/10.1007/BF03347427] [PMID: 17505154]

[99] Monteiro R, de Castro PMST, Calhau C, Azevedo I. Adipocyte size and liability to cell death. Obes Surg 2006; 16(6): 804-6.
[http://dx.doi.org/10.1381/096089206777346600] [PMID: 16756747]

[100] Cinti S, Mitchell G, Barbatelli G, *et al.* Adipocyte death defines macrophage localization and function in adipose tissue of obese mice and humans. J Lipid Res 2005; 46(11): 2347-55.
[http://dx.doi.org/10.1194/jlr.M500294-JLR200] [PMID: 16150820]

[101] Cobb WS, Burns JM, Kercher KW, Matthews BD, James Norton H, Todd Heniford B. Normal intraabdominal pressure in healthy adults. J Surg Res 2005; 129(2): 231-5.
[http://dx.doi.org/10.1016/j.jss.2005.06.015] [PMID: 16140336]

[102] Monteiro R, Calhau C, Azevedo I. Obstructive sleep apnoea and adipocyte death. Eur J Heart Fail 2007; 9(1): 103-4.
[http://dx.doi.org/10.1016/j.ejheart.2006.10.010] [PMID: 17137838]

[103] Lambert DM, Marceau S, Forse RA. Intra-abdominal pressure in the morbidly obese. Obes Surg 2005;

15(9): 1225-32.
[http://dx.doi.org/10.1381/096089205774512546] [PMID: 16259876]

[104] Tchoukalova Y, Koutsari C, Jensen M. Committed subcutaneous preadipocytes are reduced in human obesity. Diabetologia 2007; 50(1): 151-7.
[http://dx.doi.org/10.1007/s00125-006-0496-9] [PMID: 17096115]

[105] Monteiro R, Calhau C, Azevedo I. Comment on: Tchoukalova Y, Koutsari C, Jensen M (2007) Committed subcutaneous preadipocytes are reduced in human obesity. Diabetologia 50:151-157. Diabetologia 2007; 50(7): 1569.
[http://dx.doi.org/10.1007/s00125-007-0636-x] [PMID: 17356839]

[106] Hausman GJ, Richardson RL. Adipose tissue angiogenesis. J Anim Sci 2004; 82(3): 925-34.
[http://dx.doi.org/10.2527/2004.823925x] [PMID: 15032451]

[107] Wang B, Wood IS, Trayhurn P. Hypoxia induces leptin gene expression and secretion in human preadipocytes: differential effects of hypoxia on adipokine expression by preadipocytes. J Endocrinol 2008; 198(1): 127-34.
[http://dx.doi.org/10.1677/JOE-08-0156] [PMID: 18463145]

[108] Wood IS, de Heredia FP, Wang B, Trayhurn P. Cellular hypoxia and adipose tissue dysfunction in obesity. Proc Nutr Soc 2009; 68(4): 370-7.
[http://dx.doi.org/10.1017/S0029665109990206] [PMID: 19698203]

[109] Hosogai N, Fukuhara A, Oshima K, *et al.* Adipose tissue hypoxia in obesity and its impact on adipocytokine dysregulation. Diabetes 2007; 56(4): 901-11.
[http://dx.doi.org/10.2337/db06-0911] [PMID: 17395738]

[110] Negrão MR, Monteiro R, Calhau C, Soares R, Azevedo I. Comment on: Hosogai et al. (2007) Adipose tissue hypoxia in obesity and its impact on adipocytokine dysregulation. Diabetes 56:901-911, 2007. Diabetes 2008; 57(11)e15
[http://dx.doi.org/10.2337/db08-0603] [PMID: 18971432]

[111] Gunderson EP, Sternfeld B, Wellons MF, *et al.* Childbearing may increase visceral adipose tissue independent of overall increase in body fat. Obesity (Silver Spring) 2008; 16(5): 1078-84.
[http://dx.doi.org/10.1038/oby.2008.40] [PMID: 18356843]

[112] Monteiro R, Keating E, Castro P, Azevedo I. Abdominal cavity compliance: a participant more in the building up of visceral obesity. Obesity (Silver Spring) 2009; 17(5): 937.
[http://dx.doi.org/10.1038/oby.2009.34] [PMID: 19396079]

[113] Ingram KH, Hunter GR, James JF, Gower BA. Central fat accretion and insulin sensitivity: differential relationships in parous and nulliparous women. Int J Obes 2017; 41(8): 1214-7.
[http://dx.doi.org/10.1038/ijo.2017.104] [PMID: 28465610]

[114] Chanson P, Salenave S. Metabolic syndrome in Cushing's syndrome. Neuroendocrinology 2010; 92 (Suppl. 1): 96-101.
[http://dx.doi.org/10.1159/000314272] [PMID: 20829627]

[115] Jackson SE, Kirschbaum C, Steptoe A. Hair cortisol and adiposity in a population-based sample of 2,527 men and women aged 54 to 87 years. Obesity (Silver Spring) 2017; 25(3): 539-44.
[http://dx.doi.org/10.1002/oby.21733] [PMID: 28229550]

[116] Yener S, Baris M, Peker A, Demir O, Ozgen B, Secil M. Autonomous cortisol secretion in adrenal incidentalomas and increased visceral fat accumulation during follow-up. Clin Endocrinol (Oxf) 2017; 87(5): 425-32.
[http://dx.doi.org/10.1111/cen.13408] [PMID: 28656620]

[117] Incollingo Rodriguez AC, Epel ES, White ML, Standen EC, Seckl JR, Tomiyama AJ. Hypothalamic-pituitary-adrenal axis dysregulation and cortisol activity in obesity: A systematic review. Psychoneuroendocrinology 2015; 62: 301-18.
[http://dx.doi.org/10.1016/j.psyneuen.2015.08.014] [PMID: 26356039]

[118] Cansu GB, Atılgan S, Balcı MK, Sarı R, Özdem S, Altunbaş HA. Which type 2 diabetes mellitus patients should be screened for subclinical Cushing's syndrome? Hormones (Athens) 2017; 16(1): 22-32.
[PMID: 28500825]

[119] Newell-Price J, Bertagna X, Grossman AB, Nieman LK. Cushing's syndrome. Lancet 2006; 367(9522): 1605-17.
[http://dx.doi.org/10.1016/S0140-6736(06)68699-6] [PMID: 16698415]

[120] Findling JW, Raff H. DIAGNOSIS OF ENDOCRINE DISEASE: Differentiation of pathologic/neoplastic hypercortisolism (Cushing's syndrome) from physiologic/non-neoplastic hypercortisolism (formerly known as pseudo-Cushing's syndrome). Eur J Endocrinol 2017; 176(5): R205-16.
[http://dx.doi.org/10.1530/EJE-16-0946] [PMID: 28179447]

[121] Loriaux DL. Diagnosis and Differential Diagnosis of Cushing's Syndrome. N Engl J Med 2017; 376(15): 1451-9.
[http://dx.doi.org/10.1056/NEJMra1505550] [PMID: 28402781]

[122] Young EA, Abelson J, Lightman SL. Cortisol pulsatility and its role in stress regulation and health. Front Neuroendocrinol 2004; 25(2): 69-76.
[http://dx.doi.org/10.1016/j.yfrne.2004.07.001] [PMID: 15571755]

[123] Qiao S, Li X, Zilioli S, et al. Hair Measurements of Cortisol, DHEA, and DHEA to Cortisol Ratio as Biomarkers of Chronic Stress among People Living with HIV in China: Known-Group Validation. PLoS One 2017; 12(1)e0169827
[http://dx.doi.org/10.1371/journal.pone.0169827] [PMID: 28095431]

[124] Björntorp P, Holm G, Rosmond R. Hypothalamic arousal, insulin resistance and Type 2 diabetes mellitus. Diabet Med 1999; 16(5): 373-83.
[http://dx.doi.org/10.1046/j.1464-5491.1999.00067.x] [PMID: 10342336]

[125] Matthews K, Schwartz J, Cohen S, Seeman T. Diurnal cortisol decline is related to coronary calcification: CARDIA study. Psychosom Med 2006; 68(5): 657-61.
[http://dx.doi.org/10.1097/01.psy.0000244071.42939.0e] [PMID: 17012518]

[126] Bergmann N, Gyntelberg F, Faber J. The appraisal of chronic stress and the development of the metabolic syndrome: a systematic review of prospective cohort studies. Endocr Connect 2014; 3(2): R55-80.
[http://dx.doi.org/10.1530/EC-14-0031] [PMID: 24743684]

[127] Bergmann N, Ballegaard S, Krogh J, et al. Chronic psychological stress seems associated with elements of the metabolic syndrome in patients with ischaemic heart disease. Scand J Clin Lab Invest 2017; 77(7): 513-9.
[http://dx.doi.org/10.1080/00365513.2017.1354254] [PMID: 28727492]

[128] Sanghez V, Razzoli M, Carobbio S, et al. Psychosocial stress induces hyperphagia and exacerbates diet-induced insulin resistance and the manifestations of the Metabolic Syndrome. Psychoneuroendocrinology 2013; 38(12): 2933-42.
[http://dx.doi.org/10.1016/j.psyneuen.2013.07.022] [PMID: 24060458]

[129] Mason JI, Rainey WE. Steroidogenesis in the human fetal adrenal: a role for cholesterol synthesized de novo. J Clin Endocrinol Metab 1987; 64(1): 140-7.
[http://dx.doi.org/10.1210/jcem-64-1-140] [PMID: 3023427]

[130] Menzies RI, Zhao X, Mullins LJ, et al. Transcription controls growth, cell kinetics and cholesterol supply to sustain ACTH responses. Endocr Connect 2017; 6(7): 446-57.
[http://dx.doi.org/10.1530/EC-17-0092] [PMID: 28720595]

[131] Drewnowski A, Rehm CD, Solet D. Disparities in obesity rates: analysis by ZIP code area. Soc Sci Med 2007; 65(12): 2458-63.

[http://dx.doi.org/10.1016/j.socscimed.2007.07.001] [PMID: 17761378]

[132] Chetty R, Stepner M, Abraham S, *et al.* The Association Between Income and Life Expectancy in the United States, 2001-2014. JAMA 2016; 315(16): 1750-66.
[http://dx.doi.org/10.1001/jama.2016.4226] [PMID: 27063997]

[133] Villermé L. De la mortalité dans les divers quartiers de la ville de Paris, et des causes qui la rendent très différente dans plusiers d'entre eux, ansi que les divers quartiers de beaucoup de grandes villes. Annales d'Hygiène Publique et de Médecine Légale 1830; 3: 294-341.

[134] Engels F. Die Lage der arbeitenden Klasse in England. Leipzig: Wigand 1887.

[135] Virchow R, Ed. Mittheilungen über die in Oberschlesien herrschenden Typhus-Epidemie. Berlin: Reiner 1848.
[http://dx.doi.org/10.1515/9783111683898]

[136] Deaton A. On Death and Money: History, Facts, and Explanations. JAMA 2016; 315(16): 1703-5.
[http://dx.doi.org/10.1001/jama.2016.4072] [PMID: 27063421]

[137] Marmot M, Wilkinson RG, Eds. Social determinants of health. 2nd ed., Oxford: University Press 2006.

[138] Frieden TR. SHATTUCK LECTURE: The Future of Public Health. N Engl J Med 2015; 373(18): 1748-54.
[http://dx.doi.org/10.1056/NEJMsa1511248] [PMID: 26510022]

[139] Marmot MG, Smith GD, Stansfeld S, *et al.* Health inequalities among British civil servants: the Whitehall II study. Lancet 1991; 337(8754): 1387-93.
[http://dx.doi.org/10.1016/0140-6736(91)93068-K] [PMID: 1674771]

[140] Marmot MG, Bosma H, Hemingway H, Brunner E, Stansfeld S. Contribution of job control and other risk factors to social variations in coronary heart disease incidence. Lancet 1997; 350(9073): 235-9.
[http://dx.doi.org/10.1016/S0140-6736(97)04244-X] [PMID: 9242799]

[141] Seeman M, Stein Merkin S, Karlamangla A, Koretz B, Seeman T. Social status and biological dysregulation: the "status syndrome" and allostatic load. Soc Sci Med 2014; 118: 143-51.
[http://dx.doi.org/10.1016/j.socscimed.2014.08.002] [PMID: 25112569]

[142] Daly M, Boyce C, Wood A. A social rank explanation of how money influences health. Health Psychol 2015; 34(3): 222-30.
[http://dx.doi.org/10.1037/hea0000098] [PMID: 25133843]

[143] Snyder-Mackler N, Sanz J, Kohn JN, *et al.* Social status alters immune regulation and response to infection in macaques. Science 2016; 354(6315): 1041-5.
[http://dx.doi.org/10.1126/science.aah3580] [PMID: 27885030]

[144] Sapolsky RM. Proinflammatory primates. Science 2016; 354(6315): 967-8.
[http://dx.doi.org/10.1126/science.aal3170] [PMID: 27884990]

[145] García AR, Gurven M, Blackwell AD. A matter of perception: Perceived socio-economic status and cortisol on the island of Utila, Honduras. Am J Hum Biol 2017; 29(5)
[http://dx.doi.org/10.1002/ajhb.23031] [PMID: 28667791]

[146] O'Brien KM, Meyer J, Tronick E, Moore CL. Hair cortisol and lifetime discrimination: Moderation by subjective social status. Health Psychol Open 2017; 4(1)2055102917695176
[http://dx.doi.org/10.1177/2055102917695176] [PMID: 28491342]

[147] De Bucy C, Guignat L, Niati T, Bertherat J, Coste J. Health-related quality of life of patients with hypothalamic-pituitary-adrenal axis dysregulations: a cohort study. Eur J Endocrinol 2017; 177(1): 1-8.
[http://dx.doi.org/10.1530/EJE-17-0048] [PMID: 28404594]

[148] Block JP, He Y, Zaslavsky AM, Ding L, Ayanian JZ. Psychosocial stress and change in weight among US adults. Am J Epidemiol 2009; 170(2): 181-92.

[http://dx.doi.org/10.1093/aje/kwp104] [PMID: 19465744]

[149] Udo T, Grilo CM, McKee SA. Gender differences in the impact of stressful life events on changes in body mass index. Prev Med 2014; 69: 49-53.
[http://dx.doi.org/10.1016/j.ypmed.2014.08.036] [PMID: 25204986]

[150] Wardle J, Chida Y, Gibson EL, Whitaker KL, Steptoe A. Stress and adiposity: a meta-analysis of longitudinal studies. Obesity (Silver Spring) 2011; 19(4): 771-8.
[http://dx.doi.org/10.1038/oby.2010.241] [PMID: 20948519]

[151] Kubzansky LD, Bordelois P, Jun HJ, et al. The weight of traumatic stress: a prospective study of posttraumatic stress disorder symptoms and weight status in women. JAMA Psychiatry 2014; 71(1): 44-51.
[http://dx.doi.org/10.1001/jamapsychiatry.2013.2798] [PMID: 24258147]

[152] Andersen SL. Exposure to early adversity: Points of cross-species translation that can lead to improved understanding of depression. Dev Psychopathol 2015; 27(2): 477-91.
[http://dx.doi.org/10.1017/S0954579415000103] [PMID: 25997766]

[153] Chopra KK, Ravindran A, Kennedy SH, et al. Sex differences in hormonal responses to a social stressor in chronic major depression. Psychoneuroendocrinology 2009; 34(8): 1235-41.
[http://dx.doi.org/10.1016/j.psyneuen.2009.03.014] [PMID: 19386421]

[154] Sanghez V, Cubuk C, Sebastián-Leon P, et al. Chronic subordination stress selectively downregulates the insulin signaling pathway in liver and skeletal muscle but not in adipose tissue of male mice. Stress 2016; 19(2): 214-24.
[http://dx.doi.org/10.3109/10253890.2016.1151491] [PMID: 26946982]

[155] Blane D. The life course, the social gradient, and health.Social determinants of health. 2nd ed. Oxford: University Press 2006; pp. 54-77.

[156] Shaw M, Dorling D, Smith GD. Poverty, social exclusion, and minorities.Social determinants of health. 2nd ed. Oxford: University Press 2006; pp. 196-223.

[157] Seeman TE, Singer B, Wilkinson CW, McEwen B. Gender differences in age-related changes in HPA axis reactivity. Psychoneuroendocrinology 2001; 26(3): 225-40.
[http://dx.doi.org/10.1016/S0306-4530(00)00043-3] [PMID: 11166486]

[158] Lanas F, Bazzano L, Rubinstein A, et al. Prevalence, Distributions and Determinants of Obesity and Central Obesity in the Southern Cone of America. PLoS One 2016; 11(10)e0163727
[http://dx.doi.org/10.1371/journal.pone.0163727] [PMID: 27741247]

[159] Pradhan AD. Sex differences in the metabolic syndrome: implications for cardiovascular health in women. Clin Chem 2014; 60(1): 44-52.
[http://dx.doi.org/10.1373/clinchem.2013.202549] [PMID: 24255079]

[160] Murphy MO, Loria AS. Sex-specific effects of stress on metabolic and cardiovascular disease: are women at higher risk? Am J Physiol Regul Integr Comp Physiol 2017; 313(1): R1-9.
[http://dx.doi.org/10.1152/ajpregu.00185.2016] [PMID: 28468942]

[161] Möller-Leimkühler AM. Higher comorbidity of depression and cardiovascular disease in women: a biopsychosocial perspective. World J Biol Psychiatry 2010; 11(8): 922-33.
[http://dx.doi.org/10.3109/15622975.2010.523481] [PMID: 20950120]

[162] Zipursky RT, Press MC, Srikanthan P, et al. Relation of Stress Hormones (Urinary Catecholamines/Cortisol) to Coronary Artery Calcium in Men *Versus* Women (from the Multi-Ethnic Study of Atherosclerosis [MESA]). Am J Cardiol 2017; 119(12): 1963-71.
[http://dx.doi.org/10.1016/j.amjcard.2017.03.025] [PMID: 28456316]

[163] Ziaei S, Frith AL, Ekström EC, Naved RT. Experiencing Lifetime Domestic Violence: Associations with Mental Health and Stress among Pregnant Women in Rural Bangladesh: The MINIMat Randomized Trial. PLoS One 2016; 11(12)e0168103
[http://dx.doi.org/10.1371/journal.pone.0168103] [PMID: 27992478]

[164]   Jaffe A, Giveon S, Wulffhart L, *et al.* Adult Arabs have higher risk for diabetes mellitus than Jews in Israel. PLoS One 2017; 12(5)e0176661
[http://dx.doi.org/10.1371/journal.pone.0176661] [PMID: 28481942]

[165]   Oh S, Tanaka K, Noh JW, *et al.* Abdominal obesity: causal factor or simply a symptom of obesity-related health risk. Diabetes Metab Syndr Obes 2014; 7: 289-96.
[http://dx.doi.org/10.2147/DMSO.S64546] [PMID: 25050072]

[166]   Mackenbach JP. Politics is nothing but medicine at a larger scale: reflections on public health's biggest idea. J Epidemiol Community Health 2009; 63(3): 181-4.
[http://dx.doi.org/10.1136/jech.2008.077032] [PMID: 19052033]

CHAPTER 16

Breaking the Borders Between Obesity and Cancer

Pedro Coelho[1,2], **Raquel Costa**[1,2], **Susana G. Guerreiro**[1,2], **Raquel Soares**[1,2] and **Sara Andrade**[1,2,3,*]

[1] *Department of Biomedicine, Biochemistry Unit, Faculty of Medicine, University of Porto, Porto, Portugal*

[2] *i3S - Instituto de Investigação e Inovação em Saúde, University of Porto, Porto, Portugal*

[3] *Endocrine, Cardiovascular & Metabolic Research, Department of Anatomy, Multidisciplinary Unit for Biomedical Research (UMIB), ICBAS, University of Porto, Porto, Portugal*

Abstract: More than one decade ago, the International Association of Research on Cancer reported that obesity increases the risk in the development of several cancers. With the increasing epidemic rates that we face today, obesity is a major risk for cancer development. In fact, despite the increasing awareness of the public to cancer risk factors, the prevalence of several types of cancer remains high. Nevertheless, the mechanisms behind this association are not clear. Clinical and preclinical evidence indicate that obesity stands together with disturbed metabolism, insulin resistance, oxidative stress, chronic inflammation, abnormal presence of adipokines, growth factors and hormones, enhanced tissue fibrosis and imbalanced angiogenesis. Accordingly, obesity promotes a proinflammatory phenotype, characterized by a switch in M2 to M1 macrophages and exacerbated cytokine release, increased circulating levels of glucose, free fatty acids and hormones (namely insulin or leptin) and reduced circulating levels of adiponectin. All these features are often observed in neoplasia, suggesting a strong link between these two pathological conditions. This chapter highlights these putative mechanisms underlying the obesity-cancer interplay. We will tackle the processes that are imbalanced in obesity and can affect cancer development and progression, both at a systemic level as well as at local tumor environment. Identifying the features that characterize the obesity-associated cancer is mandatory for developing novel therapeutic strategies, which will definitely enhance quality of life and survival of these patients and reduce the concomitant economic burden of national healthcare systems.

Keywords: Adipocytokines, Adiposity, AMPK signaling, Angiogenesis, Cancer, Carbohydrate and lipid metabolism, Chemotherapy, Desmoplasia, Fibrosis, Glycemia, Host neighboring cell metabolism, Inflammation, Metabolic improvement therapeutic strategies, Metabolic organs adaptation, Oncology,

---

* **Corresponding author Sara Andrade:** Department of Biomedicine, Biochemistry Unit, Faculty of Medicine, University of Porto, Alameda Professor Hernâni Monteiro, 4200-319 Porto, Portugal; Tel/Fax: +351 225513624; E-mail: sandrade@med.up.pt

Rosário Monteiro and Maria João Martins (Eds.)
All rights reserved-© 2020 Bentham Science Publishers

Oxidative stress, Radiotherapy, Tumor metabolism, VEGF signaling.

INTRODUCTION

Obesity is defined by the World Health Organization (WHO) as an excessive accumulation of adipose tissue that may impair health. It results from the imbalance between caloric intake and energy expenditure, and is a consequence of the industrialization of the modern world, with increased availability of highly processed, calorie-dense foods and an overall decrease in physical activity due to a more sedentary work environment [1].

The WHO estimates that in 2014, 1.9 billion of the global adult population were overweight and, of these, 600 million were obese. A study by Ng *et al* showed that, between 1980 and 2013, the prevalence of overweight and obesity among men rose from 28.8% to 36.9%, and from 29.8% to 38.0% for women. Amongst children and adolescents, obesity is also increasing at an alarming rate [2].

Body mass index (BMI) is the most common way to access and define overweight and obesity: a patient with a BMI value below 24.9 kg/m^2 is considered normal weight, between 25.0 and 29.9 kg/m^2 is considered overweight and above 30.0 kg/m^2 is considered obese [1]. Although it is widely established, there are some concerns regarding the use of BMI especially because it fails to give information regarding the body composition and the local distribution of fat [3].

Adipose tissue (AT) may behave differently depending on its localization and on the type of adipocytes present. AT can be divided into white adipose tissue (WAT), which is involved in fat storage, and brown adipose tissue (BAT), playing a role in thermogenesis. Furthermore, the ability of some white adipocytes to turn into a brown adipocyte phenotype ("browning") has been reported [4]. These adipocytes have been named "beige" or "brite" and, like brown adipocytes, have the ability to dissipate energy as heat [5]. WAT, *per se*, has been historically considered as a mere deposit of energy in the form of lipid accumulation in adipocytes. However, it is now widely accepted that WAT is an endocrine organ, secreting a number of important molecules with different functions, such as hormones and cytokines, that are generally named adipokines [6]. With the development of overweight and obesity, AT becomes dysregulated. The chronic low-grade inflammatory state that is associated with obesity, and the consequent increase in oxidative stress of the patients, may be key factors in the development of obesity-related comorbidities.

There are several WAT depots, that differ not only in localization within the body, but that have different metabolic profiles. For instance, the visceral WAT depot (vWAT) is highly innervated and vascularized, and presents a higher infiltration of immune cells with increased production of proinflammatory cytokines than the subcutaneous depot (scWAT). While scWAT absorbs circulating free fatty acids (FFA) for storage, in the form of triglycerides, vWAT has a higher capacity to generate FFA [7]. In general, it is commonly accepted that the vWAT is more metabolically-active than the scWAT and is, thus, highly associated with metabolic disturbances and metabolic syndrome, being regarded as the main culprit behind the obesity-associated comorbidities [7].

Given its huge incidence worldwide, obesity is considered an increasing global health problem. It is widely recognized that overweight and obesity are frequently associated with several comorbidities, such as type 2 diabetes *mellitus* (T2DM), cardiovascular diseases and numerous types of cancer [8, 9], with severe personal and financial costs for the patients and the national health systems [10].

A few decades ago, the International Association of Research in Cancer reported that the development risk of a few neoplasms was related to BMI [11]. Today, the list of neoplasia that are influenced by BMI has increased dramatically [9].

A hypoxic, inflammatory and oxidative tumor environment persists in obese patients. This cluster of systemic conditions renders tumor and host neighboring cells to be more aggressive. Tumors from either obese patients or obesity animal models present increased number and size of adipocytes [12, 13]. Moreover, these conditions affect metabolic cues within tumor cells as well as host neighboring cells.

The main aim of this chapter is to focus on the epidemiological and experimental evidence that sustain a relationship between obesity and cancer, and to review the pathological mechanisms that are more likely to be responsible by this association.

EPIDEMIOLOGICAL AND EXPERIMENTAL EVIDENCE OF OBESITY-CANCER ASSOCIATION

Several epidemiological and experimental studies point towards a strong relationship between obesity and the development and progression of various types of cancer [9]. In fact, it was recently estimated that 3.6% of the total new-cancer cases diagnosed in 2012 were attributable to a high BMI. Furthermore, if the prevalence of obesity had not changed from the one recorded in 1982, one quarter of these new cancer cases could have been avoided [14].

Not all cancers are associated with obesity, and the relative risks of those which are, are not identical. Nonetheless the number of cancers that are confirmed to be associated with adiposity is increasing. It is now accepted that not only the cancers of the esophagus, colon and rectum, breast (postmenopausal), *corpus uteri* and kidney, but also, cancers of the gastric cardia, liver, gallbladder, pancreas, ovary, thyroid, meningioma and multiple myeloma are highly associated with obesity [9]. This number may be increasing with all the current research interest in this area.

Numerous experimental studies and meta-analysis have focused on the association of obesity and cancer. We will review the most important mechanisms that were proposed to act as potential mediators between these pathologies.

PATHOLOGICAL CONDITIONS INVOLVED IN THIS ASSOCIATION

Hormone Disturbances as Links between Obesity and Cancer

Nowadays, AT is considered an endocrine organ due to the production of multiple bioactive molecules. These adipose-derived secreted factors can exert effects at both local and systemic levels. The great majority of these factors are cytokines, chemokines and inflammatory mediators, some with a role in growth regulation as a new aspect of adipokines has been revealed by novel adipocyte-released molecules [15]. Deregulated production or secretion of these adipokines, caused by excess adiposity and AT dysfunction, has been linked to the pathogenesis of various obesity-linked diseases, including cancer [16, 17].

A number of biological changes associated with obesity have been identified as predictors of a poor prognosis in cancer patients, including hyperinsulinemia, insulin resistance [18, 19] and increased insulin-like growth factor 1 (IGF1) activity, changes in the production of adipokines, including increased circulating levels of leptin [20, 21] and resistin [21] and decreased circulating levels of adiponectin [18, 22]. Leptin and resistin secreted by fat tissue serve as angiogenic and mitogenic factors in many malignancies, including colorectal carcinoma, endometrial cancer and melanoma tumor growth and metastasis [20, 21, 23 - 26], while adiponectin exerts primordially antiproliferative and antiinflammatory effects [19, 27].

By binding to its receptor, leptin activates mitogen-activated protein kinase (MAPK), Phosphatidylinositol-3 kinase (PI3K) and signal transducer and activator of transcription (STAT) signaling pathways that culminate in cell proliferation and survival [28]. Thus, leptin is one potential molecule linking obesity to cancer. Recently, it has also been reported that the presence of leptin may play a particularly important role in immune dysregulation, as many immune cells express the leptin receptor. Accordingly, high circulating levels of leptin present in obese patients, impede the differentiation of T cells into regulatory T-cells and also decrease natural-killer (NK) cells activity [29]. Conversely, systemic levels of adiponectin inversely correlate with development risk of pre- and postmenopausal breast, endometrial and pancreatic cancers [30 - 32], suggesting a protective role of this hormone in cancer. Remarkably, obese patients usually present decreased adiponectin plasma levels being, therefore, predisposed to develop certain types of cancers. Although the mechanisms by which adiponectin protects against cancer development are not completely described, one possible explanation lies in the activation of the energy metabolic regulator, AMP-activated protein kinase (AMPK), since adiponectin receptors activation results in AMPK increased activity. Moreover, adiponectin also reduces reactive oxygen species (ROS) production, thus, leading to cell growth inhibition.

Interestingly, AT is a major source of endocrine activity. Visfatin and resistin are usually upregulated in visceral WAT depot. Visfatin has been reported to be overexpressed in obese patients with breast, colon, stomach and endometrial cancers. Resistin plays a proinflammatory role, being recently associated with poor prognosis in lung cancer patients [33]. The role of these hormones in cancer risk and prognosis render them putative preventive and therapeutic cancer agents in obese patients [34]. Nevertheless, more studies addressing the molecular mechanisms of these adipokines are essential.

Adiposity also influences the synthesis and bioavailability of a variety of steroid sex hormones, namely estrogen which is associated with estrogen-dependent breast cancer risk. Obesity is a risk factor for postmenopausal breast cancer. This association can be explained by the significant expression of aromatase by adipocytes, an enzyme converting adrenal androgens into estrogens [35].

In addition, higher levels of circulating insulin and IGF1 inhibit the synthesis of sex hormone-binding globulin, a protein involved in estrogen and testosterone transport in bloodstream. Deficiency of this protein, prevents hormone removal, resulting in increased estrogen bioactivity [36]. Higher expression and activity of aromatase were recently observed in undifferentiated fibroblasts, rather than mature adipocytes in breast AT [37], indicating a strong link between estrogen synthesis and fibrotic reaction, preventing hence tumor vascularization and concomitant efficient drug therapeutic delivery.

Moreover, estrogens play anti- or proinflammatory roles depending, among other reasons, on immune stimulus and on the type of estrogen receptor present in the tumor microenvironment [38, 39]. In breast cancer, estrogen receptor beta (ERβ) expression is correlated with improved therapy response and survival. On the other hand, estrogen receptor alpha (ERα) is correlated with poor prognostic and survival. *In vitro* studies reveal that obesity suppresses ERβ expression in breast cancer cells, *via* a human epidermal growth factor receptor 2 (HER2)-mediated pathway leading to poor prognosis [40]. Taking these findings into account, besides estrogen circulating levels, the local source of these hormones within tumor microenvironmental cells, particularly the presence of fibroblasts and adipocytes, plays a crucial role in breast cancer development, progression and therapy [40].

Insulin and Growth Factors

Obesity often clusters with glucose intolerance, insulin resistance and dyslipidemia [10]. Serum insulin and IGF1 are thus raised in obese people as compared to healthy lean individuals, and have been reported to increase the risk of certain types of cancer [41]. In fact, patients with cancer that have pre-existing T2DM have worse prognosis and have higher mortality rates than normoglycemic ones [42]. The mechanisms by which those molecules affect cancer are yet undetermined. However, a crosstalk between insulin and IGF1 and PI3K/ mammalian target of rapamycin (mTOR) and rat sarcoma (Ras) signaling pathways, two transduction pathways often implicated in cancer cells, was established [43], explaining their effects in inhibiting apoptosis and stimulating tumor proliferation [44]. The fact that insulin and IGF1 are overexpressed in obesity, lead us to assume that obese patients are much more predisposed to develop more aggressive tumors than lean subjects [45].

Increased circulating insulin levels will activate mitogenic pathways through its binding to its receptor (IR) and to insulin and IGF1 hybrid receptors (IR/IGF1R). The binding of the hormone to these receptors in cancer cells will eventually activate MAPK and the PI3K/protein kinase B (PKB or Akt) oncogenic pathway [46]. On the other hand, high levels of circulating insulin may also have an indirect effect in the development of cancer, through increasing IGF1, an important growth factor in cancer, that has a role regulating cellular growth and the survival of transformed cells [47] and decreasing IGF-binding proteins (IGFBPs) [48]. In fact, it is thought that the mitogenic effects of insulin are mediated by IGF1, since it is the activation of IGF1R that stimulates cell growth and proliferation.

Additionally, endocrine-mediated consequences of obesity also result in increased circulating levels of several other adipose-secreted growth factors, angiogenic modulators and inflammatory mediators. Elevated circulating levels of epidermal growth factor (EGF), transforming growth factor beta (TGFβ), hepatocyte growth factor (HGF), fibroblast growth factor 1, 2 and 21 (FGF1, FGF2 and FGF21) and platelet-derived growth factor (PDGF) have been reported in obese individuals. Adipocytes secrete numerous proangiogenic modulators including vascular endothelial growth factor (VEGF), FGF2, HGF, tumor necrosis factor alpha and beta (TNFα and TNFβ), interleukin 1 beta, 6 and 8 (IL1β, IL6 and IL8), placental growth factor (PlGF), PDGF, visfatin, resistin, neuropeptide Y, leptin and angiopoietins, as well as antiangiogenic factors thrombospondin-1, plasminogen activator inhibitor 1 (PAI1) and adiponectin, whose expression balance will determine the triggering or halting of the angiogenic switch [49 - 52]. In addition to adipocytes, AT contains diverse cell types including adipose stromal cells (ASCs) and adipose tissue macrophages (ATMs) that further contribute to angiogenesis. ASCs produce a pleiade of angiogenic factors [VEGF, HGF, granulocyte-macrophage colony-stimulating factor (GM-CSF), FGF2 and TGFβ] [53, 54], while macrophages release VEGF and the angiogenic cytokines TNFα, FGF2, IL1β, IL6 and IL8 [55]. Matrix metalloproteinases (MMPs) 2 and 9 (MMP2 and MMP9) are secreted by AT, and potentially affect preadipocyte differentiation and microvessel maturation by modulating the extracellular matrix (ECM). Moreover, MMPs release the matrix-bound VEGF and indirectly induce angiogenesis [54]. ATMs also produce an overlapping collection of cytokines, such as TNFα, IL1β, IL6, IL8, monocyte chemotactic protein 1 (MCP1) and TGFβ [55, 56].

The accumulation of adipose-derived secreted factors mentioned above can induce signal transduction upon binding to the respective receptors located on the cell surface. Overexpression of numerous G-protein-coupled receptors and receptor tyrosine kinases has long been recognized to play central roles in the metastatic phenotype of numerous malignancies [57, 58]. This in turn leads to the activation of their downstream signaling cascades, most of them converging at the PI3K/AKT and MAPK pathways. However, most malignancies already harbor constitutively activating mutations in MAPK and PI3K/AKT pathways and raise doubts about the magnitude of the effects of these adipose-derived factors in promoting carcinogenesis. However, these factors might have a greater impact in the remodeling of the tumor microenvironment. Adipose-derived angiogenic factors might be a source of premature angiogenic stimuli in the tumor microenvironment [59]. The induction of an early switch to the vascular phenotype contributes to the acceleration of tumor growth, accompanied by a deleterious impact in the disease metastatic onset in overweight individuals [60].

In summary, obesity-associated superfluous AT could be an important additional source of extracellular growth factors that provide paracrine stimulation and activation of intracellular pathways involved in proliferation, migration and invasion of tumor cells.

Oxidative Stress Promotes Cancer Development

As previously stated, obesity-derived dysregulated AT releases a panoply of molecules, such as hormones, proinflammatory cytokines, ROS and reactive nitrogen species (RNS). The excessive production of ROS, such as superoxide anions, peroxides and hydroxyl radicals, and RNS, such as nitric oxide and peroxynitrite, will imbalance the redox homeostasis and together with the depletion of antioxidant defenses will finally culminate in oxidative stress [61].

Central adiposity, in particular, is characterized by a general increase in systemic oxidative stress, in part through higher levels of ROS and RNS but also by a systemic depletion of antioxidant defenses [17, 62].

Oxidative stress, has long been recognized as an adverse event for promoting tumorigenesis and cancer progression [63, 64]. Exacerbated levels of ROS and RNS can irreversibly modify protein, lipid and DNA molecules, and permanently or temporarily change their cellular behavior, leading to the accumulation of somatic DNA mutations, activation of proto-oncogenes and induction of epigenetic alterations. Conversely, increased signaling via AKT, RAS/rapidly accelerated fibrosarcoma (RAF)/extracellular signal-regulated kinases (ERK) and nuclear factor kappa-light-chain-enhancer of activated B cells (NF-κB) pathways, constitutively activated signaling cascades in most malignant cells, stimulate endogenous ROS and RNS production, further enhancing oxidative damage within the tumor microenvironment [65, 66].

Furthermore, various types of cells present in the tumor microenvironment can generate not only ROS but also RNS. Tumor-associated macrophages are effective producers of ROS and RNS and further contribute to a prooxidant environment [67]. ROS and RNS produced from inflamed peritumoral AT and cancer-associated adipocytes also accelerate oxidative stress within tumor cells and might contribute to cancer progression in overweight patients [68].

In fact, oxidative stress has been proposed as a mechanistic link between obesity and cancer [69]. The increased oxidative burden in peritumoral AT, which is increased in the context of overweight and obesity, accelerate oxidative stress within the tumor milieu, further increasing oxidative damage to DNA, RNA, lipids and proteins, instigating carcinogenesis and sponsoring cancer progression in obese patients [70].

The Hypoxia-Angiogenesis-Inflammationo Axis

Obesity is characterized by a chronic low-grade inflammatory condition [71]. Generally, excessive lipid uptake by adipocytes results predominantly in adipocyte hypertrophy rather than an increase in the number of adipocytes. These enlarged adipocytes induce the recruitment of macrophage infiltration into AT, through the release of proinflammatory factors, such as IL1β, TNFα and MCP1.

Accordingly, obesity associates with M2 to M1 macrophage switch, a proinflammatory change. Interestingly, the AT inflammatory role varies depending on the origin of the fat depot, vWAT being the most predisposed one to inflammation by releasing a vast number of proinflammatory cytokines. Despite the presence of macrophages and other inflammatory cells is well established in AT, the reason why these cells are present it is not clear. One possible explanation lies in the fact that the vascular content of AT does not accompany adipogenesis within the same extent. A deficient vascular network results in hypoxia, and adipocytes immediately express hypoxia-induced transcription factor 1 alpha, HIF1α [72]. HIF1α, in turn, is responsible for the upregulation of angiogenic activators [VEGF, PDGF, nitric oxide synthase (NOS)] as well as of many proinflammatory cytokines, such as TNFα, MCP1 and IL1β [43, 72], leading to monocyte chemotaxis. Therefore, this hypoxia-angiogenesis-metainflammation alignment, which is initiated by the lipid metabolic disturbance in the first place, explains the proinflammatory environment that is concomitant with adiposity.

The fact that chronic inflammation can cause cancer is quite well established in many conditions. Reflux gastritis, virus-induced hepatitis and silicosis are some of the disorders that predispose to cancer [73]. Epidemiological studies also show that AT-associated inflammation is common in cancer patients, and often associates with poor prognosis and tumor aggressiveness [74 - 76]. Interestingly, it has been reported that the presence of crown-like structures, a hallmark of chronic inflammation, is considered a biomarker of increased breast cancer risk [77]. Inflammation causes mutagenesis, either directly or through exacerbated production of ROS by local macrophages and other host cells in tumor environment [78], supporting the assumption that a proinflammatory systemic and local environment favored by adiposity facilitates cancer risk.

The Metabolic-Vascular Hypothesis

Obesity is characterized by increased lipid deposition in AT but also in other organs, namely liver and skeletal muscle. These lipid accumulations are often associated and play a causative role in insulin resistance and metabolic disturbances that contributes to a variety of pathological conditions including T2DM, cardiovascular diseases and cancer [79].

The family of VEGFs comprises VEGF-A, VEGF-B, VEGF-C, VEGF-D and PlGF [80]. VEGF-A is the most potent angiogenic factor, and exerts its action through the activation of its main receptor, VEGFR2, and target proteins promoting vascularization [81, 82]. Hypoxia, inflammation and oxidative stress are among the principal angiogenic stimuli present in both obesity and cancer. In response to angiogenic stimuli, endothelial cells (ECs) proliferate and migrate to avascular areas. In this situation, ECs at the front of the migrating vessel rely on glycolysis to produce ATP for rapid generation of energy and sprouting [83]. The uptake of glucose by ECs is mediated through the activation of the PI3K/AKT pathway, promoting the expression of glucose transporters (GLUT), mainly GLUT1 [84]. It has been reported that the 6-phosphofructo-2-kinase/fructose-2,6-biphosphatase 3 (PFKFB3) enzyme expression is induced by hypoxia in avascular areas in several cell lines [85] and human cancer cells [86]. PFKFB3 is a bifunctional enzyme abundant in ECs, that plays an important role in ensuring the high glycolytic flux, essential for vessel growth [83]. Accordingly, PFKFB3 was found upregulated in organs where angiogenesis is exacerbated and downregulated whenever this process is impaired, such as in the heart of obese diabetic animals [82]. Recently, Schoors *et al* demonstrated the therapeutic potential of endothelial PFKFB3 regulation. PFKFB3 *in vitro* inhibition and PFKFB3 *in vivo* silencing induced a 30-40% decrease in the glycolytic pathway that was sufficient to reduce angiogenesis [87]. These data suggest that anti-angiogenic therapies could be based on the inhibition of this metabolic target, starving pathological vessels. Thus, PFKFB3 expression emerges as an important regulator of the endothelial phenotype, postulating that a metabolic switch induces the angiogenic switch and could be an important strategy to counteract the increased tumor vascularization.

Although belonging to the family of angiogenic factors, the signaling cascade triggered by the binding between VEGF-B and its receptor, VEGFR1, and co-receptor, neuropilin 1(NP1), has recently been associated with endothelial lipid transport and metabolism [88]. Recent research demonstrates the role of endothelium in regulating fatty acid transport and uptake into perivascular cells to be metabolized [88]. Hagberg *et al* revealed that the activation of VEGF-B/VEGFR1 pathway induces the expression of fatty acid transporter protein (FABP) 3 and FATP4, involved in the transendothelial transport of circulating FFA into tissues, such as skeletal muscle and heart, contributing to the ectopic lipid accumulation and obesity. Thus VEGF-B contributes to the lipotoxicity found in obesity. Moreover, VEGF-B is overexpressed in a variety of tumors. Mice deficient in VEGF-B showed reduced levels of fatty acid uptake and lipid accumulation in skeletal muscle, as well as in the heart and brown AT, compared to wild-type animals. A study conducted by Robciuc *et al* found improved glucose metabolism, insulin sensitivity and reduced inflammation in AT of *Vegfb*-transduced mice and in a *Vegfb* transgenic mouse model [89]. These findings suggest that targeting VEGF-B efficiently prevents lipid deposition in peripheral tissue.

Another important regulatory mechanism that mediates the transport of fatty acids across the cell membrane is the fatty acid translocase (FAT), also recognized as the scavenger receptor CD36 [90]. It is upregulated in several tissues, including liver and skeletal muscle of obese individuals, exacerbates dyslipidemia and lipotoxicity [91 - 93] and is considered as a promising therapeutic target to control lipid fluxes in the body [88, 94] and for the management of vascular derangements present in obesity and cancer.

Tumor Fibrosis - Impact on Therapeutics

The obesity-associated proinflammatory state results in immune cell infiltration, ECM remodeling and often fibrosis, three features that characterize the neoplastic tissue.

Obesity is associated with a worse prognosis in breast cancer and pancreatic ductal adenocarcinoma, among others [12, 95]. This is at least partially attributed to obesity-increased fibrosis since desmoplasia (the growth of fibrotic connective tissue surrounding tumors, with accumulation of ECM components such as collagen, fibronectin, elastin and hyaluronan) is present in tumors from obese patients [43, 95, 96].

This fibrotic tumor microenvironment is associated to poor prognostic, positively influencing tumor progression and invasion as well as hampering the efficacy of chemotherapy [12, 96, 97]. Different cell types contribute to the fibrosis stage tumor microenvironment, including fibroblasts, leucocytes (such as neutrophils, lymphocytes and macrophages) and adipocytes [43].

Increased deposition of WAT in the organs, as occurs in obesity, results in enhanced inflammation and self-interstitial fibrosis [98]. Moreover, AT hypertrophy and hyperplasia induce the release of a huge number of hormones (*e.g.* estrogens), growth factors (*e.g.* IGF1, TGFβ) and adipokines (*e.g.* adiponectin, leptin and IL6) that affect ECM dynamics, immunosurveillance and tumor cell proliferation and invasion [36, 43]. TGFβ plays a primordial role in fibrosis, being also a local immunosuppressor [78].

In obesity animal models, the levels of collagen VI are higher compared to non-obese animals; and when animals lack collagen VI, a reduction of interstitial fibrosis is observed [97, 99]. Importantly, a fragment of collagen VI, named endotrophin, associates with increased fibrosis, angiogenesis and inflammation in an animal model of breast cancer, and is held as a chemoresistance biomarker [97].

In fibrotic tumor stroma, the abnormal deposition of collagen and impairment in degradation of these proteins lead to decreased flexibility and increased stiffness and density of ECM, which lead to changes in mechanical forces and in cellular signaling, facilitating survival and migration of the cancer cells [96, 100].

Patients with pancreatic ductal adenocarcinoma (PDAC) and exhibiting high BMI present increased desmoplasia and tumor growth [12]. In addition, the same authors showed that PDAC obese mice have an increase in fibrillary collagen and hyaluronic acid in adipocyte-enriched tumor areas [12]. They also reported that increased collagen I content associates with pancreatic stellate cell activation and infiltration of neutrophils in the same mouse model [12]. Interestingly, accelerated tumor growth is prevented by depleting tumor-associated neutrophils or IL1β in these obese animals, implying a strong link between inflammation and fibrosis, in an obesity context [12]. To further investigate this, our group has been studying a series of gastric cancers from 20 T2DM and 20 non-diabetic patients. As expected, the diabetic gastric cancer patients present significantly increased glycemia than their non-diabetic counterparts. We found that fibrosis is significantly increased among the gastric cancers from diabetic patients as compared to non-diabetic ones (data in preparation). Interestingly enough, fibrosis, as evaluated by histological staining, is also significantly higher in the tumor than in normal adjacent gastric mucosa in both control and diabetic groups. These results led us to assume that obesity may affect therapeutic response as well, since fibrosis blocks drug delivery within the tumor tissue. In agreement, the association between obesity and tumor desmoplasia is accompanied by a reduction in chemotherapy response in a series of pancreatic cancer patients concomitant with a reduction in the number of perfused blood vessels [12].

Metabolism in Cancer Cells

For several years, cancer was considered a genetic disease that involved mutations in both oncogenes and tumor suppressor genes. These mutations resulted in growth advantage, potentiating migration and invasiveness capacity. Back in 1956, Warburg proposed that tumor cells metabolize glucose through glycolysis and release lactate, rather than through the whole respiratory pathway [101]. But despite this past implication of metabolic pathways in tumors, only recently metabolism has been considered a relevant cancer hallmark.

Currently, it is well established that gene mutations that characterize malignancies are intimately implicated in the reprogramming of metabolic pathways. The p53 tumor suppressor gene, the guardian of the genome, also plays a role in metabolism, activating the expression of TIGAR (TP53-induced glycolysis and apoptosis regulator), a negative mediator of glycolysis (indirectly and negatively regulating phosphofrutokinase I). P53 deleterious mutations, which are frequently found in tumors, result in the absence of this mediator, which increases glycolytic activity towards lactate production [102]. In addition, oncogenes like c-Myc, in cooperation with HIF1α, inhibit pyruvate dehydrogenase, which leads to pyruvate accumulation in the cytoplasm and its concomitant transformation in lactate what accounts for the Warburg effect [103].

Besides glucose, tumor cells depend deeply on glutamine as a fuel [104]. Glutamine plays a role in providing NADPH essential for tumor cell redox status and lipid synthesis as well as for synthesis of other amino acids and derivatives, and anaplerotic reactions [105].

In order to proliferate and migrate, tumors need to synthesize nucleotides, phospholipids and proteins in a high extent. Thus, anabolic pathways are generally activated in tumor cells, which find their building blocks in tumor microenvironment host cells. Tumor microenvironment enrolls a wide variety of host cells, including fibroblasts, several subpopulations of macrophages and other immune cells, endothelial cells, smooth muscle cells, pericytes and adipocytes [106]. Tumor environment is characterized by acidosis, chronic hypoxia, inflammation and oxidative stress [61, 107]. These features are enhanced in obesity, leading to an exacerbated metabolic reprogramming [108].

In response to tumor cell secreted factors, tumor-associated adipocytes activate lipolysis, releasing significant amounts of FFA. These, in turn, are taken up by tumor cells and are esterified to phospholipids for membrane synthesis. Part of these FFA are also internalized by host neighboring cells, as ECs, by FABP4 and oxidized to withstand angiogenesis. Saturated fatty acids released by local adipocytes bind to toll-like receptors (TLR) 2 and 4, activating hence inflammation within the tumor.

Tumor-associated adipocytes also release a panoply of adipocytokines (*e.g.* leptin, resistin, inflammatory growth factors) that play a role in tumor cell metabolism, and sustain inflammation and angiogenesis, and ECM degradation [109].

Host Cell Metabolic Changes in Cancer Patients

Metabolic reprogramming is not restricted to tumor environment. Liver, AT and muscle adapt their metabolism to the neoplastic tissue as well. The Cori cycle between tumor cells and hepatocytes will be stimulated, since tumor cell-released lactate is converted into glucose in liver and re-used by tumors. Energy for this gluconeogenic pathway is obtained from FFA that derive from AT lipolysis, which is significantly activated in cancer patients. Hepatocytes further esterify fatty acids into triglycerides and release them in very low-density lipoprotein (VLDL), which can be used by tumor cells and some neighboring host cells for energy and anabolism. Effective muscle protein degradation in cancer patients supply amino acids to tumor cell and immune cell anabolic purposes [104].

Although metabolic changes in the obese cancer patients are not clearly described, it is likely that obesity provides tumors with increased supply of energy compounds like FFA, rendering tumor cells with an excess of building blocks for cell growth. Moreover, insulin resistance that generally accompanies obesity results in catabolism activation, which provides ketone bodies and amino acids to tumors as well. Recently, a new adipokine secreted by WAT has been described. Asprosin is a WAT released polypeptide that stimulates glucose production by increasing cAMP levels and activating the protein kinase A (PKA) signaling cascade [110]. Plasma asprosin is increased in obese insulin resistant patients and animal models. Blocking asprosin protects against hyperinsulinemia associated with obesity [110]. Whether this adipocytokine plays a role in cancer patients with obesity is not known. But it is likely that it promotes cancer development by stimulating glycemia.

ROS are metabolic by-products characteristic in obesity that further contribute to the aggressiveness and progression of cancer.

PREVENTIVE AND THERAPEUTIC APPROACHES AGAINST CANCER IN OBESITY

We have been describing the role of obesity and metabolic disturbances in the various stages of tumor development and progression. Therefore, it would be expectable that with the improvement of the metabolic status of patients a beneficial effect in the carcinogenic process would be observed. In fact, the beneficial impact of caloric restriction (CR) in increasing lifespan and decreasing the incidence of cancer has been known for many years and has been reported in several studies [111 - 113]. Although the mechanisms by which this happens are not fully understood, CR appears to act on some of the aforementioned processes, such as angiogenesis, inflammation and adipokine expression [114, 115], and also possibly through epigenetic changes that suppress the activity of oncogenes and restore tumor suppression activities [116]. Improving the energy balance and consequently the metabolic status of the patient through increased physical activity appears to have the same beneficial effects as CR [117].

Furthermore, underlining the importance of the metabolic status of the patients, agents used to treat or prevent chronic metabolic diseases, such as metformin and statins, have been suggested to reduce the risk of development and progression of several types of cancer [118 - 121].

Another emerging area of interest with very exciting results is cancer-related immunity and the development of immunotherapies [122]. However, as it has been mentioned, obese patients present altered immune systems with, among other differences, a lower number and activity of CD8[+] T and NK cells [78]. The immune dysregulation is a crucial aspect to consider while developing new cancer immunotherapies for obesity-associated cancers. The proinflammatory environment present in the AT may be enhancing carcinogenesis, and should, therefore, be attenuated. On the other hand, the activation of the immune system against the tumor itself could be beneficial [123]. This means that effective immunotherapies for normal weight patients may not have the same effect in obese patients [124]. Further research focused on the immunity of obesity-related cancers is required to better characterize the involved immune populations and to define new courses of action.

Cytotoxic chemotherapy has been used as a weapon in the treatment of metastatic disease for decades. However, in obese patients, treatment planning is aggravated by a global underdosing effect. The higher adiposity interferes with drug distribution and partition in obese patients, rendering chemotherapy less effective in these scenarios. Obese patients usually have reduced dosing plans of chemotherapy, particularly in the adjuvant setting, to avoid acute toxicity and aggravation of obesity-associated comorbidities [125]. Radiotherapy is another weapon commonly employed as an adjuvant therapy modality for the majority of malignancies. However, in obese patients careful planning and dose delivery is required, which must take into account the higher BMI of obese patients. In addition to the physical constraints to dose planning and delivery, there is a shift in the delivery of external-beam ionizing radiation, resulting in the target location not receiving the full prescribed doses [126, 127]. Furthermore, recent data from our group showed that an environment rich in adipose-released factors contributes to the protection of melanoma cells from the radiation-induced damage, with a concomitant activation of the PI3K/AKT radioresistance pathway, circumventing the efficacy of radiotherapy [128].

Although scarce, the current evidence point towards an adiposity-enhanced reduced efficacy of chemo- and radiotherapy in obese patients. Further studies are of paramount importance to further elucidate the impact of obesity in cancer treatment and prognosis. Nevertheless, the current evidence already reinforces the need for the clinician to take into account whether the patient is normoponderal or overweight in treatment planning, as adiposity-associated distinct mechanisms of cancer pathogenesis might lead to worse prognosis and higher mortality rates.

CONCLUDING REMARKS

Increased attention has been payed regarding the association between obesity and cancer. Although the term "obesity paradox" proposed for cardiometabolic disorders, has also been reported in oncology, referring to the controversial fact that patients with high BMI seem to present better cancer outcomes, misinterpretation of methodological variations may be behind this concept. Moreover, increasing evidence in a vast number of cancers indicates that obesity negatively affects cancer development and progression. This chapter highlighted the main possible molecular links between these two dreadful pathological conditions, which carry together a huge burden worldwide.

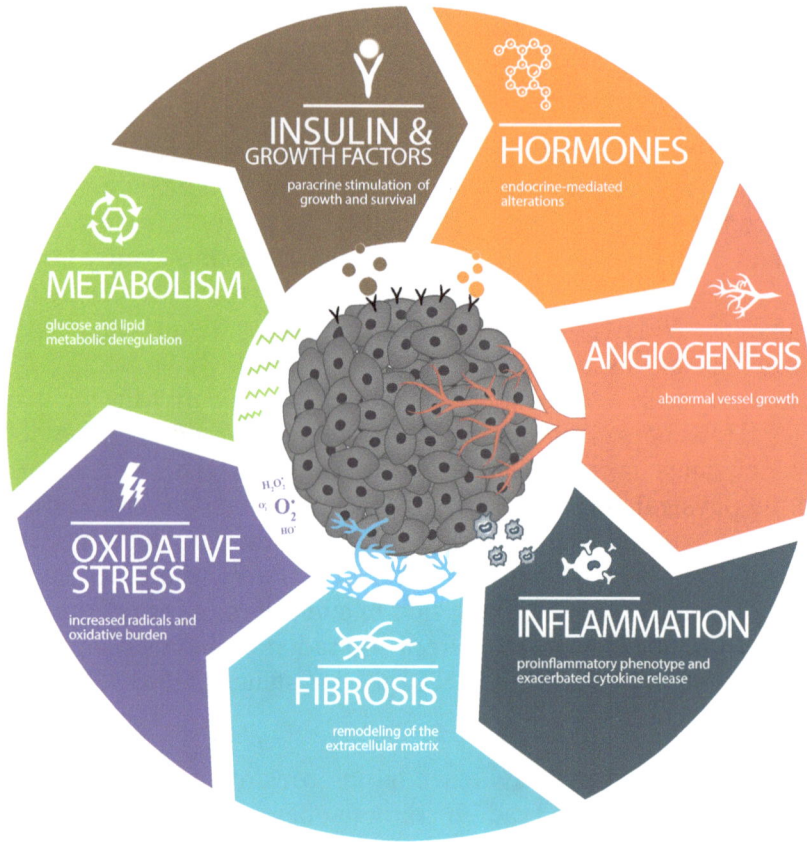

Fig. (1). Schematic diagram of the pathophysiological mechanisms that link together obesity and overall cancer development, progression and may affect therapeutic interventions.

The mechanisms involved are illustrated in Fig. (**1**), and encompass adipokines release by AT; hypoxia, which gather together with angiogenesis imbalance and metainflammation; insulin resistance and concomitant IGF family members upregulation; hyperglycemia and associated metabolism disturbance; sex steroid hormones; ROS; increased fibrosis. Altogether, these obesity-associated features can influence cancer development, progression and therapeutic interventions, rendering cancer in obese patients a distinct entity that should be addressed with particular care. Despite a lot of research is still needed, lifestyle interventions, namely metabolic (energy balance) therapeutic approaches are promising to improve cancer-related outcome in patients with high BMI.

CONSENT FOR PUBLICATION

Not applicable.

CONFLICT OF INTEREST

The authors confirm that this chapter contents have no conflict of interest.

ACKNOWLEDGEMENTS

Declared none.

REFERENCES

[1]   WHO. Fact sheet N°311. World Health Organization; Updated January 2015 [accessed 02/02/2015]..

[2]   Ng M, Fleming T, Robinson M, *et al.* Global, regional, and national prevalence of overweight and obesity in children and adults during 1980-2013: a systematic analysis for the Global Burden of Disease Study 2013. Lancet 2014; 384(9945): 766-81.
        [http://dx.doi.org/10.1016/S0140-6736(14)60460-8] [PMID: 24880830]

[3]   Okorodudu DO, Jumean MF, Montori VM, *et al.* Diagnostic performance of body mass index to identify obesity as defined by body adiposity: a systematic review and meta-analysis. Int J Obes 2010; 34(5): 791-9.
        [http://dx.doi.org/10.1038/ijo.2010.5] [PMID: 20125098]

[4]   Young P, Arch JR, Ashwell M. Brown adipose tissue in the parametrial fat pad of the mouse. FEBS Lett 1984; 167(1): 10-4.
        [http://dx.doi.org/10.1016/0014-5793(84)80822-4] [PMID: 6698197]

[5]   Lee YH, Mottillo EP, Granneman JG. Adipose tissue plasticity from WAT to BAT and in between. Biochim Biophys Acta 2014; 1842(3): 358-69.
        [http://dx.doi.org/10.1016/j.bbadis.2013.05.011] [PMID: 23688783]

[6]   Karastergiou K, Mohamed-Ali V. The autocrine and paracrine roles of adipokines. Mol Cell Endocrinol 2010; 318(1-2): 69-78.
        [http://dx.doi.org/10.1016/j.mce.2009.11.011] [PMID: 19948207]

[7]   Ibrahim MM. Subcutaneous and visceral adipose tissue: structural and functional differences. Obes Rev 2010; 11(1): 11-8.
        [http://dx.doi.org/10.1111/j.1467-789X.2009.00623.x] [PMID: 19656312]

[8]   Obesity: preventing and managing the global epidemic. Report of a WHO consultation World Health Organ Tech Rep Ser 2000; 894 i-xii, 1-253
        [PMID: 11234459]

[9]   Lauby-Secretan B, Scoccianti C, Loomis D, Grosse Y, Bianchini F, Straif K. Body Fatness and Cancer--Viewpoint of the IARC Working Group. N Engl J Med 2016; 375(8): 794-8.
        [http://dx.doi.org/10.1056/NEJMsr1606602] [PMID: 27557308]

[10]   Wang YC, McPherson K, Marsh T, Gortmaker SL, Brown M. Health and economic burden of the projected obesity trends in the USA and the UK. Lancet 2011; 378(9793): 815-25.
        [http://dx.doi.org/10.1016/S0140-6736(11)60814-3] [PMID: 21872750]

[11]   Bianchini F, Kaaks R, Vainio H. Overweight, obesity, and cancer risk. Lancet Oncol 2002; 3(9): 565-74.
[http://dx.doi.org/10.1016/S1470-2045(02)00849-5] [PMID: 12217794]

[12]   Incio J, Liu H, Suboj P, *et al.* Obesity-Induced Inflammation and Desmoplasia Promote Pancreatic Cancer Progression and Resistance to Chemotherapy. Cancer Discov 2016; 6(8): 852-69.
[http://dx.doi.org/10.1158/2159-8290.CD-15-1177] [PMID: 27246539]

[13]   Incio J, Tam J, Rahbari NN, *et al.* PlGF/VEGFR-1 Signaling Promotes Macrophage Polarization and Accelerated Tumor Progression in Obesity. Clin Cancer Res 2016; 22(12): 2993-3004.
[http://dx.doi.org/10.1158/1078-0432.CCR-15-1839] [PMID: 26861455]

[14]   Arnold M, Pandeya N, Byrnes G, *et al.* Global burden of cancer attributable to high body-mass index in 2012: a population-based study. Lancet Oncol 2015; 16(1): 36-46.
[http://dx.doi.org/10.1016/S1470-2045(14)71123-4] [PMID: 25467404]

[15]   Wang P, Mariman E, Keijer J, *et al.* Profiling of the secreted proteins during 3T3-L1 adipocyte differentiation leads to the identification of novel adipokines. Cell Mol Life Sci 2004; 61(18): 2405-17.
[http://dx.doi.org/10.1007/s00018-004-4256-z] [PMID: 15378209]

[16]   Gallagher EJ, LeRoith D. Obesity and Diabetes: The Increased Risk of Cancer and Cancer-Related Mortality. Physiol Rev 2015; 95(3): 727-48.
[http://dx.doi.org/10.1152/physrev.00030.2014] [PMID: 26084689]

[17]   Blüher M. Adipose tissue dysfunction contributes to obesity related metabolic diseases. Best Pract Res Clin Endocrinol Metab 2013; 27(2): 163-77.
[http://dx.doi.org/10.1016/j.beem.2013.02.005] [PMID: 23731879]

[18]   Antoniadis AG, Petridou ET, Antonopoulos CN, *et al.* Insulin resistance in relation to melanoma risk. Melanoma Res 2011; 21(6): 541-6.
[http://dx.doi.org/10.1097/CMR.0b013e32834b0eeb] [PMID: 21946019]

[19]   Sevim DG, Kiratli H. Serum adiponectin, insulin resistance, and uveal melanoma: clinicopathological correlations. Melanoma Res 2016; 26(2): 164-72.
[http://dx.doi.org/10.1097/CMR.0000000000000226] [PMID: 26630661]

[20]   Oba J, Wei W, Gershenwald JE, *et al.* Elevated Serum Leptin Levels are Associated With an Increased Risk of Sentinel Lymph Node Metastasis in Cutaneous Melanoma. Medicine (Baltimore) 2016; 95(11)e3073
[http://dx.doi.org/10.1097/MD.0000000000003073] [PMID: 26986135]

[21]   Malvi P, Chaube B, Pandey V, *et al.* Obesity induced rapid melanoma progression is reversed by orlistat treatment and dietary intervention: role of adipokines. Mol Oncol 2015; 9(3): 689-703.
[http://dx.doi.org/10.1016/j.molonc.2014.11.006] [PMID: 25499031]

[22]   Mantzoros CS, Trakatelli M, Gogas H, *et al.* Circulating adiponectin levels in relation to melanoma: a case-control study. Eur J Cancer 2007; 43(9): 1430-6.
[http://dx.doi.org/10.1016/j.ejca.2007.03.026] [PMID: 17512191]

[23]   Tamakoshi K, Toyoshima H, Wakai K, *et al.* Leptin is associated with an increased female colorectal cancer risk: a nested case-control study in Japan. Oncology 2005; 68(4-6): 454-61.
[http://dx.doi.org/10.1159/000086988] [PMID: 16020976]

[24]   Cymbaluk A, Chudecka-Głaz A, Rzepka-Górska I. Leptin levels in serum depending on Body Mass Index in patients with endometrial hyperplasia and cancer. Eur J Obstet Gynecol Reprod Biol 2008; 136(1): 74-7.
[http://dx.doi.org/10.1016/j.ejogrb.2006.08.012] [PMID: 17007993]

[25]   Brandon EL, Gu JW, Cantwell L, He Z, Wallace G, Hall JE. Obesity promotes melanoma tumor growth: role of leptin. Cancer Biol Ther 2009; 8(19): 1871-9.
[http://dx.doi.org/10.4161/cbt.8.19.9650] [PMID: 19713740]

[26]   Amjadi F, Mehdipoor R, Zarkesh-Esfahani H, Javanmard SH. Leptin serves as angiogenic/mitogenic factor in melanoma tumor growth Adv Biomed Res 2016; 5(127)
       [http://dx.doi.org/10.4103/2277-9175.187005] [PMID: 27563637]

[27]   Sun Y, Lodish HF. Adiponectin deficiency promotes tumor growth in mice by reducing macrophage infiltration. PLoS One 2010; 5(8)e11987
       [http://dx.doi.org/10.1371/journal.pone.0011987] [PMID: 20700533]

[28]   Zheng Q, Dunlap SM, Zhu J, *et al*. Leptin deficiency suppresses MMTV-Wnt-1 mammary tumor growth in obese mice and abrogates tumor initiating cell survival. Endocr Relat Cancer 2011; 18(4): 491-503.
       [http://dx.doi.org/10.1530/ERC-11-0102] [PMID: 21636700]

[29]   Naylor C, Petri WA Jr. Leptin Regulation of Immune Responses. Trends Mol Med 2016; 22(2): 88-98.
       [http://dx.doi.org/10.1016/j.molmed.2015.12.001] [PMID: 26776093]

[30]   Tworoger SS, Eliassen AH, Kelesidis T, *et al*. Plasma adiponectin concentrations and risk of incident breast cancer. J Clin Endocrinol Metab 2007; 92(4): 1510-6.
       [http://dx.doi.org/10.1210/jc.2006-1975] [PMID: 17213279]

[31]   Stolzenberg-Solomon RZ, Weinstein S, Pollak M, *et al*. Prediagnostic adiponectin concentrations and pancreatic cancer risk in male smokers. Am J Epidemiol 2008; 168(9): 1047-55.
       [http://dx.doi.org/10.1093/aje/kwn221] [PMID: 18801887]

[32]   Barb D, Williams CJ, Neuwirth AK, Mantzoros CS. Adiponectin in relation to malignancies: a review of existing basic research and clinical evidence. Am J Clin Nutr 2007; 86(3): s858-66.
       [http://dx.doi.org/10.1093/ajcn/86.3.858S] [PMID: 18265479]

[33]   Demiray G, Degirmencioglu S, Ugurlu E, Yaren A. Effects of Serum Leptin and Resistin Levels on Cancer Cachexia in Patients With Advanced-Stage Non-Small Cell Lung Cancer. Clin Med Insights Oncol 2017; 11(1-7)
       [http://dx.doi.org/10.1177/1179554917690144] [PMID: 28469508]

[34]   Booth A, Magnuson A, Fouts J, Foster M. Adipose tissue, obesity and adipokines: role in cancer promotion. Horm Mol Biol Clin Investig 2015; 21(1): 57-74.
       [http://dx.doi.org/10.1515/hmbci-2014-0037] [PMID: 25781552]

[35]   Calle EE, Kaaks R. Overweight, obesity and cancer: epidemiological evidence and proposed mechanisms. Nat Rev Cancer 2004; 4(8): 579-91.
       [http://dx.doi.org/10.1038/nrc1408] [PMID: 15286738]

[36]   Hefetz-Sela S, Scherer PE. Adipocytes: impact on tumor growth and potential sites for therapeutic intervention. Pharmacol Ther 2013; 138(2): 197-210.
       [http://dx.doi.org/10.1016/j.pharmthera.2013.01.008] [PMID: 23353703]

[37]   Bulun SE, Chen D, Moy I, Brooks DC, Zhao H. Aromatase, breast cancer and obesity: a complex interaction. Trends Endocrinol Metab 2012; 23(2): 83-9.
       [http://dx.doi.org/10.1016/j.tem.2011.10.003] [PMID: 22169755]

[38]   Ramos-Nino ME. The role of chronic inflammation in obesity-associated cancers. ISRN Oncol 2013; 2013(1-25)
       [http://dx.doi.org/10.1155/2013/697521] [PMID: 23819063]

[39]   Straub RH. The complex role of estrogens in inflammation. Endocr Rev 2007; 28(5): 521-74.
       [http://dx.doi.org/10.1210/er.2007-0001] [PMID: 17640948]

[40]   Bowers LW, Brenner AJ, Hursting SD, Tekmal RR, deGraffenried LA. Obesity-associated systemic interleukin-6 promotes pre-adipocyte aromatase expression via increased breast cancer cell prostaglandin E2 production. Breast Cancer Res Treat 2015; 149(1): 49-57.
       [http://dx.doi.org/10.1007/s10549-014-3223-0] [PMID: 25476497]

[41]   Pollack MN. Insulin, insulin-like growth factors, insulin resistance, and neoplasia. Am J Clin Nutr

2007; 86(3): s820-2.
[http://dx.doi.org/10.1093/ajcn/86.3.820S] [PMID: 18265475]

[42]   Barone BB, Yeh HC, Snyder CF, *et al.* Long-term all-cause mortality in cancer patients with preexisting diabetes mellitus: a systematic review and meta-analysis. JAMA 2008; 300(23): 2754-64.
[http://dx.doi.org/10.1001/jama.2008.824] [PMID: 19088353]

[43]   Fukumura D, Incio J, Shankaraiah RC, Jain RK. Obesity and cancer: an angiogenic and inflammatory link. Microcirculation 2016; 23(3): 191-206.
[http://dx.doi.org/10.1111/micc.12270] [PMID: 26808917]

[44]   Nimptsch K, Pischon T. Obesity Biomarkers, Metabolism and Risk of Cancer: An Epidemiological Perspective. Recent Results Cancer Res 2016; 208(199-217)
[http://dx.doi.org/10.1007/978-3-319-42542-9_11] [PMID: 27909909]

[45]   Vigneri R, Goldfine ID, Frittitta L. Insulin, insulin receptors, and cancer. J Endocrinol Invest 2016; 39(12): 1365-76.
[http://dx.doi.org/10.1007/s40618-016-0508-7] [PMID: 27368923]

[46]   Pollak MN, Schernhammer ES, Hankinson SE. Insulin-like growth factors and neoplasia. Nat Rev Cancer 2004; 4(7): 505-18.
[http://dx.doi.org/10.1038/nrc1387] [PMID: 15229476]

[47]   Brahmkhatri VP, Prasanna C, Atreya HS. Insulin-like growth factor system in cancer: novel targeted therapies. Biomed Res Int 2015; 2015: 1-24.
[http://dx.doi.org/10.1155/2015/538019] [PMID: 25866791]

[48]   Gallagher EJ, LeRoith D. Minireview: IGF, Insulin, and Cancer. Endocrinology 2011; 152(7): 2546-51.
[http://dx.doi.org/10.1210/en.2011-0231] [PMID: 21540285]

[49]   Coelho P, Almeida J, Prudêncio C, Fernandes R, Soares R. Effect of Adipocyte Secretome in Melanoma Progression and Vasculogenic Mimicry. J Cell Biochem 2016; 117(7): 1697-706.
[http://dx.doi.org/10.1002/jcb.25463] [PMID: 26666522]

[50]   Cao Y. Adipose tissuea angiogenesis as a therapeutic target for obesity and metabolic diseases. Nat Rev Drug Discov 2010; 9: 107-5.
[http://dx.doi.org/10.1159/000353254] [PMID: 24217609]

[51]   Han J, Lee JE, Jin J, *et al.* The spatiotemporal development of adipose tissue. Development 2011; 138(22): 5027-37.
[http://dx.doi.org/10.1242/dev.067686] [PMID: 22028034]

[52]   Lemoine AY, Ledoux S, Larger E. Adipose tissue angiogenesis in obesity. Thromb Haemost 2013; 110(4): 661-8.
[http://dx.doi.org/10.1160/TH13-01-0073] [PMID: 23595655]

[53]   Rubina K, Kalinina N, Efimenko A, *et al.* Adipose stromal cells stimulate angiogenesis via promoting progenitor cell differentiation, secretion of angiogenic factors, and enhancing vessel maturation. Tissue Eng Part A 2009; 15(8): 2039-50.
[http://dx.doi.org/10.1089/ten.tea.2008.0359] [PMID: 19368510]

[54]   Bouloumié A, Sengenès C, Portolan G, Galitzky J, Lafontan M. Adipocyte produces matrix metalloproteinases 2 and 9: involvement in adipose differentiation. Diabetes 2001; 50(9): 2080-6.
[http://dx.doi.org/10.2337/diabetes.50.9.2080] [PMID: 11522674]

[55]   Mantovani A, Sica A. Macrophages, innate immunity and cancer: balance, tolerance, and diversity. Curr Opin Immunol 2010; 22(2): 231-7.
[http://dx.doi.org/10.1016/j.coi.2010.01.009] [PMID: 20144856]

[56]   Mayi TH, Daoudi M, Derudas B, *et al.* Human adipose tissue macrophages display activation of cancer-related pathways. J Biol Chem 2012; 287(26): 21904-13.
[http://dx.doi.org/10.1074/jbc.M111.315200] [PMID: 22511784]

[57] Easty DJ, Gray SG, O'Byrne KJ, O'Donnell D, Bennett DC. Receptor tyrosine kinases and their activation in melanoma. Pigment Cell Melanoma Res 2011; 24(3): 446-61.
[http://dx.doi.org/10.1111/j.1755-148X.2011.00836.x] [PMID: 21320293]

[58] Rosero RA, Villares GJ, Bar-Eli M. Protease-Activated Receptors and other G-Protein-Coupled Receptors: the Melanoma Connection Front Genet 2016; 7: 1-6.
[http://dx.doi.org/10.3389/fgene.2016.00112] [PMID: 27379162]

[59] Nieman KM, Romero IL, Van Houten B, Lengyel E. Adipose tissue and adipocytes support tumorigenesis and metastasis. Biochim Biophys Acta 2013; 1831(10): 1533-41.
[http://dx.doi.org/10.1016/j.bbalip.2013.02.010] [PMID: 23500888]

[60] Bielenberg DR, Zetter BR. The Contribution of Angiogenesis to the Process of Metastasis. Cancer J 2015; 21(4): 267-73.
[http://dx.doi.org/10.1097/PPO.0000000000000138] [PMID: 26222078]

[61] Manna P, Jain SK. Obesity, Oxidative Stress, Adipose Tissue Dysfunction, and the Associated Health Risks: Causes and Therapeutic Strategies. Metab Syndr Relat Disord 2015; 13(10): 423-44.
[http://dx.doi.org/10.1089/met.2015.0095] [PMID: 26569333]

[62] Furukawa S, Fujita T, Shimabukuro M, *et al.* Increased oxidative stress in obesity and its impact on metabolic syndrome. J Clin Invest 2004; 114(12): 1752-61.
[http://dx.doi.org/10.1172/JCI21625] [PMID: 15599400]

[63] Fried L, Arbiser JL. The reactive oxygen-driven tumor: relevance to melanoma. Pigment Cell Melanoma Res 2008; 21(2): 117-22.
[http://dx.doi.org/10.1111/j.1755-148X.2008.00451.x] [PMID: 18384505]

[64] Fruehauf JP, Trapp V. Reactive oxygen species: an Achilles' heel of melanoma? Expert Rev Anticancer Ther 2008; 8(11): 1751-7.
[http://dx.doi.org/10.1586/14737140.8.11.1751] [PMID: 18983235]

[65] Meyskens FL Jr, Buckmeier JA, McNulty SE, Tohidian NB. Activation of nuclear factor-kappa B in human metastatic melanomacells and the effect of oxidative stress. Clin Cancer Res 1999; 5(5): 1197-202.
[PMID: 10353757]

[66] Meierjohann S. Oxidative stress in melanocyte senescence and melanoma transformation. Eur J Cell Biol 2014; 93(1-2): 36-41.
[http://dx.doi.org/10.1016/j.ejcb.2013.11.005] [PMID: 24342719]

[67] Hussein MR. Tumour-associated macrophages and melanoma tumourigenesis: integrating the complexity. Int J Exp Pathol 2006; 87(3): 163-76.
[http://dx.doi.org/10.1111/j.1365-2613.2006.00478.x] [PMID: 16709225]

[68] Wagner M, Bjerkvig R, Wiig H, *et al.* Inflamed tumor-associated adipose tissue is a depot for macrophages that stimulate tumor growth and angiogenesis. Angiogenesis 2012; 15(3): 481-95.
[http://dx.doi.org/10.1007/s10456-012-9276-y] [PMID: 22614697]

[69] Roberts DL, Dive C, Renehan AG. Biological mechanisms linking obesity and cancer risk: new perspectives. Annu Rev Med 2010; 61: 301-16.
[http://dx.doi.org/10.1146/annurev.med.080708.082713] [PMID: 19824817]

[70] Matsuda M, Shimomura I. Increased oxidative stress in obesity: implications for metabolic syndrome, diabetes, hypertension, dyslipidemia, atherosclerosis, and cancer. Obes Res Clin Pract 2013; 7(5): e330-41.
[http://dx.doi.org/10.1016/j.orcp.2013.05.004] [PMID: 24455761]

[71] Monteiro R, Azevedo I. Chronic inflammation in obesity and the metabolic syndrome. Mediators Inflamm 2010; 2010: 1-10.
[http://dx.doi.org/10.1155/2010/289645] [PMID: 20706689]

[72] Forsythe JA, Jiang BH, Iyer NV, *et al.* Activation of vascular endothelial growth factor gene transcription by hypoxia-inducible factor 1. Mol Cell Biol 1996; 16(9): 4604-13.
[http://dx.doi.org/10.1128/MCB.16.9.4604] [PMID: 8756616]

[73] Schäfer M, Werner S. Cancer as an overhealing wound: an old hypothesis revisited. Nat Rev Mol Cell Biol 2008; 9(8): 628-38.
[http://dx.doi.org/10.1038/nrm2455] [PMID: 18628784]

[74] Gucalp A, Iyengar NM, Zhou XK, *et al.* Periprostatic adipose inflammation is associated with high-grade prostate cancer. Prostate Cancer Prostatic Dis 2017; 20(4): 418-23.
[http://dx.doi.org/10.1038/pcan.2017.31] [PMID: 28653675]

[75] Vaysse C, Lomo J, Garred O, *et al.* Inflammation of mammary adipose tissue occurs in overweight and obese patients exhibiting early-stage breast cancer. NPJ Breast Cancer 2017; 3: 1-10.
[http://dx.doi.org/10.1038/s41523-017-0015-9] [PMID: 28649659]

[76] Donninelli G, Del Corno M, Pierdominici M, *et al.* Distinct Blood and Visceral Adipose Tissue Regulatory T Cell and Innate Lymphocyte Profiles Characterize Obesity and Colorectal Cancer Front Immunol 2017; 8(1-11)
[http://dx.doi.org/10.3389/fimmu.2017.00643] [PMID: 28649243]

[77] Subbaramaiah K, Morris PG, Zhou XK, *et al.* Increased levels of COX-2 and prostaglandin E2 contribute to elevated aromatase expression in inflamed breast tissue of obese women. Cancer Discov 2012; 2(4): 356-65.
[http://dx.doi.org/10.1158/2159-8290.CD-11-0241] [PMID: 22576212]

[78] Zitvogel L, Pietrocola F, Kroemer G. Nutrition, inflammation and cancer. Nat Immunol 2017; 18(8): 843-50.
[http://dx.doi.org/10.1038/ni.3754] [PMID: 28722707]

[79] Lara-Castro C, Garvey WT. Intracellular lipid accumulation in liver and muscle and the insulin resistance syndrome. Endocrinol Metab Clin North Am 2008; 37(4): 841-56.
[http://dx.doi.org/10.1016/j.ecl.2008.09.002] [PMID: 19026935]

[80] Ferrara N, Gerber HP. The role of vascular endothelial growth factor in angiogenesis. Acta Haematol 2001; 106(4): 148-56.
[http://dx.doi.org/10.1159/000046610] [PMID: 11815711]

[81] Carmeliet P. VEGF as a key mediator of angiogenesis in cancer. Oncology 2005; 69 (3): 4-10.
[http://dx.doi.org/10.1159/000088478] [PMID: 16301830]

[82] Costa R, Rodrigues I, Guardão L, *et al.* Modulation of VEGF signaling in a mouse model of diabetes by xanthohumol and 8-prenylnaringenin: Unveiling the angiogenic paradox and metabolism interplay. Mol Nutr Food Res 2017; 61(4): 1-27.
[http://dx.doi.org/10.1002/mnfr.201600488] [PMID: 27921359]

[83] De Bock K, Georgiadou M, Carmeliet P. Role of endothelial cell metabolism in vessel sprouting. Cell Metab 2013; 18(5): 634-47.
[http://dx.doi.org/10.1016/j.cmet.2013.08.001] [PMID: 23973331]

[84] Yeh WL, Lin CJ, Fu WM. Enhancement of glucose transporter expression of brain endothelial cells by vascular endothelial growth factor derived from glioma exposed to hypoxia. Mol Pharmacol 2008; 73(1): 170-7.
[http://dx.doi.org/10.1124/mol.107.038851] [PMID: 17942749]

[85] Atsumi T, Nishio T, Niwa H, *et al.* Expression of inducible 6-phosphofructo-2-kinase/fructose-2,6-bisphosphatase/PFKFB3 isoforms in adipocytes and their potential role in glycolytic regulation. Diabetes 2005; 54(12): 3349-57.
[http://dx.doi.org/10.2337/diabetes.54.12.3349] [PMID: 16306349]

[86] Bando H, Atsumi T, Nishio T, *et al.* Phosphorylation of the 6-phosphofructo-2-kinase/fructose 2,6-bisphosphatase/PFKFB3 family of glycolytic regulators in human cancer. Clin Cancer Res 2005;

11(16): 5784-92.
[http://dx.doi.org/10.1158/1078-0432.CCR-05-0149] [PMID: 16115917]

[87] Schoors S, De Bock K, Cantelmo AR, *et al.* Partial and transient reduction of glycolysis by PFKFB3 blockade reduces pathological angiogenesis. Cell Metab 2014; 19(1): 37-48.
[http://dx.doi.org/10.1016/j.cmet.2013.11.008] [PMID: 24332967]

[88] Hagberg CE, Falkevall A, Wang X, *et al.* Vascular endothelial growth factor B controls endothelial fatty acid uptake. Nature 2010; 464(7290): 917-21.
[http://dx.doi.org/10.1038/nature08945] [PMID: 20228789]

[89] Robciuc MR, Kivelä R, Williams IM, *et al.* VEGFB/VEGFR1-Induced Expansion of Adipose Vasculature Counteracts Obesity and Related Metabolic Complications. Cell Metab 2016; 23(4): 712-24.
[http://dx.doi.org/10.1016/j.cmet.2016.03.004] [PMID: 27076080]

[90] Goldberg IJ, Eckel RH, Abumrad NA. Regulation of fatty acid uptake into tissues: lipoprotein lipase- and CD36-mediated pathways J Lipid Res 2009; 50 (S86-90.).
[http://dx.doi.org/10.1194/jlr.R800085-JLR200] [PMID: 19033209]

[91] Pietka TA, Schappe T, Conte C, *et al.* Adipose and muscle tissue profile of CD36 transcripts in obese subjects highlights the role of CD36 in fatty acid homeostasis and insulin resistance. Diabetes Care 2014; 37(7): 1990-7.
[http://dx.doi.org/10.2337/dc13-2835] [PMID: 24784828]

[92] Pardina E, Ferrer R, Rossell J, *et al.* Hepatic CD36 downregulation parallels steatosis improvement in morbidly obese undergoing bariatric surgery. Int J Obes 2017; 41(9): 1388-93.
[http://dx.doi.org/10.1038/ijo.2017.115] [PMID: 28555086]

[93] Costa R, Rodrigues I, Guardao L, *et al.* Xanthohumol and 8-prenylnaringenin ameliorate diabetic-related metabolic dysfunctions in mice. J Nutr Biochem 2017; 45(39-47)
[http://dx.doi.org/10.1016/j.jnutbio.2017.03.006] [PMID: 28431322]

[94] Glatz JF, Luiken JJ, Bonen A. Membrane fatty acid transporters as regulators of lipid metabolism: implications for metabolic disease. Physiol Rev 2010; 90(1): 367-417.
[http://dx.doi.org/10.1152/physrev.00003.2009] [PMID: 20086080]

[95] Seo BR, Bhardwaj P, Choi S, *et al.* Obesity-dependent changes in interstitial ECM mechanics promote breast tumorigenesis. Sci Transl Med 2015; 7(301)301ra130
[http://dx.doi.org/10.1126/scitranslmed.3010467] [PMID: 26290412]

[96] Lu P, Weaver VM, Werb Z. The extracellular matrix: a dynamic niche in cancer progression. J Cell Biol 2012; 196(4): 395-406.
[http://dx.doi.org/10.1083/jcb.201102147] [PMID: 22351925]

[97] Park J, Morley TS, Scherer PE. Inhibition of endotrophin, a cleavage product of collagen VI, confers cisplatin sensitivity to tumours. EMBO Mol Med 2013; 5(6): 935-48.
[http://dx.doi.org/10.1002/emmm.201202006] [PMID: 23629957]

[98] Sun K, Halberg N, Khan M, Magalang UJ, Scherer PE. Selective inhibition of hypoxia-inducible factor 1α ameliorates adipose tissue dysfunction. Mol Cell Biol 2013; 33(5): 904-17.
[http://dx.doi.org/10.1128/MCB.00951-12] [PMID: 23249949]

[99] Khan T, Muise ES, Iyengar P, *et al.* Metabolic dysregulation and adipose tissue fibrosis: role of collagen VI. Mol Cell Biol 2009; 29(6): 1575-91.
[http://dx.doi.org/10.1128/MCB.01300-08] [PMID: 19114551]

[100] Frantz C, Stewart KM, Weaver VM. The extracellular matrix at a glance. J Cell Sci 2010; 123(Pt 24): 4195-200.
[http://dx.doi.org/10.1242/jcs.023820] [PMID: 21123617]

[101] Warburg O. On the origin of cancer cells. Science 1956; 123(3191): 309-14.
[http://dx.doi.org/10.1126/science.123.3191.309] [PMID: 13298683]

[102] Madan E, Gogna R, Bhatt M, Pati U, Kuppusamy P, Mahdi AA. Regulation of glucose metabolism by p53: emerging new roles for the tumor suppressor. Oncotarget 2011; 2(12): 948-57.
[http://dx.doi.org/10.18632/oncotarget.389] [PMID: 22248668]

[103] Dang CV. The interplay between MYC and HIF in the Warburg effect. Ernst Schering Found Symp Proc. 35-53.
[PMID: 18811052]

[104] Newsholme E, Leech A. Functional Biochemistry in Health and Disease ed: Wiley. 2010.

[105] Carracedo A, Cantley LC, Pandolfi PP. Cancer metabolism: fatty acid oxidation in the limelight. Nat Rev Cancer 2013; 13(4): 227-32.
[http://dx.doi.org/10.1038/nrc3483] [PMID: 23446547]

[106] Bussard KM, Mutkus L, Stumpf K, Gomez-Manzano C, Marini FC. Tumor-associated stromal cells as key contributors to the tumor microenvironment. Breast Cancer Res 2016; 18(1): 84.
[http://dx.doi.org/10.1186/s13058-016-0740-2] [PMID: 27515302]

[107] Justus CR, Sanderlin EJ, Yang LV. Molecular Connections between Cancer Cell Metabolism and the Tumor Microenvironment. Int J Mol Sci 2015; 16(5): 11055-86.
[http://dx.doi.org/10.3390/ijms160511055] [PMID: 25988385]

[108] Diedrich J, Gusky HC, Podgorski I. Adipose tissue dysfunction and its effects on tumor metabolism. Horm Mol Biol Clin Investig 2015; 21(1): 17-41.
[http://dx.doi.org/10.1515/hmbci-2014-0045] [PMID: 25781550]

[109] De Palma M, Biziato D, Petrova TV. Microenvironmental regulation of tumour angiogenesis. Nat Rev Cancer 2017; 17(8): 457-74.
[http://dx.doi.org/10.1038/nrc.2017.51] [PMID: 28706266]

[110] Romere C, Duerrschmid C, Bournat J, *et al.* Asprosin, a Fasting-Induced Glucogenic Protein Hormone. Cell 2016; 165(3): 566-79.
[http://dx.doi.org/10.1016/j.cell.2016.02.063] [PMID: 27087445]

[111] Weindruch R, Walford RL. Dietary restriction in mice beginning at 1 year of age: effect on life-span and spontaneous cancer incidence. Science 1982; 215(4538): 1415-8.
[http://dx.doi.org/10.1126/science.7063854] [PMID: 7063854]

[112] Colman RJ, Anderson RM, Johnson SC, *et al.* Caloric restriction delays disease onset and mortality in rhesus monkeys. Science 2009; 325(5937): 201-4.
[http://dx.doi.org/10.1126/science.1173635] [PMID: 19590001]

[113] Colman RJ, Beasley TM, Kemnitz JW, *et al.* Caloric restriction reduces age-related and all-cause mortality in rhesus monkeys. Nat Commun 2014; 5: 1-5.
[http://dx.doi.org/10.1038/ncomms4557] [PMID: 24691430]

[114] Meynet O, Ricci JE. Caloric restriction and cancer: molecular mechanisms and clinical implications. Trends Mol Med 2014; 20(8): 419-27.
[http://dx.doi.org/10.1016/j.molmed.2014.05.001] [PMID: 24916302]

[115] Hursting SD, Dunlap SM, Ford NA, Hursting MJ, Lashinger LM. Calorie restriction and cancer prevention: a mechanistic perspective. Cancer Metab 2013; 1(1): 10.
[http://dx.doi.org/10.1186/2049-3002-1-10] [PMID: 24280167]

[116] Supic G, Jagodic M, Magic Z. Epigenetics: a new link between nutrition and cancer. Nutr Cancer 2013; 65(6): 781-92.
[http://dx.doi.org/10.1080/01635581.2013.805794] [PMID: 23909721]

[117] Adraskela K, Veisaki E, Koutsilieris M, Philippou A. Physical Exercise Positively Influences Breast Cancer Evolution. Clin Breast Cancer 2017; 17(6): 408-17.
[http://dx.doi.org/10.1016/j.clbc.2017.05.003] [PMID: 28606800]

[118] Lee CK, Jung M, Jung I, *et al.* Cumulative Metformin Use and Its Impact on Survival in Gastric

Cancer Patients After Gastrectomy. Ann Surg 2016; 263(1): 96-102.
[http://dx.doi.org/10.1097/SLA.0000000000001086] [PMID: 25575260]

[119] Morales DR, Morris AD. Metformin in cancer treatment and prevention. Annu Rev Med 2015; 66: 17-29.
[http://dx.doi.org/10.1146/annurev-med-062613-093128] [PMID: 25386929]

[120] Demierre MF, Higgins PD, Gruber SB, Hawk E, Lippman SM. Statins and cancer prevention. Nat Rev Cancer 2005; 5(12): 930-42.
[http://dx.doi.org/10.1038/nrc1751] [PMID: 16341084]

[121] Vallianou NG, Kostantinou A, Kougias M, Kazazis C. Statins and cancer. Anticancer Agents Med Chem 2014; 14(5): 706-12.
[http://dx.doi.org/10.2174/18715206136666131129105035] [PMID: 24295174]

[122] Yang Y. Cancer immunotherapy: harnessing the immune system to battle cancer. J Clin Invest 2015; 125(9): 3335-7.
[http://dx.doi.org/10.1172/JCI83871] [PMID: 26325031]

[123] Conroy MJ, Dunne MR, Donohoe CL, Reynolds JV. Obesity-associated cancer: an immunological perspective. Proc Nutr Soc 2016; 75(2): 125-38.
[http://dx.doi.org/10.1017/S0029665115004176] [PMID: 26567898]

[124] Mirsoian A, Murphy WJ. Obesity and cancer immunotherapy toxicity. Immunotherapy 2015; 7(4): 319-22.
[http://dx.doi.org/10.2217/imt.15.12] [PMID: 25917623]

[125] Lyman GH, Sparreboom A. Chemotherapy dosing in overweight and obese patients with cancer. Nat Rev Clin Oncol 2013; 10(8): 451-9.
[http://dx.doi.org/10.1038/nrclinonc.2013.108] [PMID: 23856744]

[126] Strom SS, Kamat AM, Gruschkus SK, *et al.* Influence of obesity on biochemical and clinical failure after external-beam radiotherapy for localized prostate cancer. Cancer 2006; 107(3): 631-9.
[http://dx.doi.org/10.1002/cncr.22025] [PMID: 16802288]

[127] Wang LS, Murphy CT, Ruth K, *et al.* Impact of obesity on outcomes after definitive dose-escalated intensity-modulated radiotherapy for localized prostate cancer. Cancer 2015; 121(17): 3010-7.
[http://dx.doi.org/10.1002/cncr.29472] [PMID: 26033633]

[128] Coelho P, Silva L, Faria I, *et al.* Adipocyte Secretome Increases Radioresistance of Malignant Melanocytes by Improving Cell Survival and Decreasing Oxidative Status. Radiat Res 2017; 187(5): 581-8.
[http://dx.doi.org/10.1667/RR14551.1] [PMID: 28362167]

Recent Advances in Obesity Research, 2020, Vol. 1, 425-464 425

CHAPTER 17

Obesity: A Bad Partner for the Elderly

Henrique Almeida[1,2] and **Delminda Neves**[1,2,*]

[1] *Department of Biomedicine, Experimental Biology Unit, Faculty of Medicine, University of Porto, Porto, Portugal*

[2] *i3S - Instituto de Investigação e Inovação em Saúde, University of Porto, Porto, Portugal*

Abstract: Ageing is an unavoidable process that along time conduces to the loss of function of cells and tissues. Age-related modifications culminate in disease and death of the organisms. Life expectancy of humans has steadily increased in the last 50 years and the incidence of age-associated disease has increased too. Among the time-dependent changes that afflict the aged individuals, obesity has gained a great importance. Adiposity increases in older individuals and tends to accumulate in visceral space, creating a metabolic threat that, together with senescence-related cell modifications, results in tissue degeneration increment and disease. In this chapter, the contribution of obesity to the ageing phenotype is discussed with a special focus on the senescence of adipose cells. In the final part of the chapter, strategies directed to mitigate the effects of obesity in old individuals that include bariatric surgery, nutritional and pharmacological interventions are presented.

Keywords: Adipokines, Adipose tissue, Adiposity assessment, Antidiabetic drugs, Brown adipose tissue, Energy restriction mimetics, Epidemiology of obesity, Epigenetics of ageing and obesity, Genetics of ageing and obesity, Human ageing, Menopause, MicroRNAs, Obesity paradox, Senescent cells, Telomere attrition, Visceral white adipose tissue.

INTRODUCTION

As human life expectancy increases, the exposure of humans to the health hazards increases too. For these reasons, age-related signs and symptoms become apparent to evidence the organism's degenerative changes; in addition, the continued exposure to extrinsic, harmful, human-related or environmental factors threatens health, may cause disease and accelerate death.

---

* **Corresponding author Delminda Neves:** Department of Biomedicine, Experimental Biology Unit, Faculty of Medicine, University of Porto, Al. Prof. Hernâni Monteiro, 4200-319 Porto, Portugal; Tel: +351 225513600; Fax: +351 225513601; E-mail: delmagal@med.up.pt

Rosário Monteiro and Maria João Martins (Eds.)

Increased weight is one of those factors. It has been generally categorized as overweight (also preobesity), considered as the state of body mass index (BMI) in the range of 25.0 and 29.9 kg/m^2, and obesity, referring to BMI of $\geq$ 30.0 kg/m^2 with additional specific classes [1]. It is implicit that the elevated BMI results from the increase of adipose tissue in the body as «overweight and obesity are defined as abnormal or excessive fat accumulation that may impair health» [2]. As a consequence, elevated BMI has been used to identify individuals who are at greater health risk on account of enhanced body content in adipose tissue.

Increased weight, and obesity in particular, has become a worldwide public health issue due to recognized direct implications. In fact, in just 10 years' time, from 2005 to 2015, obesity-attributed deaths and disability-adjusted life years (DALYs, a measure of the burden imposed by a disorder on the individuals' ability to be active) increased about 20% [3].

OVERWEIGHT AND OBESITY EPIDEMICS

The worldwide increasing prevalence of obesity has been referred as a pandemic; it likely started in the 1970s and 1980s in developed countries and extended to developing countries in the following years [4, 5]. Despite this global involvement, differences can be identified when specific countries or population groups are compared [5, 6]. For example, in a 2013 survey, the prevalence of excess weight was 4% in Ethiopian male adults and 88.3% in Tonga female adults [5].

Excepting for cases that are the result of individual's genetic constitution, the rise in obesity observed in the last four decades is consequent to environmental factors and stems at the increase in wealth experienced in most countries, the widespread mechanization/motorization of human activities and the enlargement of urban areas. As these changes were rapidly made available to an increasing number of people, they allowed the establishment of factors, referred as drivers of the obesity epidemic, such as the easy and fast provision of low-cost, palatable, energy-dense and processed foods as well as the refinement of marketing techniques aiming at food consumption [4].

The condition of excess of weight shows peculiar patterns when children and adolescents or adults are compared and when men and women are contrasted. Clearly, the prevalence of children and adolescents with weight excess is higher in developed countries, which parallels the prevalence of weight excess in adults, also higher in developed countries.

The prevalence of obesity among children and adolescents grew consistently along the past 40 years and even experienced an increase in the rate by the mid-

1990s [5]. Surprisingly, since the early 2000s, the rate reduced so that the prevalence of obesity stabilized in many parts of the world, and even decreased in selected regions [6]. These promising findings are more notorious in children and adolescents, compared to the adults, and although the reasons are not clear, it is possible that a decrement in the incidence and the duration of the condition have both contributed.

There are sexual differences in children and adolescents; interestingly, boys tend to have excess weight in developed countries whereas girls are more frequently overweight in developing countries [5]. However, the differences are slight when they are compared to adults. In developed countries, the excess of weight is substantially more prevalent in males compared to females, a finding that reverses in developing countries where the prevalence of excess weight in females is clearly higher. Furthermore, when overt obesity is considered (BMI $\geq$ 30 kg/m^2), the higher prevalence in females is now observed at all ages, irrespective of the social and economic condition of the country of origin [5].

An important aspect to highlight is the prevalence of weight excess and of obesity along ageing assessed by BMI. The social and economic characteristics of the countries also count and show that, again, excess weight is more prevalent in developed countries. Similarly to the sexual differences, global surveys show that higher prevalence of excess weight and obesity are observed in males from developed countries and in females from developing countries, with a peak at the end of the 7th decade of life and a decrement thereafter [5].

Between 1990 and 2015, a period that coincides with a remarkable increase in weight excess prevalence, there was a global expansion of the population exposure to the effects of high BMI; the increase was 38.7% and 34.4% for men and women respectively. In a time when other major health risks, as poor sanitation or children undernutrition decreased around 30% in prevalence, such substantial increment was only surpassed by the occupational exposure to some hazards [3].

Not surprisingly, in the period between 2005 and 2015 there was a 19.5% increase of deaths attributable to excess weight and a global 22.0% increase in DALYs [3]. Such figures are even more impressive when one considers the relative position of high BMI as a global risk factor for DALYs. In fact, for both sexes it was ranked 13th in 1990, jumped to 8th in 2005 and reached the 4th position in 2015 [3]. This trend indicates a clear shift of the importance of obesity, further emphasized by the finding that two other metabolism-associated risk factors (high blood pressure and elevated fasting blood glucose) occupied the top five positions as DALYs risk factors [3]. Additional refinement of the data shows that excess weight is number one risk factor for DALYs in small countries of the South Pacific and the Caribbean, but also in populated countries of the North Africa and the Middle East [3].

Obesity is an important risk factor for the development of chronic and deadly disorders as cardiovascular diseases (CVDs) *per se*, type 2 diabetes *mellitus* and its associated morbidities, and cancer [7 - 10]. Moreover, the relative risk of death from all causes and from CVDs increases steadily in association with excess weight measured by BMI from the age of 30 up to 74 [7]. Interestingly, for the same BMI, the relative risk decreases along ageing [7].

Therefore, in time, the exposure of the population to excess weight results in a permanent burden of morbidity that is imposed on the patients, their families and the health services. The issue is specifically relevant in children and adolescents because becoming obese at those earlier ages results in more intense and lasting harmful health consequences, including death [11]. Altogether, the increase in obesity prevalence «represents a truly staggering change in human physic and functional capacity» and is «possibly the greatest driver to change that public health has ever met» [12].

In this setting, the concerns on the global weight excess rise cannot be overlooked at all and are indeed an issue of major medical and social importance.

ADIPOSE TISSUE PROPERTIES

The adipose tissue is distributed throughout the body. Structural and functional properties underlie a major distinction between brown and white adipose tissue [13]. Firstly, we will focus on white adipose tissue referred as WAT. It comprises a subcutaneous component, including the breast-related WAT, and the visceral WAT, that envelopes the abdominal viscera and heart, fills the spaces between muscles and surrounds vessels in their trajectories [13].

Irrespective of the localization, the WAT is mainly composed of adipocytes, characterized by their impressive content in cytoplasmic triglyceride (TG) containing lipid droplets. However, specialization in accumulation and breakdown of TG when needed is not the single role of adipocytes. In fact, the WAT has endocrine characteristics, on account of the variety of adipokines it synthesizes and secretes to the circulation to act at distant sites. In addition, the WAT includes other cells, as vascular cells, monocytes, macrophages and lymphocytes that support the view that it is also involved in inflammatory responses [10].

Among the adipokines stands the WAT-exclusive adiponectin [14], which is secreted by differentiated adipocytes and functions as a positive modulator of insulin by affecting glucose uptake and fatty acid mobilization in conditions of insulin resistance; interestingly, the transductive pathway, that is activated following adiponectin binding to receptors in liver and muscle, enhances the expression of adaptor protein, phosphotyrosine interacting with PH domain and leucine zipper 1 (APPL1), a protein that intervenes in the insulin transductive pathway. Serum adiponectin is reduced in established metabolic syndrome [15, 16]. In contrast, circulating adiponectin level increases with age and, significantly, in nonagerians and centenarians [17]; in addition, when obese individuals lose weight adiponectin increase is noticed [18].

Leptin is another important modulator originated mostly at the subcutaneous WAT, which acts centrally through receptors localized at the hypothalamus; when these receptors are activated, satiety is perceived. In general, serum leptin levels appear to parallel BMI along ageing and do not change significantly, unless weight changes occur. Centenarians, who have low weight, exhibit the lowest levels of leptin [19], whereas in obese individuals, the leptin values tend to be higher [20].

The WAT is also source of adipsin, a protease involved in the complement system activation [21], and other important proteins as angiotensinogen, plasminogen activator inhibitor type 1 (PAI1), tumor necrosis factor alpha (TNFα), interleukin 6 (IL6) and retinol-binding protein 4 (RBP4). They target a variety of biological processes that include satiety, energy and metabolism regulation, angiogenesis and coagulation [22, 23].

Most cells present in the WAT are thus adipocytes, but an important proportion of them are preadipocytes, which appear to derive from multipotent mesenchymal stem cells [24]. Preadipocytes proliferate in response to unknown stimuli that involves the activation of the peroxisome proliferator-activated receptor gamma, in a fashion that relates to local WAT conditions and particular preadipocytes properties [24]. In addition, preadipocytes differentiate into the TG-containing adipocytes as a result of stimulation by insulin-like growth factor 1 (IGF1) and other signals [25].

Based on imagiological patterns and topographical criteria, body WAT has been classified as subcutaneous and internal [26]. The majority of the internal WAT is composed of visceral WAT that surrounds the abdominal hollow organs and extends to the mesentery, the omentum and the WAT accompanying the retroperitoneal space. The subcutaneous WAT refers largely to the superficial WAT; on the subcutaneous compartment, it is also frequent to refer an upper body (abdominal) and a lower body (gluteofemoral) WAT [26].

The distinction between superficial and deep subcutaneous WAT is not only topography-related; the data referred above support the view that such anatomical differences reflect functional aspects.

In fact, in men and women with normal weight, visceral WAT stores dietary fatty acids more efficiently than abdominal subcutaneous WAT, and even more efficiently when comparing with gluteal and femoral compartments [24]. In individuals who are obese, those differences in storage ability are more marked, as occurs in women whose lower body depots are more important targets for fatty acid storage and WAT expansion [27]. In fasting periods, fatty acid release from the WAT is greater in the upper body compartment compared to the lower body. When insulin is administered, the fatty acid release suppression is stronger at the lower body, compared to the upper body, whereas visceral WAT appears to resist insulin antilipolytic effect, thus resulting in enhanced TG breakdown and fatty acid release to the circulation [24, 27].

Adipocytes in the visceral WAT are larger than adipocytes from other locations; they also exhibit decreased secretion of adiponectin [28], synthesis of adiponectin receptor protein 1 (AdipoR1) [29] and leptin [30]. In contrast, there is enhanced expression of proinflammatory cytokines (such as IL6) [31] likely as a result of the higher macrophage concentration in the visceral WAT compared to the subcutaneous compartment [32].

Differences between visceral and subcutaneous WAT may result from different ontological characteristics. In general, cells originated from the subcutaneous WAT proliferate more extensively than those collected from the omentum, eventually because of the presence of a higher % of rapidly replicating cells [33] or the individual variation and different experimental conditions [24]. Fast replicating cells also exhibit higher ability to express adipogenic transcripts [24].

In conditions of overfeeding, the enlargement of the WAT is the likely consequence of cell proliferation instead of hypertrophic accumulation of fat tissue, although both conditions and regional differences may occur. For example, following WAT expansion, in abdominal subcutaneous WAT, the preadipocyte number accompanies the change several fold [34]; moreover, abdominal subcutaneous differentiated adipocytes tend to enlarge whereas thigh differentiated adipocytes preferentially proliferate [35].

In old age, compared to younger individuals, there is a decline in preadipocytes ability to proliferate, which limits expansion of WAT [36], and to perform adipogenesis [37]; in contrast, more inflammatory cytokines are expressed [38], notably IL6 [39], particularly when the metabolic syndrome is present. In this condition, adipocytes from older people have enhanced secretion of C-reactive protein (CRP), IL6, TNFα and leptin as well as reduced adiponectin synthesis

[16]. The inflammatory condition is further intensified in visceral WAT by the enhanced presence of macrophages [40]. The enlargement of adipocytes is also facilitated in elderly owning to the decrease in collagen in the extracellular matrix [41]. In these conditions, the ectopic deposition of fat in tissues, such as muscle or liver, is incremented, which is particularly deleterious in the old individuals [42].

The properties of the WAT at older ages may show unexpected features in individuals undergoing weight variations. In fact, during weight gain, the increase in WAT is substantially higher compared to the increase in lean tissue; during weight loss, the reduction is not as profound as the loss of lean mass [43]. In other words, gaining weight in old age is mostly a gain in WAT whereas losing weight involves lean mass considerably.

Assessing Adiposity

Since long time ago, BMI has been employed to perform a stratification of individuals, distinguishing those who have normal or increased weight. This assessment has worldwide use because it employs simple, easily collectable, biometrical data that one may perceive when looking at the individual under assessment.

As a means to diagnose obesity, BMI would measure the WAT; however, an elevated BMI cannot distinguish between, for example, a non-obese athlete with well-developed muscular tissue, who would have a high BMI. Because it employs two sets of data (weight and height) BMI is also likely to overestimate adiposity of shorter people and to underestimate adiposity in taller people [44]. In addition, a reduction in BMI may reflect skeletal muscle mass loss, and a no-change may associate to muscle mass replacement by WAT [45, 46]. Either the reduction of the stature and the loss of muscle mass are conditions not unusual in old people.

Moreover, it should be emphasized that the commonly used cut-off criteria to categorize BMI have been set mainly to Caucasians and Africans, whereas different cut-offs were proposed for Asian populations [1]. Not unexpectedly, although the specificity may reach values as high as 0.9, the sensitivity was estimated around 0.5 [47].

In the search for another simple method, the measurement of waist circumference (WC) has been credited as more predictive of total body and intra-abdominal adiposity [12, 48, 49]. To refine the assessment of visceral WAT, blood TG determination was further added to WC measurement [50].

In contrast to the standard BMI measurement, that may show a decline after the 7th decade but is likely to underestimate the presence of WAT, the WC measurement continues to increase to peak at 75-80 years of age in men and 70 years in women [51, 52]; such change is accompanied by a decrease of the skinfold thickness in a variety of sites, including the abdomen of both women and men [53].

Age-related WC trend parallels closely the notorious age-related visceral/subcutaneous WAT ratio increase along ageing, from the 3rd to the 8th decades [10]. This finding points to WC as a simple procedure to measure total body and abdominal WAT accumulation [12] although concerns exist regarding the lack of consensus on the precise way to measure it [54].

The implication of the age-related WC and abdominal fat increasing trends, together with the occupation by fat of new territories as the bone marrow, muscle and the liver [22], has important implications, mostly because of the relation between visceral fat and the development of elevated plasma glucose and TG levels, appearance of insulin resistance and the establishment of metabolic disorders [53, 55 - 58]. Reliable data having prognostic value is thus of utmost importance in the assessment of WAT.

Differently from the BMI determination, WAT distribution is a better discriminator in predicting metabolic disorders [23] and, in this context, visceral WAT stands as cause for abdominal obesity-related metabolic risk even in non-obese subjects [59, 60]. Individuals with increased visceral and deep subcutaneous WAT have a poorer insulin response upon stimulation with glucose [61]. Additional features usually associated to insulin resistance were observed in association with the deep subcutaneous WAT in contrast to superficial WAT further suggesting the similarity with visceral WAT [61].

To estimate body composition and WAT distribution, quantitative methods were proposed. They may be simple biometrical measurements as those underlying BMI, or may be technologically complex or time-consuming assessments, as those employing computerized tomography, magnetic resonance imaging, underwater weighing, deuterium dilution, dual-energy X-ray absorptiometry and bioelectrical impedance analysis. Unfortunately, most of these procedures cannot be applied on a large scale basis and a 'gold-standard' reference method has not yet been established [54]. So, in this setting, WC measurement remains a better predictor of metabolic risk, compared with BMI [10, 62].

While a large amount of studies associate obesity or overweight with the risk to develop a variety of metabolic disorders and their morbid features, a report in the late 1990s showed that in patients with chronic kidney disease on dialysis, overweight associated with reduced 1-year mortality, compared to those who had «healthy» weight [63]. Similar associations were found in other disorders as cancer, heart failure, coronary artery disease and hypertension, which led to the coinage of the expression «obesity paradox» [64].

These puzzling observations are controversial and have been the subject of much attention. Part of the explanation for the finding may stem at the controversy regarding the value of BMI to assess one's WAT and resulting metabolic risk, referred above in this text. It has been noticed that a number of individuals, whose prevalence is estimated in ~8%, who have BMI at the normal range have «unhealthy» metabolic markers as elevated blood pressure, plasma TG, fasting plasma glucose and CRP values; in contrast, other individuals (~28% of prevalence) are considered «metabolically healthy» although they are classified as overweight or obese according to the BMI criteria [65].

In another explanation, it was suggested that some excess of WAT, *i.e.*, cell TG might provide some protection. In fact, manipulated yeast strains with increased TG content presented an extended chronological lifespan [66] by a mechanism apparently independent of energy metabolism. Lipid droplets, where TG are stored, physically interact with organelles involved in the elimination of reactive oxygen species (ROS) and their radicalized derivatives; thus, their presence endows cells with a conserved prosurvival mechanism to cope with age-related oxidative damage by acting as a «radical sink» [66].

An important part of the criticism on the results supporting the «obesity paradox» relates to inadequate sampling of patients. In the case of old patients, a reduction in weight to normal range may be part of a decline in weight that frequently is noticed in older people before death because of the progress of an underlying disease [67].

Recent assessments were not able to further clarify this controversy. In a meta-analysis of studies comprising near 3 million individuals, higher mortality was found in grades 2 and 3 of obesity (BMI ≥ 35 kg/m^2), but not in grade 1 (BMI of 30 to < 35 kg/m^2), when compared to normal weight; interestingly, overweight (BMI of 25 to < 30 kg/m^2) associated to lower mortality [9]. In another study with near 4 million individuals from various parts of the world, with a follow-up of weight variation for 5 years and exclusion of smokers, there was a positive association of overweight and obesity to all-cause mortality [67].

Apart from maintaining the controversy, the studies evidence two important aspects under current discussion: the questionable value of BMI in the prognostic assessment of overweight and obesity, and the need to carefully set the criteria for patient recruitment.

The Peculiar Case of Menopause

Menopause, the last menses episode, is an event that results from the cessation of the ovulation, itself consequent to critical reduction of ovarian follicles. The median age at menopause in white women of western industrialized societies is between 50 and 52 years [68], a time that is well behind what one usually calls ageing but, in fact, it is the result of the reproductive ageing. An important additional change is the lack of cyclical estradiol synthesis and secretion by granulosa cells consequent to follicle loss.

A recurrent issue is whether menopause causes increase in weight or induces obesity. To ascertain that would require the verification of a postmenopausal notorious increase in weight, compared to a time immediately antedating menopause. That is not the case [5] and the increase in weight by that age should be regarded as part of the BMI trend along ageing.

Nevertheless, there is an important change in the body composition. Similarly to ageing that associates to an increase in visceral adiposity, menopause is accompanied by an increase in overall adiposity [69] at the expense of lean mass [44]. Menopause is thus peculiar in the sense that WAT composition can change without major net effect on the body weight or BMI.

Another menopause-related modification is the WAT pattern distribution. In reproductive age women there is a preponderance of WAT in gluteal and femoral areas irrespective of changes in BMI [70], which contrasts with men who tend to accumulate WAT in the abdomen [71]. Gluteofemoral WAT in women has smaller adipocytes, compared to visceral WAT, uptakes more free fatty acids and synthesizes more TG, thus resulting in gluteofemoral fat growth [44]; the finding of an important expression of Homeobox family genes involved in cell differentiation was reported in the gluteofemoral WAT, suggesting the existence of a local regulation of WAT [72]. Interestingly, population studies indicated that the gluteofemoral WAT does not contribute to an adverse metabolic profile; actually, it associates with a protective role [73, 74].

By menopause and the following time, there is a change in the external habit implying a shift in predominance from the previous gluteofemoral WAT into abdominal WAT. In fact, imagiological studies provide support to such change, that it is irrespective of the previous weight [75 - 78]. There is thus the acquisition of an android external habit and an age-related increase of adipocyte size [10].

Beyond a variety of genetic or environmental or lifestyle conditions contributing to the postmenopausal changes in WAT, a major factor is the reduction in estrogen synthesis and secretion to the circulation [79]. Estrogen is a recognized regulator of the WAT. Its level in the premenopausal women has been inversely associated to BMI [80], which is likely related to the effect on the WAT: inhibition of transcription of genes that favor lipid storage and activation of enzymes involved in lipolysis that lead to adipocyte size reduction [81]. Interestingly, the consequences of substantial reduction of estrogen may be noticed in the setting of transsexual change. When a female-to-male change occurs, administration of testosterone that adds to the estrogen reduction, results in redistribution from the gluteofemoral to abdominal areas [82]. Moreover, the use of estrogen replacement therapy for menopause, by itself does not cause weight increase [44, 83]; in contrast, it may have beneficial effects on the body WAT composition and mitigate the risk of progress of CVDs [84 - 86] already noticed in pre-menopausal women [87].

Genetics of Obesity and Longevity

Genetic variants may contribute to life expectancy and particularly to exceptional longevity [88]. The most convincing correlation (negative correlation) was found between increased longevity and carriers of apolipoprotein E4 (*APOE*4) allele, which strongly decreases the prevalence of cardiovascular and Alzheimer diseases [89]. In addition, longitudinal analysis demonstrated an association between increased longevity in humans and genetic variation in the TERC locus of the telomerase gene, and in the genes that codify Mn-superoxide dismutase and glutathione peroxidase (GPx) 1. For these genes, encoding proteins protecting against ROS, a synergistic effect was observed for specific polymorphisms [90, 91]. Other gene variants were also reported to be associated with human longevity but studies across populations failed to demonstrate consistent replication of results.

Obesity, on the other hand, is mainly associated with the excessive ingestion of high-fat and high-sugar diets together with sedentarism. However, genetic factors contribute to the variability in BMI. In a recently published genome-wide association study, which enrolled nearly 340000 individuals, 97 BMI-associated *loci* were identified, 56 of which for the first time. These *loci* may account for 2.7% of the individual variation in BMI in a cumulative fashion, which suggests that as much as 21% of BMI variation can be justified by genetic features [92]. Conversely, 5 genetic *loci* associated with lean body mass were also identified [93].

Effects of Obesity in Senescent Cells

The process of ageing of tissues depends not only of senescence of the cells that constitute the tissues, but also of stem cell exhaustion and altered cellular communication [94]. Senescent cells present common features, including genomic instability, telomere attrition, epigenetic alterations and loss of mechanisms of proteostasis and autophagy, resulting in the accumulation of damaged DNA and dysfunctional proteins. In a setting of obesity, these mechanisms suffer modifications that often accelerate age-related dysfunction and that seriously intervene in the regulation of the whole organisms.

Autophagy

DNA, especially of long-lived postmitotic cells, tends to accumulate damage along ageing caused by the exposure to oxidative conditions that affect mitochondrial and nuclear genomes, and by exogenous contributors, such as ultra-violet radiation or mutagenic molecules. Damage persists because DNA repair mechanisms and autophagic activity loose efficiency in senescent cells [95, 96]. Autophagy, the mechanism of intracellular digestion of damaged molecules, essential in the cell survival in conditions of nutrient restriction, is also affected by obesity. The link between autophagy and obesity is complex and tissue-specific. Indeed, the repression of autophagy, by knock-down of gene *Atg*7 in the hypothalamus, leads to the development of obesity and type 2 diabetes *mellitus*, but impedes obesity progression when deleted in adipose tissue of mice [97]. Interestingly, in *Atg*7-/- animals, WAT presents cells with features of brown adipocytes [98], which contribute to an elevated rate of fatty acid beta-oxidation and an increment in lean body mass. Corroborating this duality in the crosstalk between autophagy and obesity, it was demonstrated that autophagy in adipocytes of obese men in the 5th and 6th decades of life was upregulated comparatively to controls [99], but impaired in skeletal muscle of aged overweight individuals (BMI of 28 kg/m^2 in average). Overweight also associated with an increase in endoplasmic reticulum stress in these patients [100]. Taken together, these findings suggest that the role of obesity on the regulation of autophagy is age and tissue-dependent and that downregulation of autophagy in WAT intervenes in the regulation of obesity.

Epigenetics

Epigenetic modifications refer to mechanisms not related to DNA nucleotide sequence that intervene in the regulation of gene expression at the transcriptional level. These modifications that include DNA methylation, post-translational histone modifications and non-coding microRNAs (miRNAs), are often heritable by cell division but are potentially affected by environmental factors and modified along life. Many factors, such as nutritional, inflammatory, level of physical activity and age-induced changes influence the epigenome. In addition, the fact that epigenetic alterations are not permanent, may vary among tissues and may either be causal or arise as a consequence of disease, needs to be considered.

Along ageing epigenetic marks modify, a process named epigenetic drift. Epigenetic drift is variable among individuals of the same age, including siblings, and in the same individual occurs in a cell- and tissue-specific manner [101]. The crosstalk between ageing and obesity in each group of epigenetic modifications is discussed below.

DNA Methylation

DNA methylation is an easily accessible epigenetic marker and several studies demonstrated that methylation pattern varies with age and obesity. Most of them were carried out in white blood cells, but despite the tissue-specificity of the epigenome, Ronn *et al* demonstrated that methylation biomarkers in blood mirror those found in adipose tissue [102, 103].

Ageing leads to modification in DNA methylation with a generalized decrease in genome-wide methylated bases, and a disproportional methylation of the CpG islands, which represses expression of genes regulated by this type of promoters (that include most of the house-keeping genes essential for normal cell functions). In fact, it was demonstrated that near 90% of the studied CpG sites showed a positive correlation between methylation level and age in the adipose tissue of 96 men [102]. In addition, along ageing the variability of methylation pattern of the genome tends to increase. Data regarding association between obesity (BMI) and methylation pattern did not match variation with age, particularly when focused on single CpG site hypo- or hypermethylation events [102]. On the other hand, Nevailen *et al* demonstrated that obesity accelerates epigenetic ageing in blood cells until middle-age, based on simultaneous analysis of multiple CpG sites [104], and Horvath *et al* found that obesity accelerates ageing of liver in average 3.3 years for 10 BMI units, based on DNA methylation analysis [105]. A recently published epigenome-wide association study of BMI demonstrated that the alterations found in DNA methylation in individuals with high BMI are predominantly the consequence of adiposity rather than the cause [103] the authors found that with enhanced adiposity, the methylation *loci* are enriched for functional genomic features in multiple tissues and mainly in genes involved in lipid and lipoprotein metabolism, substrate transport and inflammatory pathways. For the majority of tissues, however, the effect of obesity in DNA methylation appears to have less impact than ageing, but is still a contributor [106, 107]. In fact, in the same individuals, bariatric surgery results in variation of methylation markers in blood, liver and adipose tissue [108 for review], which agrees with previous evidence that nutritional intervention, such as energy restriction, or exercise mediate epigenetic modulation [109].

On the other hand, in special conditions, methylation pattern changes may be the cause of the obesity phenotype whereby methylation of a specific region of chromosome 15 is likely to induce sporadic Prader-Willi syndrome cases, characterized by insatiable-hyperphagia and obesity [110].

The activity of DNA methyltransferase (Dnmt) 1, the enzyme that catalyzes maintenance methylation of C bases, decreases in senescent cells while other Dnmts involved in *de novo* methylation of bases may increase their activity, justifying reduced genome-wide methylation associated with regional or gene-localized hypermethylation in ageing cells [111]. A study carried out in a large sample of european individuals demonstrated that the expression of both Dnmt1 and Dnmt3b (a *de novo* methyltransferase) decline with ageing in peripheral blood mononuclear cells. A positive correlation between Dnmt3b expression and BMI was found in this study [112].

Post-Translational Histone Modifications

Histones are basic proteins that with DNA double-helix chain assist the formation of nucleosomes. Each nucleosome includes two copies of each of the four histones H2A, H2B, H3 and H4. Histones possess peptide tails that protrude from nucleosome core and often suffer post-translational modifications, such as methylation, acetylation and phosphorylation, catalyzed by enzymes so distinct as histone methyltransferases, histone demethylases, histone acetyltransferases or histone deacetylases. Histone modifications are copied from one cell generation to the next and modify the accessibility of genes, and respective regulatory sequences, to the enzymes that catalyze their transcription. Despite the overall age-related effect on histone modifications is far from being clarified, a specific decrease of lysine methylation in H3 and an increase in methylation and acetylation of H4 have been associated with ageing. These modifications impair transcription and DNA repair and contribute to age-related chromosome instability [94]. Interestingly, some of these age-dependent histone post-translational modifications were identified in hepatic cellular senescence pathways genes in a diet-induced obesity rat model when treated with high-fat diet [113]. On the other hand, it was demonstrated that mice deficient in JHDM2A (JmjC-domain-containing histone demethylase 2A) present high-levels of histone H3 methylated in lysine 9 (that decreases along ageing) and manifest obesity and metabolic dysfunction [114]. These data evidence that epigenetic markers, including histone post-translational modifications, affect gene expression in a complex pattern that results from the intervention of multiple factors.

Sirtuins

Among the enzymes that intervene in the post-translational modifications of histones, mammalian sirtuins (SIRT1–7) play an important role. SIRTs are members of the class III of NAD$^+$-dependent deacetylases and belong to a family of seven enzyme orthologs of the silent information regulator 2 (Sir2) of the yeast [115]. In the yeast, Sir2 extends replicative lifespan, silences genes by histone deacetylation and enables DNA repair. In mammals, expression of sirtuins is tissue-specific [116], presents differentiated cellular locations and affects a broad range of cellular functions, but, so far, no role in lifespan regulation for any sirtuin was found, excepting for SIRT3, considered an important tumor suppressor in human cancers [117].

SIRT1, 2, 3 and 6 are those that catalyze deacetylation of histones, promoting the formation of heterochromatin and the repression of gene expression [118, 119 for review]. Histone H4 acetylated in lysine 16 (H4K16ac) is a chief substrate for the SIRT1 and the age-related generalized increase of H4K16ac reflects the decrease in deacetylation activity.

Interestingly, novel evidence suggests that the mammalian sirtuins crosstalk inside the cells and cooperate in the molecular responses to spontaneous acetylations in organelles and in the responses to the nutritional status [120]. In fact, SIRT1, 2, 3 and 6 are upregulated in conditions of nutrient deprivation [119]. Energy restriction is a well-recognized non-pharmacological intervention to prolong lifespan [119], in part through SIRT1 activation. Moreover, by transcriptional analysis of genes included in the functional categories of mitochondrial energy metabolism, inflammation and ribosomal structure it was recently demonstrated that SIRT3 intervenes in a mechanism to delay ageing and reduce age-related disease vulnerability. This transcriptional signature is reversed with consumption of a high-fat diet, obesity and metabolic diseases [121].

Among the anti-ageing, protective actions of sirtuins, both SIRT6 and 1 intervene in DNA repair contributing to the maintenance of genomic stability [122, 123]. Additionally, SIRT1 positively regulates autophagy [124] and induces post-translational modification of transcription factors, such as those of FOXO family, which regulate responses to oxidative stress [125, 126]. Moreover, both SIRT2 and 3 participate in the regulation of antioxidant defenses [127]. SIRT3, in particular, reduces free radical levels, improves thermogenesis regulation [128] and upregulates the mitochondrial glutathione antioxidant defense system [129], Mn-superoxide dismutase [130] and catalase [131]. Concerning cell survival and senescence, SIRT1 down-regulates p53, what increases cell survival [132] and deacetylates NF-κB (what in turn suppresses the ability of NF-κB to activate pro-inflammatory transcriptional targets), and even promotes cell apoptosis in stressful conditions [133].

The whole expression of SIRT1 presents an age-dependent tissue related pattern.

In particular, SIRT1 activity tends to decrease with ageing in liver, heart, kidney and lung of the rat owing to the decreased bioavailability of NAD^+ [134]. As well, obesity strongly affects the expression of sirtuins in adipose-derived stem cells in visceral WAT, considering that in obese patients a significant down-regulation of all the sirtuins, excepting SIRT7, was found [135]. This finding is consistent with protective effects of sirtuins, including SIRT3, against visceral obesity and inflammation. In addition, SIRT1 apparently protects from brown adipose tissue degeneration that causes diet-induced obesity and insulin resistance in mouse [136] and inhibits hyperplasia of adipocytes [137].

The NAD^+ dependence of sirtuins strongly links their activity to the metabolic state of the cell, creating thus an intricate connection between acetylation/deacetylation, energetic state and gene expression [138]. It was recently demonstrated that SIRT1 affects DNA methylation in genes responsive to the nutritional status [139], suggesting a crosstalk between DNA methylation and histone modifications in the dietary- and age- dependent regulatory mechanisms.

Non-coding MicroRNAs

Non-coding miRNAs are a class of endogenous, 21 to 25 nucleotides long and single-stranded RNA molecules that constitute an additional mechanism of post-transcriptional regulation of gene expression.

Maturation of miRNAs is a multistep process: after being transcribed in the nucleus by RNA polymerase II or III, the primary transcripts are recognized and processed by the Drosha complex that contains a RNase III enzyme and the resultant 70 nucleotide excised hairpins are delivered to the cytosol by a process mediated by exportin-5. In the cytosol the precursors of functional miRNAs suffer an additional cleavage by the Dicer complex before integrating the RNA-induced silencing complex (RISC) and targeting the specific mRNAs to silence [140]. The base pairing between target mRNA and miRNA takes place mainly in the mRNA's 3'-untranslated region (UTR) but sometimes also occurs in coding regions or 5'-UTR. Base-pairing leads to translation repression, mRNA degradation or both, depending on both the miRNA that binds and its concentration. Each mRNA transcription can be regulated by multiple miRNAs and also each miRNA can base-pair with several mRNAs strongly increasing the complexity of the regulation of gene expression mediated by this epigenetic mechanism [140].

Globally, miRNAs expression is decreased during cellular senescence [141]. Considering that the main function of miRNAs is to repress the translation of target mRNAs, this may contribute to protein accumulation during cellular senescence. Several miRNAs are differentially expressed across various tissues during ageing [140] and also in response to diet or obesity [142 - 144], but the specific functions of many of these miRNAs are still unknown. Among the miRNAs that vary with ageing, Kim *et al* selected six (miRNA-16-5p, miRNA-130a-3p, miRNA-17-5p, miRNA-103-3p, miRNA-30c-5p, and miRNA-21a-5p), normally down-regulated in blood and liver in the elderly, and transfected old mice with them. The authors observed a reversed regulation of ageing-associated pathways, demonstrating the importance of miRNAs in the ageing mechanisms [145]. MiRNAs can affect other mechanisms of epigenetic regulation, as recently suggested after demonstration that miRNA-217 modulates human skin fibroblast senescence by directly targeting Dnmt1 [146].

Although most of the miRNAs are downregulated, miRNA-34 is upregulated in ageing [140] and in the liver of high-fat induced obese mice [147]. The authors also demonstrated that miRNA-34 reduces bioavailability of NAD^+ and SIRT1 activity and expression [140], which contributes to the ageing phenotype of the individuals.

The evidence for an association between miRNA variation with obesity and ageing is weak, not only because of the small number of studies, particularly in humans, but also because of the intervention of each miRNA in several mechanisms. Thus, currently miRNAs are considered biomarkers of ageing or disease, but not yet potential therapeutic targets.

Telomere Attrition

The shortening of the telomeres, specialized non-coding repetitive DNA-protein structures found at the ends of eukaryotic chromosomes, is a consequence of the successive cell divisions, considering that the replication of the lagging strand of the DNA of each chromosome is incomplete in the absence of active telomerase. Somatic cells in general do not possess it and thus divide a limited number of times before entering in replicative senescence. Telomere attrition is a marker of senescent cells that proportionally increase in the tissues of aged individuals [94]. Besides ageing, several diseases characterized by an increase in oxidative stress and inflammation, including obesity, aggravate loss of telomeres [148, 149]. In fact, the extension of the telomeres is inversely correlated with adiposity and BMI [150] and additionally an inverse association between visceral adiposity and presence of other partners of metabolic syndrome and telomerase activity was demonstrated in blood cells of women [151]. Corroborating this finding, the obesity phenotype has been associated with shorter telomeres in women [152].

In sum, telomere length is a biological marker for age and for stress-related conditions. Another conclusion that one can take on this evidence is that obesity may accelerate the ageing process through the shortening of the telomeres.

INTERVENTION FOR OBESITY IN ELDERLY

Among the interventions available to mitigate effects of obesity in the elderly summarized in Table **1**, the best strategy is a balanced diet, with an appropriated content of macro- and micronutrients adjusted to each individual, as well as a special concern with the health problems that often develop along ageing and prudent use of the medication prescribed for their control. Nutritional intervention could avoid the onset and progression of obesity, especially if associated with regular practice of physical exercise [153 for review].

Table 1. Interventions for obesity in elderly.

Intervention /compound	Food	Outcomes in cells/animals	Outcomes in humans	Ref.
Avoidance of added sugars	Artificially sweetened foods	Added sugars lead to: ⇑ Oxidative stress ⇑Glycation of proteins ⇑Inflammation Dyslipidemia Insulin resistance ⇑Age-associated diseases	Added sugars lead to: ⇑Glycation of proteins ⇑Inflammation Dyslipidemia Insulin resistance ⇑Age-associated diseases	[154]
Avoidance of dietary AGE	High-temperature cooked foods, caramel, cola and other browned foods	AGE from food lead to: ⇑Oxidative stress ⇑Glycation of proteins ⇑Inflammation Age-associated diseases	AGE from food lead to: ⇑Oxidative stress ⇑Glycation of proteins ⇑Inflammation Age-associated diseases	[155, 156]
Bariatric surgery	-	-	⇓Body weight	[159]
Resveratrol	Grapes, red wine, peanuts, berries	⇓Adipocyte differentiation Inhibits adipogenesis Induction of WAT browning Regulate BAT activity ⇑Sirtuin 1 expression Delay in mice's mortality ⇓Ectopic adiposity in mice	No effect in BMI in humans	[169, 174, 175, 204, 205]

(Table 1) cont.....

Intervention /compound	Food	Outcomes in cells/animals	Outcomes in humans	Ref.
Curcumin	Turmeric	Inhibits adipogenesis Induction of WAT browning ⇑Body temperature of mice Mechanisms independent of those activated by energy restriction	No effect in BMI in humans	[169, 187]
EGCG	Green tea	Inhibits DNA methyl transferases activity	⇓BMI and waist circumference of elderly patients ⇓Lipid peroxidation	[181, 183 - 185]
Isoflavones/ Genistein	Soy beans, broad beans	⇑Sirtuin 1 expression Inhibits adipogenesis Regulates BAT activity	⇓Body weight, fat mass and waist circumference Ameliorates blood lipid profile when combined with soy proteins	[169, 189, 190]
Quercetin	Apple, broccoli, onion, leafy vegetable, asparagus, capers, lovage, grapes	Increments thermogenesis in mice Activates sirtuin 1 ⇓Adiposity in mice	⇓BMI and in waist circumference in (APOE)3/3 individuals	[169, 177, 180]
Capsinoids	Chili pepper	Induction of WAT browning	⇑Energy expenditure in BAT- positive individuals under cold exposure	[169]
Cinnamaldehyde	Cinammon	⇓Visceral fat deposition	-	[169]
Fucoxanthin	Brown alga	Ameliorates progression of obesity	Ameliorate progression of obesity	[169]
Metformin	-	Improves healthspan and lifespan ⇓AGE	⇓All-cause mortality in diabetic patients ⇓BMI	[193 - 195, 197]
Pioglitazone	-	⇓AGE Activates telomerase ⇑Sirtuin 1 expression	⇑Subcutaneous body fat, but not visceral fat	[195, 198 - 200]
NDGA	-	⇑Longevity in mice ⇓Body weight in mice	-	[202, 203]
Magnesium	Natural mineralized water, spinach, chard, banana, black beans	Magnesium deficiency increases central obesity in aged rats	Improvement in metabolic parameters and blood pressure	[192]
Beta3-adrenoceptor agonists	-	Induction of WAT browning	-	[165]

(Table 1) cont.....

Intervention /compound	Food	Outcomes in cells/animals	Outcomes in humans	Ref.
Irisin	-	-	Activation of BAT	[166]
FGF21	-	-	Activation of BAT	[166]
Liraglutide	-	Induction of WAT browning ⇩AGE	⇩BMI ⇩Cardiovascular disease risk in type 2 diabetes *mellitus*	[167, 168, 201]

AGE - advanced glycation end-products; BAT - brown adipose tissue; BMI - body mass index; EGCG - epigallocatechin gallate; FGF21 - fibroblast growth factor 21; NDGA - meso-nordihydroguaiaretic acid; Ref - reference; WAT - white adipose tissue.

Nutritional Adjustment

For old people it is not only recommended the inclusion of all the essential nutrients in the diet, preferentially in the form of nutrient-rich foods and not supplements, but also the avoidance of excessive energy intake, to prevent body weight gain, and of foods that contribute to the acceleration of the ageing process. Among these foods, added sugars are particular deleterious [154], considering their intervention in the increase of oxidative stress, protein glycation, inflammation and metabolic dysfunction. The same is true for the consumption of dietary advanced glycation end-products (AGEs) that despite not contributing directly to obesity strongly lead to molecular deterioration in cells. Besides endogenously formed AGEs, diet also represents an important source of these substances, especially if preparation of food was carried out at high temperatures. Browned or caramelized foodstuffs, such as coffee or cola drinks, also have high levels of AGEs that are incorporated into foods for intensifying the natural flavors. In fact, the AGEs content of the Western diet significantly increased in the last 50 years, together with sugars and lipids. This is deleterious to the population, particularly for the older individuals, because it is believed that AGEs from the diet are absorbed and moved into the circulation. In this setting, a strong correlation between AGE consumption and serum levels was demonstrated [155]. Dietary AGEs together with those that form slowly in chronological ageing by non-enzymatic reaction between sugars and proteins accumulate progressively in tissues. AGE modifications occur predominantly on the long-lived proteins, such as those that exist in extracellular matrix that present a slow turnover [156 for review]. It is believed that carbonylated protein and AGE formation are likely to be implicated in the molecular basis of ageing and age-related diseases as suggested by *in silico* approaches [157].

Bariatric Surgery

One of the interventions to treat obesity is bariatric surgery. According to a report of Dorman in 2009, the number of patients aged 65 years or more undergoing bariatric surgery, accounted for 4.8% of total bariatric surgeries in several hospitals in USA [158]. In addition, elderly patients did not experience higher risk of major complications for either open or laparoscopic procedures [159]. Moreover, after body weight reduction, they experienced the equivalent benefits to those observed in younger patients.

Increment in Brown Adipose Tissue

Albeit in low amount in adult and aged individuals, the cells of brown adipose tissue (BAT), also called brite or beige cells, remain in six anatomically distinct depots: cervical, supraclavicular, axillary, paraspinal, mediastinal, and abdominal [160]. They are characterized by multiple lipid droplets and large numbers of mitochondria that use lipids to generate heat. BAT is protective but its responsiveness decreases with obesity and ageing [161]. BAT thermogenesis has been demonstrated to prevent obesity, as observed by Lowell *et al* that generated a model of obese mice after destruction of brown adipocytes [162]. Thus, a possible strategy to mitigate age-associated diseases including obesity would be to increase BAT in old patients and to increase its thermogenic activity. BAT formation can be induced in WAT depots upon cold stimulation [163] and also by administration of an adrenergic stimulant [164]. Therefore, it may be possible to prevent the age-related decrease of BAT content with exogenous interventions, such as treatment with beta3-adrenoceptor agonists [165], irisin, fibroblast growth factor 21 (FGF21) [166] and the glucagon-like peptide 1 (GLP1) analogue liraglutide [167]. Nevertheless, safety of administration of these drugs concomitantly with others, frequently prescribed to old patients, should be carefully considered. Liraglutide seems to have particularly beneficial effects in the prevention of age-associated diseases including obesity [168].

Other strategies, including treatments with natural compounds present in plants used as foods, some of them with potential capability to promote WAT to BAT conversion [169], or drugs, could be employed to control obesity while slowing ageing mechanisms. The plant-derived compounds often possess antioxidant and anti-inflammatory properties, which directly counteract the prooxidant and proinflammatory conditions of the ageing process. In addition, for some of these compounds, stimulatory effect on sirtuins or antiobesity effects, including inhibition of adipocyte differentiation, were demonstrated [119].

Energy Restriction Mimetics

Energy restriction (ER) is an efficient antiobesity and anti-ageing non-pharmacological intervention, however hard to maintain in humans owing to the discomfort and hungry that causes [119]. Thus, researchers identified a group of drugs and natural compounds considered ER mimetics. ER mimetics intervene in the major pathways affected by ER with the intention of obtaining its benefits while avoiding the undesirable side effects of this nutritional regimen. In fact, the ideal ER mimetic should produce metabolic, hormonal and physiological effects similar to those of ER without reducing the food intake and provide beneficial effects on mortality and age-associated diseases [170]. ER mimetics act through different mechanisms, such as weight loss or stimulation of sirtuin activity and epigenetic modifications. We will focus on mimetics that conduce to the decrease in BMI and have potential to be used in elderly patients. Some of them are naturally present in foods and referred as activators of SIRT1, such as unsaturated fatty acids and the polyphenolic compounds quercetin and resveratrol.

Sirtuin Activity Stimulators

Resveratrol

Resveratrol is a polyphenolic phytochemical (3,5,4'-trihydroxystilbene) that occurs naturally in foods, including grapes and red wine [171]. It is a sirtuin activator that increases the secretion of GLP1, and has antidiabetogenic, antiobesity and CVD protective effects [172, 173]. Resveratrol increases longevity and health in mice fed with high-energy diet [174]; however, in humans, the clinical trials employing resveratrol-based treatments have been disappointing, considering the absence of effects on body weight particularly in non-obese individuals [175]. In line, a recently conducted placebo-controlled pilot study that enrolled 32 aged obese patients failed to demonstrate beneficial effects of 300 or 1000 mg/day during 12 weeks in either body weight or metabolic outcomes [176], despite the good tolerance found for resveratrol supplement.

Further studies with a higher number of participants and longer treatment duration with resveratrol are necessary to certify its effects in human age-related diseases and obesity.

Quercetin

Quercetin is a flavonol abundantly found in plant products, such as capers, lovage, apples, onions and grapes, and presents antiadipogenic properties in high-fat treated animals [177]. Similarly to resveratrol, clinical trials failed to demonstrate a clear antiobesity effect of quercetin supplementation either in normal-weight or in overweight and obese subjects [178, 179]. Only a moderate but significant reduction in BMI and in WC was found in homozygous individuals for apolipoprotein E (*APOE*) 3/3 but not in *APOE*4, demonstrating the importance of the genotype in the responsiveness to nutritional modulation [180].

Other Natural Compounds

Cathechins

Catechins are polyphenolic flavonoids that exist in green tea, an infusion prepared from dried leaves of the plant *Camellia sinensis* (Theaceace). Epigallocatechin gallate (EGCG) is the most abundant catechin, and besides being an inhibitor of Dnmt1 [181], reportedly has antiobesity and antiadipogenic effects [119 for review].

The effects of catechins in the control of obesity in human are far from being established. Green tea consumption may contribute to inhibition of the appetite, reducing the ingestion of food and could also intervene in the decreased absorption of nutrients in the gastrointestinal tract, particularly of carbohydrates and probably fat [182]. Despite the benefits in the control of obesity this effect could be deleterious in the aged individuals. In addition, a decrease in the BMI and WC of elderly patients with metabolic syndrome were reported after consumption of green tea for 2 or 3 months [183, 184]. EGCG also led to a reduction in lipid peroxidation [185], indicating amelioration on the oxidative processes characteristic of the ageing phenotype.

Curcumin

Curcumin is a naturally-occurring polyphenol (dyferuloylmethane) found in the Indian spice turmeric that presents very low toxicity.

Concerning human trials, no demonstration of significant influence of curcumin in BMI or total body fat tissue exists [186]. Interestingly, curcumin effect in the organism does not superimpose on the effect of ER [187].

Isoflavones

Isoflavones, such as daidzein, genistein and glycitein, are found in soy and soy products, and could have a beneficial effect on obesity in animals and humans.

Most of the clinical trials were conducted in postmenopausal women, considering the resemblance of isoflavones to endogenous estrogen [188]. It has been demonstrated that soy protein-based meals with high concentration of isoflavones (and not isoflavones alone) not only decrease body weight, fat mass and WC, but also ameliorate the blood lipid profile [189, 190].

Antiobesity Effects of Magnesium

A deficient magnesium status is frequently associated with obesity and with elderly [191]. In fact, a negative association between magnesium intake and central obesity, body fat percentage and BMI was verified in type 2 diabetes *mellitus* patients with 65 years or older [191].

In addition, it was demonstrated that magnesium supplementation leads to an improvement of metabolic disorders and blood pressure, however without decrement in BMI [192]. Despite this, the full extension of the magnesium role in cell and organism metabolisms remains to be elucidated.

Pharmacological Interventions

Obesity is a complex problem, particularly in the elderly. Owing to the lack of clinical studies in this age group and the concomitant diseases that affect old people, the efficacy and safety of supplement or drugs use for weight loss have not been demonstrated in older adults. Thus, the strategies for weight loss should be carefully individualized, and the administration of supplements or drugs must be strictly monitorized for potential toxicity or undesirable effects. Among the drugs that could be safely prescribed to obese aged patients are the oral antidiabetics.

Antidiabetic Drugs

Metformin is currently the oral biguanide most frequently prescribed to hyperglycemic patients. Besides its effects in blood glucose lowering, it was recently demonstrated that metformin improves healthspan and lifespan in mice [193]. In addition, it was reported that metformin is more effective than insulin in reducing all-cause mortality and diabetes-related endpoints in diabetic patients, providing cardiovascular protection independently of its hypoglycemic effects [194]. By reducing glucose in blood, metformin decreases the formation of AGEs [195], a hallmark of cells and tissues in the elderly. Moreover, metformin activates autophagy, a common feature of all ER mimetics [196]. One of the side-effects of metformin treatment is the decrease of body weight, which is of great advantage to obese patients [197].

Pioglitazone is a member of the family of thiazolidinedione compounds used in the treatment of diabetes. Similarly to metformin, it sensitizes peripheral tissues to insulin and inhibits glycation reducing AGEs formation in tissues [195], being thus considered an anti-ageing drug. In addition, pioglitazone activates aortic telomerase [198] and increases mRNA levels of SIRT1 in nondiabetic subjects treated with combined pioglitazone, ephedrine and caffeine [199]. Regarding body weight, pioglitazone increased subcutaneous body fat, but not visceral fat, which implies a metabolic benefit [200].

A new generation of antidiabetics, incretin-related drugs, that include GLP1 analogues, emerges as potential strategies to ameliorate age-related diseases, including obesity [168]. Based on data of the clinical trial (LEADER) that enrolled 9340 type 2 diabetes *mellitus* patients with 50 years or more with high-risk of CVD (that is the main cause of death in the elderly), the authors concluded that liraglutide significantly protects against CV events [201], in part through its anti-glycative effect. As far as we know, GLP1 analogues benefits in aged people remain to be elucidated, but these drugs seem to be promising.

Other Anti-ageing Drugs

One of the anti-ageing novel class of drugs is the group of meso-nordihydroguaiaretic acid (NDGA), a lignin present at high concentrations in *Larrea tridentate*. Besides NDGA effect in the increment of lifespan of male mice [202], a dose-dependent reduction in mice body weight was also evident without change in food intake [203]. While NDGA was not overtly toxic at its therapeutic dosage, less toxic derivatives of NDGA need to be developed for potential use as anti-ageing and antiobesity therapeutics in humans.

CONCLUDING REMARKS

In modern societies, development has mitigated, or even eliminated, previous important health risks, as poor sanitation and nutritional insufficiencies, that still exist in many parts of the world. However, the various aspects of society transition and its accompanying lifestyles may have led to the rise of excess weight and overt obesity. Such finding includes both sexes and all ages because obesity expansion starts in childhood and continues throughout adulthood and old age. While facing these fast growing challenges, objective knowledge is required on both the ageing mechanisms and the consequences of obesity for the individual health, especially on account of life expectancy continued expansion.

Ageing is the accumulation of metabolic errors that results in cell and tissue dysfunction and organism frailty. The effects of ageing in the cells and tissues result in various biological process changes, some of which intensified in the presence of obesity.

Another consequence is the enhancement of metabolism-related disorders; unfortunately, in the coming decades, as the number of obese children increases, modern societies will face enhanced related morbidity when children become adults and these become old individuals.

Functional modulators or therapeutic options have been sought and are under intense assessment. While waiting for their results, actions towards excess weight control are much recommended following middle age, because this is a time when body composition changes considerably due to increment in adipose tissue.

Nowadays, those actions mean the implementation of appropriate physical exercise and nutritional programs. Eventually, they may be the sole approach without significant side effects.

CONSENT FOR PUBLICATION

Not applicable.

CONFLICT OF INTEREST

The authors confirm that this chapter contents have no conflict of interest.

ACKNOWLEDGEMENTS

Declared none.

REFERENCES

[1]   World Health Organization[http://www.who.int/en/]. Health Topics. Body Mass Index – BMI. [cited: September 5th 2017] Available from http://www.who.int/en/http://www.euro.who.int/en/health-topics /disease-prevention/nutrition/a-healthy-lifestyle/body-mass-index-bmi

[2]   World Health Organization[http://www.who.int/en/]. WHO Media Centre. Fact Sheets: Obesity and Overweight. . [cited: September 5th 2017] (Updated June 2016). Available from http://www.who.int/en/http://www.who.int/mediacentre/factsheets/fs311/en/

[3]   Global, regional, and national comparative risk assessment of 79 behavioural, environmental and occupational, and metabolic risks or clusters of risks, 1990-2015: a systematic analysis for the Global Burden of Disease Study 2015. Lancet 2016; 388(10053): 1659-724.
        [http://dx.doi.org/10.1016/S0140-6736(16)31679-8] [PMID: 27733284]

[4]   Swinburn BA, Sacks G, Hall KD, *et al*. The global obesity pandemic: shaped by global drivers and local environments. Lancet 2011; 378(9793): 804-14.
        [http://dx.doi.org/10.1016/S0140-6736(11)60813-1] [PMID: 21872749]

[5]   Ng M, Fleming T, Robinson M, *et al*. Global, regional, and national prevalence of overweight and obesity in children and adults during 1980-2013: a systematic analysis for the Global Burden of Disease Study 2013. Lancet 2014; 384(9945): 766-81.
        [http://dx.doi.org/10.1016/S0140-6736(14)60460-8] [PMID: 24880830]

[6]   Rokholm B, Baker JL, Sørensen TI. The levelling off of the obesity epidemic since the year 1999--a review of evidence and perspectives. Obes Rev 2010; 11(12): 835-46.
        [http://dx.doi.org/10.1111/j.1467-789X.2010.00810.x] [PMID: 20973911]

[7]   Stevens J, Cai J, Pamuk ER, Williamson DF, Thun MJ, Wood JL. The effect of age on the association between body-mass index and mortality. N Engl J Med 1998; 338(1): 1-7.
        [http://dx.doi.org/10.1056/NEJM199801013380101] [PMID: 9414324]

[8]   Guh DP, Zhang W, Bansback N, Amarsi Z, Birmingham CL, Anis AH. The incidence of co-morbidities related to obesity and overweight: a systematic review and meta-analysis. BMC Public Health 2009; 9: 88.
        [http://dx.doi.org/10.1186/1471-2458-9-88] [PMID: 19320986]

[9]   Flegal KM, Kit BK, Orpana H, Graubard BI. Association of all-cause mortality with overweight and obesity using standard body mass index categories: a systematic review and meta-analysis. JAMA 2013; 309(1): 71-82.
[http://dx.doi.org/10.1001/jama.2012.113905] [PMID: 23280227]

[10]   Tchernof A, Després JP. Pathophysiology of human visceral obesity: an update. Physiol Rev 2013; 93(1): 359-404.
[http://dx.doi.org/10.1152/physrev.00033.2011] [PMID: 23303913]

[11]   Must A, Jacques PF, Dallal GE, Bajema CJ, Dietz WH. Long-term morbidity and mortality of overweight adolescents. A follow-up of the Harvard Growth Study of 1922 to 1935. N Engl J Med 1992; 327(19): 1350-5.
[http://dx.doi.org/10.1056/NEJM199211053271904] [PMID: 1406836]

[12]   Han TS, Tajar A, Lean ME. Obesity and weight management in the elderly. Br Med Bull 2011; 97: 169-96.
[http://dx.doi.org/10.1093/bmb/ldr002] [PMID: 21325341]

[13]   Cohen P, Spiegelman BM. Cell biology of fat storage. Mol Biol Cell 2016; 27(16): 2523-7.
[http://dx.doi.org/10.1091/mbc.e15-10-0749] [PMID: 27528697]

[14]   Ruan H, Dong LQ. Adiponectin signaling and function in insulin target tissues. J Mol Cell Biol 2016; 8(2): 101-9.
[http://dx.doi.org/10.1093/jmcb/mjw014] [PMID: 26993044]

[15]   Lim S, Yoon JW, Choi SH, *et al.* Combined impact of adiponectin and retinol-binding protein 4 on metabolic syndrome in elderly people: the Korean Longitudinal Study on Health and Aging. Obesity (Silver Spring) 2010; 18(4): 826-32.
[http://dx.doi.org/10.1038/oby.2009.232] [PMID: 19661959]

[16]   Stenholm S, Koster A, Alley DE, *et al.* Adipocytokines and the metabolic syndrome among older persons with and without obesity: the InCHIANTI study. Clin Endocrinol (Oxf) 2010; 73(1): 55-65.
[PMID: 19878507]

[17]   Atzmon G, Pollin TI, Crandall J, *et al.* Adiponectin levels and genotype: a potential regulator of life span in humans. J Gerontol A Biol Sci Med Sci 2008; 63(5): 447-53.
[http://dx.doi.org/10.1093/gerona/63.5.447] [PMID: 18511746]

[18]   Yang WS, Lee WJ, Funahashi T, *et al.* Weight reduction increases plasma levels of an adipose-derived anti-inflammatory protein, adiponectin. J Clin Endocrinol Metab 2001; 86(8): 3815-9.
[http://dx.doi.org/10.1210/jcem.86.8.7741] [PMID: 11502817]

[19]   Baranowska B, Bik W, Baranowska-Bik A, *et al.* Neuroendocrine control of metabolic homeostasis in Polish centenarians. J Physiol Pharmacol 2006; 57 (Suppl. 6): 55-61.
[PMID: 17228087]

[20]   Isidori AM, Strollo F, Morè M, *et al.* Leptin and aging: correlation with endocrine changes in male and female healthy adult populations of different body weights. J Clin Endocrinol Metab 2000; 85(5): 1954-62.
[http://dx.doi.org/10.1210/jcem.85.5.6572] [PMID: 10843181]

[21]   Schleinitz D. Genetic Determination of Serum Levels of Diabetes-Associated Adipokines. Rev Diabet Stud 2015; 12(3-4): 277-98.
[http://dx.doi.org/10.1900/RDS.2015.12.277] [PMID: 26859657]

[22]   Tchkonia T, Morbeck DE, Von Zglinicki T, *et al.* Fat tissue, aging, and cellular senescence. Aging Cell 2010; 9(5): 667-84.
[http://dx.doi.org/10.1111/j.1474-9726.2010.00608.x] [PMID: 20701600]

[23]   Wronska A, Kmiec Z. Structural and biochemical characteristics of various white adipose tissue depots. Acta Physiol (Oxf) 2012; 205(2): 194-208.
[http://dx.doi.org/10.1111/j.1748-1716.2012.02409.x] [PMID: 22226221]

[24]   Tchkonia T, Thomou T, Zhu Y, *et al.* Mechanisms and metabolic implications of regional differences among fat depots. Cell Metab 2013; 17(5): 644-56.
[http://dx.doi.org/10.1016/j.cmet.2013.03.008] [PMID: 23583168]

[25]   Cristancho AG, Lazar MA. Forming functional fat: a growing understanding of adipocyte differentiation. Nat Rev Mol Cell Biol 2011; 12(11): 722-34.
[http://dx.doi.org/10.1038/nrm3198] [PMID: 21952300]

[26]   Shen W, Wang Z, Punyanita M, *et al.* Adipose tissue quantification by imaging methods: a proposed classification. Obes Res 2003; 11(1): 5-16.
[http://dx.doi.org/10.1038/oby.2003.3] [PMID: 12529479]

[27]   Guo Z, Hensrud DD, Johnson CM, Jensen MD. Regional postprandial fatty acid metabolism in different obesity phenotypes. Diabetes 1999; 48(8): 1586-92.
[http://dx.doi.org/10.2337/diabetes.48.8.1586] [PMID: 10426377]

[28]   Drolet R, Bélanger C, Fortier M, *et al.* Fat depot-specific impact of visceral obesity on adipocyte adiponectin release in women. Obesity (Silver Spring) 2009; 17(3): 424-30.
[http://dx.doi.org/10.1038/oby.2008.555] [PMID: 19219061]

[29]   Rasmussen MS, Lihn AS, Pedersen SB, Bruun JM, Rasmussen M, Richelsen B. Adiponectin receptors in human adipose tissue: effects of obesity, weight loss, and fat depots. Obesity (Silver Spring) 2006; 14(1): 28-35.
[http://dx.doi.org/10.1038/oby.2006.5] [PMID: 16493120]

[30]   Van Harmelen V, Reynisdottir S, Eriksson P, *et al.* Leptin secretion from subcutaneous and visceral adipose tissue in women. Diabetes 1998; 47(6): 913-7.
[http://dx.doi.org/10.2337/diabetes.47.6.913] [PMID: 9604868]

[31]   Fontana L, Eagon JC, Trujillo ME, Scherer PE, Klein S. Visceral fat adipokine secretion is associated with systemic inflammation in obese humans. Diabetes 2007; 56(4): 1010-3.
[http://dx.doi.org/10.2337/db06-1656] [PMID: 17287468]

[32]   Ferrante AW Jr. The immune cells in adipose tissue. Diabetes Obes Metab 2013; 15 (Suppl. 3): 34-8.
[http://dx.doi.org/10.1111/dom.12154] [PMID: 24003919]

[33]   Tchkonia T, Tchoukalova YD, Giorgadze N, *et al.* Abundance of two human preadipocyte subtypes with distinct capacities for replication, adipogenesis, and apoptosis varies among fat depots. Am J Physiol Endocrinol Metab 2005; 288(1): E267-77.
[http://dx.doi.org/10.1152/ajpendo.00265.2004] [PMID: 15383371]

[34]   Kirkland JL, Hollenberg CH, Kindler S, Gillon WS. Effects of age and anatomic site on preadipocyte number in rat fat depots. J Gerontol 1994; 49(1): B31-5.
[http://dx.doi.org/10.1093/geronj/49.1.B31] [PMID: 8282974]

[35]   Tchoukalova YD, Votruba SB, Tchkonia T, Giorgadze N, Kirkland JL, Jensen MD. Regional differences in cellular mechanisms of adipose tissue gain with overfeeding. Proc Natl Acad Sci USA 2010; 107(42): 18226-31.
[http://dx.doi.org/10.1073/pnas.1005259107] [PMID: 20921416]

[36]   Schipper BM, Marra KG, Zhang W, Donnenberg AD, Rubin JP. Regional anatomic and age effects on cell function of human adipose-derived stem cells. Ann Plast Surg 2008; 60(5): 538-44.
[http://dx.doi.org/10.1097/SAP.0b013e3181723bbe] [PMID: 18434829]

[37]   Hotta K, Bodkin NL, Gustafson TA, Yoshioka S, Ortmeyer HK, Hansen BC. Age-related adipose tissue mRNA expression of ADD1/SREBP1, PPARgamma, lipoprotein lipase, and GLUT4 glucose transporter in rhesus monkeys. J Gerontol A Biol Sci Med Sci 1999; 54(5): B183-8.
[http://dx.doi.org/10.1093/gerona/54.5.B183] [PMID: 10361996]

[38]   Cartwright M, Tchkonia T, Lenburg M, *et al.* Aging, fat depot origin, and fat cell progenitor expression profiles: setting the stage for altered fat tissue function. J Gerontol 2010; 65: 242-51.
[http://dx.doi.org/10.1093/gerona/glp213]

[39]   Starr ME, Evers BM, Saito H. Age-associated increase in cytokine production during systemic inflammation: adipose tissue as a major source of IL-6. J Gerontol A Biol Sci Med Sci 2009; 64(7): 723-30.
[http://dx.doi.org/10.1093/gerona/glp046] [PMID: 19377014]

[40]   Gabrielsson BG, Johansson JM, Lönn M, *et al.* High expression of complement components in omental adipose tissue in obese men. Obes Res 2003; 11(6): 699-708.
[http://dx.doi.org/10.1038/oby.2003.100] [PMID: 12805391]

[41]   Divoux A, Clément K. Architecture and the extracellular matrix: the still unappreciated components of the adipose tissue. Obes Rev 2011; 12(5): e494-503.
[http://dx.doi.org/10.1111/j.1467-789X.2010.00811.x] [PMID: 21366833]

[42]   Slawik M, Vidal-Puig AJ. Lipotoxicity, overnutrition and energy metabolism in aging. Ageing Res Rev 2006; 5(2): 144-64.
[http://dx.doi.org/10.1016/j.arr.2006.03.004] [PMID: 16630750]

[43]   Newman AB, Lee JS, Visser M, *et al.* Weight change and the conservation of lean mass in old age: the Health, Aging and Body Composition Study. Am J Clin Nutr 2005; 82(4): 872-8.
[http://dx.doi.org/10.1093/ajcn/82.4.872] [PMID: 16210719]

[44]   Leeners B, Geary N, Tobler PN, Asarian L. Ovarian hormones and obesity. Hum Reprod Update 2017; 23(3): 300-21.
[http://dx.doi.org/10.1093/humupd/dmw045] [PMID: 28333235]

[45]   Baumgartner RN. Body composition in healthy aging. Ann N Y Acad Sci 2000; 904: 437-48.
[http://dx.doi.org/10.1111/j.1749-6632.2000.tb06498.x] [PMID: 10865787]

[46]   Rolland Y, Lauwers-Cances V, Cristini C, *et al.* Difficulties with physical function associated with obesity, sarcopenia, and sarcopenic-obesity in community-dwelling elderly women: the EPIDOS (EPIDemiologie de l'OSteoporose) Study. Am J Clin Nutr 2009; 89(6): 1895-900.
[http://dx.doi.org/10.3945/ajcn.2008.26950] [PMID: 19369381]

[47]   Okorodudu DO, Jumean MF, Montori VM, *et al.* Diagnostic performance of body mass index to identify obesity as defined by body adiposity: a systematic review and meta-analysis. Int J Obes 2010; 34(5): 791-9.
[http://dx.doi.org/10.1038/ijo.2010.5] [PMID: 20125098]

[48]   Lean ME, Han TS, Deurenberg P. Predicting body composition by densitometry from simple anthropometric measurements. Am J Clin Nutr 1996; 63(1): 4-14.
[http://dx.doi.org/10.1093/ajcn/63.1.4] [PMID: 8604668]

[49]   Visscher TLS, Seidell JC, Molarius A, van der Kuip D, Hofman A, Witteman JCM. A comparison of body mass index, waist-hip ratio and waist circumference as predictors of all-cause mortality among the elderly: the Rotterdam study. Int J Obes Relat Metab Disord 2001; 25(11): 1730-5.
[http://dx.doi.org/10.1038/sj.ijo.0801787] [PMID: 11753597]

[50]   Lemieux I, Poirier P, Bergeron J, *et al.* Hypertriglyceridemic waist: a useful screening phenotype in preventive cardiology? Can J Cardiol 2007; 23 (B): 23B-31B.
[http://dx.doi.org/10.1016/S0828-282X(07)71007-3]

[51]   Vlassopoulos A, Combet E, Lean ME. Changing distributions of body size and adiposity with age. Int J Obes 2014; 38(6): 857-64.
[http://dx.doi.org/10.1038/ijo.2013.216] [PMID: 24247373]

[52]   Tanamas SK, Shaw JE, Backholer K, Magliano DJ, Peeters A. Twelve-year weight change, waist circumference change and incident obesity: the Australian diabetes, obesity and lifestyle study. Obesity (Silver Spring) 2014; 22(6): 1538-45.
[http://dx.doi.org/10.1002/oby.20704] [PMID: 24436317]

[53]   Hughes VA, Roubenoff R, Wood M, Frontera WR, Evans WJ, Fiatarone Singh MA. Anthropometric assessment of 10-y changes in body composition in the elderly. Am J Clin Nutr 2004; 80(2): 475-82.

[http://dx.doi.org/10.1093/ajcn/80.2.475] [PMID: 15277173]

[54]   Tanamas SK, Lean MEJ, Combet E, Vlassopoulos A, Zimmet PZ, Peeters A. Changing guards: time to move beyond body mass index for population monitoring of excess adiposity. QJM 2016; 109(7): 443-6.
[http://dx.doi.org/10.1093/qjmed/hcv201] [PMID: 26527773]

[55]   Kannel WB, Cupples LA, Ramaswami R, Stokes J III, Kreger BE, Higgins M. Regional obesity and risk of cardiovascular disease; the Framingham Study. J Clin Epidemiol 1991; 44(2): 183-90.
[http://dx.doi.org/10.1016/0895-4356(91)90265-B] [PMID: 1995775]

[56]   Després JP, Moorjani S, Lupien PJ, Tremblay A, Nadeau A, Bouchard C. Regional distribution of body fat, plasma lipoproteins, and cardiovascular disease. Arteriosclerosis 1990; 10(4): 497-511.
[http://dx.doi.org/10.1161/01.ATV.10.4.497] [PMID: 2196040]

[57]   Yang YK, Chen M, Clements RH, Abrams GA, Aprahamian CJ, Harmon CM. Human mesenteric adipose tissue plays unique role versus subcutaneous and omental fat in obesity related diabetes. Cell Physiol Biochem 2008; 22(5-6): 531-8.
[http://dx.doi.org/10.1159/000185527] [PMID: 19088435]

[58]   Sparrow D, Borkan GA, Gerzof SG, Wisniewski C, Silbert CK. Relationship of fat distribution to glucose tolerance. Results of computed tomography in male participants of the Normative Aging Study. Diabetes 1986; 35(4): 411-5.
[http://dx.doi.org/10.2337/diab.35.4.411] [PMID: 3956878]

[59]   Matsuzawa Y. The role of fat topology in the risk of disease. Int J Obes 2008; 32 (Suppl. 7): S83-92.
[http://dx.doi.org/10.1038/ijo.2008.243] [PMID: 19136997]

[60]   Goodpaster BH, Krishnaswami S, Harris TB, *et al*. Obesity, regional body fat distribution, and the metabolic syndrome in older men and women. Arch Intern Med 2005; 165(7): 777-83.
[http://dx.doi.org/10.1001/archinte.165.7.777] [PMID: 15824297]

[61]   Kelley DE, Thaete FL, Troost F, Huwe T, Goodpaster BH. Subdivisions of subcutaneous abdominal adipose tissue and insulin resistance. Am J Physiol Endocrinol Metab 2000; 278(5): E941-8.
[http://dx.doi.org/10.1152/ajpendo.2000.278.5.E941] [PMID: 10780952]

[62]   Lean ME, Han TS, Morrison CE. Waist circumference as a measure for indicating need for weight management. BMJ 1995; 311(6998): 158-61.
[http://dx.doi.org/10.1136/bmj.311.6998.158] [PMID: 7613427]

[63]   Fleischmann E, Teal N, Dudley J, May W, Bower JD, Salahudeen AK. Influence of excess weight on mortality and hospital stay in 1346 hemodialysis patients. Kidney Int 1999; 55(4): 1560-7.
[http://dx.doi.org/10.1046/j.1523-1755.1999.00389.x] [PMID: 10201023]

[64]   Bosello O, Donataccio MP, Cuzzolaro M. Obesity or obesities? Controversies on the association between body mass index and premature mortality. Eat Weight Disord 2016; 21(2): 165-74.
[http://dx.doi.org/10.1007/s40519-016-0278-4] [PMID: 27043948]

[65]   Wildman RP, Muntner P, Reynolds K, *et al*. The obese without cardiometabolic risk factor clustering and the normal weight with cardiometabolic risk factor clustering: prevalence and correlates of 2 phenotypes among the US population (NHANES 1999-2004). Arch Intern Med 2008; 168(15): 1617-24.
[http://dx.doi.org/10.1001/archinte.168.15.1617] [PMID: 18695075]

[66]   Li X, Handee W, Kuo MH. The slim, the fat, and the obese: guess who lives the longest? Curr Genet 2017; 63(1): 43-9.
[http://dx.doi.org/10.1007/s00294-016-0617-z] [PMID: 27230908]

[67]   Di Angelantonio E, Bhupathiraju ShN, Wormser D, *et al*. Body-mass index and all-cause mortality: individual-participant-data meta-analysis of 239 prospective studies in four continents. Lancet 2016; 388(10046): 776-86.
[http://dx.doi.org/10.1016/S0140-6736(16)30175-1] [PMID: 27423262]

[68]   Gold EB. The timing of the age at which natural menopause occurs. Obstet Gynecol Clin North Am 2011; 38(3): 425-40.
[http://dx.doi.org/10.1016/j.ogc.2011.05.002] [PMID: 21961711]

[69]   Tchernof A, Poehlman ET. Effects of the menopause transition on body fatness and body fat distribution. Obes Res 1998; 6(3): 246-54.
[http://dx.doi.org/10.1002/j.1550-8528.1998.tb00344.x] [PMID: 9618130]

[70]   Gallagher D, Kuznia P, Heshka S, *et al.* Adipose tissue in muscle: a novel depot similar in size to visceral adipose tissue. Am J Clin Nutr 2005; 81(4): 903-10.
[http://dx.doi.org/10.1093/ajcn/81.4.903] [PMID: 15817870]

[71]   Shay CM, Secrest AM, Goodpaster BH, Kelsey SF, Strotmeyer ES, Orchard TJ. Regional adiposity and risk for coronary artery disease in type 1 diabetes: does having greater amounts of gluteal-femoral adiposity lower the risk? Diabetes Res Clin Pract 2010; 89(3): 288-95.
[http://dx.doi.org/10.1016/j.diabres.2010.03.028] [PMID: 20413171]

[72]   Karastergiou K, Fried SK, Xie H, *et al.* Distinct developmental signatures of human abdominal and gluteal subcutaneous adipose tissue depots. J Clin Endocrinol Metab 2013; 98(1): 362-71.
[http://dx.doi.org/10.1210/jc.2012-2953] [PMID: 23150689]

[73]   Pandzic Jaksic V, Sucic M. Multiple symmetric lipomatosis - a reflection of new concepts about obesity. Med Hypotheses 2008; 71(1): 99-101.
[http://dx.doi.org/10.1016/j.mehy.2008.01.028] [PMID: 18367347]

[74]   Fox CS, Massaro JM, Hoffmann U, *et al.* Abdominal visceral and subcutaneous adipose tissue compartments: association with metabolic risk factors in the Framingham Heart Study. Circulation 2007; 116(1): 39-48.
[http://dx.doi.org/10.1161/CIRCULATIONAHA.106.675355] [PMID: 17576866]

[75]   Panotopoulos G, Ruiz JC, Raison J, Guy-Grand B, Basdevant A. Menopause, fat and lean distribution in obese women. Maturitas 1996; 25(1): 11-9.
[http://dx.doi.org/10.1016/0378-5122(96)01119-X] [PMID: 8887304]

[76]   Panotopoulos G, Raison J, Ruiz JC, Guy-Grand B, Basdevant A. Weight gain at the time of menopause. Hum Reprod 1997; 12 (Suppl. 1): 126-33.
[http://dx.doi.org/10.1093/humrep/12.suppl_1.126] [PMID: 9403329]

[77]   Phillips GB, Jing T, Heymsfield SB. Does insulin resistance, visceral adiposity, or a sex hormone alteration underlie the metabolic syndrome? Studies in women. Metabolism 2008; 57(6): 838-44.
[http://dx.doi.org/10.1016/j.metabol.2008.01.029] [PMID: 18502268]

[78]   Abdulnour J, Doucet E, Brochu M, *et al.* The effect of the menopausal transition on body composition and cardiometabolic risk factors: a Montreal-Ottawa New Emerging Team group study. Menopause 2012; 19(7): 760-7.
[http://dx.doi.org/10.1097/gme.0b013e318240f6f3] [PMID: 22395454]

[79]   Kozakowski J, Gietka-Czernel M, Leszczyńska D, Majos A. Obesity in menopause - our negligence or an unfortunate inevitability? Przegl Menopauz 2017; 16(2): 61-5.
[http://dx.doi.org/10.5114/pm.2017.68594] [PMID: 28721132]

[80]   Freeman EW, Sammel MD, Lin H, Gracia CR. Obesity and reproductive hormone levels in the transition to menopause. Menopause 2010; 17(4): 718-26.
[PMID: 20216473]

[81]   D'Eon TM, Souza SC, Aronovitz M, Obin MS, Fried SK, Greenberg AS. Estrogen regulation of adiposity and fuel partitioning. Evidence of genomic and non-genomic regulation of lipogenic and oxidative pathways. J Biol Chem 2005; 280(43): 35983-91.
[http://dx.doi.org/10.1074/jbc.M507339200] [PMID: 16109719]

[82]   Elbers JM, Asscheman H, Seidell JC, Gooren LJ. Effects of sex steroid hormones on regional fat depots as assessed by magnetic resonance imaging in transsexuals. Am J Physiol 1999; 276(2): E317-

25.
[PMID: 9950792]

[83] Norman RJ, Flight IH, Rees MC. Oestrogen and progestogen hormone replacement therapy for peri-menopausal and post-menopausal women: weight and body fat distribution. Cochrane Database Syst Rev 2000; 2(2)CD001018
[PMID: 10796730]

[84] Santen RJ, Allred DC, Ardoin SP, *et al.* Postmenopausal hormone therapy: an Endocrine Society scientific statement. J Clin Endocrinol Metab 2010; 95(7) (Suppl. 1): s1-s66.
[http://dx.doi.org/10.1210/jc.2009-2509] [PMID: 20566620]

[85] Manson JE, Chlebowski RT, Stefanick ML, *et al.* Menopausal hormone therapy and health outcomes during the intervention and extended poststopping phases of the Women's Health Initiative randomized trials. JAMA 2013; 310(13): 1353-68.
[http://dx.doi.org/10.1001/jama.2013.278040] [PMID: 24084921]

[86] Manson JE, Kaunitz AM. Menopause management–getting clinical care back on track. N Engl J Med 2016; 374(9): 803-6.
[http://dx.doi.org/10.1056/NEJMp1514242] [PMID: 26962899]

[87] Pascot A, Lemieux S, Lemieux I, *et al.* Age-related increase in visceral adipose tissue and body fat and the metabolic risk profile of premenopausal women. Diabetes Care 1999; 22(9): 1471-8.
[http://dx.doi.org/10.2337/diacare.22.9.1471] [PMID: 10480511]

[88] Ferrario A, Villa F, Malovini A, Araniti F, Puca AA. The application of genetics approaches to the study of exceptional longevity in humans: potential and limitations. Immun Ageing 2012; 9(1): 7.
[http://dx.doi.org/10.1186/1742-4933-9-7] [PMID: 22524405]

[89] Schächter F, Faure-Delanef L, Guénot F, *et al.* Genetic associations with human longevity at the APOE and ACE loci. Nat Genet 1994; 6(1): 29-32.
[http://dx.doi.org/10.1038/ng0194-29] [PMID: 8136829]

[90] Soerensen M, Christensen K, Stevnsner T, Christiansen L. The Mn-superoxide dismutase single nucleotide polymorphism rs4880 and the glutathione peroxidase 1 single nucleotide polymorphism rs1050450 are associated with aging and longevity in the oldest old. Mech Ageing Dev 2009; 130(5): 308-14.
[http://dx.doi.org/10.1016/j.mad.2009.01.005] [PMID: 19428448]

[91] Soerensen M, Thinggaard M, Nygaard M, *et al.* Genetic variation in TERT and TERC and human leukocyte telomere length and longevity: a cross-sectional and longitudinal analysis. Aging Cell 2012; 11(2): 223-7.
[http://dx.doi.org/10.1111/j.1474-9726.2011.00775.x] [PMID: 22136229]

[92] Locke AE, Kahali B, Berndt SI, *et al.* Genetic studies of body mass index yield new insights for obesity biology. Nature 2015; 518(7538): 197-206.
[http://dx.doi.org/10.1038/nature14177] [PMID: 25673413]

[93] Zillikens MC, Demissie S, Hsu YH, *et al.* Large meta-analysis of genome-wide association studies identifies five loci for lean body mass. Nat Commun 2017; 8(1): 80.
[http://dx.doi.org/10.1038/s41467-017-00031-7] [PMID: 28724990]

[94] López-Otín C, Blasco MA, Partridge L, Serrano M, Kroemer G. The hallmarks of aging. Cell 2013; 153(6): 1194-217.
[http://dx.doi.org/10.1016/j.cell.2013.05.039] [PMID: 23746838]

[95] Rossi DJ, Bryder D, Seita J, Nussenzweig A, Hoeijmakers J, Weissman IL. Deficiencies in DNA damage repair limit the function of haematopoietic stem cells with age. Nature 2007; 447(7145): 725-9.
[http://dx.doi.org/10.1038/nature05862] [PMID: 17554309]

[96] Terman A, Gustafsson B, Brunk UT. Autophagy, organelles and ageing. J Pathol 2007; 211(2): 134-

43.
[http://dx.doi.org/10.1002/path.2094] [PMID: 17200947]

[97]   Zhang Y, Goldman S, Baerga R, Zhao Y, Komatsu M, Jin S. Adipose-specific deletion of autophagy-related gene 7 (atg7) in mice reveals a role in adipogenesis. Proc Natl Acad Sci USA 2009; 106(47): 19860-5.
[http://dx.doi.org/10.1073/pnas.0906048106] [PMID: 19910529]

[98]   Singh R, Xiang Y, Wang Y, *et al.* Autophagy regulates adipose mass and differentiation in mice. J Clin Invest 2009; 119(11): 3329-39.
[http://dx.doi.org/10.1172/JCI39228] [PMID: 19855132]

[99]   Kovsan J, Blüher M, Tarnovscki T, *et al.* Altered autophagy in human adipose tissues in obesity. J Clin Endocrinol Metab 2011; 96(2): E268-77.
[http://dx.doi.org/10.1210/jc.2010-1681] [PMID: 21047928]

[100] Potes Y, de Luxán-Delgado B, Rodriguez-González S, *et al.* Overweight in elderly people induces impaired autophagy in skeletal muscle. Free Radic Biol Med 2017; 110: 31-41.
[http://dx.doi.org/10.1016/j.freeradbiomed.2017.05.018] [PMID: 28549989]

[101] Li Y, Tollefsbol TO. Age-related epigenetic drift and phenotypic plasticity loss: implications in prevention of age-related human diseases. Epigenomics 2016; 8(12): 1637-51.
[http://dx.doi.org/10.2217/epi-2016-0078] [PMID: 27882781]

[102] Rönn T, Volkov P, Gillberg L, *et al.* Impact of age, BMI and HbA1c levels on the genome-wide DNA methylation and mRNA expression patterns in human adipose tissue and identification of epigenetic biomarkers in blood. Hum Mol Genet 2015; 24(13): 3792-813.
[http://dx.doi.org/10.1093/hmg/ddv124] [PMID: 25861810]

[103] Wahl S, Drong A, Lehne B, *et al.* Epigenome-wide association study of body mass index, and the adverse outcomes of adiposity. Nature 2017; 541(7635): 81-6.
[http://dx.doi.org/10.1038/nature20784] [PMID: 28002404]

[104] Nevalainen T, Kananen L, Marttila S, *et al.* Obesity accelerates epigenetic aging in middle-aged but not in elderly individuals. Clin Epigenetics 2017; 9: 20.
[http://dx.doi.org/10.1186/s13148-016-0301-7] [PMID: 28289477]

[105] Horvath S, Erhart W, Brosch M, *et al.* Obesity accelerates epigenetic aging of human liver. Proc Natl Acad Sci USA 2014; 111(43): 15538-43.
[http://dx.doi.org/10.1073/pnas.1412759111] [PMID: 25313081]

[106] van Dijk SJ, Molloy PL, Varinli H, Morrison JL, Muhlhausler BS. Members of EpiSCOPE. Epigenetics and human obesity. Int J Obes 2015; 39(1): 85-97.
[http://dx.doi.org/10.1038/ijo.2014.34]

[107] Mansego ML, Milagro FI, Zulet MÁ, Moreno-Aliaga MJ, Martínez JA. Differential DNA Methylation in Relation to Age and Health Risks of Obesity. Int J Mol Sci 2015; 16(8): 16816-32.
[http://dx.doi.org/10.3390/ijms160816816] [PMID: 26213922]

[108] Sala P, de Miranda Torrinhas RSM, Fonseca DC, Ravacci GR, Waitzberg DL, Giannella-Neto D. Tissue-specific methylation profile in obese patients with type 2 diabetes before and after Roux-en-Y gastric bypass. Diabetol Metab Syndr 2017; 9: 15.
[http://dx.doi.org/10.1186/s13098-017-0214-4] [PMID: 28250848]

[109] Miyamura Y, Tawa R, Koizumi A, *et al.* Effects of energy restriction on age-associated changes of DNA methylation in mouse liver. Mutat Res 1993; 295(2): 63-9.
[http://dx.doi.org/10.1016/0921-8734(93)90002-K] [PMID: 7680421]

[110] Goldstone AP. Prader-Willi syndrome: advances in genetics, pathophysiology and treatment. Trends Endocrinol Metab 2004; 15(1): 12-20.
[http://dx.doi.org/10.1016/j.tem.2003.11.003] [PMID: 14693421]

[111] Lopatina N, Haskell JF, Andrews LG, Poole JC, Saldanha S, Tollefsbol T. Differential maintenance

and de novo methylating activity by three DNA methyltransferases in aging and immortalized fibroblasts. J Cell Biochem 2002; 84(2): 324-34.
[http://dx.doi.org/10.1002/jcb.10015] [PMID: 11787061]

[112]   Ciccarone F, Malavolta M, Calabrese R, *et al.* Age-dependent expression of DNMT1 and DNMT3B in PBMCs from a large European population enrolled in the MARK-AGE study. Aging Cell 2016; 15(4): 755-65.
[http://dx.doi.org/10.1111/acel.12485] [PMID: 27169697]

[113]   Zhang X, Zhou D, Strakovsky R, Zhang Y, Pan YX. Hepatic cellular senescence pathway genes are induced through histone modifications in a diet-induced obese rat model. Am J Physiol Gastrointest Liver Physiol 2012; 302(5): G558-64.
[http://dx.doi.org/10.1152/ajpgi.00032.2011] [PMID: 22194422]

[114]   Inagaki T, Tachibana M, Magoori K, *et al.* Obesity and metabolic syndrome in histone demethylase JHDM2a-deficient mice. Genes Cells 2009; 14(8): 991-1001.
[http://dx.doi.org/10.1111/j.1365-2443.2009.01326.x] [PMID: 19624751]

[115]   Landry J, Sutton A, Tafrov ST, *et al.* The silencing protein SIR2 and its homologs are NAD-dependent protein deacetylases. Proc Natl Acad Sci USA 2000; 97(11): 5807-11.
[http://dx.doi.org/10.1073/pnas.110148297] [PMID: 10811920]

[116]   Michishita E, Park JY, Burneskis JM, Barrett JC, Horikawa I. Evolutionarily conserved and nonconserved cellular localizations and functions of human SIRT proteins. Mol Biol Cell 2005; 16(10): 4623-35.
[http://dx.doi.org/10.1091/mbc.e05-01-0033] [PMID: 16079181]

[117]   Bellizzi D, Rose G, Cavalcante P, *et al.* A novel VNTR enhancer within the SIRT3 gene, a human homologue of SIR2, is associated with survival at oldest ages. Genomics 2005; 85(2): 258-63.
[http://dx.doi.org/10.1016/j.ygeno.2004.11.003] [PMID: 15676284]

[118]   Vaquero A, Scher M, Lee D, Erdjument-Bromage H, Tempst P, Reinberg D. Human SirT1 interacts with histone H1 and promotes formation of facultative heterochromatin. Mol Cell 2004; 16(1): 93-105.
[http://dx.doi.org/10.1016/j.molcel.2004.08.031] [PMID: 15469825]

[119]   Neves D, Martins MJ, dos Passos E, Tomada I. To eat or not to eat.Anti-ageing nutrientes Evidence-based prevention of age-associated diseases. UK: Wiley-Blackwell 2015; pp. 33-132.
[http://dx.doi.org/10.1002/9781118823408.ch2]

[120]   Osborne B, Bentley NL, Montgomery MK, Turner N. The role of mitochondrial sirtuins in health and disease. Free Radic Biol Med 2016; 100: 164-74.
[http://dx.doi.org/10.1016/j.freeradbiomed.2016.04.197] [PMID: 27164052]

[121]   Barger JL, Anderson RM, Newton MA, *et al.* A conserved transcriptional signature of delayed aging and reduced disease vulnerability is partially mediated by SIRT3. PLoS One 2015; 10(4)e0120738
[http://dx.doi.org/10.1371/journal.pone.0120738] [PMID: 25830335]

[122]   Oberdoerffer P, Michan S, McVay M, *et al.* SIRT1 redistribution on chromatin promotes genomic stability but alters gene expression during aging. Cell 2008; 135(5): 907-18.
[http://dx.doi.org/10.1016/j.cell.2008.10.025] [PMID: 19041753]

[123]   Wang RH, Sengupta K, Li C, *et al.* Impaired DNA damage response, genome instability, and tumorigenesis in SIRT1 mutant mice. Cancer Cell 2008; 14(4): 312-23.
[http://dx.doi.org/10.1016/j.ccr.2008.09.001] [PMID: 18835033]

[124]   Lee IH, Cao L, Mostoslavsky R, *et al.* A role for the NAD-dependent deacetylase Sirt1 in the regulation of autophagy. Proc Natl Acad Sci USA 2008; 105(9): 3374-9.
[http://dx.doi.org/10.1073/pnas.0712145105] [PMID: 18296641]

[125]   Brunet A, Sweeney LB, Sturgill JF, *et al.* Stress-dependent regulation of FOXO transcription factors by the SIRT1 deacetylase. Science 2004; 303(5666): 2011-5.
[http://dx.doi.org/10.1126/science.1094637] [PMID: 14976264]

[126] Alcendor RR, Gao S, Zhai P, *et al.* Sirt1 regulates aging and resistance to oxidative stress in the heart. Circ Res 2007; 100(10): 1512-21.
[http://dx.doi.org/10.1161/01.RES.0000267723.65696.4a] [PMID: 17446436]

[127] Wang F, Nguyen M, Qin FX, Tong Q. SIRT2 deacetylates FOXO3a in response to oxidative stress and caloric restriction. Aging Cell 2007; 6(4): 505-14.
[http://dx.doi.org/10.1111/j.1474-9726.2007.00304.x] [PMID: 17521387]

[128] Shi T, Wang F, Stieren E, Tong Q. SIRT3, a mitochondrial sirtuin deacetylase, regulates mitochondrial function and thermogenesis in brown adipocytes. J Biol Chem 2005; 280(14): 13560-7.
[http://dx.doi.org/10.1074/jbc.M414670200] [PMID: 15653680]

[129] Someya S, Yu W, Hallows WC, *et al.* Sirt3 mediates reduction of oxidative damage and prevention of age-related hearing loss under caloric restriction. Cell 2010; 143(5): 802-12.
[http://dx.doi.org/10.1016/j.cell.2010.10.002] [PMID: 21094524]

[130] Qiu X, Brown K, Hirschey MD, Verdin E, Chen D. Calorie restriction reduces oxidative stress by SIRT3-mediated SOD2 activation. Cell Metab 2010; 12(6): 662-7.
[http://dx.doi.org/10.1016/j.cmet.2010.11.015] [PMID: 21109198]

[131] Sundaresan NR, Gupta M, Kim G, Rajamohan SB, Isbatan A, Gupta MP. Sirt3 blocks the cardiac hypertrophic response by augmenting Foxo3a-dependent antioxidant defense mechanisms in mice. J Clin Invest 2009; 119(9): 2758-71.
[http://dx.doi.org/10.1172/JCI39162] [PMID: 19652361]

[132] Luo J, Nikolaev AY, Imai S, *et al.* Negative control of p53 by Sir2alpha promotes cell survival under stress. Cell 2001; 107(2): 137-48.
[http://dx.doi.org/10.1016/S0092-8674(01)00524-4] [PMID: 11672522]

[133] Yeung F, Hoberg JE, Ramsey CS, *et al.* Modulation of NF-kappaB-dependent transcription and cell survival by the SIRT1 deacetylase. EMBO J 2004; 23(12): 2369-80.
[http://dx.doi.org/10.1038/sj.emboj.7600244] [PMID: 15152190]

[134] Braidy N, Guillemin GJ, Mansour H, Chan-Ling T, Poljak A, Grant R. Age related changes in NAD+ metabolism oxidative stress and Sirt1 activity in wistar rats. PLoS One 2011; 6(4)e19194
[http://dx.doi.org/10.1371/journal.pone.0019194] [PMID: 21541336]

[135] Mariani S, Di Rocco G, Toietta G, Russo MA, Petrangeli E, Salvatori L. Sirtuins 1-7 expression in human adipose-derived stem cells from subcutaneous and visceral fat depots: influence of obesity and hypoxia. Endocrine 2017; 57(3): 455-63.
[http://dx.doi.org/10.1007/s12020-016-1170-8] [PMID: 27844208]

[136] Xu F, Zheng X, Lin B, *et al.* Diet-induced obesity and insulin resistance are associated with brown fat degeneration in SIRT1-deficient mice. Obesity (Silver Spring) 2016; 24(3): 634-42.
[http://dx.doi.org/10.1002/oby.21393] [PMID: 26916242]

[137] Abdesselem H, Madani A, Hani A, *et al.* SIRT1 Limits Adipocyte Hyperplasia through c-Myc Inhibition. J Biol Chem 2016; 291(5): 2119-35.
[http://dx.doi.org/10.1074/jbc.M115.675645] [PMID: 26655722]

[138] Finkel T, Deng CX, Mostoslavsky R. Recent progress in the biology and physiology of sirtuins. Nature 2009; 460(7255): 587-91.
[http://dx.doi.org/10.1038/nature08197] [PMID: 19641587]

[139] Guarente L, Picard F. Calorie restriction--the SIR2 connection. Cell 2005; 120(4): 473-82.
[http://dx.doi.org/10.1016/j.cell.2005.01.029] [PMID: 15734680]

[140] Smith-Vikos T, Slack FJ. MicroRNAs and their roles in aging. J Cell Sci 2012; 125(Pt 1): 7-17.
[http://dx.doi.org/10.1242/jcs.099200] [PMID: 22294612]

[141] Zhu Y, Xiong K, Shi J, Cui Q, Xue L. A potential role of microRNAs in protein accumulation in cellular senescence analyzed by bioinformatics. PLoS One 2017; 12(6)e0179034

[http://dx.doi.org/10.1371/journal.pone.0179034] [PMID: 28591170]

[142] Micó V, Berninches L, Tapia J, Daimiel L. NutrimiRAging: Micromanaging Nutrient Sensing Pathways through Nutrition to Promote Healthy Aging. Int J Mol Sci 2017; 18(5)E915
[http://dx.doi.org/10.3390/ijms18050915] [PMID: 28445443]

[143] Schroen B, Heymans S. Small but smart--microRNAs in the centre of inflammatory processes during cardiovascular diseases, the metabolic syndrome, and ageing. Cardiovasc Res 2012; 93(4): 605-13.
[http://dx.doi.org/10.1093/cvr/cvr268] [PMID: 21994347]

[144] Guglielmi V, D'Adamo M, Menghini R, *et al.* MicroRNA 21 is up-regulated in adipose tissue of obese diabetic subjects. Nutr Healthy Aging 2017; 4(2): 141-5.
[http://dx.doi.org/10.3233/NHA-160020] [PMID: 28447068]

[145] Kim JH, Lee BR, Choi ES, *et al.* Reverse Expression of Aging-Associated Molecules through Transfection of miRNAs to Aged Mice. Mol Ther Nucleic Acids 2017; 6: 106-15.
[http://dx.doi.org/10.1016/j.omtn.2016.11.005] [PMID: 28325277]

[146] Wang B, Du R, Xiao X, *et al.* Microrna-217 modulates human skin fibroblast senescence by directly targeting DNA methyltransferase 1. Oncotarget 2017; 8(20): 33475-86.
[http://dx.doi.org/10.18632/oncotarget.16509] [PMID: 28380423]

[147] Choi SE, Fu T, Seok S, *et al.* Elevated microRNA-34a in obesity reduces NAD+ levels and SIRT1 activity by directly targeting NAMPT. Aging Cell 2013; 12(6): 1062-72.
[http://dx.doi.org/10.1111/acel.12135] [PMID: 23834033]

[148] Valdes AM, Andrew T, Gardner JP, *et al.* Obesity, cigarette smoking, and telomere length in women. Lancet 2005; 366(9486): 662-4.
[http://dx.doi.org/10.1016/S0140-6736(05)66630-5] [PMID: 16112303]

[149] Tzanetakou IP, Katsilambros NL, Benetos A, Mikhailidis DP, Perrea DN. "Is obesity linked to aging?": adipose tissue and the role of telomeres. Ageing Res Rev 2012; 11(2): 220-9.
[http://dx.doi.org/10.1016/j.arr.2011.12.003] [PMID: 22186032]

[150] Lee M, Martin H, Firpo MA, Demerath EW. Inverse association between adiposity and telomere length: The Fels Longitudinal Study. Am J Hum Biol 2011; 23(1): 100-6.
[http://dx.doi.org/10.1002/ajhb.21109] [PMID: 21080476]

[151] Epel ES, Lin J, Wilhelm FH, *et al.* Cell aging in relation to stress arousal and cardiovascular disease risk factors. Psychoneuroendocrinology 2006; 31(3): 277-87.
[http://dx.doi.org/10.1016/j.psyneuen.2005.08.011] [PMID: 16298085]

[152] Nordfjäll K, Eliasson M, Stegmayr B, Melander O, Nilsson P, Roos G. Telomere length is associated with obesity parameters but with a gender difference. Obesity (Silver Spring) 2008; 16(12): 2682-9.
[http://dx.doi.org/10.1038/oby.2008.413] [PMID: 18820651]

[153] Tomada I, Andrade JP. Evidence-based retardation of ageing.Anti-ageing nutrientes Evidence-based prevention of age-associated diseases. UK: Wiley-Blackwell 2015; pp. 335-90.

[154] Gatineau E, Polakof S, Dardevet D, Mosoni L. Similarities and interactions between the ageing process and high chronic intake of added sugars. Nutr Res Rev 2017; 30(2): 191-207.
[http://dx.doi.org/10.1017/S0954422417000051] [PMID: 28511733]

[155] Semba RD, Ang A, Talegawkar S, *et al.* Dietary intake associated with serum versus urinary carboxymethyl-lysine, a major advanced glycation end product, in adults: the Energetics Study. Eur J Clin Nutr 2012; 66(1): 3-9.
[http://dx.doi.org/10.1038/ejcn.2011.139] [PMID: 21792213]

[156] Neves D. Advanced glycation end-products: a common pathway in diabetes and age-related erectile dysfunction. Free Radic Res 2013; 47(S1) (Suppl. 1): 49-69.
[http://dx.doi.org/10.3109/10715762.2013.821701] [PMID: 23822116]

[157] Baraibar MA, Liu L, Ahmed EK, Friguet B. Protein oxidative damage at the crossroads of cellular

senescence, aging, and age-related diseases. Oxid Med Cell Longev 2012; 2012919832
[http://dx.doi.org/10.1155/2012/919832] [PMID: 23125894]

[158] Dorman RB, Abraham AA, Al-Refaie WB, Parsons HM, Ikramuddin S, Habermann EB. Bariatric surgery outcomes in the elderly: an ACS NSQIP study. J Gastrointest Surg 2012; 16(1): 35-44.
[http://dx.doi.org/10.1007/s11605-011-1749-6] [PMID: 22038414]

[159] Yoon J, Sherman J, Argiroff A, *et al.* Laparoscopic sleeve gastrectomy and gastric bypass for the aging population. Obes Surg 2016; 26(11): 2611-5.
[http://dx.doi.org/10.1007/s11695-016-2139-7] [PMID: 26983631]

[160] Leitner BP, Huang S, Brychta RJ, *et al.* Mapping of human brown adipose tissue in lean and obese young men. Proc Natl Acad Sci USA 2017; 114(32): 8649-54.
[http://dx.doi.org/10.1073/pnas.1705287114] [PMID: 28739898]

[161] Mattson MP. Perspective: Does brown fat protect against diseases of aging? Ageing Res Rev 2010; 9(1): 69-76.
[http://dx.doi.org/10.1016/j.arr.2009.11.004] [PMID: 19969105]

[162] Lowell BB, S-Susulic V, Hamann A, *et al.* Development of obesity in transgenic mice after genetic ablation of brown adipose tissue. Nature 1993; 366(6457): 740-2.
[http://dx.doi.org/10.1038/366740a0] [PMID: 8264795]

[163] Wu J, Boström P, Sparks LM, *et al.* Beige adipocytes are a distinct type of thermogenic fat cell in mouse and human. Cell 2012; 150(2): 366-76.
[http://dx.doi.org/10.1016/j.cell.2012.05.016] [PMID: 22796012]

[164] Bartelt A, Heeren J. Adipose tissue browning and metabolic health. Nat Rev Endocrinol 2014; 10(1): 24-36.
[http://dx.doi.org/10.1038/nrendo.2013.204] [PMID: 24146030]

[165] Ghorbani M, Claus TH, Himms-Hagen J. Hypertrophy of brown adipocytes in brown and white adipose tissues and reversal of diet-induced obesity in rats treated with a beta3-adrenoceptor agonist. Biochem Pharmacol 1997; 54(1): 121-31.
[http://dx.doi.org/10.1016/S0006-2952(97)00162-7] [PMID: 9296358]

[166] Lee P, Linderman JD, Smith S, *et al.* Irisin and FGF21 are cold-induced endocrine activators of brown fat function in humans. Cell Metab 2014; 19(2): 302-9.
[http://dx.doi.org/10.1016/j.cmet.2013.12.017] [PMID: 24506871]

[167] Zhu E, Yang Y, Zhang J, *et al.* Liraglutide suppresses obesity and induces brown fat-like phenotype via Soluble Guanylyl Cyclase mediated pathway in vivo and in vitro. Oncotarget 2016; 7(49): 81077-89.
[http://dx.doi.org/10.18632/oncotarget.13189] [PMID: 27835589]

[168] Mancini MC, de Melo ME. The burden of obesity in the current world and the new treatments available: focus on liraglutide 3.0 mg. Diabetol Metab Syndr 2017; 9: 44.
[http://dx.doi.org/10.1186/s13098-017-0242-0] [PMID: 28580018]

[169] Azhar Y, Parmar A, Miller CN, Samuels JS, Rayalam S. Phytochemicals as novel agents for the induction of browning in white adipose tissue. Nutr Metab (Lond) 2016; 13: 89.
[http://dx.doi.org/10.1186/s12986-016-0150-6] [PMID: 27980598]

[170] Ingram DK, Zhu M, Mamczarz J, *et al.* Calorie restriction mimetics: an emerging research field. Aging Cell 2006; 5(2): 97-108.
[http://dx.doi.org/10.1111/j.1474-9726.2006.00202.x] [PMID: 16626389]

[171] Hu Y, Liu J, Wang J, Liu Q. The controversial links among calorie restriction, SIRT1, and resveratrol. Free Radic Biol Med 2011; 51(2): 250-6.
[http://dx.doi.org/10.1016/j.freeradbiomed.2011.04.034] [PMID: 21569839]

[172] Dao TM, Waget A, Klopp P, *et al.* Resveratrol increases glucose induced GLP-1 secretion in mice: a mechanism which contributes to the glycemic control. PLoS One 2011; 6(6)e20700

[http://dx.doi.org/10.1371/journal.pone.0020700] [PMID: 21673955]

[173] Park SJ, Ahmad F, Philp A, *et al.* Resveratrol ameliorates aging-related metabolic phenotypes by inhibiting cAMP phosphodiesterases. Cell 2012; 148(3): 421-33.
[http://dx.doi.org/10.1016/j.cell.2012.01.017] [PMID: 22304913]

[174] Baur JA, Pearson KJ, Price NL, *et al.* Resveratrol improves health and survival of mice on a high-calorie diet. Nature 2006; 444(7117): 337-42.
[http://dx.doi.org/10.1038/nature05354] [PMID: 17086191]

[175] Yoshino J, Conte C, Fontana L, *et al.* Resveratrol supplementation does not improve metabolic function in nonobese women with normal glucose tolerance. Cell Metab 2012; 16(5): 658-64.
[http://dx.doi.org/10.1016/j.cmet.2012.09.015] [PMID: 23102619]

[176] Anton SD, Embry C, Marsiske M, *et al.* Safety and metabolic outcomes of resveratrol supplementation in older adults: results of a twelve-week, placebo-controlled pilot study. Exp Gerontol 2014; 57: 181-7.
[http://dx.doi.org/10.1016/j.exger.2014.05.015] [PMID: 24866496]

[177] Jung CH, Cho I, Ahn J, Jeon TI, Ha TY. Quercetin reduces high-fat diet-induced fat accumulation in the liver by regulating lipid metabolism genes. Phytother Res 2013; 27(1): 139-43.
[http://dx.doi.org/10.1002/ptr.4687] [PMID: 22447684]

[178] Egert S, Boesch-Saadatmandi C, Wolffram S, Rimbach G, Müller MJ. Serum lipid and blood pressure responses to quercetin vary in overweight patients by apolipoprotein E genotype. J Nutr 2010; 140(2): 278-84.
[http://dx.doi.org/10.3945/jn.109.117655] [PMID: 20032478]

[179] Knab AM, Shanely RA, Jin F, Austin MD, Sha W, Nieman DC. Quercetin with vitamin C and niacin does not affect body mass or composition. Appl Physiol Nutr Metab 2011; 36(3): 331-8.
[http://dx.doi.org/10.1139/h11-015] [PMID: 21574787]

[180] Pfeuffer M, Auinger A, Bley U, *et al.* Effect of quercetin on traits of the metabolic syndrome, endothelial function and inflammation in men with different APOE isoforms. Nutr Metab Cardiovasc Dis 2013; 23(5): 403-9.
[http://dx.doi.org/10.1016/j.numecd.2011.08.010] [PMID: 22118955]

[181] Fang MZ, Wang Y, Ai N, *et al.* Tea polyphenol (-)-epigallocatechin-3-gallate inhibits DNA methyltransferase and reactivates methylation-silenced genes in cancer cell lines. Cancer Res 2003; 63(22): 7563-70.
[PMID: 14633667]

[182] Hsu TF, Kusumoto A, Abe K, *et al.* Polyphenol-enriched oolong tea increases fecal lipid excretion. Eur J Clin Nutr 2006; 60(11): 1330-6.
[http://dx.doi.org/10.1038/sj.ejcn.1602464] [PMID: 16804556]

[183] Vieira Senger AE, Schwanke CH, Gomes I, Valle Gottlieb MG. Effect of green tea (Camellia sinensis) consumption on the components of metabolic syndrome in elderly. J Nutr Health Aging 2012; 16(9): 738-42.
[http://dx.doi.org/10.1007/s12603-012-0081-5] [PMID: 23131813]

[184] Suliburska J, Bogdanski P, Szulinska M, Stepien M, Pupek-Musialik D, Jablecka A. Effects of green tea supplementation on elements, total antioxidants, lipids, and glucose values in the serum of obese patients. Biol Trace Elem Res 2012; 149(3): 315-22.
[http://dx.doi.org/10.1007/s12011-012-9448-z] [PMID: 22581111]

[185] Basu A, Sanchez K, Leyva MJ, *et al.* Green tea supplementation affects body weight, lipids, and lipid peroxidation in obese subjects with metabolic syndrome. J Am Coll Nutr 2010; 29(1): 31-40.
[http://dx.doi.org/10.1080/07315724.2010.10719814] [PMID: 20595643]

[186] Mohammadi A, Sahebkar A, Iranshahi M, *et al.* Effects of supplementation with curcuminoids on dyslipidemia in obese patients: a randomized crossover trial. Phytother Res 2013; 27(3): 374-9.

[http://dx.doi.org/10.1002/ptr.4715] [PMID: 22610853]

[187] Wang J, Vanegas SM, Du X, *et al.* Caloric restriction favorably impacts metabolic and immune/inflammatory profiles in obese mice but curcumin/piperine consumption adds no further benefit. Nutr Metab (Lond) 2013; 10(1): 29.
[http://dx.doi.org/10.1186/1743-7075-10-29] [PMID: 23531279]

[188] Martin PM, Horwitz KB, Ryan DS, McGuire WL. Phytoestrogen interaction with estrogen receptors in human breast cancer cells. Endocrinology 1978; 103(5): 1860-7.
[http://dx.doi.org/10.1210/endo-103-5-1860] [PMID: 570914]

[189] Allison DB, Gadbury G, Schwartz LG, *et al.* A novel soy-based meal replacement formula for weight loss among obese individuals: a randomized controlled clinical trial. Eur J Clin Nutr 2003; 57(4): 514-22.
[http://dx.doi.org/10.1038/sj.ejcn.1601587] [PMID: 12700612]

[190] Deibert P, König D, Schmidt-Trucksaess A, *et al.* Weight loss without losing muscle mass in pre-obese and obese subjects induced by a high-soy-protein diet. Int J Obes Relat Metab Disord 2004; 28(10): 1349-52.
[http://dx.doi.org/10.1038/sj.ijo.0802765] [PMID: 15303108]

[191] Huang JH, Lu YF, Cheng FC, Lee JN, Tsai LC. Correlation of magnesium intake with metabolic parameters, depression and physical activity in elderly type 2 diabetes patients: a cross-sectional study. Nutr J 2012; 11: 41.
[http://dx.doi.org/10.1186/1475-2891-11-41] [PMID: 22695027]

[192] Rodríguez-Moran M, Guerrero-Romero F. Oral magnesium supplementation improves the metabolic profile of metabolically obese, normal-weight individuals: a randomized double-blind placebo-controlled trial. Arch Med Res 2014; 45(5): 388-93.
[http://dx.doi.org/10.1016/j.arcmed.2014.05.003] [PMID: 24830937]

[193] Martin-Montalvo A, Mercken EM, Mitchell SJ, *et al.* Metformin improves healthspan and lifespan in mice. Nat Commun 2013; 4: 2192.
[http://dx.doi.org/10.1038/ncomms3192] [PMID: 23900241]

[194] Kirpichnikov D, McFarlane SI, Sowers JR. Metformin: an update. Ann Intern Med 2002; 137(1): 25-33.
[http://dx.doi.org/10.7326/0003-4819-137-1-200207020-00009] [PMID: 12093242]

[195] Rahbar S, Natarajan R, Yerneni K, Scott S, Gonzales N, Nadler JL. Evidence that pioglitazone, metformin and pentoxifylline are inhibitors of glycation. Clin Chim Acta 2000; 301(1-2): 65-77.
[http://dx.doi.org/10.1016/S0009-8981(00)00327-2] [PMID: 11020463]

[196] Xie Z, Lau K, Eby B, *et al.* Improvement of cardiac functions by chronic metformin treatment is associated with enhanced cardiac autophagy in diabetic OVE26 mice. Diabetes 2011; 60(6): 1770-8.
[http://dx.doi.org/10.2337/db10-0351] [PMID: 21562078]

[197] Paolisso G, Amato L, Eccellente R, *et al.* Effect of metformin on food intake in obese subjects. Eur J Clin Invest 1998; 28(6): 441-6.
[http://dx.doi.org/10.1046/j.1365-2362.1998.00304.x] [PMID: 9693934]

[198] Werner C, Gensch C, Pöss J, Haendeler J, Böhm M, Laufs U. Pioglitazone activates aortic telomerase and prevents stress-induced endothelial apoptosis. Atherosclerosis 2011; 216(1): 23-34.
[http://dx.doi.org/10.1016/j.atherosclerosis.2011.02.011] [PMID: 21396644]

[199] Bogacka I, Gettys TW, de Jonge L, *et al.* The effect of beta-adrenergic and peroxisome proliferator-activated receptor-gamma stimulation on target genes related to lipid metabolism in human subcutaneous adipose tissue. Diabetes Care 2007; 30(5): 1179-86.
[http://dx.doi.org/10.2337/dc06-1962] [PMID: 17351280]

[200] Smith SR, De Jonge L, Volaufova J, Li Y, Xie H, Bray GA. Effect of pioglitazone on body composition and energy expenditure: a randomized controlled trial. Metabolism 2005; 54(1): 24-32.

[http://dx.doi.org/10.1016/j.metabol.2004.07.008] [PMID: 15562376]

[201] Marso SP, Daniels GH, Brown-Frandsen K, *et al.* Liraglutide and Cardiovascular Outcomes in Type 2 Diabetes. N Engl J Med 2016; 375(4): 311-22.
[http://dx.doi.org/10.1056/NEJMoa1603827] [PMID: 27295427]

[202] Strong R, Miller RA, Astle CM, *et al.* Nordihydroguaiaretic acid and aspirin increase lifespan of genetically heterogeneous male mice. Aging Cell 2008; 7(5): 641-50.
[http://dx.doi.org/10.1111/j.1474-9726.2008.00414.x] [PMID: 18631321]

[203] Spindler SR, Mote PL, Lublin AL, Flegal JM, Dhahbi JM, Li R. Nordihydroguaiaretic Acid Extends the Lifespan of Drosophila and Mice, Increases Mortality-Related Tumors and Hemorrhagic Diathesis, and Alters Energy Homeostasis in Mice. J Gerontol A Biol Sci Med Sci 2015; 70(12): 1479-89.
[http://dx.doi.org/10.1093/gerona/glu190] [PMID: 25380600]

[204] Timmers S, Konings E, Bilet L, *et al.* Calorie restriction-like effects of 30 days of resveratrol supplementation on energy metabolism and metabolic profile in obese humans. Cell Metab 2011; 14(5): 612-22.
[http://dx.doi.org/10.1016/j.cmet.2011.10.002] [PMID: 22055504]

[205] Poulsen MM, Vestergaard PF, Clasen BF, *et al.* High-dose resveratrol supplementation in obese men: an investigator-initiated, randomized, placebo-controlled clinical trial of substrate metabolism, insulin sensitivity, and body composition. Diabetes 2013; 62(4): 1186-95.
[http://dx.doi.org/10.2337/db12-0975] [PMID: 23193181]

SUBJECT INDEX

A

ABC transporters 280
Ability 9, 68, 69, 70, 124, 128, 129, 133, 136, 137, 138, 142, 238, 325, 328, 401, 430
  metabolism disruption 142
  preadipocytes 430
  predictive 9
  thyroid hormone-disrupting 128
Absorption 160, 126, 160, 195, 221, 255, 256, 272, 277, 278, 279, 280, 284, 326, 335
  acyclovir 160
  anthocyanin 278
  anthocyanin glycoside 279
  dermal 126
  fat-soluble vitamin 160
  gastric 278
  intestinal calcium 255
  polyphenol 277
  reduced lipid 221
  systemic 195
Acetyl-CoA carboxylase (ACC) 287
Acid, pantothenic 325
Acid-derived endocannabinoids 239
Actinobacteria 324
Activation 67, 69, 70, 86, 88, 112, 128, 129, 286, 287, 346, 351, 404, 405, 406, 407, 408, 409, 411, 413, 429
  catabolism 413
  complement system 429
  ligand 287
  mitigated obesity-induced adipose tissue 351
  obesity-induced inflammasome 112
  of AMP-activated protein kinase 286
   pancreatic stellate cell 411
Activity 83, 86, 128, 132, 198, 238, 272, 326, 345, 346, 351, 376, 380, 403, 404, 411, 413, 438, 440, 441
  antioxidant 272
  carbonic anhydrase 198
  glycolytic 411
  lipolytic 238

parasympathetic 380
phagocytic 351
progenitor 345
respiratory 376
restore tumor suppression 413
telomerase 441
Adenosine triphosphate 58
Adipocyte hypertrophy 62, 63, 66, 69, 100, 106, 107, 110, 113, 130, 137, 346
  restricting 69
Adipocyte(s) 55, 58, 59, 60, 61, 62, 63, 64, 65, 66, 69, 81, 82, 83, 84, 85, 86, 106, 130, 136, 138, 141, 285, 345, 346, 374, 379, 383, 401, 405, 412, 428, 430, 440
  apoptotic signaling 346
  autophagy 346
  dysfunction 66, 81, 82, 136, 138
  glucose homeostasis 141
  hyperplasia 55, 61, 62, 63, 130, 440
  hyperplasic 66
  hypertrophic 63, 64, 66, 82, 374
  hypertrophied 69
  mature epididymal 347
  tumor-associated 412
Adipocytokines 400, 412, 413
Adipogenesis 64, 65, 68, 87, 88, 285, 286, 287, 326, 328, 344, 345, 442, 443
  activating 328
  enhancing 326
  inhibiting 286
Adipogenic transcripts 430
Adipokines 55, 62, 66, 81, 82, 83, 88, 90, 131, 352
  anti-inflammatory 62, 66, 81, 82, 83, 88
  chemotactic 82
  ideal biomarkers 90
  inflammatory 131
  novel anti-inflammatory 88
  pathological 81
  proinflammatory 82, 83, 352
  secretion 55
Adiponectin synthesis 131, 348, 430
  reduced 430
Adipose 345, 406